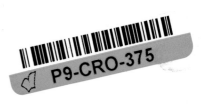

INTRODUCTION TO DIAGNOSTIC RADIOLOGY

INTRODUCTION TO DIAGNOSTIC RADIOLOGY

Editor-in-Chief

Khaled M. Elsayes, MD
Associate Professor of Diagnostic Radiology
Department of Diagnostic Radiology
The University of Texas MD Anderson Cancer Center
Houston, Texas

Sandra A. A. Oldham, MD
Professor of Radiology, Chief, Section of Thoracic Imaging
Vice Chairman for Education, Department of Diagnostic and Interventional Imaging
The University of Texas Health Science Center, Houston, Texas

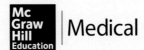

New York   Chicago   San Francisco   Athens   London   Madrid   Mexico City   New Delhi
San Juan   Singapore   Sydney   Toronto

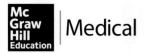

Introduction to Diagnostic Radiology

1 2 3 4 5 6 7 8 9 0 CTP/CTP 18 17 16 15 14

MHID 0-07-180180-4
ISBN 978-0-07-180180-5

This book was set in Minion by MPS.
The editors were Michael Weitz and Christie Naglieri.
The production supervisor was Richard Ruzycka.
Project management was provided by Vipra Fauzdar at MPS.
The cover designer was Anthony Landi.
The index was prepared by Edwin Durbin.
China Translation & Printing Services, Ltd. was printer and binder.

This book is printed on acid-free paper.

Library of Congress Cataloging-in-Publication Data
Introduction to diagnostic radiology (Elsayes)
  Introduction to diagnostic radiology / editor-in-chief, Khaled Elsayes, Sandra Oldham.
      p. ; cm.
  Includes bibliographical references and index.
  ISBN 978-0-07-180180-5 (casebound : alk. paper)—ISBN 0-07-180180-4
  I. Elsayes, Khaled, editor of compilation. II. Oldham, Sandra, editor of compilation. III. Title.
  [DNLM: 1. Diagnostic Imaging. WN 180]
  RC78.7.D53
  616.07'543—dc23
                                                           2013032867

McGraw-Hill books are available at special quantity discounts to use as premiums and sales promotions, or for use in corporate training programs. To contact a representative, please visit the Contact Us pages at www.mhprofessional.com.

To the memory of my parents
To my wife and children
Dr Khaled M. Elsayes

All my thanks and appreciation
to my children, Christine and Patrick
Dr Sandra A. A. Oldham

Contents

Contributors

Mohammed Al-Natour, MD
Senior Resident, Radiology Department, The University of Toledo Medical Center, Toledo, Ohio

Behrang Amini, MD, PhD
Assistant Professor of Diagnostic Radiology, Department of Diagnostic Radiology, The University of Texas MD Anderson Cancer Center, Houston, Texas

Bilal Anwer, MD
Graduate Resident, Department of Diagnostic and Interventional Imaging, The University of Texas Medical School at Houston, Houston, Texas

Eliana Bonfante, MD
Assistant Professor of Radiology, Department of Diagnostic and Interventional Imaging, The University of Texas Health Science Center, Houston, Texas

David C. Brandon, MD
Assistant Professor, Division of Nuclear Medicine, Emory University, Health Care, Atlanta, Georgia

Jennifer Caero, MD
Resident, Department of Diagnostic Radiology, Baylor University Medical Center, Dallas, Texas

Haitham Elsamaloty, MD
Professor and Vice Chairman, Radiology Department, University of Toledo Medical Center, Toledo, Ohio

Khaled M. Elsayes, MD
Associate Professor of Diagnostic Radiology, Department of Diagnostic Radiology, The University of Texas MD Anderson Cancer Center, Houston, Texas

Nakul Gupta, MD
Fellow, Section of Body Imaging, Department of Diagnostic and Interventional Imaging, The University of Texas Health Science Center, Houston, Texas

Tara Hagopian, DO
Fellow, Diagnostic Neuroradiology Section, Mallinckrodt Institute of Radiology, Washington University School of Medicine, St. Louis, Missouri

Neda Haswah, MD
Senior Resident, Radiology Department, The University of Toledo Medical Center, Toledo, Ohio

Stephanie Holz, MD
Assistant Professor of Clinical Radiology and Imaging Sciences, Indiana University, Indianapolis, Indiana

Robert Klinglesmith, MD, PsyD
Staff Radiologist, Singleton Associates, PA, Houston, Texas

Michael Mahlmann, MD
Senior Resident, Department of Diagnostic and Interventional Imaging, The University of Texas Health Science Center, Houston, Texas

Patrick Marcin, MD
Fellow, Department of Diagnostic Radiology, The University of Texas MD Anderson Cancer Center, Houston, Texas

Eduardo J. Matta, MD
Assistant Professor of Diagnostic and Interventional Imaging, Department of Radiology, The University of Texas Medical School at Houston, Houston, Texas

Zeyad A. Metwalli, MD
Fellow, Vascular and Interventional Radiology, Department of Radiology, Northwestern University, Chicago, Illinois

Ajaykumar C. Morani, MD
Assistant Professor of Diagnostic Radiology, Department of Diagnostic Radiology, The University of Texas MD Anderson Cancer Center, Houston, Texas

Sandra A. A. Oldham, MD
Professor of Radiology, Chief, Section of Thoracic Imaging, Vice Chairman for Education, Department of Diagnostic and Interventional Imaging, The University of Texas Health Science Center, Houston, Texas

Gregory C. Ravizzini, MD
Assistant Professor, Department of Nuclear Medicine, The University of Texas MD Anderson Cancer Center, Houston, Texas

Usama Salem, MD
Department of Diagnostic Radiology, The University of Texas MD Anderson Cancer Center, Houston, Texas

Assistant Lecturer, Department of Diagnostic Radiology, National Cancer Institute, Cairo University, Cairo, Egypt

Santosh Shah, MD
Clinical Assistant in Radiology at Harvard Medical School, Department of Neuroradiology, Massachusetts General Hospital, Boston, Massachusetts

Megan Speer, MD
Department of Diagnostic and Interventional Imaging, The University of Texas Health Science Center, Houston, Texas

Aaron J. Thomas
Medical Student, The University of Texas Medical School at Houston, Houston, Texas

Ayda Youssef, MD
Lecturer of radio diagnosis Department of Diagnostic Radiology, National Cancer Institute, Cairo University, Cairo, Egypt

Navid F. Zaer, MD
Graduate Resident from the Department of Diagnostic Radiology and Interventional Imaging, The University of Texas Medical School at Houston, Houston, Texas

Acknowledgments

I take this opportunity to extend my appreciation to those individuals who have been instrumental in my career in radiology and those who have inspired me to complete this project:

   To my mentors, friends, and all colleagues in:

–MD Anderson Cancer Center, especially Chusilp Charnsangavej, Marshall Hicks, Joel Dunnington, Vikas Kundra, Randy Ernst, and Aliya Qayyum

–University of Michigan, especially Isaac Francis, Melvyn Korobkin, Joel Platt, Reed Dunnick, James Ellis, Rich Cohan, and Hero Hussain

–Egypt, especially Hazem Moharram, Mamdouh Mahfouz, Tarek Eldiasty, Ikram Hamed, Ahmed Samy, Mohamed Moustafa, Hatem Ghonim, Moustafa Ismail, Omar Moawyah, Ihab Fathy, and Amr Nasef

–Mallinckrodt Institute of Radiology, especially Jeffrey J. Brown, Vamsidhar R. Narra, Jay Heiken, and Christine Menias

–Elsewhere, especially John Leyendecker (Wake Forest), Rich Baron (Chicago), Mosleh Al-Raddadi (KSA), Haitham Elsamaloty (Toledo), and Akram Shaaban (Utah)

   To the great teacher, my coeditor Dr Sandra A. A. Oldham
   To Mike Weitz and Christie Naglieri (editor: McGraw-Hill)
   To the great medical illustrator David Bier
   To all contributors of this book
   To all of my medical students and residents

Khaled M. Elsayes

Preface

Recent growth in the field of diagnostic radiology has dramatically increased the complexity of this field. Diagnostic imaging has become widely available and plays an increasing role in clinical diagnosis and therapy. However, in most practices, miscommunication between radiologists and other physicians occurs frequently mainly because physicians often are not completely familiar with the role of radiology in patient care. This misunderstanding leads to the ordering of incorrect imaging studies, duplication of orders, unnecessary requests for follow-up imaging, too many exam orders, and other problems. In addition, inappropriate use of imaging is increasing because referring clinicians are often unsure what tests to order and when. These problems are costly and can delay diagnosis and therapy (thus decreasing patient throughput) and expose patients to unnecessary ionizing radiation. Appropriateness criteria for imaging tests are available but are not widely known or easily applied by nonradiologists, who also may interpret images incorrectly. Furthermore, nonradiologists who do not have a good knowledge about radiology often cannot communicate well with radiologists.

Addressing these problems starts with medical students, the forgotten members of the academic radiology community. Despite sporadic efforts, there is no standardized national diagnostic radiology curriculum to teach medical students not only basic radiology but also the role radiology currently plays in diagnosis, treatment, and overall patient care; radiation protection; and the importance of good communication between nonradiologist clinicians and radiologists. The availability of radiology clerkships and electives is highly variable among medical schools, and many clerkship/elective directors are limited in time and academic resources. Among the institutions that do provide some training in diagnostic radiology, the training differs significantly in scope, detail, and presentation methods.

The book is written, with medical students in mind, as an alternative to the traditionally large (and hard to learn) reference textbooks. We believe that trainees should learn the essentials before delving into the subjects in depth. This up-to-date book contains practical and concise descriptions and high-quality illustrations. State-of-the-art techniques and the most common types of clinical cases encountered in daily practice are discussed.

This book handles diagnoses from a practical point of view. Our book takes cases from the emergency room and physician offices and uses a practical approach to reach an accurate diagnosis. The cases walk the reader through a radiology expert's analysis. The cases are presented progressively, with the expert's thinking process described in detail. Comments at the end of each case tie up loose ends and provide references and additional relevant factual material. The cases are discussed in regards to clinical presentation, clinical suspicion, modality of choice and radiological technique, and pertinent imaging features of common disease processes.

The purpose of this book is to provide a quick, portable reference for improving basic knowledge of diagnostic radiology of medical students, beginner radiologists, and nonradiologists so that they can order correct radiological examinations, improve image interpretation through a distillate of clinically useful information, and enhance their interpretation of various radiological manifestations. This book does not detail the literature of all disease processes. Instead, we focus on the most common clinical scenarios encountered in daily practice. We also discuss practical imaging techniques and protocols used to address common problems, and we give readers easily accessible tools to aid in reaching a specific diagnosis by reviewing our simple relevant case scenarios.

This book is divided into several chapters. The first two chapters provide basic information regarding various diagnostic radiology techniques and contrast agents. Each of the following chapters discuss imaging of a specific organ system, starting with a description of the pertinent clinical presentation or suspicion and continuing with a description of the imaging modalities of choice and illustration of relevant features to help simplify the differential diagnosis. Based on the effect of similar material we use with our graduating medical students, we believe that the practical emphasis of this text will be useful to medical students, beginner radiology residents, family practitioners, and any nonradiologist physician wishing to better understand diagnostic radiology.

Chapter 1

Overview of Diagnostic Modalities and Contrast Agents

By Navid F. Zaer, Behrang Amini, and Khaled M. Elsayes

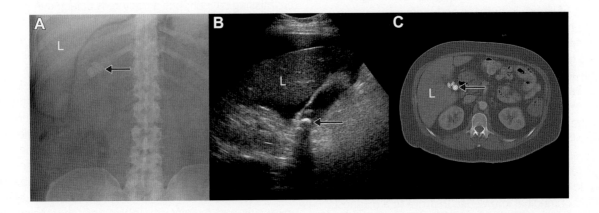

INTRODUCTION

Every day, millions of people undergo imaging evaluations to assess a wide range of medical conditions. When the power of imaging technology is appropriately expanded, these studies yield a wealth of useful medical information. However, like all medical procedures, most imaging studies are associated with risks to patients and costs to patients and society as a whole. These drawbacks are made more significant when the studies fail to yield useful information, such as when an inappropriate study is ordered or when an imaging study is not indicated. Knowledge of the different imaging modalities and their relative costs and benefits is vital to proper management of patients.

WHAT IS DIAGNOSTIC RADIOLOGY?

The foundations of diagnostic imaging were laid over the course of a few years, starting with the discovery of x-rays by Wilhelm Conrad Röntgen in 1895, radioactivity by Henri Becquerel in 1896, and radium by Marie and Pierre Curie in 1898 [3]. *Radiology*, or the study of radiation, is an anachronistic term still in use that recalls the years before sound waves and nuclear magnetic resonance were harnessed as ultrasound (US) and magnetic resonance imaging (MRI) for medical use. Today, diagnostic imaging encompasses the use of various imaging technologies for the diagnosis of illness in humans and animals.

Medical physicists, imaging technologists, and radiologists collaborate to use this technology to answer questions raised by referring clinicians, with the ultimate goal of providing accurate and specific diagnoses to the patient. Medical physicists ensure the optimal and safe use of technology in patients. Imaging technologists are expertly trained in the use of specific imaging equipment used for acquisition of medical images.

Radiologists are physicians with specialized training in the interpretation of medical images. The radiologist must combine knowledge of imaging physics and anatomy with a broad fund of medical knowledge to arrive at a diagnosis relevant to the patient's clinical presentation. In this capacity, the radiologist serves as a consultant to referring physicians. Therefore, effective communication between the referring clinician and the radiologist is vital in all stages of imaging. This communication ideally starts even before a diagnostic study is ordered, when the optimal imaging study can be chosen for the patient based on the clinical question after consideration of the strengths and weaknesses of the different imaging modalities available.

THE ART OF IMAGE INTERPRETATION

Like other aspects of clinical medicine, image interpretation combines subjective and objective information to reach a diagnosis. In some cases, this results in a single diagnosis.

In most cases, however, there is a list of diagnoses that must be arranged in the order of likelihood, and require additional imaging, clinical, or pathological evaluation.

A firm grasp of the capabilities of the image storage and display system (PACS [picture archiving and communication system]) and ideally computer systems in general is a prerequisite for modern image interpretation. The ability to easily manipulate image settings and apply special software algorithms is essential. Knowledge of computer programming is not a requirement, but it can make interpretation more efficient by allowing the radiologist to create personalized solutions for the many deficiencies inherent in modern PACS software. At its most basic level, image interpretation requires identification of abnormalities on images. The radiologist must have a thorough understanding of the relevant anatomy and how it manifests on various imaging modalities in various states of disease and health (see Fig. 1.1). The radiologist also must have an organized system for image interpretation, in the form of a mental checklist of all anatomical structures that must be assessed for a given study. This is so the radiologist does not fall prey to a "satisfaction of search" error: stopping the checklist once a diagnosis is reached. This error results in missed ancillary findings, some of which may be relevant to the primary diagnosis (eg, missing metastases once the primary tumor is detected), or represent important unrelated diagnoses (eg, missing cancer once a fracture is detected in a trauma patient). The easiest thing one can do to become a better radiologist is to look at all the images. This may be an obvious statement, but time pressures often lead to shortcuts that can be disastrous.

Information derived from diagnostic imaging is then combined with patient information (eg, age, history and chief complaint, physical examination findings, and laboratory values) and a broad fund of medical knowledge to solve the clinical puzzle and reach a conclusion relevant to the patient and her physician. The art of image interpretation, then, is a subjective assessment of all available data and relies heavily on communication between referring physicians and radiologists. In this way, an imaging study differs from most laboratory studies, which yield objective results in a vacuum of clinical information. Appropriate

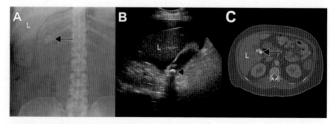

Fig. 1.1 Examples of the liver and gallstones on (A) radiography, (B) ultrasound, and (C) CT. L, liver. The liver edge has been outlined in panel A.

clinical history not only improves clinical decision making by the radiologist, but also affects perception in interpreting the images in the first place by focusing the attention of the radiologist on relevant anatomy and physiology [4, 5]. As seen in Fig. 1.2, a diagnosis of soft-tissue sarcoma became much less likely when a history of recent cat scratch was provided.

Unfortunately, this clinical information is often lacking. Electronic medical record systems have gone a long way to address the issue; however, multiple hurdles often prevent efficient access to patient data. These obstacles include lack of integration with PACS, poor user interface, slow network access, and lack of uniformity across different hospital systems and clinics.

The cycle of communication is completed either by direct discussion between the radiologist and the clinician, as is appropriate for urgent or unexpected findings, or through the written radiology report for more routine matters. Thus, another important role of the radiologist is as a medical communication expert who generates concise and accurate reports, avoiding ambiguity and outdated or confusing terminology. To that end, professional societies in radiology have proposed lexicons for the standardized reporting of imaging findings. The most successful of these has been the Breast Imaging Reporting and Data System (BI-RADS) of the American College of Radiology (ACR), which will be described in more detail in chapter 10.

Artifacts

An *artifact* is an imaging finding that does not directly correspond to the reality of the patient and may mimic a clinical feature, degrade image quality, or obscure anatomy. They can be related to the patient, hardware, or software (and their use by the operator). Some artifacts can be seen across different modalities (eg, patient motion in radiography, computed tomography [CT], MRI, and nuclear medicine), while others are specific to the technology being used (eg, susceptibility artifact in MRI). Knowledge of artifacts specific to each modality is vital in accurate interpretation of the provided images.

IMAGE CONTRAST

Image contrast is the difference in brightness between an area of interest and its surroundings. The larger the difference in brightness between different tissue types, the easier it is to differentiate them from each other. Figure 1.3 shows examples of images with different levels of contrast.

In diagnostic imaging, image contrast depends not only on tissue characteristics, but also on modality-specific

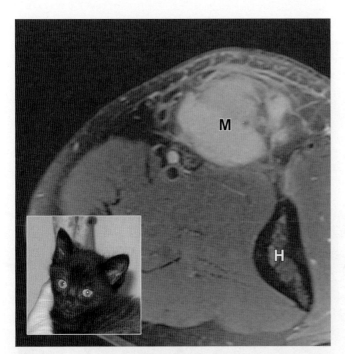

Fig. 1.2 45-year-old man with a lump at the elbow. MR image shows an enhancing soft-tissue mass (M) proximal to the elbow joint (H=humerus). Based on the provided history of "soft tissue mass, medial aspect of the elbow," the radiologist diagnosed the lesion as a soft-tissue sarcoma. The patient was referred to a national cancer referral center, where further questioning of the patient prompted the recollection of a scratch or bite on his arm by his cat (inset) a month prior to the MRI. Given the history, the soft-tissue lump was identified as an inflamed lymph node), and the patient was successfully treated with antibiotics.

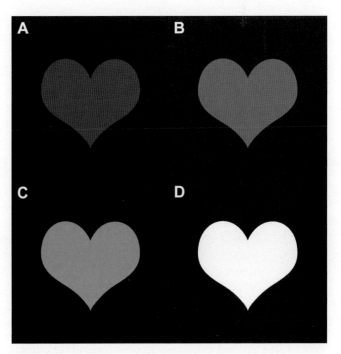

Fig. 1.3 Images with increasing contrast between the area of interest and background. (A) Image with low contrast. (D) Image with high contrast.

factors that will be discussed in subsequent sections later in this chapter.

PLANAR VERSUS CROSS-SECTIONAL IMAGING

Imaging studies can be broadly divided into planar and cross-sectional. In their simplest form, planar images are shadows of complex three-dimensional objects. These images compress a large amount of information into a two-dimensional image; however, as would be expected, important anatomical relationships can be obscured in this fashion (Fig. 1.4A,B). The best-known planar imaging technique is radiography (eg, chest x-rays and mammography), which seems to be a required prop in all movie depictions of hospitals and doctor's offices.

Cross-sectional imaging techniques address the three-dimensional reality of human anatomy by creating a detailed composite analysis of two-dimensional "slices" (Fig. 1.4C-E), and include CT, ultrasound, and MRI. Depending on the modality, images can be acquired in two or three dimensions. The unit elements of an image are referred to as *pixels* (picture elements) for two-dimensional images, and *voxels* (volume elements) for three-dimensional images. The images can be mathematically manipulated to obtain two-dimensional images in different planes (Fig. 1.4E) or three-dimensional images highlighting specific regions or anatomy. The mathematical algorithms and detailed physics remain beyond the scope of this text. It is important to note that these technologies have revolutionized the field of radiology in terms of highly specific diagnostic capability as well as high volume data acquisition, manipulation, and storage.

COST

Progressive reliance on diagnostic radiology as an integral part of a patient's clinical evaluation has resulted in marked growth in the number of studies performed. Continued research and technologic advancements provide the clinician with a range of imaging modalities and examinations to choose from. In addition to judicious selection based on the clinical scenario, one must not forget the practical impact of these choices with regard to the financial responsibilities of the patient, payers, and society as a whole. Due to the enormous variability in reimbursement rates across and within nations, it is impossible to provide an absolute cost for each modality and type of examination that exists. However, it is imperative that one acquires a general idea

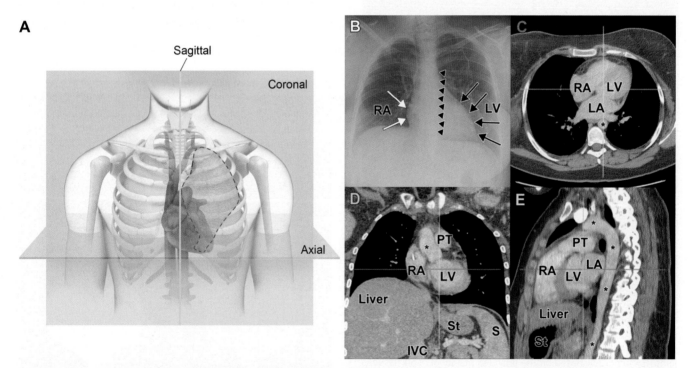

Fig. 1.4 Cross-sectional Imaging. (A) Diagram of the chest with "slices" through the heart. (B) Planar radiograph of the chest showing the margins of the right atrium (RA, white arrows), left ventricle (LV, black arrows), and descending thoracic aorta (small black arrowheads). (C) Axial CT image of the chest with pixel values adjusted for visualization of the soft tissues, showing the RA, left atrium (LA), LV, and aorta (*). The blue and yellow lines show the levels of the coronal (D) and sagittal (E) reformations, respectively. (D) Coronal reformation showing the RA, LV, and aorta (*), in addition to the pulmonary trunk (PT), liver, spleen (S), stomach (St), and inferior vena cava (IVC). The red and yellow lines show the levels of the axial (C) and sagittal (E) reformations, respectively. (E) Sagittal reformation of the chest showing the RA, LV, LA, PT, aorta (*), liver, and stomach. The red and blue lines show the levels of the axial and coronal reformations, respectively.

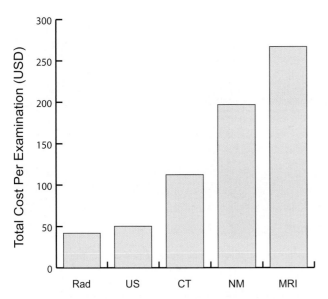

Fig. 1.5 Relative costs for various diagnostic imaging examinations. Although these are only relative values, they serve to provide a tangible reference point when considering advanced imaging for a patient. Rad, radiography; US, ultrasound; CT, computed tomography; NM, nuclear medicine, excluding PET and PET/CT; MRI, magnetic resonance imaging. Data from [1].

of the relative cost of one modality compared to another (Fig. 1.5) [1].

The sections that follow will cover some of the more commonly used imaging modalities used in diagnostic imaging and discuss how images are acquired and interpreted, the strengths and weaknesses of each modality, and issues of safety and cost. The literature cited will be to helpful review articles rather than to primary sources, and the interested reader is advised to consult these papers for a more thorough coverage of the subjects included in this chapter.

RADIOGRAPHY

Radiography is the oldest of the imaging modalities used in diagnostic radiology. Strictly speaking, *radiography* is the use of x-rays to generate images. This definition would include projectional radiography (eg, chest x-rays) and CT; however, in common usage, the words x-ray, plain film, radiograph, and conventional radiograph are used interchangeably to refer to projectional radiography. *Fluoroscopy* is an application of projectional radiography that allows real-time observation of the internal structures of a patient and is used predominantly in gastrointestinal imaging, interventional radiology, and musculoskeletal radiology.

This section will provide a brief overview of radiography and fluoroscopy, and an introduction to radiation dose measurements and radiation safety.

IMAGE FORMATION

Radiographs are produced by passing an x-ray beam generated by an x-ray tube (see the "Equipment" section) through a patient and using one of many methods of capturing the attenuated beam. The image produced represents a "shadow" of the structures the x-ray beam passed through.

Image Contrast

Image contrast in radiography is produced by the ability of different materials to attenuate (weaken) the x-ray beam. For example, x-rays passing through a patient's chest will encounter little resistance passing through the air in the lungs, and the resulting transmitted x-ray beam will not be significantly attenuated. Bones, on the other hand, result in substantial attenuation of the x-ray beam, while soft tissues (such as the heart and mediastinum) result in intermediate attenuation of the x-ray beam. Attenuation of the x-ray beam for a given tissue is quantified in a single parameter, the mass attenuation coefficient, which is expressed as cm^2/g. Several physical characteristics of a tissue contribute to a tissue's mass attenuation coefficient. A detailed description of these physical characteristics is beyond the scope of this book; however, a familiarity with mass attenuation coefficient is important for understanding the basis of image contrast in radiography and CT (see the "Computed Tomography" section), and understanding how liquids like iodinated contrast agents can have higher attenuation than solids like cortical bone. The interested reader is referred to the excellent review by Bushberg [6] for more comprehensive coverage of this topic.

Contrast Agents. A variety of substances are available to enhance the contrast between different anatomical structures. Contrast media can be classified as positive or negative. Positive contrast agents result in increased attenuation of x-rays and show up as white on the conventional method of visualizing x-rays (Fig. 1.6A,B). Negative contrast agents, on the other hand, result in decreased attenuation of x-rays and show up as black or gray (Fig. 1.6C). Barium and iodinated agents are positive contrast agents used in radiography, while negative agents include air and carbon dioxide.

> **Barium Sulfate:** This inexpensive contrast agent is utilized in both fluoroscopic and CT examinations to opacify (make whiter) the gastrointestinal tract. It can be given orally as well as rectally and is excreted unchanged in the feces. It is generally well tolerated and can be formulated to various viscosities as needed for the level of mucosal coating desired. Mucosal coating is important in fluoroscopic examinations for assessment details of the endoluminal surface of the gastrointestinal tract. Adverse reactions are infrequent and often mild. Constipation, nausea, and diarrhea are several known side effects and are typically self-limiting. Allergic reactions have been reported but are

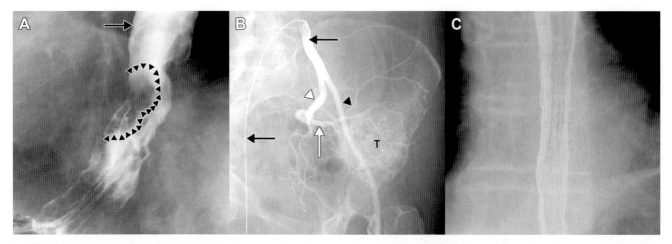

Fig. 1.6 Positive and negative contrast agents. (A) Double (CO_2 and barium) contrast esophagography showing positive contrast outlining the proximal esophagus (black arrow), as well as a tumor (arrowheads). (B) Intravascular use of contrast material in a left common iliac artery angiogram. The tip of the catheter (black arrows) is located in the proximal right common iliac artery. Injected contrast opacifies the internal (white arrowhead) and external (black arrowhead) iliac arteries, showing that the blood supply to the tumor (T) is predominantly from branches of the superior gluteal artery (white arrow). (C) Double contrast esophagogram in another patient after passage of barium into the stomach shows mucosal detail outlined by barium in an esophagus that is a distended by CO_2 gas.

exceedingly rare. The foremost risk of barium sulfate is peritonitis if spilled into the abdominal cavity in a patient with bowel perforation. The barium forms fibrinous deposits and a chemical irritation that leads to marked third-spacing of fluid and subsequent hypovolemia. Nearly half of all affected patients progress to sepsis and eventual death. If bowel perforation is suspected, water-soluble iodinated agents are used.

Iodinated Agents: These agents can be used for gastrointestinal or intravascular administration. In the gastrointestinal tract, they are considered inferior to barium for the purposes of fluoroscopic gastrointestinal studies because of opacification by passive filling rather than mucosal coating and are mainly used in the setting of suspected bowel perforation. Water-soluble iodinated agents are quickly absorbed by the peritoneal surface if spilled into the peritoneal cavity and will not cause peritonitis. Intravascular use of these contrast agents will be discussed in more detail in the CT section.

Gases: Carbon dioxide gas in the form of effervescent powder or tablet is activated in the presence of water and is an effective means of distending the stomach for fluoroscopic evaluation. Air injected via nasogastric or rectal tube is also efficient for gastric or colonic distension, respectively.

EQUIPMENT

X-Ray Tube

A complete description of the technology and physics of the modern x-ray tube and housing is beyond the scope of this book; however, a brief description is provided to help conceptualize the device. The x-ray tube is an evacuated

chamber containing a cathode and an anode, across which an electric potential is applied (Fig. 1.7). The cathode contains a high-melting point metal filament, such as tungsten, that is heated, liberating electrons in a process called thermionic emission. The amount of heating, and thus the number of electrons "boiling off" the filament, is controlled by the milliampere (mA) setting on the x-ray control panel. The electric potential applied between the cathode and anode draws the electrons toward the anode, where they strike the anode disk, generating x-rays as well as a large amount of heat (approximately 99% of the energy of the electrons is lost as heat). The energy of the generated x-rays depends on the speed of the electrons as they travel from the cathode to the anode. The speed of the electrons, in turn, depends on the strength of the electric potential

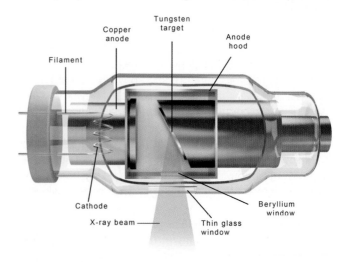

Fig. 1.7 The x-ray tube.

between the cathode and the anode. This is controlled by the kilovoltage peak (kVp) setting on the x-ray control panel. Higher kVp settings are used when high-energy x-ray beams are needed, such as when imaging thicker and/or denser anatomic parts.

From Film to Digital

The x-ray beam traverses the patient and is attenuated based on the characteristics of the tissues in its path. Several technologies are available for making the radiographic image. The three main technological solutions currently in use are conventional (film-based) radiography, computed radiography (CR), and direct radiography (DR).

Modern conventional radiography involves the use of a screen-film combination to capture the image information. X-ray photons strike one or two intensifying screens, which convert x-ray energy into visible light. This clean-film system is housed in a light-proof cassette, where the visible light generated by the intensifying screen(s) exposes the radiographic film to generate the image. The cassette is then taken to a film processor, which develops the film for visual interpretation. The main advantages of these systems are high spatial resolution of film, high sensitivity, easy handling, and low cost. The main disadvantage is the coupling of image acquisition and storage in the form of the film, high storage costs, and narrow dynamic range (the range of x-ray intensities a detector can differentiate between).

Computed radiography and direct radiography are digital radiography techniques that at some stage use a digital data format in acquiring, processing, displaying, or managing an x-ray image [7]. The main advantage of digital radiography techniques is the ability to separate image acquisition, processing, and display, which allows for optimization of each of these stages, as well as the ability to digitally manipulate acquired images [7]. Computed radiography involves acquiring the image on a filmless cassette containing an image sensor that temporarily stores information about the x-ray beam. The image sensor consists of a thin plate coated with tiny crystals of photostimulable phosphor (also called the image plate), which store the energies of the absorbed x-rays. After acquisition of the image, the cassette is inserted into a CR scanner, which automatically opens the cassette and scans the image plate with a laser (the readout process). The information is displayed on a small monitor, where the technologist can check the image quality for positioning and technical errors, as well as image artifacts. The digital image can then be sent to the PACS for storage and interpretation by the radiologist [8].

In contrast to both CR and conventional radiography, DR does not require a physical cassette for image acquisition. Direct radiography is a cassetteless system where the x-ray energy is converted to electrical energy, either directly using a photoconductor that converts x-ray photons into

electrical charge or indirectly by a scintillator that emits light when exposed to x-rays, after which the light is converted into an electrical charge [9]. This image can then be sent to the PACS in the same manner as in CR.

Fluoroscopy

Fluoroscopy involves a mobile x-ray tube that generates a continuous, adjustable x-ray beam, allowing for real-time visualization of anatomic structures. The x-ray beams strike a fluorescing screen coupled to an image intensifier that can transmit the images to a monitor [10]. Single images or a series of images can be stored for future review. Coupled with intravenous or enteric contrast administration, this modality provides a wide array of diagnostic and therapeutic options in multiple radiologic subspecialties. For example, intravenous contrast can be used to visualize vessels (Fig. 1.6B) and enteric contrast is commonly used in gastrointestinal evaluation, such as barium swallow studies (Fig. 1.6A,C).

IMAGE INTERPRETATION

Image interpretation in radiography depends on a thorough understanding of the three-dimensional anatomy of the region under evaluation and how it is compressed into two dimensions under different projection techniques. For example, the cardiac silhouette ("heart shadow") can change size depending on the position of the patient in relationship to the x-ray source and the cassette (or image detector in direct radiography). In the standard posteroanterior (PA) projection, the x-ray source is behind the patient and the cassette is in front, closer to the heart. Therefore, the size of the shadow cast by the heart is fairly close to the actual size (Fig. 1.8A). In contrast, the anteroposterior (AP) projection used in portable studies places the cassette behind the patient, with the x-ray source in front. This projection results in a larger shadow being cast by the heart, a phenomenon that is referred to as magnification (Fig. 1.8B). In addition, the radiologist must know the strengths and weaknesses of different projections. For example, cervical spine radiographs typically consist of anteroposterior, lateral, and odontoid views. The lateral view allows for an assessment of the alignment of the spine, prespinal soft tissues, and vertebral body and disc space heights (Fig. 1.8C). When pathology involving the neural foramina is sought (eg, for initial assessment of radiculopathy), oblique views are obtained, allowing assessment of the bony configuration of the neural foramina (Fig. 1.8D).

Another important concept is the attenuation characteristics of different tissues, introduced in theoretical form earlier in the section Image Contrast. In practice, differences in attenuation mean that bone, metal, and contrast agents appear white on images, soft tissues and fat appear

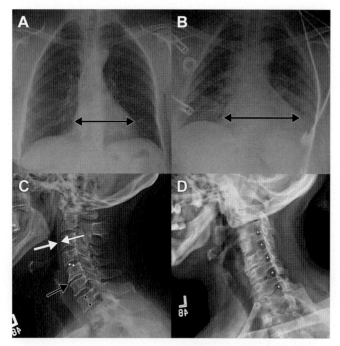

Fig. 1.8 Importance of projection in image interpretation. (A) Posteroanterior (PA) chest radiograph obtained by placing the x-ray source behind the patient. The heart shadow is indicated by the double-headed arrow and is normal. (B) Anteroposterior projection (AP) results in apparent enlargement of the heart, a phenomenon known as magnification. (C) Lateral radiograph of the cervical spine is used to assess the alignment of the spine, thickness of the prevertebral soft tissues (between white arrows), and heights of the vertebral bodies (double black arrow) and discs (double white arrow), to name a few. In this patient, disc space narrowing is present at C5-C6 (black arrow). (D) The oblique view of the cervical spine highlights the bony contours of the neural foramina (*).

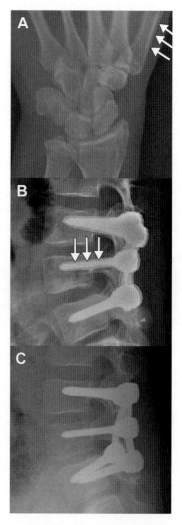

Fig. 1.9 Artifacts in radiography. (A) Patient motion can affect all techniques of radiography and results in a blurry image and doubling of cortical lines, best seen in the radial cortex of the thumb metacarpal (arrows). (B) The Uberschwinger (overswing or rebound) artifact results in a lucent halo around metal or at interfaces where there are sudden large difference in image density (ie, at areas of high spatial frequency). This postprocessing (software) artifact seen in computed and direct radiography is most pronounced with high degrees of edge enhancement. (C) Radiograph in the same patient without edge enhancement removes the artifact.

as varying shades of gray, and gas appears black. Normal anatomy and pathology can then be identified based on their composition and anatomic location.

Artifacts

Artifacts can be seen in conventional, computed, and direct radiography. Some artifacts, such as patient motion (Fig. 1.9) and dust particles, can affect all techniques of radiography, while others are specific to one or more of the three methods. Ultimately, it is important for the radiologist to have an understanding of common artifacts in order to prevent errors in interpretation. The interested reader may refer to papers by Shetty, et al [11] and Walz-Flannigan, et al [12] for a review of artifacts in computed and digital radiography, respectively.

SAFETY
Radiation

We are exposed to radiation from a multitude of different natural sources at all times. Ionizing radiation can damage living cells by causing undesired chemical reactions and altering the structure of macromolecules in cells. In imaging modalities that produce ionizing radiation (radiography, CT, and nuclear medicine), this potential harm can affect physicians, technologists, patients, and sometimes their families (in the case of nuclear medicine). Children, young adults, and women of reproductive age are particularly vulnerable. Therefore, it is important to critically weigh the risks and benefits of any study before recommending it for a patient.

The concept of ALARA (as low as reasonably achievable) in relationship to radiation dose is an extension of the oath to do no harm. In practice, this means using the lowest radiation exposure that is reasonably achievable to perform a study, weighing the risk of the adverse effects of radiation (see Biological Effects of Radiation) against the benefit of a diagnosis that can influence treatment. Dose minimization is the responsibility of every health care professional involved in the care of the patient, including the clinician who orders the study, the radiologist who determines how the study should be performed, the medical physicist who optimizes the imaging parameters, and the technologist who performs the study. The ALARA principle begins at the moment an imaging study is considered, by selecting the appropriate imaging study. An examination should only be requested if it directly influences patient. Unfortunately, imaging is sometimes inappropriately performed to satisfy academic curiosity, as a medicolegal strategy, or at the behest of patients.

Biological Effects of Radiation. The biological effects of radiation can be conceptualized as either deterministic or stochastic. Deterministic effects are thought to occur only once a certain threshold of exposure has been exceeded and are generally seen with higher doses of radiation. Biologically, these effects are caused by significant cell damage or death that overwhelms the physiological ability of the affected organ to repair itself. Adverse events resulting in deterministic effects are rare in diagnostic imaging, but tend to make headlines in the popular press when they do occur [13]. Examples include skin damage (erythema, necrosis, and epilation), cataracts, sterility, radiation sickness, teratogenesis, and fetal death. Teratogenic effects can occur with large doses of radiation and include growth restriction, microcephaly, and mental retardation. The risk of central nervous system injury with radiation is greatest when the exposure occurs between 8 and 15 weeks of gestation, with no proven risk above or below this range [14]. The National Council on Radiation Protection has recommended that cumulative dose to the fetus remain less than 50 mSv during the course of gestation.

Unlike deterministic effects, which do not occur below a certain threshold of radiation exposure, stochastic effects are thought to follow a linear, no-threshold model. It is thought that stochastic effects occur as a result of ionizing radiation causing symmetrical translocations that occur during cell division, with the most important consequence being cancer. This risk is most pronounced in children in general, and specifically in rapidly dividing tissues, such as reproductive organs and breasts in young women.

The linear, no-threshold model is based on fitting the data from Japanese survivors of the atomic bomb attacks with a linear model [2]. This is seen as the thick line in Fig. 1.10. At levels below 100 mSv, which is the range of doses of most medical imaging studies, any increase in radiation-induced cancers is thought to be too small to be distinguishable from the background cancer incidence

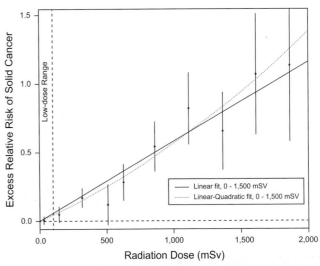

Fig. 1.10 Relationship between radiation-induced solid cancer risk and administered dose. The solid line shows the fit of the linear model to the data, while the dotted line shows the fit of a linear-quadratic model. For solid cancer incidence, the linear-quadratic model did not offer a statistically significant improvement in fit. Data in the low-dose range is more limited, and the difference between the two models illustrated is small in this region. Some have advocated the application of other models to fit the data in this region. Graph modified from [2].

due to other causes [15]. However, application of the linear model to these low doses may result in the overestimation of the risk of low-dose radiation, and other models have been proposed. The linear, no-threshold model is prudent for establishing radiation protection standards for members of the public and people whose occupations expose them to radiation [16]. However, overestimation of risks for medically indicated imaging procedures can stimulate sensationalistic reports in the popular press and result in fear and anxiety of imaging examinations and cancellation or deferral of vital imaging studies [15].

Quantification of Radiation Dose. Radiation exposure can be conceptualized as absorbed dose and effective dose. Absorbed dose (expressed in Grays, Gy) is a measurement of the total radiation energy absorbed per volume of tissue exposed and provides little information on the biologic effects of radiation. Effective dose, on the other hand, applies a weighting factor to absorbed dose for each exposed tissue based on its tendency to develop stochastic effects, and gives a measure of the risk for stochastic effects in the whole patient. For example, the weighting factor for the breast is 0.12, while that for the brain is 0.01. Therefore, the same amount of absorbed dose will result in different effective doses for these organs [17]. The effective dose is measured in Sieverts (Sv). A helpful way to conceptualize radiation doses for beginners is the background equivalent radiation time (BERT), which compares a given radiation dose to the exposure of the entire population from sources of natural ionizing radiation. This exposure comes from a variety of sources, such as cosmic radiation and natural uranium and thorium (and their indirect decay product, radon gas). This natural "background" effective dose is approximately 3 mSv per year, although the exact number varies by location and altitude [18, 19]. Using the BERT system, the radiation received from a given source is expressed in terms of a certain number of days or years of background radiation [17]. For example, a PA and lateral chest radiograph is equivalent to a background exposure of between 7 and 19 days, while an abdominal series is equivalent to a background exposure of between 3 and 4 months [17].

STRENGTHS AND WEAKNESSES

Radiography is widely available and inexpensive, has high spatial resolution, and exposes patients to lower doses of radiation than studies such as CT. In addition, it offers excellent visualization of bones for the purpose of tumor characterization and fracture identification, sometimes superior or complementary to MRI. The main disadvantage of radiography is the collapse of complex three-dimensional structures into a two-dimensional image, which can lead to uncertainty about the location of lesions in space and decreased sensitivity in detection of lesions hidden behind higher attenuation structures. In addition, the contrast resolution of radiography is inferior to CT and MRI.

COMPUTED TOMOGRAPHY (CT)

The introduction of computed tomography in the early 1970s is heralded as the greatest advance in the field of radiology since the discovery of x-rays. It provided a means by which x-rays could be utilized to create cross-sectional images and thereby allowed physicians to identify a greater range of abnormalities within the human body.

Allan M. Cormack was a South African physicist who discovered that changes in radiation therapy dose distributions within the body were related to differences in the tendency of various tissues to attenuate x-rays. He surmised that these differences could be used to create projection imaging using gray-scale models. His research went relatively unnoticed but its concepts later emerged independently in the work of Sir Godfrey Hounsfield, a British engineer. Hounsfield's experiments with an x-ray tube resulted in data acquisition and processing times of 9 hours and 2½ hours, respectively; far too long for effective clinical use. The first clinical application of the CT scanner was in October 1971 at Atkinson Morley Hospital in London where a brain scan revealed a frontal lobe brain tumor in a 41-year-old woman. In 1979, Hounsfield and Cormack shared the Nobel Prize for Medicine for their

contributions to the realization of projection imaging. Modifications in technique have reduced data acquisition and processing times to minutes [20].

IMAGE FORMATION

The components of a CT system are housed within the donut-shaped gantry, which contains the radiation source (x-ray tube) and detectors (Fig. 1.11). The examination table carries the patient through the donut hole of the gantry. The images are obtained by rapid rotations of the x-ray tube around the patient. Essentially, a narrow beam of x-rays passes through a section of the patient and sensitive detectors measure the radiation transmitted directly across the beam. Computer processing of the data results in cross-sectional images of the body.

Image Contrast

Image contrast in CT relies on the same principles as radiography: the difference in attenuation (weakening) of the x-ray beam as its passes through different substances. In

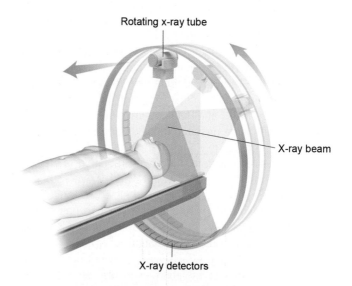

Rotating x-ray tube

X-ray beam

X-ray detectors

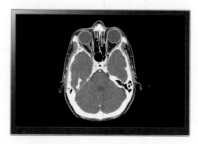

Fig. 1.11 Image acquisition in a modern CT scanner. In this example of a multidetector CT (MDCT) operating in helical mode, the rotating x-ray tube acquires images as it moves along the body part of interest (the head in this case).

CT, this difference is reproducibly quantifiable. As mentioned previously, each CT slice is composed of a matrix of volume elements or voxels. Each voxel has a value that represents the attenuation of x-ray photons that traverse that portion of tissue during the scan. The voxels are converted for display into a corresponding matrix of picture elements or pixels. Each pixel is assigned a numerical value (CT number) representing the average of the attenuation values in the voxel from which it was derived. Their values are given interpretive meaning on the Hounsfield

Table 1.1 Range of HU for Different Tissues

Tissue	HU
Lungs	−600 to −400
Fat	−100 to −30
Water	0 to 20
Soft tissue	40 to 80

unit (HU) scale which is named in honor of the inventor of CT. The numbers are, by convention, compared to the average attenuation value of water. Water is assigned a value of 0 HU. The scale ranges from approximately −1000 HU (black) for air to greater than +1000 HU (white) for metal. Important HU values for interpretation of images are shown in Table 1.1 and illustrated in Fig. 1.12A [21].

Contrast Agents. As described earlier, image contrast can be enhanced by the addition of agents that (most commonly) result in increased attenuation of the x-ray beam. Iodine and barium are commonly used agents that result in increased attenuation of the x-ray beam. Contrast agents can be administered through any cavity (natural or iatrogenic) and enhance differences between tissues that would normally have similar attenuation. The primary routes of delivery for CT are intravascular (venous) and enteric (oral and rectal). The use of contrast media is nearly ubiquitous in modern imaging, and its optimal use

Box 1.1 – TERMINOLOGY

There is often disregard for the difference between the terms *attenuation* and *density* in CT. However, the terms have specific and distinct meanings, and confusion of the two signals a lack of knowledge of or disregard for the physics of CT. **Attenuation** refers to the ability of a tissue to weaken the x-ray beam that passes through it, and is the correct term to use to refer to how bright a structure is on CT. **Density** refers to the mass per unit volume of a substance.

While attenuation of x-ray beams is usually related to the density of a substance, this is not always the case. For example, liquid iodinated contrast agents result in significant attenuation of x-ray beams, sometimes more so than solid bone.

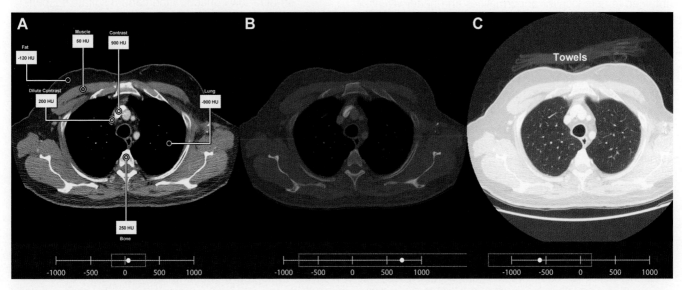

Fig. 1.12 (A) CT image with pixel values optimized for assessment of the soft tissues ("soft tissue windows"). Inset at bottom shows the range of pixel values centered at 55, with a width of 500. Attenuation values of various tissues on CT: Lung (−900 HU), subcutaneous fat (−120 HU), pectoralis major muscle (50 HU), iodinated contrast material in the superior vena cava diluted by circulation (200 HU), bone marrow (250 HU), and undiluted contrast in the brachiocephalic vein (900 HU). (B) CT image with pixel values optimized for assessment of bones ("bone windows"), centered at 750, with a width of 3000. Please note that the attenuation values for the various structures are the same as in A. Only the pixel values chosen for display are changed. (C) CT image with pixel values optimized for assessment of lungs ("lung windows") centered at −600, with a width of 1500. Note that using this window, there is better visualization of the lung parenchyma, as well as the towels placed on the patient for comfort.

has been carefully studied in order to tailor CT protocols for specific clinical questions.

Intravascularly administered agents are iodinated material that move quickly into the extracellular fluid. No significant metabolism or transformation occurs. Excretion is primarily through the kidneys. In patients with compromised renal function there is greater excretion through the biliary system and gastrointestinal tract. Dynamic contrast-enhanced imaging refers to precise timing of the injection of intravascular agents coupled with image acquisition spaced in time. This technique can help identify and classify abnormalities by taking advantage of the difference in contrast enhancement among different tissues across time (see Image Interpretation on page 14). For example, a lesion can have the same attenuation as its surroundings on noncontrast and delayed images, but will have intense enhancement on arterial phase images (image obtained when most of the contrast enhancement is in the arterial system) (see chapter 5, case 6).

CT angiography also makes use of precise contrast timing to image vascular anatomy. This is helpful because vessels often have the same or similar attenuation as their surroundings and because emboli and thrombi often have the same attenuation as blood. With the injection of intravascular contrast, bland (nontumorous) emboli and thrombi retain their soft-tissue attenuation while the surrounding blood has higher attenuation due to the injected contrast. Coronal and sagittal reformations are commonly obtained to help localize abnormalities and better visualize anatomy.

Intravascular Agents. Water-soluble iodinated contrast agents can be used intravenously in CT for visualization of hypervascular tissues (eg, tumor) and vascular structures (they can also be used for improved image contrast in the gastrointestinal tract, as will be discussed in the next section). The various iodinated contrast agents do not differ significantly from one another in terms of imaging capabilities when similar concentrations, administration rates, and volumes are utilized. They do, however, show important differences in adverse-reaction profiles primarily based on their charge, osmolality, and viscosity when administered intravenously.

First Generation Agents: The initial iodinated contrast agents were high-osmolar ionic compounds. These agents are very hypertonic—5 to 8 times the osmolality of blood. This high osmolality was shown to cause greater reported incidents of pain or discomfort when injected intravenously. Additionally, blood volume

expansion caused by osmotic differences was a cause for concern in volume-overloaded patients such as those with heart failure. As a result, these agents have fallen out of favor for intravascular administration. They do retain utility in gastrointestinal or retrograde urological procedures (eg, cystography) because they can provide safe and adequate imaging at low cost.

Second Generation Agents: Low osmolality nonionic compounds demonstrated fewer adverse reactions and were more tolerable in terms of intravascular administration. Common agents include iohexol (Omnipaque), ioversol (Optiray), and iopamidol (Isovue).

Third Generation Agents: The nonionic iso-osmolar dimer iodixanol (Visipaque) has found use in patients at elevated risk for contrast induced nephrotoxicity (more in the following section) due to its unique chemical properties and hydrophilic nature. Due to its higher cost, it is typically reserved for patients at elevated risk of renal insult.

Gastrointestinal Agents

Barium Sulfate: As discussed, barium sulfate mixtures are used to opacify the bowel. For CT imaging, the patient ingests the barium sulfate suspension approximately 1½ to 2 hours prior to imaging to allow for appropriate transit within the bowel. As noted earlier, if bowel perforation is suspected, water-soluble iodinated agents are preferred.

An ultra-low concentration barium sulfate suspension (VoLumen) has been developed for special use in CT. This formulation contains sorbitol, a nonabsorbable sugar alcohol that promotes gastrointestinal distension by limiting resorption of water across the small bowel wall. Unlike conventional positive contrast agents that result in increased attenuation of x-rays, this agent provides negative contrast by filling the bowel with low-attenuation fluid. Consequently, it provides excellent evaluation of the bowel wall and is being used extensively in CT enterography. The use of a negative enteric contrast such as water or VoLumen coupled with intravenous contrast highlights hypervascular lesions as well as bowel wall thickening or abnormal enhancement and enables evaluation of bowel wall thickness and perienteric fat and vasculature [22].

Water-Soluble Iodinated Agents: As mentioned in the radiography section, these agents are used in patients with suspected bowel perforation to avoid complications of peritonitis. Dilute solutions are routinely used for oral and rectal contrast administration. A mild laxative effect may be seen due to the high osmolality.

EQUIPMENT

Image Acquisition

The first commercially utilized CT scanner became available in 1972. There was a rapid push by multiple companies to produce innovations in its design. Four generations of CT scanners evolved over the short period of four years with continued reduction in scan times. Most modern scanners make use of a combination of technologies to allow rapid acquisition of high-quality images at radiation doses lower than what was possible with earlier generations of scanners.

First Generation. Hounsfield's Mark I scanner employed an x-ray tube and detector which were linked in opposing positions. A narrow, pencil-width beam passed through the patient to the detectors, while the tube-detector assembly rotated incrementally around the patient for a total of 180°. The patient was then moved through the gantry by a small increment, and the process repeated. This "step-and-shoot" incremental sequence is referred to as translation-rotation. This geometry resulted in an average scan time of five to six minutes. Because these long scan times required multiple breath holds, patient motion was a major source of image degradation [23].

Second Generation. These units generated multiple narrow fan-shaped beams that passed through the patient to multiple detectors using the original translation-rotation motion for scanning. The arrangement of multiple detectors reduced the number of translations required, resulting in a nearly three-fold reduction in scan time. The mechanical complexity of the rotate-translate mechanism remained a limiting factor [23].

Third Generation. In order to reduce scan times, the translation-rotation mechanism was changed to a purely rotational system with a large fan-beam of x-rays, which covered the entire width of the patient. A large array of detectors was utilized to measure data across the entire width of the beam. The tube and detectors continue to rotate together in what can be termed rotation-rotation motion. The design was very successful and a scan could be performed in less than 10 seconds [23].

Fourth Generation. A new design emerged employing a large, stationary ring of detectors with only the x-ray tube undergoing rotation around the patient. A disadvantage of the system was its size, owing to the fact that the tube had to rotate within the ring of detectors rather than in the same rotational path.

With the exception of minor improvements, CT technology remained relatively stable until 1987. Delays between each translation-rotation or rotation-rotation sequence (interscan delay) were the limiting factor in the existing systems. This was because after each 360° rotation of the tube-detector assembly, the power cables connected to the tube and detectors had to be respun in the opposite direction before the next rotation. Therefore, each complete rotation was followed by braking and then reversal before the next scan, resulting in long procedure times. This problem was solved by the invention of the "slip ring," which passes power to the rotating components without a fixed connection. The innovative technology allowed for continuous rotation and data acquisition leading to dramatically reduced procedure times [23].

Helical (Spiral) CT. Slip ring technology allows the patient to be moved through the gantry at a constant speed while being continuously scanned. The complete elimination of interscan delay allows certain studies to be completed with just a single breath hold. It has also reduced artifacts caused by patient breathing/motion and allows for more precisely timed scanning. The continuous volume of image data acquisition made multiplanar reformations and detailed three-dimensional imaging feasible options [23].

Multidetector CT (MDCT). This system uses the principles of helical scanning but incorporates multiple rows of detector rings rather than a single row. Commercially available units have evolved from 4- to 256-detector row systems, which has significantly reduced scan time by increasing the area of the patient covered by x-ray beams. Additionally, because of superior gantry rotation speeds, some scanners are at least eight times faster than single-detector CTs. Other benefits include improved resolution, reduced motion, and more detailed image reformations [24].

Image Display and Manipulation

The human eye cannot effectively differentiate between the shades of gray that make up the full spectrum of attenuation values in a CT image. Therefore, a clinically useful gray scale is established by limiting the number of Hounsfield units being displayed by setting the "window width" and "window level." The window width sets parameters by which only CT numbers of the tissues of interest are included. Pixel values above and below the window width limits are displayed as white and black, respectively. The window level represents the middle value of the numbers within the window width (insets, Fig. 1.12A-C). The ability to display images using these parameters on radiology workstations is critical to the complete examination of all anatomic structures contained in the study.

Contemporary CT imaging allows the acquisition of images with near-isotropic voxels, which means that the sides of each voxel are of the same size, allowing display of images in any anatomic plane, without significant loss in image resolution. Standard views for most modern CT examinations include coronal and sagittal reformations. Coronal reformations divide the body from front to back, while sagittal reformations divide it from left to right. Oblique reformations can also be generated. These reformations supplement the information contained in axial images and allow for easier evaluation of complex structures, such as the spine or vessels (Fig. 1.13A,B).

As mentioned earlier, each CT slice contains pixels whose values represent the average of the attenuation values in the voxel from which it was derived. Instead of assigning the average value to a pixel, images can be derived where pixel values represent the maximum or minimum of the attenuation values in the voxel from which they were derived. These result in maximum intensity projections (MIP) and minimum-intensity projections (mIP). The MIP method displays only the highest value in each voxel and is very useful in evaluating the vasculature (Fig. 1.13C). The mIP method only displays the minimum value of each voxel and is used in assessing the airway and structures with inherently low attenuation.

Finally, data can be reformatted into three-dimensional images, providing information regarding orientation and surface characteristics of various organs (Fig. 1.14). Three-dimensional rendering creates realistic two-dimensional images that intuitively convey three-dimensional relationships and also help communicate complex imaging findings to nonradiologists. The two main modes of generating these images are surface rendering and volume rendering. **Surface rendering** (Fig. 1.14A) is an older and less computationally intense method that treats the object of interest as if it were only composed of the voxels at its surface. Images derived from this method are useful for evaluating bone surfaces and surfaces of tubular structures such as the colon (virtual colonoscopy) or airways (virtual bronchoscopy). **Volume rendering** (Fig. 1.14B) is a newer and more computationally intense process that incorporates all of the data contained in the volume of interest. Volume rendered images can show multiple overlying objects.

IMAGE INTERPRETATION

Rapid advances in CT technology coupled with research in its clinical application have resulted in continued improvement in diagnostic accuracy and have made CT an indispensable tool for clinicians of every specialty. The radiologist in a busy practice is routinely tasked with interpreting a large volume of CT scans, which often contain multiple reformations and specific sequences which the interpreter must evaluate in an accurate and efficient manner.

Axial images remain the plane of primary interpretation. This remnant of the days of nonisometric CT may be supplanted in the future as radiologists become more familiar with primary interpretation in other planes [25].

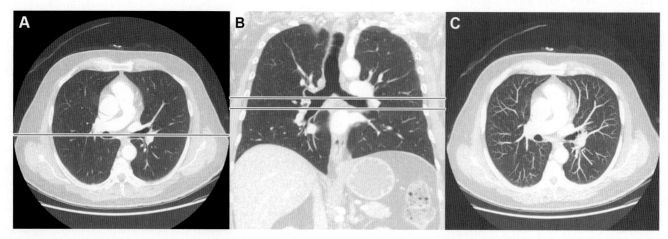

Fig. 1.13 Reformations (A) CT image in lung windows showing an axial image in the subcarinal region. (B) A coronal reformation through the mid-portion of the airway, at the level shown by the line at (A). (C) Maximum intensity projection with pixel values in this image derived from the maximum of each voxel between the lines in (B). Note that vessels are seen in more complete detail.

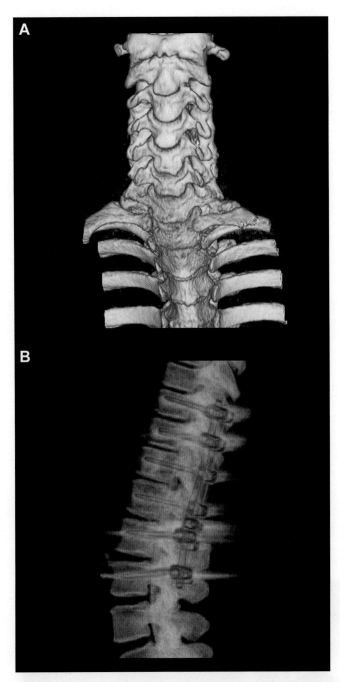

Fig. 1.14 Three-dimensional techniques. (A) Surface rendering in of the spine. (B) Volume rendering in the thoracic spine showing hardware (red). Please note that surface and volume rendering refer to techniques and not necessarily to the appearance of the images. For example, an image highlighting the surface features of a structure, such as seen in panel A, can be generated with surface rendering or volume rendering techniques. On the other hand, images showing internal characteristics of a structure can only be generated using volume rendering techniques.

An axial CT image is conventionally displayed as if standing at the patient's feet, with the right side of the image representing the left side of the patient (Fig. 1.12). Most modern radiology practices use computers for image display ("soft-copy" as opposed to "hard copy" film). The images are viewed sequentially (scrolling) multiple times in order to appropriately evaluate multiple structures using different window settings.

As mentioned in the introduction, it is helpful to develop a checklist for reading studies which one adheres to for every exam. For example, on a CT of the abdomen and pelvis one may first look at the soft tissues of the body wall, followed by the bones, vessels, solid organs, gastrointestinal tract, etc. The order in which structures are evaluated is not relevant. Rather, it is essential that one performs a mental checklist in the same manner for every similar study in order to avoid missing important findings. Remember that the mind does not know what the eye does not see.

An important component of CT image interpretation involves taking advantage of the standardized attenuation values of tissues of interest. For example, a renal lesion with fat attenuation most likely represents angiomyolipoma. A renal lesion demonstrating water attenuation (0 to 10-20 HU) is most likely a renal cyst. A higher attenuation renal lesion may represent a hemorrhagic cyst or neoplasm (see chapter 6, case 7). In the setting of traumatic brain injury or subarachnoid hemorrhage, a noncontrast head CT can reveal high-attenuation (60–80 HU) blood (see chapter 3, case 3).

The pattern and time course of contrast enhancement is also an important part of CT image interpretation. Dynamic contrast-enhanced (multi-phase) CT refers to acquiring multiple images of the same region in different phases of contrast enhancement. This is most commonly used in liver, adrenal, and pancreatic imaging, as well as CT arteriography and venography. For example, a hepatic hemangioma has a characteristic pattern of peripheral stippled enhancement early (arterial images), with progressive central filling on subsequent phases of contrast enhancement. In this setting, an unenhanced scan is obtained prior to contrast administration. The first (arterial) phase highlights the hepatic arterial system and is scanned 20 seconds after initiation of contrast injection. The second (parenchymal) phase is scanned after a 35-second delay and provides maximal enhancement of certain hypervascular neoplasms. The third (portal venous) phase is performed after a 60-second delay, at which point hepatic parenchymal enhancement is highlighted. Scan delays vary based on CT systems and institutional preferences, but the aforementioned values are a reasonable approximation.

Artifacts

Knowledge of the artifacts specific to CT is vital for accurate interpretation. Some artifacts relate to the technology (eg, single-detector versus multidetector, helical versus "step-and-shoot"). Three of the more common artifacts are presented here. A full review of these artifacts is beyond the scope of this chapter. The interested reader is referred to the excellent review by Barrett and Keat [26].

Motion Artifact: Patient motion, either voluntary or involuntary, can cause blurring of images or irregularities between interfaces of different attenuation (Fig. 1.15A).

Streak Artifact: This is a type of beam hardening artifact that appears as dark bands or streaks between two dense objects (Fig. 1.15B). Beam hardening refers to the loss of low-energy photons as an x-ray beam passes through an object (the beam becomes strengthened or "hardened"). In very heterogeneous cross sections of the body, portions of the beam that pass through one of the objects at one tube position is hardened less than when the beam passes through both objects at another tube position.

Stair-Step Artifact: This artifact occurs when thick images are used for generating reformations. The appearance is that of stair steps around the edges of structures (Fig. 1.15C).

SAFETY

Contrast Media

Safety issues relating to contrast media can be related to the initial injection (air embolism, extravasation) or related to systemic effects of the contrast (nephrotoxicity, contrast reactions).

Air Embolism. Air can enter the venous system during injection of intravenous contrast. This is more common during hand injection, and usually of little to no clinical significance if the amount of air is small. This is usually seen incidentally as small air bubbles or air-fluid levels in the intrathoracic veins, main pulmonary artery, or right ventricle [27]. Clinically significant venous air embolism is rare but can be fatal. The air bubble can migrate to the systemic circulation and result in neurological deficits in patients with right-to-left intracardiac shunts or pulmonary arteriovenous malformations. Treatment includes administration of 100% oxygen and positioning the patient with her left side down. This maneuver places the right ventricular outflow tract inferior to the right ventricle, preventing air from migrating to an obstructing position [28].

Contrast Extravasation. Extraluminal (extravasated) iodinated contrast materials are toxic to soft tissues and result in an acute local inflammatory response that is usually limited to adjacent skin and subcutaneous tissues. The response can peak 24 to 48 hours after the initial event, and this must be explained to the patient prior to discharge with clear instructions to seek medical care if there is any worsening of symptoms. Severe manifestations can result in permanent injury to the patient in the form of skin ulceration, tissue necrosis, and compartment syndrome. Compartment syndrome is the result of mechanical compression from the edema incited by the contrast material and is more common with extravasation of larger volumes of contrast media and/or with extravasation into smaller compartments such as the hand or wrist [27].

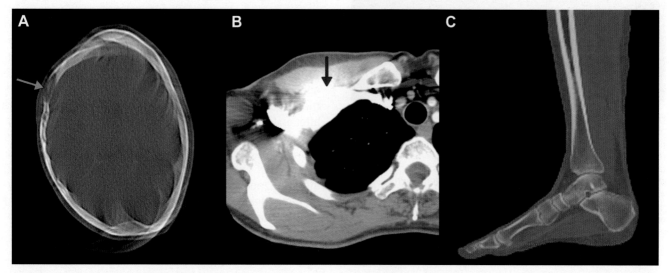

Fig. 1.15 Artifacts in CT. (A) Motion artifact due to respiration, which limits evaluation of the right frontal skull lesion (white arrow). (B) Streak artifact from contrast material in the right subclavian vein (black arrow). (C) Stair-step artifact in a sagittal reformation obtained from thick slices of the ankle and foot.

Because initial signs and symptoms of compartment syndrome can be relatively mild, several hours of close clinical observation are needed prior to discharge of the patient. Surgical consultation may be needed in the setting of progressive swelling or pain, altered tissue perfusion, change in sensation in the affected limb, and skin ulceration or blistering [27].

Treatment protocols vary, can be contradictory, and have not been validated in controlled studies. Elevation of the affected limb is thought to decrease capillary hydrostatic pressure and may promote resorption of the contrast material. Warm and cold compresses are used in different institutions. Those who advocate the use of the former posit that warm compresses improve absorption of the contrast material and improve blood flow, while those who favor the latter report that cold compresses help relieve pain at the injection site [27].

Contrast Reactions

Most contrast reactions are mild and do not require treatment. Severe contrast reactions to high-osmolarity iodinated contrast materials occur in 0.1% to 0.2% of patients compared to 0.04% with low-osmolarity contrast materials [29]. For the purposes of management, contrast reactions are graded as mild, moderate, and severe. Recognition of key symptoms is important to making the appropriate management decisions, which range from reassurance to calling a code. For specific treatment recommendations, please refer to the ACR Manual on Contrast Media, available online at: http://www.acr.org/Quality-Safety/Resources/Contrast-Manual.

Box 1.3 – TERMINOLOGY

There has been debate in the literature about whether an antigen-antibody response occurs in contrast reactions (ie, whether contrast reactions are anaphylactic reactions). Nevertheless, some contrast reactions appear identical to and are treated just like anaphylactic reactions, and are referred to as "anaphylactoid," "allergiclike," or "idiosyncratic" reactions.

Mild Reaction: Most mild reactions are not allergiclike reactions and simply represent physiologic response to injection of the contrast material. Common symptoms include nausea, vomiting, or longer than expected duration of warmth or flushing. Patients may also develop allergiclike reactions like urticaria and mild angioedema (eg, scratchy throat, slight swelling of the tongue or face, and paroxysmal sneezing). While antihistamines may be given for mild symptomatic allergiclike

reactions, most cases of allergiclike and nonallergiclike reactions do not require treatment beyond reassurance. Monitoring of the patient's vital signs and clinical status for 30 minutes is commonly recommended to ensure that symptoms do not progress [27].

Moderate Reaction: These are not life-threatening but often require treatment because some may progress in severity. Manifestations include allergiclike reactions like severe urticaria or erythema, bronchospasm, moderate swelling of the tongue and face, and transient hypotension with tachycardia, as well as nonallergiclike reactions such as severe vasovagal reactions. These require close monitoring of the patient until resolution of symptoms [27].

Severe Reaction: Although rare, these occur rapidly and unpredictably, requiring trained personnel at hand for immediate treatment. These are usually allergiclike reactions and can present with diffuse erythema, altered mental status, seizures, severe bronchospasm, laryngeal edema, severe hypotension, or sudden cardiac arrest. Severe nonallergiclike reactions include severe vasovagal reactions, pulmonary edema, and seizures [27]. A conservative estimate of 0.9 fatalities for every 100,000 injections of low osmolality contrast has been made [30].

Severe reactions are sporadic and unpredictable. The most important risk factor for an allergiclike reaction is a prior allergiclike reaction to contrast material; however, this is not an absolute predictor, with only ~1/3 of patients with a prior history of an allergiclike reaction having a recurrent reaction. The available data support the use of non-ionic contrast material to lower the risk of adverse events in patients with prior reactions [31, 32]. In addition, various premedication strategies with corticosteroids and antihistamines have been proposed and are in wide use for patients at higher risk for contrast reactions. These aim to reduce the incidence of life-threatening reactions; however, the quality of data supporting their use is surprisingly poor, especially given the known risks associated with corticosteroid use (gastrointestinal ulcers, mood disturbances, relative immunodeficiency, and hyperglycemia). It is important from a medicolegal and risk management point of view to be knowledgeable about and adhere to the pretreatment protocol(s) at your institution; however, it is important from a patient care point of view to be aware that contrast reactions can occur despite the use of premedication. In addition, while 12-hour premedication protocols have shown a small benefit in decreasing mild reactions, none have been shown to make a statistically significant difference in the rate of *severe* contrast reactions [32]. Therefore, premedication should not lull one into a state of complacency, and emergency management skills are as important as prophylaxis in protecting your patients [31]. In addition, emergent studies should not be delayed for steroid premedication when the results of the imaging study can have an important influence in patient management [32]. As in all aspects of radiology, communication between the radiologist and referring clinician, with thorough evaluation of the risks and benefits of a study, is needed to ensure optimal management of the patient.

Nephrotoxicty. Contrast-induced nephrotoxicity (CIN) is defined as acute renal dysfunction that is seen 2 to 3 days after intravenous administration of iodinated contrast material. One definition is an absolute increase in baseline serum creatinine of at least 0.5 mg/dL [27].

Contrast-induced nephrotoxicity is either very rare or nonexistent. This undertainty is due to the fact that most studies on this subject have not included a control group, and those that have included a control group have found that the physiologic variation in serum creatinine accounts for most, if not all, cases of "contrast-induced nephrotoxicity" [27]. For example, one study found that the incidence of post-CT elevation of serum creatinine was equal between patients who did and did not receive intravenous contrast [33].

Most radiology practices, however, screen patients for the presence of risk factors for contrast-induced nephrotoxicity, in order to exclude high-risk patients from receiving intravascular iodinated contrast material. Because the most important risk factor for contrast-induced nephrotoxicity is preexisting renal insufficiency, various thresholds for renal function have been advanced beyond which intravascular iodinated contrast medium is not administered. There is, however, great variability amongst radiology practices in this regard, and no single threshold in serum creatinine or estimated glomerular filtration rate (eGFR) has sufficient data to advocate its use [27]. Familiarity with your institution's screening protocols and exclusion thresholds for the administration of iodinated contrast material is important for medicolegal reasons.

The situation is slightly different in patients with acute renal injury, where it is prudent to avoid additional nephrotoxicity, however small [27].

Metformin. A very rare side effect of the anti-hyperglycemic agent metformin in patients with renal failure is lactic acidosis, with 50% of patients progressing to death. Patients taking metformin who then experience contrast-induced nephropathy would therefore have increased susceptibility to developing lactic acidosis. For this reason, the United States Food and Drug Administration recommends withholding metformin temporarily for patients receiving iodinated intravascular contrast [27]. The ACR recommends that patients taking metformin be classified into three categories for the purposes of determining proper management when administering intravenous contrast. Patients with normal renal function and no known comorbidities (as defined in [27]) do not need to discontinue metformin prior receiving intravenous contrast. Patients

with multiple comorbidities with apparently normal renal function should discontinue metformin at the time of the examination for 48 hours. Renal function can be followed prior to restarting metformin, but this is left to the discretion of the radiologist and the patient's physician. In patients with known renal dysfunction, metformin should be stopped prior to administration of intravenous contrast and renal function carefully followed up until metformin can be safely reinstituted [27].

Radiation

The concepts of radiation dose measurements and radiation biology summarized in the radiography section apply to CT; however, because of the geometry and usage of CT, specific parameters have been developed for radiation dose in CT [34]. In radiography, measures of exposure are based on a source from one or two locations. The geometry of CT image acquisition leads to an exposure pattern that is more or less continuous around the patient. In addition, the fact that CT covers a volume leads to multiple exposures along the length of a patient. The radiation dose from CT, then, depends on many factors, including patient factors such as size and region being scanned, as well as machine parameters such as the energy and geometry of the beam [34]. The CT dose index (CTDI, mGy) is the average dose imparted to a phantom (physical model that is meant to simulate the body) under specific acquisition parameters for a single slice of data acquisition, and is often modified to reflect different acquisition parameters, complete descriptions of which are beyond the scope of this book [34]. One important modification of the CTDI is the $CTDI_{vol}$, which takes into account the parameters specific to the imaging protocol being used. The dose length product (DLP, mGy-cm) is an estimate of the radiation exposure during the entire sequence of image acquisition. Most modern CT scanners can be configured to give an estimate of patient dose for a given study. This is usually in terms of DLP which is obtained by multiplying the $CTDI_{vol}$ by the length irradiated, sometimes with a correction factor for helical scanning, as was done in the example shown in Fig. 1.16 [35]. Familiarity with the dose reports from scanners used at your institution will not only help in understanding your patient's radiation exposure, but may be a required part of the radiology report in the future. This has already been put into law in California [36].

Dose Minimization. CT accounted for almost half of the collective dose from radiologic and nuclear medicine procedures in the United States in 2006 [37]. Discretion with CT is especially warranted when dynamic contrast-enhanced examinations such as a dedicated liver or pancreatic CT are considered and in young and pregnant patients. In the latter case, ultrasonography or MRI can be

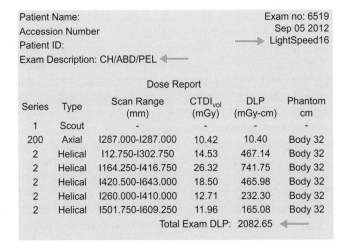

Patient Name:				Exam no: 6519	
Accession Number				Sep 05 2012	
Patient ID:				⟶ LightSpeed16	
Exam Description: CH/ABD/PEL ◀—					

Dose Report

Series	Type	Scan Range (mm)	CTDI$_{vol}$ (mGy)	DLP (mGy-cm)	Phantom cm
1	Scout	-	-	-	-
200	Axial	I1287.000-I1287.000	10.42	10.40	Body 32
2	Helical	I112.750-I1302.750	14.53	467.14	Body 32
2	Helical	I1164.250-I1416.750	26.32	741.75	Body 32
2	Helical	I1420.500-I1643.000	18.50	465.98	Body 32
2	Helical	I1260.000-I1410.000	12.71	232.30	Body 32
2	Helical	I1501.750-I1609.250	11.96	165.08	Body 32
			Total Exam DLP:	2082.65 ◀—	

Fig. 1.16 Sample General Electric CT Dose Report from a CT of the chest, abdomen, and pelvis. The dose report contains information about the patient (deleted), type of scan (long arrow) and the machine used (short arrow). It also lists the series number (first column), imaging mode (axial vs helical, second column), the length of the scan (scan range, third column, in this case as table "I" positions, which are subtracted to get the length of the scan), the CTDI$_{vol}$, (4th column), DLP (5th column), and the phantom used for dose estimation (in this case a 32-cm body phantom). The first row represents the scout images, which are acquired in projection mode (similar to radiography). The absence of CTDI and DLP values does not mean that the patient was not exposed to radiation, simply that the CTDI method does not apply to this type of image acquisition. The second row (series 200) represents the images obtained during real-time contrast tracking. This involves scanning a single slice of the patient continuously (in this case the abdominal aorta) and initiating additional scans based on the arrival of contrast. This is done to optimize contrast enhancement. The third through seventh rows show the different acquisitions that were placed into series 2 of this study. These included CT of the chest (third row), CT of the abdomen and pelvis (4th and 5th rows), delayed images through the kidneys to show excretion of contrast into the renal pelvis and proximal ureters (6th row), and delayed images through the pelvis to show excreted contrast in the urinary bladder (last row). The DLPs are summed and the total exam DLP generated. In this case the patient was exposed to 2802.65 mGy-cm.

used as alternate imaging in the appropriate clinical setting. For pregnant women, lead shielding of the fetus and low-dose techniques should be employed. Close collaboration with medical physicists and technologists can result in significant reductions in patient exposure without compromising image quality. The myriad dose reduction techniques are beyond the scope of this book. The interested reader is referred to the excellent review by McCollough et and colleagues [38].

STRENGTHS AND WEAKNESSES

Computed tomography has a multitude of strengths which make it a mainstay of radiological imaging across the world. Some of these include:

1. Speed: The ability to provide very rapid acquisition of images with a large area of coverage has made CT indispensable in assessment of patients with severe/multisystem acute trauma.
2. Good contrast resolution between different tissues: Allows for superior evaluation of abnormalities involving hemorrhage, calcium, or gas.
3. Postprocessing: The ability to obtain reformations in multiple planes and advanced 3D rendering can eliminate the need for invasive procedures such as colonoscopy and arteriography.

Radiation exposure is the main limitation of CT, which often delivers multiple times the dose of conventional radiography, especially with dynamic imaging protocols that require multiple scans of the same area. This is being addressed with technological advances that allow for low-dose image acquisition with minimal or no loss in image quality [38].

Adverse reactions and potential nephrotoxicity from iodinated contrast materials must also be included as a potential weakness of CT. In cases where intravenous iodinated contrast materials cannot be safely administered, alternate modalities can be considered. For example, MR angiography (see next section) can be performed without intravenous contrast, and can be used in patients with renal insufficiency.

FUTURE DIRECTIONS

Current innovation in CT technology is focused on continuing to reduce scan times and overall radiation dose to the patient while improving imaging quality. Major progress is being made in areas such as cardiac imaging with new geometric modifications such as dual source CT, which uses two x-ray tubes within the gantry positioned 90 degrees to each other. Each tube rotates 180 degrees, which effectively cuts the scan time in half. Dual source CT can also be used with different energies of x-rays generated from each source (dual-energy CT). Taking advantage of differential change in attenuation of biological tissues at different energy levels, data from dual-energy CT can then be processed to subtract certain material from images. This has been used in imaging uric acid crystals in gout and removing iodine in postcontrast imaging to determining the enhancement characteristics of a lesion.

ULTRASOUND (US)

The term ultrasound describes high-frequency inaudible sound waves over 20 kHz that are utilized by mammals such as dolphins and bats to communicate and locate food. The first serious experiments to evaluate the existence of ultrasound in nature were performed on bats by an

Italian priest and physiologist named Lazzaro Spallanzani (1729-1799) [39]. He discovered that blindfolded bats could maneuver obstacles normally, but bumped into their environment when their mouths were covered. He concluded that their ears were a more sensitive navigational instrument than their eyes. This was later proven when ultrasound was found to emanate from the mouth of a bat in flight. The ultrasound waves reflected off objects in the environment with the echoes providing "audible" information concerning size and distance. This phenomenon is termed *echolocation*.

Echolocation was initially used for nautical purposes. Reginald Fessenden patented and built the first working SONAR (sound navigation and ranging) system based on the principles of echolocation. This was built and utilized shortly after the sinking of the *Titanic* in 1912, in part to help prevent similar catastrophes, and could detect an iceberg up to two miles away. A French physicist named Paul Langevin and a Russian scientist Constantin Chilowsky then developed an underwater sonar device for submarines called the "hydrophone." These techniques were refined and gained widespread use during both world wars [40].

Many pioneers were involved in the application of ultrasound principles to the medical field. Karl Dussik, a neurologist from the University of Vienna, began using ultrasound to try and locate brain tumors and the cerebral ventricles as early as 1942 [41]. Professor Ian Donald of Glasgow after being exposed to radar and sonar technology during his time in the Royal Air Force, utilized ultrasound to visualize pelvic masses and eventually detect early pregnancies. John J. Wild, an English-born American physician who has been described as the "father of medical ultrasound" made important contributions to the detection of intestinal and breast malignancies [40]. Ultrasound equipment and techniques have evolved rapidly and have found wide diagnostic (and growing therapeutic) utility in many specialties including obstetrics, cardiology, and emergency medicine, to name a few.

IMAGE FORMATION

At its most basic level, medical ultrasound consists of passing sound waves into tissues and analyzing the reflected waves (echoes). Sound passing through tissue undergoes attenuation, or loss of energy. Sound waves at tissue interfaces undergo reflection and refraction, the proportions of which depend on the difference in the acoustic impedances of each medium. Large differences result in more reflection and less refraction [42].

To understand image generation in ultrasound, imagine a sound wave being generated and passed through the skin in a simplified model consisting of different materials

(Fig. 1.17, top panel). The sound is generated by the transducer (see Equipment on the next page), passes through the first material until it comes to the fist interface. At this point, portions of the sound wave are reflected back toward the skin, and portions are refracted and pass through the second material. The process repeats, with loss of energy at each interface [42].

If we were listening at the skin (Fig. 1.17, bottom panel), we would hear our generated pulse, then a gap followed by the echo reflected at first interface. The plot of the amplitudes of these echoes represents A-mode ultrasound (Box 1.4). The gap-echo pair repeats at each interface, until there is so much energy loss that the echoes are no longer heard. We can use the times between the generated sound pulse and the echoes to determine the depth of each interface, and we can use the information about the strength of the sound wave to determine information about the tissue interfaces and the tissues the sound waves passed through. The combination of multiple such lines of data results in the gray-scale (B-mode) ultrasound image [42].

An important aspect of modern ultrasonography is the use of Doppler analysis to characterize blood flow. Sound waves reflecting off of moving objects can have their frequencies increased or decreased based on the direction of flow. The information about the direction and speed of the moving objects can be overlaid on the gray-scale ultrasound image or analyzed separately to quantify the dynamics of the flow waveform.

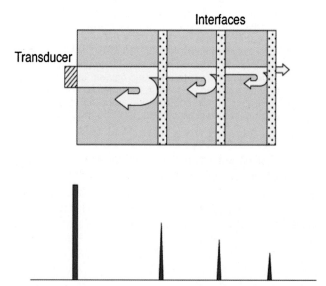

Fig. 1.17 The basic concept of ultrasound. Top panel: There is reflection and progressive loss of energy at each interface encountered. Bottom: The reflected wavefronts are recorded as signals of varying amplitudes. Upper panel modified with permission from Hagan AD, DeMaria AN. *Clinical Applications of Two-Dimensional Echocardiography and Cardiac Doppler*. Boston, MA: Little Brown; 1989.

Image Contrast

Contrast in ultrasound images is based on the reflection of sound waves at the interfaces of different types of tissues. Each pixel ranges from black to white based on the energy of the returning echoes. The ability of an object to generate echoes is referred to as echogenicity. By convention, objects that result in no echoes are colored black (anechoic), while those that result in strong echoes are colored white (hyperechoic).

Contrast Agents. Doppler ultrasonography provides valuable information regarding the presence, direction, and velocity of blood flow. It cannot, however, accurately determine the pattern of blood flow within small vessels to determine tissue perfusion. Contrast enhanced ultrasound (CEUS) refers to the use of microbubble contrast agents coupled with specialized subtraction imaging techniques to characterize blood flow and tissue perfusion. Microbubble contrast agents are typically 1 to 4 micrometers in diameter, making them smaller than red blood cells and allowing for unhindered flow through microcirculation. They are composed of a gas core and an outer shell. These microbubbles produce a high degree of echogenicity and enhance the Doppler signal of flowing blood. Specialized imaging techniques suppress the background tissue to highlight the signal from the blood pool [43].

There are only two second-generation FDA approved microbubble contrast agents, Optison (GE Healthcare) and Definity (Lantheus Medical Imaging), which are limited to cardiac imaging and are typically used to enhance the contrast between tissue and blood to provide clearer images of critical structures.

EQUIPMENT

The basic ultrasound machine consists of a transducer, console, and the central processing unit (CPU) (Fig. 1.18). The transducer generates the ultrasound waves and listens for the echoes generated at tissue interfaces. The console has a number of controls that allow for real-time manipulation of the signal generated by the transducer and how the signal received by the transducer is processed by the CPU.

Transducer

The transducer is the site of interaction between the ultrasound machine and the patient. The transducer has an array of multiple *piezoelectric* crystals (Fig. 1.19) that allows it to function as both a transmitter and a receiver. These crystals convert electrical signals from the CPU into sound waves to generate the ultrasound pulse and convert reflected sound waves into electrical signals that are sent to the CPU.

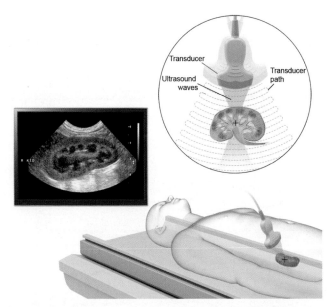

Fig. 1.18 Components of an ultrasound machine. The transducer (probe) is the handheld unit that both transmits and receives sound waves. The CPU (not shown) analyzes the sound waves being received and processes the information into images that are displayed on the monitor. The console has controls that can modulate the ultrasound waves being emitted and adjust display parameters.

The design of the transducer will determine the shape and the field-of-view of the ultrasound image. For example, linear array transducers (Fig. 1.20A) result in rectangular images and are used for imaging anatomy close to the transducer (just under the skin surface). Phased-array transducers (Fig. 1.20B) result in images that have the appearance of a pizza slice and are used for imaging organs from tight spaces (eg, between the ribs). Curved array transducers (shown in Figs. 1.18 and 1.20D) are a hybrid of linear and phased-array transducers and are wide with a gentle curve. An intracavitary transducer (Fig. 1.20C) has a curved face like the curved array probe, but is typically of a higher frequency (8-13 MHz) and is elongated to allow insertion into a cavity (most commonly the vagina).

An important concept in ultrasound is probe resolution, which refers to the ability to distinguish two closely situated objects as separate entities. The two types of resolution in ultrasonography are *axial* and *lateral* resolution. Axial resolution is the ability to differentiate two objects lying in a plane parallel to the ultrasound beam (depth), whereas lateral resolution refers to objects located perpendicular to the beam.

Axial resolution is based on duration of the emitted pulse—shorter pulse lengths result in better axial resolution. Higher beam frequencies result in shorter pulse lengths and, consequently, high-frequency probes provide the best axial resolution.

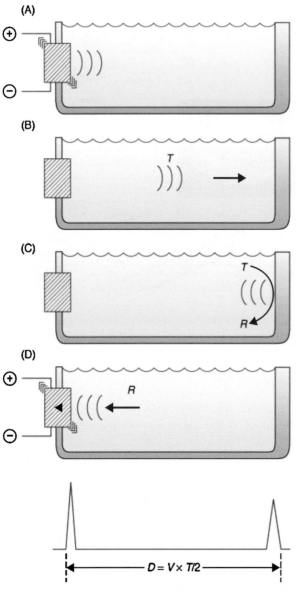

(A)

(B)

(C)

(D)

$$D = V \times T/2$$

Fig. 1.19 The piezoelectric crystals. The crystal is activated by passing a current through it, producing a transmitted pulse (T), which reflects off the interface. The reflected pulse (R) excites the crystal, producing an electric current. Because the velocity of the pulse is constant, distance can be calculated based on the transit time. (Because the pulse must travel back and forth from the interface, the time is divided by 2.) Modified with permission from Weyman AW. Physical principles of ultrasound. In: Weyman AE, ed. *Principles and Practice of Echocardiography.* 2nd ed. Philadelphia, PA: Lea & Febiger; 1994:3–28.

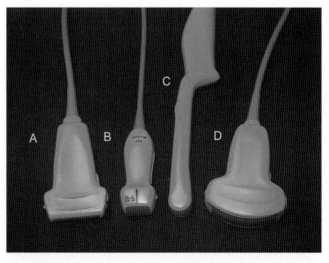

Fig. 1.20 Common ultrasound transducers. (A): Linear small parts probe (soft tissue probe). (B): Phased array. (C): Intracavitary curved array. (D): Curved array. Reproduced with permission from Stone CK, Humphries RL, eds. *Current Diagnosis & Treatment in Emergency Medicine,* 7th. McGraw-Hill, Inc. Copyright 2011. Fig. 6-1.

Box 1.4 – HISTORICAL JOURNEY

You may occasionally hear the term "B-mode" used in relation to ultrasound. This is a remnant from the early days of ultrasound where B-mode was a major technological advance over A-mode.

A-mode (Amplitude mode) was a simple line plot display, consisting of a horizontal axis representing the time taken for an echo to return while the vertical axis represents the amplitude of the echo.

B-mode (Brightness mode) is the workhorse of modern US imaging combining the pulse-echo approach with a brightness mode image display. It generates the familiar gray-scale ultrasound images and is commonly referred to as 2D scanning. More recent advances have resulted in 3D imaging, which are obtained by processing multiple 2D data sets, and 4D imaging, which is 3D with the addition of the time dimension to capture movement. These modes are most commonly used to create pictures for expectant parents and grandparents, and may help in assessing anatomically complex congenital malformations.

Lateral resolution is inversely related to beam width, which varies with distance from the probe (Fig. 1.21). The beam can be divided into a *near field, focal zone,* and *far field.* The near field is the nondivergent part of the beam closer to the probe, while the far field diverges with distance from the probe. The focal zone is the narrowest part of the beam providing the area of highest lateral resolution.

The distance of the focal zone from the transducer can be adjusted to control the areas highest lateral resolution. Two objects that are closer together than the beam width cannot be distinguished as separate objects.

High-frequency probes can create narrower beam widths and consequently have better lateral resolution. Low-frequency probes have improved tissue penetration

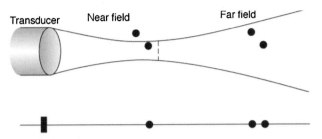

Fig. 1.21 The ultrasound beam. The transducer emits an ultrasonic beam that has a near field (where the beam is relatively focused) and a far field (where the beam width increases). Lower panel: In the near field, the beam reflects off only one of two objects in close proximity to each other. In the far field, however, two similarly positioned objects are both within the beam width. Therefore, lateral resolution is compromised, and the objects' positions are misrepresented. Reproduced with permission from Fuster V, Walsh RA, Harrington RA, et al. *Hurst's The Heart*, 13th ed. McGraw-Hill, Inc. Copyright 2011. Fig 18-4.

at the expense of both axial and lateral resolution. These probes are therefore favored for imaging deeper structures of greater size.

Regardless of their design, all transducers require a coupling medium for optimal function. Recall that the degree of reflection of sound waves at an interface is proportional to the difference in the acoustic impedances between the two materials. If the transducer were placed directly on the body, the large difference in acoustic impedance between air and skin would result in the vast majority of the beam reflecting back toward the transducer. Ultrasound gel is used as an acoustic coupling agent in order to provide an air-free path for the sound waves to be transmitted into tissue.

The transducer has a ridge or groove on one side to assist with orientation. By convention, this ridge is directed toward the patient's head or right side. Under this convention, an axial image will have the right side of the patient on the left side of the image, and coronal and sagittal images will have the head of the patient on the left of the image.

The Console

The ultrasound machine is controlled from the console for optimization and real-time manipulation of images. The most common control features will be discussed here and are common across all manufacturers. The implementation of each feature, however, may vary from machine to machine.

Depth: This function controls the distance that one is imaging into the far-field. It is beneficial to start with greater depth in order to make sure that no important findings are excluded from view. The depth can then be lowered to include only the relevant structures and improve resolution and magnification in the near-field. It is important not to waste the image space with excessive depth—increased depth results in longer

echo return times, which can degrade image quality. The area of interest is typically kept in the top two-thirds of the screen.

Gain: The gain controls how the probe listens for the returning echoes. Increasing the gain amplifies the strength of returning echoes and helps compensate for signal loss caused by tissue attenuation. The overall result is a brighter image. Conversely, decreasing the gain will darken the image as needed. In addition to overall gain adjustments, the time-gain compensation (TGC) function can be utilized to selectively control gain at different depths. A series of sliding knobs allows for a stepwise amplification of signal, progressively increasing with depth, in order to offset the greater attenuation of waves returning from deeper structures. The gain should ideally be set at a level that delivers a clear image that is neither too bright nor too dark. Certain machines have image optimization buttons that work to automatically adjust gain appropriately throughout the image.

Focus: Adjustment of the focal zone allows for optimal lateral resolution at a given depth by changing the location of the narrowest point of the beam. A small marker or arrow on the screen indicates where the focal zone is being placed.

Frequency: Allows the probe frequency to be changed for specific transducers with variable frequencies within a narrow range. A lower frequency setting chosen for deeper penetration may be changed to higher frequency for better near-field resolution on the same probe.

M-Mode: Activates motion-mode acquisition, which generates time-motion graphs for analysis of moving structures, such as the heart (Fig. 1.22).

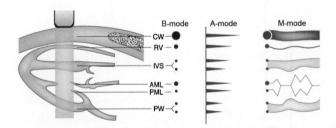

Fig. 1.22 Formation of A-mode, B-mode, and M-mode echocardiograms. The transducer emits an ultrasound beam, which reflects at each anatomic interface. The reflected wavefronts can be represented as dots (B mode) or spikes (A mode). The dot brightness and spike magnitude vary with the amplitude of the reflected wave. If the B-mode scan is swept from left to right with time, an M-mode image is produced. AML, anterior mitral leaflet; CW, chest wall; IVS, interventricular septum; PML, posterior mitral leaflet; PW, posterior wall; RV, right ventricle. Modified with permission from Hagan AD, DeMaria AN. *Clinical Applications of Two-Dimensional Echocardiography and Cardiac Doppler*. Boston, MA: Little Brown; 1989.

Doppler: Activates Doppler mode, which is used to visualize blood flow. The movement of blood toward or away from the probe is differentiated based on the frequency of the returning echoes. By convention, blood flowing toward the probe is displayed as red while blood flowing away is blue. It is important to remember that this information only relates to the direction of blood flow based on probe positioning/angulation and is not necessarily a reliable indicator of whether an isolated vessel is an artery or vein based on color mapping.

Power Doppler: Similar to Doppler but without information regarding the direction of flow. Shades of a single color, usually orange, are assigned to represent the intensity of signal. Power Doppler is more sensitive for identifying low flow, but is more susceptible to motion artifact.

Continuous-Wave and Pulsed-Wave Doppler: In clinical practice, Doppler shift data is obtained from a small, specifically selected area for measurement of flow velocity over time (Fig. 1.23). Continuous-wave (CW) Doppler is older technology and is good for measuring high blood velocities accurately, making it useful in detection of valvular and congenital heart disease. Pulsed-wave (PW) systems represent more advanced technology, and are preferred when Doppler data needs to be measured from a small segment along the ultrasound beam [44].

Central Processing Unit (CPU)

We have discussed both the generation of ultrasound waves as well as their modulation as they pass through the body and return to their source. The final part in this sequence is the interpretation of the returning echoes and their conversion into a digital image. The CPU receives information regarding both the time taken for an echo to return after transmission, as well as the strength of the echo (Fig. 1.17). Using this data, the CPU determines the values to assign to each pixel in the image. Longer return times correspond to deeper structures and strong echoes correspond to brighter pixels (hyperechoic). In this way, data points are plotted in two-dimensional space to create a composite digital image. This image can be manipulated and annotated using the console and transmitted to PACS for storage and interpretation.

IMAGE INTERPRETATION

Unlike other modalities in diagnostic imaging, reaching a diagnosis in ultrasound requires facility in both acquisition and interpretation of images, and it involves close interaction between technologists and interpreting radiologists. The technologist is skilled in a wide variety of sonographic techniques and guides the patient through a study while obtaining the necessary diagnostic images. Image acquisition is typically followed by a discussion between the technologist and radiologist regarding relevant findings and potential problems with the study. The ultimate responsibility for providing

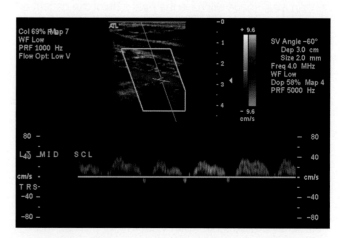

Fig. 1.23 Pulsed-wave (PW) and continuous-wave (CW) Doppler. Left panel: With PW, a single pulse of ultrasound energy is emitted, and its reflection from a sample volume is received before the following pulse is transmitted. CW is the older method and involves continuous transmission and reception of ultrasound energy. Right panel: A combined gray-scale, color Doppler, and PW image investigating flow in the subclavian vein (SCL). Part A Reproduced with permission from Fuster V, Walsh RA, Harrington RA, et al. *Hurst's The Heart*. 13th ed. McGraw-Hill, Inc. Copyright 2011. Fig 18-27.

diagnostic-quality and clinically relevant images rests on the radiologist, who must be able determine whether the images are of diagnostic quality, quickly identify findings that require closer inspection, and be able to scan the patient to trouble-shoot problems in real-time. Once diagnostic-quality images are acquired, image interpretation begins by assessing structures based on their internal echogenicity, shape, presence of characteristic artifacts (Fig. 1.24 is discussed in more detail as you read further), and appearance on Doppler imaging.

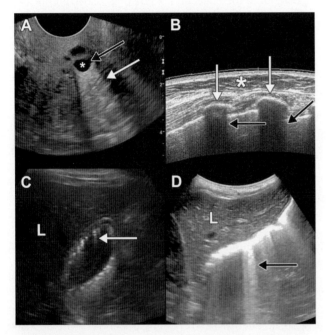

Fig. 1.24 Common ultrasound artifacts. (A) Increased through-transmission (arrow) is seen deep to a Nabothian cyst (*) in the cervix. (B) Shadowing (black arrows) is seen deep to two ribs (white arrows) in this composite image of the chest wall, which also shows subcutaneous edema (*). (C) Comet tail artifacts (arrow) in a patient with adenomyomatosis of the gallbladder. L, liver. (D) Ring down artifact (arrow) from gas in bowel. L, liver.

One of the greatest strengths of ultrasound is its ability to differentiate cysts from solid lesions, making it a useful problem-solving tool for further evaluation of cystic lesions incidentally noted on CT. A *simple cyst* is typically anechoic with thin walls and demonstrates increased through-transmission (hyperechoic area deep to the cyst in Fig. 1.24A). Simple cysts are commonly encountered in the liver, kidneys, and ovaries.

A *complex cyst* is one that has a certain degree of internal echogenicity due to its fluid content containing particulate matter such as blood, mucin, or proteinaceous substances. Ultrasound characteristics that can help distinguish complex cysts from solid masses include layering and swirling of fluid if the lesion is compressed or repositioned.

Homogeneity of the internal echoes can sometimes suggest the diagnosis of a complex cyst, although this is not always the case (see chapter 10, case 16). Once a diagnosis of a solid lesion is made, evaluation moves to biopsy or other imaging modalities, as ultrasound is generally not specific enough to make a histological diagnosis in the vast majority of cases.

The internal echogenicity of solid organs can also be used to determine the presence of disease. Solid organs have a speckled pattern of echogenicity or texture ("echotexture") that is fairly characteristic, either in isolation or in comparison with adjacent reference organs. For example, normal liver and kidney are similar in echogenicity whereas the pancreas is normally more hyperechoic than both these organs. These observations can help identify diffuse pathology such as fatty infiltration of the liver [45].

Solid lesions can be hypo- or hyperechoic or blend in with the surrounding organ (Fig. 1.25A,B). Focal deviation from the expected echotexture of an organ can be used to detect subtle lesions (Fig. 1.25C). Space-occupying lesions can also alter the normal surface contours of an organ and result in bulging or nodularity (Fig. 1.25D).

Doppler imaging can either be used as a problem-solving part of an ultrasound study or as the main component of a dedicated study of flow dynamics. The main

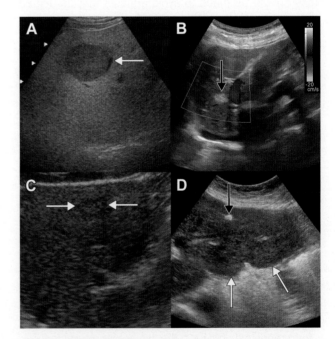

Fig. 1.25 Various liver lesions. (A) Focal nodular hyperplasia in the liver presenting as a hypoechoic lesion (arrow). (B) Hemangioma with characteristic hyperechoic appearance. Although hemangiomas are vascular lesions, they usually demonstrate no flow on Doppler, possibly due to multidirectional or low-velocity flow. (C) Hepatic adenoma manifesting as subtle deviation from the normal echotexture of the liver. (D) Widespread hepatic metastases, manifesting as lobulated contour of the deep surface of the liver (white arrows). A hemangioma (black arrow) is also present.

problem-solving use of Doppler imaging is its use in differentiation of simple and complex cysts from solid lesions, and in diagnosis of vascular abnormalities, such as aneurysms or thrombi. Regarding the distinction between cystic and solid lesions, the presence of flow rules out a simple or complex cyst; however, the converse is not true (the absence of flow does not exclude a solid lesion), because hypovascular solid lesions can present without detectable flow on Doppler imaging. The degree of flow in a solid lesion is also not helpful in differentiating benign and malignant lesions because of significant overlap in flow characteristics of inflammation and certain benign lesions with those of malignant lesions [46].

Doppler imaging can also be the major component of a dedicated study of flow dynamics. A common application in this setting is the setting of symptomatic internal carotid artery stenosis, where a combination of gray scale and color and pulsed-wave Doppler ("duplex ultrasound") is used to stratify patients into those who would and would not be expected to benefit from carotid endarterectomy (see chapter 23, case 24) [47].

Artifacts

While ultrasound is unique among diagnostic imaging modalities in the extent that artifacts are used for diagnosis, efforts should be made to avoid artifacts that do degrade images and obscure pathology [48].

Enhancement (Increased through-transmission): When the ultrasound beam encounters a poorly attenuating object such as a cyst, the echoes returning from regions deep to the object are of higher amplitude. This results in posterior enhancement, displayed as a bright band extending from the posterior aspect of the weak attenuator. This artifact is helpful when trying to distinguish a simple cyst from a hypoechoic lesion (Fig. 1.24A).

Shadowing: Conversely, if the ultrasound beam encounters a strongly attenuating or highly reflective surface, the returning echoes posterior to the structure are decreased in amplitude. The result is a dark or hypoechoic band posterior to the object. Consequently deeper structures may be obstructed. This artifact is helpful in identifying gallstones, renal stones, or metallic objects, to name a few (Fig. 1.24B).

Reverberation: The presence of two highly reflective surfaces causes the primary echo to bounce back and forth repeatedly between the two before returning to the transducer. The initial echo after a single reflection is displayed in the appropriate position, while the sequential reflected echoes manifest as repeating bands of decreasing intensity at regularly spaced intervals further from the transducer. Comet tail artifact is a special case of reverberation, where the close proximity of the two reflective surfaces results in blending of the successive echoes, and a tapered, triangular shaped artifact (Fig. 1.24C). Comet tail artifact can be caused by cholesterol crystals in Rokitansky-Aschoff sinuses and is diagnostic of adenomyomatosis [48].

Ring Down: This artifact is caused by induced vibration of fluid trapped between air bubbles, which results in a continuous source of sound energy being sent back to the transducer. This artifact appears as a continuous echogenic line or series of parallel bands posterior to the collection of gas (Fig. 1.24D). This artifact was erroneously thought to represent a variant of the comet tail artifact due to superficial similarity of their appearances [48].

SAFETY

Absence of ionizing radiation makes ultrasound the safest of the imaging modalities in common use; however, diagnostic ultrasound does transmit energy to the patient, and there is continuing examination of potential biological effects of ultrasound in order to ensure the safety of existing and future technology [49]. The intensity of the ultrasound beam is seen as the critical factor in producing thermal and mechanical bio-effects, with special attention given to fetal and embryonic exposure due to concerns about increased susceptibility during this period.

The biological effects of ultrasound can be divided into thermal and nonthermal effects. Thermal effects of ultrasound refer to tissue heating as a result of deposition of acoustic energy. Tissue heating depends on the acoustic power and the duration of exposure. This is quantified by the thermal index (TI), which is defined as the ratio of the emitted acoustic power to the power required to raise the temperature of tissue by 1°C.

The main mechanical effect of ultrasound relates to the interaction of ultrasound fields with very small pockets of gas, which can result in expansion and violent collapse of gas bubbles, creating a shock wave that causes local damage. This power is harnessed to break up renal calculi through shock wave lithotripsy. The mechanical index (MI) serves as a helpful guide for estimating the likelihood of mechanical bioeffects like cavitation and is related to the amplitude of the ultrasound pulse.

Safety guidelines have been established in terms of TI and MI to ensure safe operation of diagnostic ultrasound during the prenatal and postnatal period and continue the impressive safety profile of this modality. Nevertheless, even relatively safe procedures such as ultrasound should only be performed when there is a valid medical indication in order to limit unnecessary exposure.

STRENGTHS AND WEAKNESSES

Ultrasonography is a mainstay of diagnostic imaging for a myriad of reasons. Some of its strengths include

1. Wide availability and relatively low cost of the equipment
2. Portability, which allows for bedside examination and rapid guidance for interventional procedures, such as ultrasound-guided biopsy
3. Excellent safety profile due to absence of ionizing radiation and nephrotoxicity
4. Patient comfort and hands-on operation, allows for positive patient-physician interaction
5. Real-time imaging, allowing for evaluation of moving structures such as muscles and tendons
6. Superb superficial spatial resolution, allowing for visualization of soft tissue structures
7. Availability of Doppler, allowing for evaluation of blood flow

Some of the weaknesses in the technology include

1. Inherent dependence on operator skill, which can range from excellent to abysmal
2. Limited evaluation of deep structures, which leads to poor image quality in large patients
3. Inability to evaluate structures deep to gas collections, which limits evaluation of organs such as lungs and pancreas (located deep to the stomach or colon)

FUTURE DIRECTIONS

Ultrasound technology continues to evolve in both technological sophistication as well as clinical applications. Recent advancements include expanding the application of microbubbles, and advanced computational methods to allow for co-registration of ultrasound images with MRI and CT.

In addition to their use in echocardiography and vascular imaging, microbubbles have been investigated for use in demonstrating tissue perfusion patterns in liver lesions very similar to the standard arterial, portal venous, and delayed phases of contrast-enhanced CT and MRI. The technology shows promising application for the evaluation of pathology in other organs and there is growing support for eventual FDA approval of these agents in abdominal imaging. Several distinct advantages include the absence of nephrotoxicity, overall cost-effectiveness, and the ability to perform these studies at bedside if necessary [43].

Another application is the use of microbubbles is for targeted delivery of therapeutic agents. Microbubbles are injected into the circulation. The area of interest is exposed to a high-intensity ultrasound field so that passing microbubbles implode in the desired location. The imploding microbubbles create shockwaves that can be used to kill cancer cells. They can also be filled with therapeutic agents to allow for localized delivery of highly toxic chemicals or for gene therapy [50].

Advanced computational methods have been applied to ultrasound. The V-Nav system (GE Healthcare), for example, imports a patient's CT or MRI data into an ultrasound machine and co-registers the images with real-time ultrasound imaging using common anatomic landmarks. This process fuses the modalities and allows for a dynamic comparison of the MRI or CT images with real-time ultrasound scanning. The main benefit is in performing biopsies of lesions that are not well-visualized with ultrasound, but which would be challenging or costly to biopsy under CT or MRI guidance [51].

MAGNETIC RESONANCE IMAGING (MRI)

Nuclear magnetic resonance refers to the behavior of certain atomic nuclei, which, when placed in a static magnetic field and stimulated by an oscillating magnetic field, can re-emit some of the absorbed energy in the form of radio waves. This principle is used in nuclear spectroscopy to not only study the structure of chemicals, as well as the static and dynamic interactions between atomic nuclei. This technique found important applications in analytical and physical chemistry following its discovery in the 1930s and 1940s [52]. Further refinements allowed this chemical information to be localized in space, forming the foundation for nuclear magnetic resonance imaging (NMRI). The "nuclear" was later dropped as a marketing strategy, leaving MRI, which is currently an indispensable part of patient care in almost all areas of medicine, including neurology (early detection of cerebral ischemia), sports medicine (characterization of ligamentous and tendinous injuries), and oncology (detection, characterization, and follow-up of neoplasms). New technical developments will continue to expand the role of this modality.

IMAGE FORMATION

The underlying physics of MRI are complicated and rely on unsatisfying analogies to spinning tops, compass needles, runners on a track, and rooms full of talking people; they are beyond the scope of this book. The interested reader is encouraged to study the excellent review by Pooley for the basic concepts of MRI physics [53].

At its most basic level, an MRI machine is a strong magnet that manipulates the polarity of hydrogen atoms (protons) in the human body. The strength of the magnet is defined in terms of the SI unit, Tesla (T). The magnitude of the earth's magnetic field at the surface of our planet is between 25 and 65 μT (microteslas). By way of comparison, most MRI machines in use today are 1.5T or 3T devices. MRIs with 4 to 9.4T magnets are being used in experimental settings, and low-field strength MRIs (0.2–0.3T) are used as "open" machines for claustrophobic patients and as small in-office devices for the convenience of patients and for self-referral benefits of physicians [54].

With the protons aligned by the large static magnet, the MRI machine generates a second magnetic field oscillating in the radiofrequency range (RF pulses) that passes through these nuclei at a specific frequency in order for resonance to occur (the *R* in MRI). The energy the nuclei emit in response to the RF pulse (the "echo") is then measured and localized in space to generate an image. The following sections will provide a practical overview of image formation and point the interested reader to references for more detailed study.

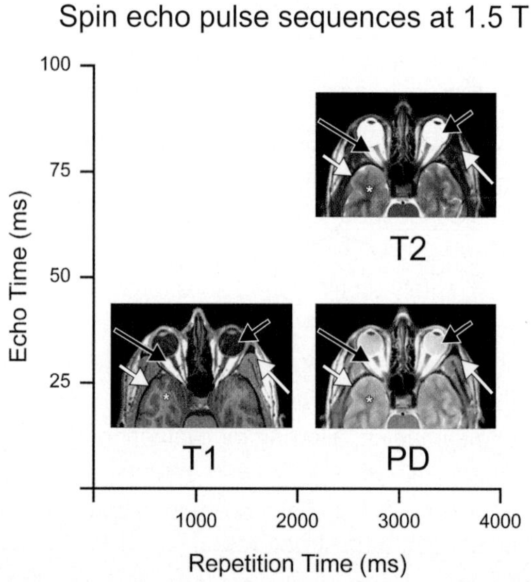

Image Contrast

Image contrast in MRI depends on intrinsic characteristics of the tissue and extrinsic factors controlled by the MRI machine. The main intrinsic factors are the density of hydrogen nuclei (protons) in the tissue (proton density), the interaction of the protons with surrounding tissue (spin-lattice relaxation time, or T1 relaxation), and the interaction of the protons with each other (spin-spin relaxation time, or T2 relaxation). Extrinsic factors can be manipulated by altering the settings on the MRI device, generating different "pulse sequences" (read further). These pulse sequences result in specific interactions of protons in tissue with the magnetic fields and electromagnetic pulses and generate images that highlight different characteristics of tissues. Different vendors have proprietary techniques and names for various pulse sequences; familiarity with the names used in your institution is helpful.

The workhorse of MR imaging is the spin echo pulse sequence and its relative, fast (turbo) spin echo. By setting certain parameters called echo time (TE) and repetition time (TR), T1-, T2-, and proton density weighted images can be generated. Examples of these basic pulse sequences are shown in Fig. 1.26. T1-weighted image will highlight fat as bright, muscle as intermediate, and water as dark. White matter and gray matter have intermediate signal intensity, but with gray matter darker than white matter. A T2-weighted image on modern MRIs will highlight water as bright, fat as slightly less bright, and muscle as intermediate. White matter (Fig. 1.26, indicated by *) and gray matter (Fig. 1.26, small arrowhead) have intermediate signal intensity, but with white matter darker than gray matter (opposite of T1-weighted images). A proton density image (PD) will be between T1- and T2-weighted images, with the specific imaging characteristics depending on the TR and TE values used [53].

Inversion recovery (IR) pulse sequences are used to generate T1-, T2-, or PD-weighted images while suppressing

Fig. 1.26 Spin echo pulse sequences at 1.5T. T1-weighted, T2-weighted, and proton density (PD) weighted images can be generated with spine echo pulse sequences by defining repetition and echo times (TR and TE, respectively). The specific numbers will vary based on the strength of the MRI. Representative numbers for a 1.5T MRI are depicted. T1-weighted images typically have short TR (<1000 ms) and short TE (<30 ms). T2-weighted images typically have long TR (>2000 ms) and long TE (>80 ms). PD-weighted images typically have long TR (>2000 ms) and short TE (<30 ms). Long black arrow, orbital fat; short black arrow, aqueous humor (mostly water); long white arrow, muscle; short white arrow, gray matter; *, white matter.

signal from specific tissues. Most commonly, this is used to suppress water (FLAIR, fluid attenuated inversion recovery) and fat (STIR, short tau inversion recovery) [53]. Examples of these pulse sequences and the corresponding non-IR images are shown in Fig. 1.27A-D. **Inversion recovery** for fat suppression (STIR, Fig. 1.27C,D) can be used with low-field strength MRIs and allows for homogeneous and global fat suppression in the face of field inhomogeneities (such as hardware, see the "Artifacts," section), but is not always specific for fat.

In addition to IR, two other methods exist for suppression of fat signal (fat suppression): fat saturation ("fat sat" in radiology slang) and opposed-phase imaging. Fat suppression is primarily used to improve visualization of lesions on postcontrast imaging and to characterize specific lesions, such as adrenal adenomas (see chapter 6, case 12) [55]. **Fat saturation** (Fig. 1.27E,F) can be used to suppress macroscopic fat signal and is good for acquisition of contrast-enhanced images, but it suffers from sensitivity to magnetic field inhomogeneities and is unreliable with low-field strength MRIs. **Opposed-phase imaging** (Fig. 1.27G,H) is predominantly used to detect lesions that contain small amounts of

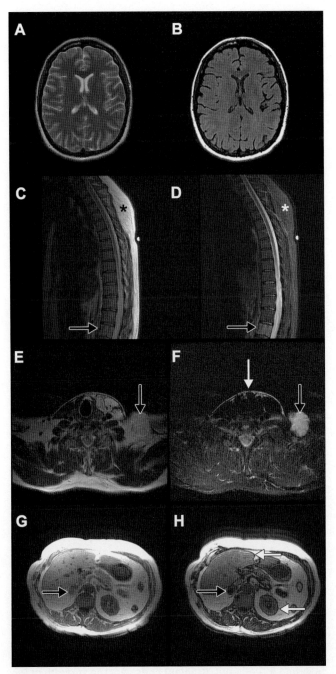

intracellular lipid, but is not ideal for detection of small tumors embedded in fatty tissue [55].

Gradient recalled echo (GRE) sequences can acquire images much faster than traditional pulse sequences. While T1- and PD-weighted images can be obtained with GRE techniques, T2-weighted images are not possible. Instead, GRE pulse sequences generate T2* (T2 star) images, which are similar in appearance to T2-weighted images, but are more susceptible to magnetic field inhomogeneities (see "Artifacts," section). The main strength of the GRE technique is its speed, which allows imaging of areas susceptible to respiratory motion (eg, chest and upper abdomen), and isotropic three-dimensional acquisition in imaging times that can be tolerated by patients [56]. Various fat suppression techniques can be applied to GRE sequences.

Diffusion-weighted imaging (DWI) is based on the random motion of water molecules in the body, which is normally restricted in biologic tissues because of cell membranes and macromolecules [57]. Diseases that result in restricted diffusion of water molecules result in increased signal on DW images. It is important to note that another component of signal on DW images is the inherent T2 signal in the tissue. This T2 signal can "shine through" to the DW images and give the appearance of restricted diffusion. To overcome this potential pitfall, the data is processed to create an apparent diffusion coefficient (ADC) map, which is a calculated image that maps areas of true restricted diffusion to low values [57]. The main use of DWI and ADC maps has been in neuroradiology, where restricted diffusion is an early sign of cerebral ischemia (see chapter 3, case 1). More recent attempts have been made to use DWI in oncological imaging, with varying levels of success [57].

Contrast Agents. Most MRI contrast agents are chelates of the rare-earth element gadolinium and produce increased signal ("positive contrast") on T1-weighted images (the effect on T2-weighted images is generally negligible).

Fig. 1.27 Examples of inversion recovery and fat suppression techniques. (A,B) T2 and FLAIR pairs are often used in brain MRIs. The FLAIR image (B) suppresses the signal from water (note the dark cerebrospinal fluid). (C,D) T2 and STIR. STIR sequences are often obtained when there is concern for heterogeneity in the magnetic field, such as in patients with hardware, or when imaging large areas such as the thoracic spine shown here. Note the T2-hyperintense lesion (arrow) that is seen better when the normal fat in the vertebral body is suppressed. Also note the homogeneous suppression of subcutaneous fat (*). (E,F) T2 and fat saturation. Note the lesion in the subcutaneous fat of the left lower neck (black arrows), which is seen more easily with fat saturation (F). Also note loss of fat suppression due to magnetic field inhomogeneity in the anterior neck (white arrow) in an area of sharp variation in anatomic structures. (G,H) The opposed phase technique is most commonly used in abdominal imaging, and results in a pair of images. The in-phase image (G) shows a small nodule in the lateral limb of the right adrenal gland (black arrow). The opposed-phase image (H) shows loss of signal in the lesion (black arrow), indicating the presence of fat, and a diagnosis of an adrenal adenoma. Opposed-phase image can be recognized by the typical black outline of organs against intra-abdominal fat (white arrows). This is the so-called "India ink" artifact, which results from loss of signal in voxels that contain both fat and nonfat components.

Negative MRI contrast agents, such as superparamagnetic iron oxide (SPIO), are not currently in widespread use (see Future Directions).

Gadolinium-based contrast agents can be classified by their primary use as well as their chemical structure. The latter can be helpful in determining the safety profile of gadolinium-based agents and will be discussed later (see Safety). For practical purposes, gadolinium contrast agents can be classified as extracellular, blood pool, or hepatobiliary.

Extracellular Agents: These are the most commonly used agents. They are typically small molecular weight compounds with nonspecific distribution in blood and extracellular space of the body and are used in inthe imaging of tumors and inflammation, as well as in magnetic resonance angiography (MRA) [58]. They can also be used as intra-articular agents in magnetic resonance arthrography (also MRA, but not confused with magnetic resonance angiography due to the context). It must be noted that intra-articular use of gadolinium agents is considered off-label in the United States.

Blood Pool Agents: These agents are used almost exclusively in magnetic resonance angiography. While the aforementioned extracellular agents are commonly used, image timing must be precise to capture the first pass of these agents in the arterial system. Blood-pool contrast agents, on the other hand, have longer intravascular half-lives, allowing the imaging time to be extended far beyond the short arterial first-pass phase [59]. These agents are further subdivided as macromolecular and low-molecular weight agents. Macromolecular agents are currently not in clinical use. The most important of the low-molecular weight agents is Gadofosveset trisodium (Ablavar, formerly Vasovist), a monomer which noncovalently binds to albumin in human plasma, making it a blood pool agent [59].

Hepatobiliary Agents: These agents were designed to improve the discrimination and diagnosis of focal hepatic lesions, and include gadobenate dimeglumine (Gd-BOPTA, MultiHance) and Gadoxetic acid (Gd-EOB-DTPA, Eovist, Primovist). Gd-BOPTA has a lipophilic moiety that allows uptake through the sinusoidal and canalicular side of hepatocytes. Its hepatic uptake is less than 5% of the injected dose, which can be highlighted on delayed images, at which point the intravascular component has mostly been excreted by the kidneys. Therefore, in the first few minutes after administration, Gd-BOPTA acts as a conventional extracellular agent; however, there is a marked and long-lasting enhancement of normal liver parenchyma 40 to 120 minutes after administration, at which point focal hepatic lesions will stand out as dark lesions in contrast to the enhancing normal liver. The obvious downside is having to wait 40 minutes to obtain diagnostic images [58].

EQUIPMENT

The MRI scanner (Fig. 1.28) is made up of a strong magnet that aligns the protons in the human body along its magnetic field. Most modern MRI scanners use superconducting electromagnets, which require liquid helium to reach superconducting temperatures and can produce strong, homogeneous magnetic fields. Low-field strength MRIs,

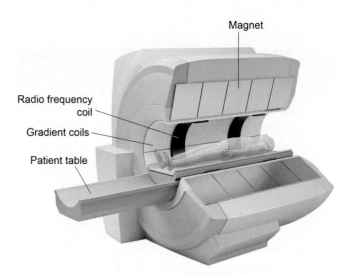

Fig. 1.28 Cut-away view of a modern MRI machine. Please see text for description.

on the other hand, have either resistive electromagnets or permanent magnets, both of which produce weaker magnetic fields and have poor field homogeneity [54].

The patient is placed into this static magnetic field (designated B_0) and bombarded with magnetic fields oscillating in the radiofrequency (RF) range (RF pulses) from **RF coils** built into the magnet. **Gradient coils** vary the strength of the main magnetic field in three directions (x, y, and z) and allow the machine to localize signals from various tissues in three-dimensional space [54]. A receiver coil (the antenna) reads the signals emitted by the body in response to the RF pulses in a process called "read-out." This coil can be the same as the RF coil; however, surface coils can be placed closer to the area of interest to get better reception.

IMAGE INTERPRETATION

Because of its superior contrast resolution, MRI is predominantly used as a problem-solving modality when there are

Table 1.2 Appearance of Various Tissue Types on Modern MRI

Tissue	T1	T2
Fat	Bright*	Bright
Water/edema	Dark	Bright
Protein-rich fluid	Bright	variable
Melanin	Bright	Dark
Calcium	Very dark	Very dark
Gadolinium	Bright	Minimally dark
Fibrous tissue	Intemediate	Dark
Muscle	Intermediate	Intermediate
Intracranial blood		
Hyperacute (<24 h)	Intermediate*	Bright
Acute (1-3 d)	Intermediate*	Dark
Early subacute (3-7 d)	Bright	Dark
Late subacute (7-30 d)	Bright	Bright
Chronic (>30 d)	Dark	Dark

*The words dark and bright used in the table are simplified ways of referring to the amount of signal (low or high, respectively) by the tissues.

questions about the tissue composition of specific lesions. Image interpretation in this context relies on understanding how the chemical composition of various tissues manifests on the many MRI pulse sequences available. Additional imaging characteristics, such as appearance of tissues in response to the various available contrast agents (Table 1.2), is beyond the scope of this chapter, but will be discussed further in the chapters that follow (see chapter 5, case 23).

Because various soft tissue structures such as intervertebral disks, muscles, ligaments, and tendons can have similar attenuation characteristics on CT, MRI is used as a primary diagnostic modality in musculoskeletal and spine imaging. Image interpretation in this context requires knowledge of the normal appearance of these structures on various pulse sequences (see chapter 7, case 17, for example).

Box 1.5 – TERMINOLOGY

Image brightness on MRI is described in terms of intensity: high signal intensity (hyperintense), intermediate signal intensity, and low signal intensity (hypointense). These words are sometimes incorrectly used in isolation. When using these terms, you must always indicate what you are comparing the intensity to: "isointense to gray matter," or "hypointense to muscle."

Finally, as in all fields of radiology, image interpretation depends on an understanding of artifacts, some of which can actually be used in image interpretation.

Artifacts

Artifacts on MR images can be related to the patient, the MRI system, the image reconstruction process, or a combination of these. Some of the more common MRI artifacts are introduced in this section. The interested reader is referred to the excellent review by Zhuo and Gullapalli [60].

Motion Artifact. Patient motion, whether voluntary or involuntary, can cause blurring of the image as well as "ghosting" in one axis of the image (the phase-encoding direction). Respiration (Fig. 1.29A) is a common involuntary motion that can be mitigated by decreasing the time for an individual sequence (eg, single breath-hold sequences). Patient discomfort can also be a source of motion, given that an MRI examination can last between 20 minutes to more than 1 hour. Decreasing total examination time by eliminating unnecessary sequences can help in this regard. Another source of motion is the pulsation of vessels, which can result in ghosting of round objects that can mimic lesions (Fig. 1.29B) or obscure important anatomy.

Susceptibility Effects. Magnetization of tissue slightly alters the magnetic field in the local area and causes field inhomogeneity at tissue boundaries. This results in geometric distortion and areas of low signal intensity on images. These can be seen at air-tissue interfaces (Fig. 1.29C), as well as near metallic hardware (Fig. 1.29D). This effect is particularly pronounced on gradient-echo images, and is used to diagnostic advantage in detecting small amounts of hemosiderin. The effect is known as "blooming," which refers to apparent enlargement of an area of low signal on T2* images when compared to T2-weighted images (Fig. 1.29E,F; see chapter 7, case 6).

Aliasing (Wraparound) Artifact. Aliasing occurs when the imaging field of view is smaller than the anatomy being imaged and appears as a part of the image wrapping around to the other side (Fig. 1.29G) with or without an interference pattern called the moiré or fringe artifact (Fig. 1.29H).

SAFETY

MRI safety issues can be caused by gadolinium-based intravenous contrast agents (specifically, nephrogenic systemic fibrosis) or by machine-related processes having to do with the large static magnetic field of the scanner, the time-varying magnetic fields generated by the gradient coils, or the energy generated by the RF coils.

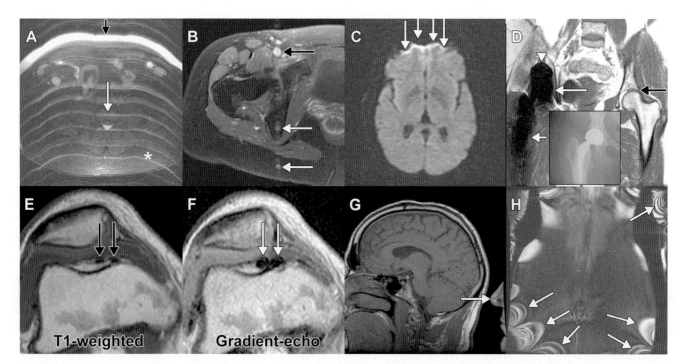

Fig. 1.29 MRI artifacts. See text for details. (A) Respiratory motion results in ghosting (white arrow shows one example) of the moving anterior abdominal wall (black arrow). Also note loss of fat saturation anteriorly due to loss of field homogeneity (the subcutaneous fat here should be dark like the rest of the subcutaneous fat in this patient, which is indicated by *). (B) Pulsation artifact is another manifestation of motion artifact. Here, the pulsating right femoral artery (black arrow), results in multiple ghosts, which can mimic lesions in bone (white arrow) and soft tissue (white arrowhead). The key is to recognize that connecting these ghosts leads to the femoral artery. (C) Susceptibility effect in a diffusion weighted image of the brain near the frontal sinuses results in distortion of the image and the appearance of a concave margin to the frontal lobes (white arrows). (D) Susceptibility effect due to hardware (inset). There is loss of signal where the right hip hardware is located (short white arrow). In addition, there is distortion of the image, with the position of the acetabular component shifted cephalad (white arrowhead) compared to its actual location (long white arrow) in line with the left acetabulum (black arrow). (E,D) Susceptibility effect due to hemosiderin in a patient with pigmented villonodular synovitis. This is termed "blooming" and is used to identify hemosiderin. The T1-weighted image (E) shows the location of small foci of low signal (black arrows), which could represent any of the low T1 tissues listed in Table 1.2. The structures enlarge ("bloom") on the GRE image (white arrows, F), suggesting the presence of hemosiderin. (G) Aliasing (wraparound) artifact, with the patient's nose (white arrow) located behind his head. (H) Aliasing (wraparound) artifact with an interference pattern known as the Moiré effect (white arrows).

The main issues with time-varying magnetic fields generated by gradient coils are the potential for peripheral nerve stimulation and acoustic noise, both of which have been addressed by manufacturers adhering to relevant international and national safety standards [60]. The remaining safety concerns will be briefly discussed in the following section. The interested reader is referred to the excellent review by Zhuo and Gullapalli [60], Price [61], and Shellock and Crues [62] for more complete coverage of this important topic.

Nephrogenic Systemic Fibrosis (NSF)

Nephrogenic systemic fibrosis (NSF) is a rare systemic disorder of unknown etiology with high morbidity and mortality rates, which is almost exclusively seen in patients with impaired renal function [63]. While it is often discussed in the setting of gadolinium-based contrast agents, it is important to note that the diagnosis does not require a history of exposure to these agents [64]. Renal impairment,

however, is an important predisposing factor, and almost all cases of NSF have been seen in patients with stage IV or V chronic kidney disease or those with acute renal injury [63]. When associated with gadolinium-based contrast agents, NSF usually presents between 2 and 10 weeks after administration and is more common with a particular class of gadolinium-based contrast agents.

As noted earlier, gadolinium-based contrast agents can be classified based on their primary use as intravascular, blood pool, or hepatobiliary. For purposes of safety profile, however, it is helpful to categorize them based on their ligand characteristic as macrocyclic, linear ionic, and linear nonionic (Table 1.3). The macrocyclic agents are shaped like cages around the gadolinium ion and have a lower probability of releasing free gadolinium. They are considered more stable than other contrast agents and have a lower risk of NSF. The linear nonionic agents are the least stable, and the linear ionic agents have intermediate stability [63]. For example, the vast majority of patients with NSF have been exposed to the linear nonionic agent, Omniscan (gadodiamide), even though it only has about 15% of the worldwide market share of gadolinium-based contrast agents [63].

Table 1.3 Ligand Characteristics of Gadolinium-Based Contrast Agents

Contrast Agent Trade Name (Generic Name)	Class
Gadovist (Gadobutrol)	Macrocyclic
Dotarem (Gadoterate meglumine)	Macrocyclic
ProHance (Gadoteridol)	Macrocyclic
MultiHance (Gadobenate dimeglumine)	Linear, ionic
Eovist Primovist (Gadoxetate disodium)	Linear, ionic
Ablavar /Vasovist (Gadofosveset trisodium)	Linear, ionic
Omniscan (Gadodiamide and caldiamide)	Linear, nonionic
OptiMARK (Gadoversetamide and calversetamide)	Linear, nonionic

The diagnosis of NSF is based on a clinicopathological scoring system described in more detail by Girardi, et al [64]. The typical presentation is acute to subacute onset of limb edema that is accompanied by cutaneous papules and plaques overlying fibrosis of the cutaneous and subcutaneous fat [63]. Muscles can also be affected, including those underlying the skin changes, as well as diaphragmatic and esophageal muscles. The end result of progressive disease can range from joint contractures and loss of mobility in the extremities to death from respiratory failure. However, the disease can also be transient with clinical improvement [63].

Different clinical and laboratory algorithms have been developed to limit the chance of NSF in patients receiving gadolinium-based contrast agents. These vary among institutions, but in all cases begin with an assessment of the need for intravenous contrast. There are several options for patients on hemodialysis, peritoneal dialysis, or those with acute renal injury: they may either not get intravenous contrast, be considered for alternate imaging studies, receive a lower dose of contrast, or be examined using one of the macrocyclic agents. Patients not on dialysis or without acute renal injury can be screened based on the risk for reduced renal function (eg, older than 60, history of diabetes mellitus, hypertension, renal disease, solitary kidney, renal transplant, or renal neoplasm). These patients may then undergo serum testing for estimation of glomerular filtration rate (eGFR). Usually, those patients with eGFR<30 will not receive intravenous gadolinium-based contrast agents, and those with eGFR between 30 and 60 will receive a study with the more expensive macrocyclic agents or with half the usual dose, or both [63].

Static Magnetic Field

The large static magnetic field generated by modern MRI scanners can be deadly if appropriate care is not taken to prevent metallic objects being taken within a certain distance from the scanner. Such objects can easily turn into projectiles and harm the patient on the imaging table [60]. Certain electrical devices, such as pacemakers can become disabled or malfunction if in close enough proximity to the main magnet. It is important to read and obey signs posted at various distances from the MRI scanner to ensure the safety of patients and medical personnel (Fig. 1.30).

In addition, patient screening is vital to avoid damage from motion of metal objects inside the patient, such as metallic fragments in the eye and older intracerebral aneurysm clips. Modern aneurysm clips are made of titanium and titanium alloys and are safe for patients undergoing MR imaging [65]. Intravascular coils, filters, and stents tend to

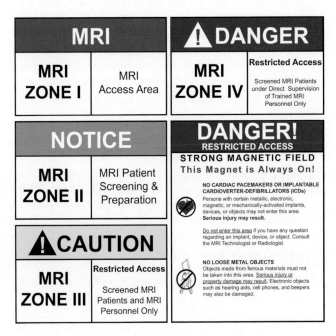

Fig. 1.30 MRI safety signs. The danger signs are placed at the 5-Gauss exclusion zone (5 G = 0.0005T) to limit access of individuals with cardiac pacemakers into high-magnetic-field areas. In addition to signage, physical barriers are employed to exclude access by the general public.

become firmly incorporated into the vessel wall after about 6 weeks and should be safe in the static magnetic field [61]. In any case, patients should always be screened for the presence of foreign objects and not be imaged unless definitive proof supporting the safety of the device can be produced [61]. A great resource is Dr Frank G. Shellock's web site on the safety of devices for use in MRI at http://mrisafety.com/.

Finally, intentional or accidental sudden loss superconductivity of the magnet can cause the liquid helium coolant to rapidly boil off ("quenching"). This can occur with destructive force and present a direct danger to anyone in proximity to the scanner. In addition, the helium gas can present a suffocation hazard. Safeguards have been designed to limit this risk, including venting systems that direct helium gas out of the building ("quench pipe") and oxygen monitors in MRI scanner rooms. The proper procedure in a quenching event is to evacuate the MRI scanner room as quickly as possible. The two most common reasons for intentional quenching are to free someone who has been pinned to the magnet by a large metallic object or in the case of fire, to allow fire personnel to enter the room.

RF Coils

Prolonged exposure of biologic tissues to RF energy can cause tissue heating. The U.S. Food and Drug Administration has established guidelines for allowable RF energy deposition to keep maximum tissue heating less than 1°C. Even when operated within these guidelines, RF energy can cause burns under specific conditions; these include presence of conductive material (eg, leads on the skin, jewelry), conductive loops (eg, skin-to-skin contact from touching body parts), direct patient contact with the transmit RF coil, and system failure (eg, RF surface coil decoupling) [62].

STRENGTHS AND WEAKNESSES

The strengths of MRI include its superior soft-tissue contrast and lack of ionizing radiation. The major weaknesses of MRI include its relatively high cost (Fig. 1.5), and long scan times (30-60 minutes).

FUTURE DIRECTIONS

Major developments will continue in development and refinement of MRI pulse sequences to increase speed with little or no loss in diagnostic image quality. Molecular imaging techniques are also being developed for use in MRI, with contrast agents targeting the reticuloendothelial system (eg, superparamagnetic iron oxide (SPIO) intravenous contrast material) and important biologic parameters of cancer, such as hypoxia (eg, trifluoroethoxy-misonidazole).

REFERENCES

1. Saini S, Seltzer SE, Bramson RT, et al. Technical cost of radiologic examinations: analysis across imaging modalities. *Radiology.* 2000;216(1):269-272.

2. Committee to Assess Health Risks from Exposure to Low Levels of Ionizing Radiation. *Health Risks from Exposure to Low Levels of Ionizing Radiation: BEIR VII—Phase 2.* Washington, DC: The National Academies Press; 2006.

3. Mould RF. The discovery of x-rays and radioactivity. In: Thomas AMK, ed. *The Invisible Light: 100 Years of Medical radiology.* London: Blackwell Science; 1995:1.

4. Berbaum KS, Franken EA Jr, Dorfman DD, et al. Influence of clinical history on perception of abnormalities in pediatric radiographs. *Acad Radiol.* 1994;1(3):217-223.

5. Leslie A, Jones AJ, Goddard PR. The influence of clinical information on the reporting of CT by radiologists. *Br J Radiol.* 2000;73(874):1052-1055.

6. Bushberg JT. The AAPM/RSNA physics tutorial for residents. X-ray interactions. *Radiographics.* 1998;18(2):457-468.

7. James JJ, Davies AG, Cowen AR, O'Connor PJ. Developments in digital radiography: an equipment update. *Eur Radiol.* 2001;11(12):2616-2626.

8. Lee KR, Siegel EL, Templeton AW, Dwyer SJ III, Murphey MD, Wetzel LH. State-of-the-art digital radiography. *Radiographics.* 1991;11(6):1013-1125; discussion 1026.

9. Körner M, Weber CH, Wirth S, Pfeifer KJ, Reiser MF, Treitl M. Advances in digital radiography: physical principles and system overview. *Radiographics.* 2007;27(3):675-686.

10. Wang J, Blackburn TJ. The AAPM/RSNA physics tutorial for residents: x-ray image intensifiers for fluoroscopy. *Radiographics.* 2000;20(5):1471-1477.

11. Shetty CM, Barthur A, Kambadakone A, Narayanan N, Kv R. Computed radiography image artifacts revisited. *AJR.* 2011;196(1):W37-W47.

12. Walz-Flannigan A, Magnuson D, Erickson D, Schueler B. Artifacts in digital radiography. *AJR.* 2012;198(1):156-161.

13. Bogdanich W. Radiation overdoses point up dangers of CT scans. *New York Times.* October 15, 2009. http://www.nytimes.com/2009/10/16/us/16radiation.html?_r=0. Accessed September 25, 2013.

14. Donadieu J, Piguet C, Bernard F, et al. A new clinical score for disease activity in Langerhans cell histiocytosis. *Pediatr Blood Cancer.* 2004;43(7):770-776.

15. Hendee WR, O'Connor MK. Radiation risks of medical imaging: separating fact from fantasy. *Radiology.* 2012;264(2):312-321.

16. Wrixon AD. New ICRP recommendations. *J Radiol Prot.* 2008;28(2):161-168.

17. Nickoloff EL, Lu ZF, Dutta AK, So JC. Radiation dose descriptors: BERT, COD, DAP, and other strange creatures. *Radiographics.* 2008;28(5):1439-1450.

18. Thorne MC. Background radiation: natural and man-made. *J Radiol Prot.* 2003;23(1):29-42.

19. National Council on Radiation Protection and Measurements. Ionizing Radiation Exposure of the Population of the United States. *NCRP Report No. 160;* 2009.

20. Hendee WR. Cross sectional medical imaging: a history. *Radiographics.* 1989;9(6):1155-1180.

21. Hounsfield GN. Computed medical imaging. Nobel lecture, December 8, 1979. *J Comput Assist Tomogr.* 1980;4(5): 665-674.

22. Paulsen SR, Huprich JE, Fletcher JG, et al. CT enterography as a diagnostic tool in evaluating small bowel disorders: review of clinical experience with over 700 cases. *Radiographics.* 2006;26(3):641-657; discussion 657-662.

23. Goldman LW. Principles of CT and CT technology. *J Nucl Med Technol.* 2007;35(3):115-128; quiz 129-130.

24. Rydberg J, Buckwalter KA, Caldemeyer KS, et al. Multisection CT: scanning techniques and clinical applications. *Radiographics.* 2000;20(6):1787-1806.

25. Sebastian S, Kalra MK, Mittal P, Saini S, Small WC. Can independent coronal multiplanar reformatted images obtained using state-of-the-art MDCT scanners be used for primary interpretation of MDCT of the abdomen and pelvis? A feasibility study. *Eur J Radiol.* 2007;64(3):439-446.

26. Barrett JF, Keat N. Artifacts in CT: recognition and avoidance. *Radiographics.* 2004:24(6):1679-1691.

27. American College of Radiology Committee on Drugs and Contrast Media. *ACR Manual on Contrast Media.* 2012:Version 8.

28. Orebaugh SL. Venous air embolism: clinical and experimental considerations. *Crit Care Med.* 1992;20(8):1169-1177.

29. Katayama H, Yamaguchi K, Kozuka T, Takashima T, Seez P, Matsuura K. Adverse reactions to ionic and nonionic contrast media. A report from the Japanese Committee on the Safety of Contrast Media. *Radiology.* 1990;175(3):621-628.

30. Caro JJ, Trindade E, McGregor M. The risks of death and of severe nonfatal reactions with high- vs low-osmolality contrast media: a meta-analysis. *AJR.* 1991;156(4):825-832.

31. Meth MJ. Maibach HI. Current understanding of contrast media reactions and implications for clinical management. *Drug Saf.* 2006;29(2):133-141.

32. Schabelman E, Witting M. The relationship of radiocontrast, iodine, and seafood allergies: a medical myth exposed. *J Emerg Med.* 2010;39(5):701-707.

33. Bruce RJ, Djamali A, Shinki K, Michel SJ, Fine JP, Pozniak MA. Background fluctuation of kidney function versus contrast-induced nephrotoxicity. *AJR.* 2009;192(3):711-718.

34. McNitt-Gray MF. AAPM/RSNA physics tutorial for residents: topics in CT. Radiation dose in CT. *Radiographics.* 2002;22(6):1541-1553.

35. van der Molen AJ, Geleijns J. Overranging in multisection CT: quantification and relative contribution to dose—comparison of four 16-section CT scanners. *Radiology.* 2007;242(1): 208-216.

36. California Senate. *Bill 1237.* California. February 19, 2010. http://www.leginfo.ca.gov/pub/09-10/bill/sen/sb_1201-1250/sb_1237_bill_20100929_chaptered.html. Accessed September 25, 2013.

37. Mettler FA Jr, Bhargavan M, Faulkner K, et al. Radiologic and nuclear medicine studies in the United States and worldwide: frequency, radiation dose, and comparison with other radiation sources—1950-2007. *Radiology.* 2009;253(2):520-531.

38. McCollough CH, Bruesewitz MR, Kofler JM Jr. CT dose reduction and dose management tools: overview of available options. *Radiographics.* 2006;26(2):503-512.

39. Cheeke JDN. *Fundamentals and Applications of Ultrasonic Waves.* 2nd ed. Boca Raton, FL: CRC Press; 2012.

40. Kane, D, Grassi W, Sturrock R, Balint PV. A brief history of musculoskeletal ultrasound: "From bats and ships to babies and hips." *Rheumatology.* 2004;43(7):931-933.

41. Dussik KT. On the possibility of using ultrasound waves as a diagnostic aid. *Neurol Psychiat.* 1942;174:153-168.

42. Hangiandreou NJ. AAPM/RSNA physics tutorial for residents. Topics in US: B-mode US: basic concepts and new technology. *RadioGraphics.* 2003;23(4):1019-1033.

43. Wilson SR, Greenbaum LD, Goldberg BB. Contrast-enhanced ultrasound: what is the evidence and what are the obstacles? *AJR.* 2009;193(1):55-60.

44. Boote EJ, AAPM/RSNA physics tutorial for residents: topics in US: Doppler US techniques: concepts of blood flow detection and flow dynamics. *Radiographic.* 2003;23(5):1315-1327.

45. Hamer OW, Aguirre DA, Casola G, Lavine JE, Woenckhaus M, Sirlin CB. Fatty liver: imaging patterns and pitfalls. *Radiographics.* 2006;26(6):1637-1653.

46. Fleischer AC, Rodgers WH, Kepple DM, Williams LL, Jones HW III, Gross PR. Color Doppler sonography of benign and malignant ovarian masses. *Radiographics.* 1992;12(5):879-885.

47. Hathout GM, Fink JR, El-Saden SM, Grant EG. Sonographic NASCET index: a new doppler parameter for assessment of internal carotid artery stenosis. *AJNR.* 2005;26(1):68-75.

48. Feldman MK, Katyal S, Blackwood MS. US artifacts. *RadioGraphics.* 2009;29(4):1179-1189.

49. Fowlkes JB. American Institute of Ultrasound in Medicine consensus report on potential bioeffects of diagnostic ultrasound: executive summary. *J Ultrasound Med.* 2008;27(4):503-515.

50. Unnikrishnan S, Klibanov AL. Microbubbles as ultrasound contrast agents for molecular imaging: preparation and application. *AJR.* 2012;199(2):292-299.

51. Jung EM, Friedrich C, Hoffstetter P, et al. Volume navigation with contrast enhanced ultrasound and image fusion for percutaneous interventions: first results. *PLOS ONE.* 2012;7(3):e33956.

52. Lindley D. Landmarks: NMR—Grandmother of MRI. *Physical Review Focus.* 2006;18:18.

53. Pooley RA. AAPM/RSNA physics tutorial for residents: fundamental physics of MR imaging. *RadioGraphics.* 2005;25(4):1087-1099.

54. Jacobs MA, Ibrahim TS, Ouwerkerk R. AAPM/RSNA physics tutorials for residents: MR imaging: brief overview and emerging applications. *Radiographics.* 2007;27(4):1213-1229.

55. Delfaut EM, Beltran J, Johnson G, Rousseau J, Marchandise X , Cotton A. Fat suppression in MR imaging: techniques and pitfalls. *Radiographics*. 1999;19(2):373–382.

56. Price RR. The AAPM/RSNA physics tutorial for residents. Contrast mechanisms in gradient-echo imaging and an introduction to fast imaging. *Radiographics*. 1995;15(1):165-178; quiz 149-150.

57. Koh DM, Collins DJ. Diffusion-weighted MRI in the body: applications and challenges in oncology. *AJR*. 2007;188(6):1622-1635.

58. Burtea C, Laurent S, Vander Elst L, Muller RN. Contrast agents: magnetic resonance. *Handb Exp Pharmacol*. 2008(185, pt 1):135-165.

59. Nielsen YW, Thomsen HS. Contrast-enhanced peripheral MRA: technique and contrast agents. *Acta Radiol*. 2012;53(7):769-777.

60. Zhuo J, Gullapalli RP. AAPM/RSNA physics tutorial for residents: MR artifacts, safety, and quality control. *Radiographics*. 2006;26(1):275-297.

61. Price RR. The AAPM/RSNA physics tutorial for residents. MR imaging safety considerations. *RadioGraphics*. 1999;19(6):1641-1651.

62. Shellock FG, Crues JV. MR procedures: biologic effects, safety, and patient care. *Radiology*. 2004;232(3):635-652.

63. Kaewlai R, Abujudeh H. Nephrogenic systemic fibrosis. *AJR*. 2012;199(1):W17-W23.

64. Girardi M, Kay J, Elston DM, Leboit PE, Abu-Alfa A, Cowper SE. Nephrogenic systemic fibrosis: clinicopathological definition and workup recommendations. *J Am Acad Dermatol*. 2011;65(6):1095-1106 e7.

65. Shellock FG, Tkach JA, Ruggieri PM, Masaryk TJ, Rasmussen PA. Aneurysm clips: evaluation of magnetic field interactions and translational attraction by use of "long-bore" and "short-bore" 3.0-T MR imaging systems. *AJNR*. 2003;24(3):463-471.

Chapter 2

Introduction to Nuclear Medicine

By David C. Brandon, Aaron J. Thomas, and Gregory C. Ravizzini

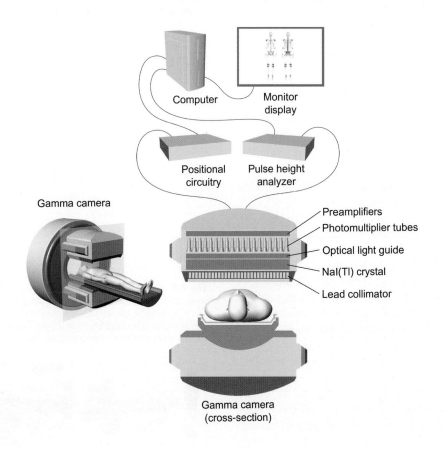

Computer

Monitor display

Positional circuitry

Pulse height analyzer

Gamma camera

Preamplifiers
Photomultiplier tubes
Optical light guide
NaI(Tl) crystal
Lead collimator

Gamma camera (cross-section)

WHAT IS NUCLEAR MEDICINE?

Nuclear medicine uses radioactive compounds called radiopharmaceuticals or radiotracers that interrogate physiologic or pathologic processes at a molecular level and provide targeted therapy for a variety of diseases. Nuclear medicine studies are clinically used to assess most organ systems with almost 100 different types of studies or therapies performed in the United States. Many more radiotracers play a crucial role in research.

When used as an imaging agent to evaluate organ function, metabolism, or membrane receptor characteristics, the amount of radiotracer administered is in the picomolar or nanomolar range, which avoids disturbing the process under evaluation while still yielding data that are quantifiable and comparable to normative standards. As functional deficits arise before morphological changes in many diseases, nuclear medicine studies can detect disease in early stages when curative or more effective palliative treatment choices may be an option. This chapter reviews the fundamentals of imaging generation for gamma and positron-emitting radiopharmaceuticals and common nuclear medicine procedures based on the organ system.

IMAGE GENERATION

Radiopharmaceuticals contain radioactive atoms that are unstable and produce ionizing radiation when they decay. High-energy rays produced by the decay interact with special light-producing crystals in nuclear medicine cameras to create the images. The types of imaging rays from radioisotope decay can be broadly placed in two categories: gamma rays or positron emission.

When gamma ray emitters such as technetium-99m decay, rays are emitted of a specific energy typically reported in kiloelectron volts (keV). For example, the workhorse of gamma imaging, technetium-99m, decays to produce a single 140 keV ray for imaging. Some radioisotopes give off several imaging rays, and gamma cameras are able to distinguish between the specific energy rays allowing for simultaneous imaging of two or more radiotracers.

Gamma cameras fundamentally are composed of 4 main parts: the collimator, a crystal, photomultiplier tubes, and electronics for processing the data (Fig. 2.1). A collimator is a sheet of lead with holes designed to reduce scatter when placed between the patient and the crystal. After interacting with the gamma rays that passed through the collimator, the sodium iodide doped with thallium crystal NaI(Tl) emits faint light, which is then detected by the photomultiplier tubes and processed into viewable nuclear images or scintigrams. The two dimensional images obtained are termed "planar" (Fig. 2.2). Because the gamma rays are coming from within the patient as opposed to from an external source as in conventional imaging, the change

in the position of the camera alters the image dramatically as the tissue attenuation changes. Figure 2.3 depicts the steps necessary to obtain images of a patient injected with

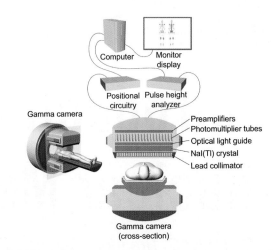

Fig. 2.1 The main components of a gamma camera responsible for imaging acquisition, processing, and display.

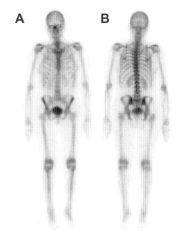

Fig. 2.2 A 52-year-old female with breast cancer, referred for evaluation of osseous metastases. Anterior (A) and posterior (B) whole-body planar images obtained 2 to 4 hours after the intravenous administration of 25 mCi of Tc-99m MDP demonstrate no evidence of bone metastases.

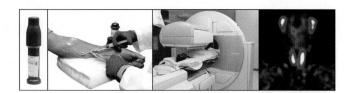

Fig. 2.3 Serial photographs, from left to right, illustrate the steps necessary to obtain images of a patient injected intravenously with a radiopharmaceutical. The syringe containing the radiopharmaceutical is provided from the radiopharmacy in a lead-shielded container called a unit dose pig. After the radiotracer is injected intravenously, the patient lies on a table under the gamma camera and images are obtained according to specific protocols.

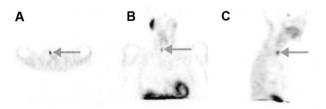

Fig. 2.4 SPECT images reconstructed in the axial (A), coronal (B), and sagittal (C) planes to further localize a lesion adjacent to the inferior pole of the right thyroid lobe (arrows).

a radiopharmaceutical intravenously. Imaging protocols vary depending on the type of radiopharmaceutical utilized, route of administration, and clinical question.

When the gamma camera is rotated around the patient, a three-dimensional data set is collected in a process termed single photon emission computed tomography (SPECT) and displayed in a multiplanar format—axial, coronal, and sagittal (Fig. 2.4). SPECT images allow for better localization of findings on planar images and can aid in the visualization of lesions obscured by overlying tracer activity just as chest CT can help evaluate a lung nodule seen on a chest radiograph. Increasingly, gamma cameras are equipped with an integrated CT scanner allowing for SPECT-CT studies. The merging of functional and anatomic data allows precise localization and appears to improve study interpretation, although the literature currently has few studies to support this. Table 2.1 lists commonly used single photon radionuclides in nuclear medicine and their physical characteristics.

Decay of positron emitters such as fluorine-18 leads to a matter-antimatter reaction, which produces a pair of 511 keV gamma rays that travel 180° apart (Fig. 2.5). A positron emission tomography (PET) machine uses a ring of crystals to take advantage of the two rays and requires near-simultaneous detection of the rays. The result is better

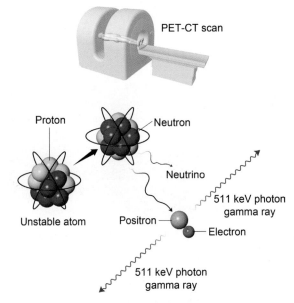

Fig. 2.5 The basic principle of electron-positron annihilation in PET imaging. When particles and antiparticles meet, they annihilate each other, releasing their combined mass as energy in the form of photons used to produce images.

image spatial resolution (4 mm) than gamma cameras can achieve (as low as 7 mm for SPECT). PET studies are three-dimensional data sets typically displayed in the axial, sagittal, and coronal planes. Today, PET machines have an integrated CT scanner that provides anatomic images and quick attenuation correction (Fig. 2.6). The anatomic data provided by the CT complements the functional data leading to a higher specificity and some improvement in sensitivity in detection of many cancers. PET-MRI machines have recently come into the commercial market, and their clinical role is still being defined. Table 2.2 lists commonly used positron-emitting radionuclides in PET imaging and their physical characteristics.

Table 2.1 Commonly Used Single-Photon Radionuclides and Their Physical Characteristics

Radionuclide	Principal Mode of Decay	Physical Half-Life	Principal Photon Energy (keV) and Abundance	Production Method
67Gallium	Electron capture	78.3 h	93 (37%) 185 (20%) 300 (17%) 395 (5%)	Cyclotron
99Molybdenum	Beta minus	2.8 d	740 (12%) 780 (4%)	Reactor
99mTechnetium	Isomeric transition	6 h	140 (89%)	Generator (99Molybdenum)
111Indium	Electron capture	2.8 d	171 (90%) 245 (94%)	Cyclotron
123Iodine	Electron capture	13.2 h	159 (83%)	Cyclotron
131Iodine	Beta minus	8 d	364 (81%)	Reactor

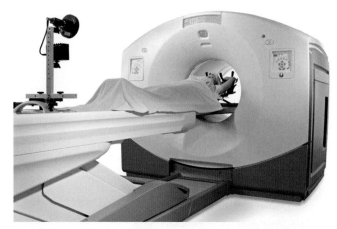

Fig. 2.6 State-of-the art PET-CT scanner manufactured by GE Healthcare, Milwaukee, WI. The PET scanner is assembled in tandem with a CT scanner and covered by a single gantry housing. The typical imaging protocol for combined PET-CT imaging includes obtaining first a CT topogram, then a spiral CT scan, followed by a PET scan.

Table 2.2 Positron-Emitting Radionuclides and Their Physical Characteristics

Radionuclide	Physical Half-Life (min)	Positron Energy (MeV)	Range in Soft tissue (mm)	Production Method
^{11}Carbon	20.4	0.96	4.1	Cyclotron
^{13}Nitrogen	9.96	1.19	5.4	Cyclotron
^{15}Oxygen	2.03	1.73	7.3	Cyclotron
^{18}Flourine	109.7	0.64	2.4	Cyclotron
^{68}Gallium	68	1.9	8.1	Generator (^{68}Germanium)
^{82}Rubidium	1.3	3.15	15	Generator (^{82}Strontium)
^{124}Iodine	4.18 d	2.1	10	Cyclotron

As nuclear medicine studies use ionizing radiation, the amount of radiopharmaceutical prescribed for a study should be the lowest dose able to create diagnostic images for the expected patient population of a department, termed the "as low as reasonably achievable" principle (ALARA). However, the radiation dose to the patient for many nuclear medicine studies is at the higher end of diagnostic imaging (Table 2.3). When ordering any study, the risks and benefits should be weighed. In the United States, the dose of a radiopharmaceutical is prescribed in millicuries (mCi) or microcuries (μCi). The curie is based on the number of disintegrations of 1 g of radium and is set at 3.7×10^{10} disintegrations per second. Internationally, the becquerel (Bq), defined as 1 disintegration per second, is used, and diagnostic radiopharmaceuticals doses are typically in the megabecquerel (MBq) range. One millicurie

Table 2.3 Typical Effective Radiation Dose From Common Radiological and Nuclear Medicine Studies

Exam	Effective Dose mSv (mrem)
Chest	0.1 (10)
Cervical spine	0.2 (20)
Thoracic spine	1.0 (100)
Lumbar spine	1.5 (150)
Pelvis	0.7 (70)
Mammogram (2 views)	0.36 (36)
Skull	0.1 (10)
Hand or foot	0.005 (0.5)
Barium enema	7.0 (700)
Abdomen (KUB)	0.7 (70)
CT head	2.0 (200)
CT chest	7.0 (700)
CT abdomen/pelvis	10.0 (1,000)
Brain (perfusion) ^{99m}Tc HMPAO	6.9 (690)
Bone ^{99m}Tc MDP	6.3 (630)
Kidney ^{99m}Tc DTPA	1.8 (180)
Kidney ^{99m}Tc MAG3	2.2 (220)
Tumor/Infection ^{67}Ga	2.5 (250)
Heart (stress-rest) ^{99m}Tc sestamibi	9.4 (940)
Heart (stress-rest) ^{201}Tl chloride	41.0 (4,100)
Heart (stress-rest) ^{99m}Tc tetrofosmin	11.0 (1,100)
Various PET Studies ^{18}FDG	14.0 (1,400)

equals 37 million Bq or 37 MBq. Prescribing of radiopharmaceuticals is restricted to physicians who have undergone specialized training and fulfilled the requirements for an authorized user (AU) set out by the Nuclear Regulatory Commission (NRC) and the states. As you read about many types of nuclear medicine studies on the following pages, note the significant role nuclear medicine studies play in patient care when used for an appropriate indication.

ENDOCRINE

THYROID

As the thyroid actively transports iodine in to make the hormones T3 and T4, several isotopes of iodine (radioiodine) have been employed to diagnose and treat benign and malignant thyroid diseases. When nuclear reactor by-product iodine-131 (I-131) became available after World War II, the radioisotope was quickly brought into clinical use and helped spur the development of nuclear medicine.

Hyperthyroid Conditions

Hyperthyroidism is a common disease in the United States with an incidence up to 1.3%, though the majority of cases are subclinical. Etiologies include Graves' disease, toxic multinodular goiter, and toxic nodule. Graves' disease has an autoimmune origin with a peak occurrence during the third to fifth decades of life and a female predominance. Toxic multinodular goiter predominantly occurs in elderly people, and the thyrotoxic state can notably worsen comorbidities. Toxic nodules are typically solitary, account for 2% to 5% of hyperthyroid patients, and arise from a mutation in the thyroid stimulating hormone (TSH) receptor signaling pathway resulting in cells that are constantly turned on and functioning independently of the normal pituitary-thyroid control mechanism. Toxic nodules need to reach approximately 3 cm in diameter before they become clinically apparent.

As iodine is an integral component of thyroid hormones, radioiodines are ideal radiopharmaceuticals as they are actively transported, trapped, and organified in the same manner as nonradioactive iodine, providing clinically relevant thyroid function data. While I-131 was initially used for imaging, the damaging beta particle emission in addition to the high-energy gamma limits the amount that can be safely used resulting in suboptimal images. Today, iodine-123 (I-123) is used for hyperthyroid imaging as there are no particulate emissions and the primary gamma emission of 159 keV is in an appropriate range for gamma cameras. Technetium-99m (Tc-99m) pertechnetate can also be used to image the thyroid as pertechnetate is trapped in the thyroid, but organification does not occur, leading to rapid washout. Due to a lower radiation dose to the thyroid, Tc-99m pertechnetate is preferentially used in children.

Hyperthyroid imaging consists of two parts—thyroid uptake and thyroid scintigraphy. The goal of thyroid uptake is to determine the percent of the radiopharmaceutical administered that was trapped in the thyroid. This uptake can be compared to normalized values for the local populations (iodine 10%-30% at 24 hours, Tc-99 pertechnetate 0.3%-4.5%). Also, the uptake can be used to calculate the dose for I-131 therapy of hyperthyroid patients, better tailoring the dose to their condition. I-123 uptake uses a separate device called an uptake probe consisting of a single-hole collimator coupled to a Na-I crystal to take readings of the neck as well as the thigh to allow background counts to be factored in (Fig. 2.7). Tc-99m pertechnetate uptake employs a camera-based technique that is less accurate.

Thyroid scintigraphy is performed on a gamma camera with a pinhole collimator (large cone-shaped collimator with a single hole used to magnify structures) for I-123 and a parallel hole collimator for T-99m pertechnetate. Unlike the anatomic detail that thyroid ultrasound provides, thyroid scintigraphy details the function of the entire thyroid. In a normal thyroid, the tracer activity will be fairly

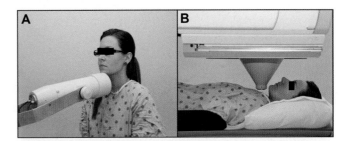

Fig. 2.7 (A) A thyroid uptake probe used to calculate the radiotracer activity concentrating in the thyroid gland in relation to the administered dose. (B) A pinhole collimator assembled in a gamma camera for thyroid imaging.

homogeneous throughout the gland. In Graves' disease, the tracer activity is also homogeneous, though more intense reflecting the greater uptake, but the contour of the thyroid becomes convex reflecting the goitrous anatomy. Multinodular goiter, both toxic and nontoxic, has rounded areas with lower uptake than a normal thyroid (photopenic areas) that corresponded to hypofunctioning thyroid nodules, rounded areas with normal uptake (or supranormal in the case of toxic multinodular), and areas of homogeneous uptake that correspond to thyroid tissue without nodules. In the case of a toxic nodule, the nodule has significant uptake while the remainder of the thyroid uptake is low to absent reflecting the suppression of the normal thyroid tissue in response to low TSH levels (Fig. 2.8).

In patients with thyroiditis, thyroid hormone levels may be elevated and the TSH suppressed, however the tracer activity in the gland will be minimal to absent. Thyroid uptake will be very low, reflecting the reduced function of the inflamed thyroid gland (Fig. 2.9). A large dose of exogenous iodine demonstrates thyroid uptake and scan findings indistinguishable from thyroiditis. Therefore, a thorough history detailing diet, medication use, and recent imaging studies should be obtained from the patient. If intravenous CT contrast has recently been administered, an iodine washout period of at least 6 weeks should be observed before thyroid scintigraphy. In rare cases, hyperthyroid patients may have suppressed cervical thyroid tissue due to hyper-functioning thyroid tissue in an ovarian teratoma (struma ovarii). Imaging over the pelvis including SPECT-CT may aid in the diagnosis.

Thyroid Nodule

Thyroid nodules are found with a greater frequency today as they are incidentally picked up on conventional imaging studies. Whether detected by physical exam or incidentally, thyroid nodules larger than 1 cm should be evaluated by ultrasound and/or biopsy unless the TSH is suppressed. In the case of TSH suppression, thyroid uptake and scan is the most cost-effective strategy to determine whether the thyroid nodule is the etiology for the thyrotoxicosis. A

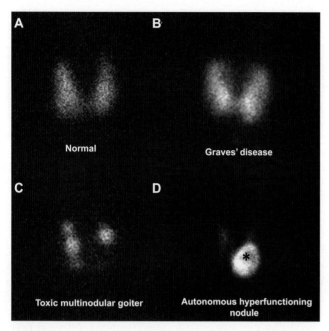

Fig. 2.8 Common imaging patterns seen in thyroid scintigraphy. (A) Anterior pinhole image of the thyroid gland in a patient with normal thyroid profile demonstrating physiologic radiotracer activity. The 24-hour radioiodine uptake was calculated to be approximately 15% (normal range is 10%-30%). (B) Anterior pinhole image in a patient with Graves' disease demonstrating diffuse increased radiotracer activity in the thyroid gland and elevated 24-hour radioiodine uptake of 77%. (C) Anterior pinhole image in a patient with thyrotoxicosis and an enlarged thyroid gland demonstrating areas of decreased radiotracer uptake interspersed between areas of normal and increased radiotracer activity, consistent with a toxic multinodular goiter. The 24-hour radioiodine uptake was calculated to be approximately 25%. (D) Anterior pinhole image shows increased radiotracer activity in the inferior portion of the left thyroid lobe, which corresponded to a palpable nodule on physical examination, compatible with an autonomous hyperfunctioning thyroid nodule (asterisk). The remaining portions of the thyroid gland are suppressed and have relatively decreased radiotracer uptake.

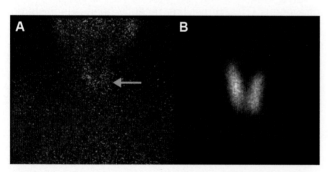

Fig. 2.9 A 41-year-old female who presented with thyrotoxicosis 2 weeks after a viral illness. (A) Anterior planar image of the neck and chest demonstrates diffuse decreased radiotracer activity in the thyroid gland, compatible with subacute thyroiditis (arrow). The 24-hour radioiodine uptake in the neck was approximately 0.3% (normal range is 10%-30%). (B) Anterior pinhole image of the thyroid gland obtained 2 months after image A demonstrates normal radiotracer activity in the thyroid gland, consistent with interval improvement.

photopenic nodule on thyroid scintigraphy has a 5% to 10% chance of being malignant and should be referred for ultrasound and fine needle aspiration (FNA) biopsy. Thyroid scintigraphy can also play a role after biopsy of a concerning nodule returns indeterminate results; the next step would be hemithyroidectomy. If the nodule has activity similar to or greater than the normal thyroid, the nodule has such a low likelihood of being thyroid cancer that it can safely be monitored with ultrasound, sparing the patient from undergoing unnecessary surgery.

Radioiodine Therapy of Hyperthyroidism

For Graves' disease, antithyroid medications such as methimazole and propylthiouracil (PTU) are initially given, often in conjunction with beta-blockers for symptomatic relief. However, the antithyroid medications have significant side effects that limit their long-term use. Thyroidectomy as treatment for Graves' disease is uncommon in the United States but more widely used in iodine-deficient areas where concomitant nodules are frequently found.

Since the 1950s, I-131 has been used to effectively treat Graves' disease, frequently with a single treatment. As the thyroid avidly accumulates most of the I-131 administered, the thyroid receives a very high dose of radiation while the remaining dose delivers a much lower dose to the rest of the body, and the unorganified I-131 washes quickly out of the body. The beta particle of I-131 has a short range, sparing surrounding tissue from high radiation doses. In the past, attempts were made to make the patient euthyroid, but the result was fluctuation between hypothyroid, euthyroid, and hyperthyroid states and multiple I-131 treatments. As the natural history of Graves' disease ends in hypothyroidism as the gland burns out, currently I-131 doses are targeted for the rapid onset of hypothyroidism by 6 months after therapy. To plan patient-specific doses, the percent uptake from the thyroid uptake and scan and the estimated gland size from palpation are needed. After therapy, patients follow radiation safety precautions discussed in the section Thyroid Cancer for several days to reduce the dose to members of the public. The endocrinologist will monitor the TSH for hypothyroidism, typically 3 to 6 months after therapy, and then place the patient on lifelong thyroid hormone replacement therapy.

Toxic multinodular goiter and toxic adenomas are more resistant to I-131 therapy, and empiric doses from 25 to 30 mCi are frequently used. The side effects of I-131 therapy are minimal. Nausea may occur initially prior to the digestion of the pill but resolves within several hours. Pain and swelling of the thyroid are uncommon. While there has been a concern about second cancers induced by the radiation, large studies have only demonstrated a small rise in leukemia in patients treated for Graves' disease.

Thyroid Cancer

The incidence of well-differentiated thyroid cancer in the United States has roughly doubled since 1990, due in part to the increased utilization of conventional imaging leading to detection of asymptomatic nodules. Most thyroid cancers occur in the young with only one-third of cases occurring after age 55. Well-differentiated thyroid carcinomas such as papillary and follicular carcinomas retain the ability to concentrate iodine, though at a lower rate than normal thyroid tissue. Anaplastic thyroid cancer is too dedifferentiated to concentrate iodine, and medullary thyroid carcinoma arises from parafollicular cells that do not concentrate iodine.

Surgical removal of the thyroid and local lymph nodes is the initial step in treatment. If the thyroid cancer is 1 cm or less in size with no lymph node metastases, further therapy with I-131 has not demonstrated a survival advantage or reduction in relapse rate. Larger thyroid cancers and those with metastases can benefit from I-131 therapy.

Approximately 6 weeks after thyroidectomy, while the patient is on a low iodine diet, a whole-body study with I-131 or I-123 surveys the body for metastases and allows uptake measurements of the neck to be obtained to ensure that significant amounts of thyroid tissue that could interfere with I-131 therapy do not remain (Fig. 2.10). The dose of I-131 prescribed by an authorized user is based on the

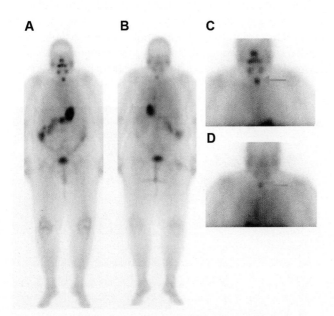

Fig. 2.10 A 69-year-old female with differentiated thyroid carcinoma status post total thyroidectomy. (A) Anterior and (B) posterior whole-body planar images and (C) anterior and (D) posterior spot images of the neck and thorax, obtained 72 hours after the oral administration of 5 mCi of sodium I-131, demonstrate a focus of increased radiotracer activity in the left thyroid bed (arrows), compatible with residual thyroid tissue. Physiologic activity is seen in the nasal region, salivary glands, stomach, bowel, and urinary bladder. The radioiodine uptake in the thyroid bed was 0.8% and the patient was subsequently administered 100 mCi of I-131 orally for thyroid remnant ablation.

pathologic features of the tumor including size and extracapsular spread, lymph node metastases, and extranodal metastases (lung, bone). For less complex cases, an empiric set of doses ranging from 75 to 200 mCi is frequently used. For more complex cases, the whole-body scan can be used to determine a higher dose of I-131 that does not give excessive radiation to the bone marrow.

Patients undergoing I-131 therapy need to follow radiation safety precautions to reduce the dose to themselves and others for 1 to 2 weeks. Most patients can safely be released after therapy, but some patients need to be admitted for several days to a lead-lined room in the hospital as their home situation does not allow for release. As I-131 is excreted in the fluids of the body, particularly the urine, patients are instructed to drink enough fluids to void every couple of hours, thereby reducing the dose to the bladder and clearing the circulating iodine from the body. For the duration of the precautions, patients should use a bathroom and shower separate from the rest of the household. Patients should maintain their distance from other people, especially children, who are more radiosensitive. As the dose of radiation falls off with the square of the distance, relatively small changes in distance result in large reductions in radiation doses. Women who are pregnant cannot be treated with I-131 due to the radiation exposure to the fetus and the possible damage to the fetal thyroid. It is not recommended that the patient become pregnant for at least 6 months after treatment.

Seven days after therapy, the patient returns for whole-body imaging using the I-131 remaining in the body after therapy to survey for metastases (Fig. 2.11). After the I-131 dose has destroyed the remaining normal thyroid tissue and hopefully treated any metastatic disease, the blood level of thyroglobulin, a protein made by thyroid tissue, is followed as it is a sensitive marker for thyroid cancer recurrence. If the thyroglobulin rises, ultrasound of the neck can be used to detect cervical lymph node metastases. Whole body scans with radioiodine can also be used to assess for metastases. Patients can receive multiple doses of I-131

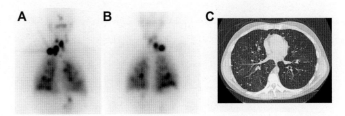

Fig. 2.11 (A) Anterior and (B) posterior planar images obtained 7 days after the oral administration of 200 mCi of sodium I-131 to a patient with metastatic papillary thyroid carcinoma. There are multiple foci of increased radiotracer uptake in the neck, mediastinum, and lungs bilaterally, compatible with radioiodine avid metastases. (C) Axial CT image demonstrating multiple pulmonary nodules bilaterally, consistent with lung metastases.

for treatment of thyroid cancer, though if above a lifetime dose of 600 mCi, the incidence of leukemia increases. The thyroid cancer can dedifferentiate over time, losing the ability to concentrate iodine and becoming refractory to I-131 therapy. When the cancer becomes iodine negative on the whole body scan, F-18 fluorodeoxyglucose (FDG) PET-CT is useful in assessing the extent of disease and the presence of FDG-avid thyroid cancer is an independent risk factor for poor prognosis.

PARATHYROID SCINTIGRAPHY

Hyperparathyroidism is generally discovered on routine lab work in asymptomatic patients as opposed to the late symptomatic presentations in the past. Primary hyperparathyroidism accounts for 80% of the cases, and 85% of patients with primary hyperparathyroidism have adenomas as the etiology. Parathyroid scintigraphy is directed at detecting adenomas as normal and hyperplastic glands are too small to reliably imaged. Secondary and tertiary hyperparathyroidism arise in the setting of severe renal dysfunction that leads to parathyroid hyperplasia and eventually autonomous function. Surgery is the treatment of choice.

Several radiopharmaceuticals have been used over the years to image parathyroid adenomas. Currently, a protocol using Tc-99m sestamibi imaged at 10 minutes and 2 hours is employed. On early images, both the thyroid and parathyroid tissue demonstrate uptake, but the thyroid activity washes out by 2 hours. Planar images must include the area from the parotid glands to the top of the heart as ectopic parathyroid adenomas found within this range are the cause of the hyperparathyroidism in less than 5% of cases. The sensitivity for adenomas 300 mg or more in size (roughly 10 times the weight of a normal gland) is greater than 85%. SPECT-CT is frequently performed to increase sensitivity and to aid in surgical planning (Fig. 2.12).

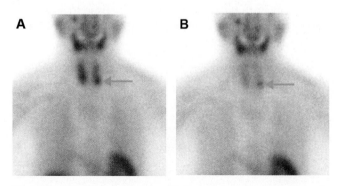

Fig. 2.12 A 79-year-old female with hypercalcemia and increased serum parathyroid hormone (PTH). (A) Immediate anterior planar image demonstrates a focus of increased radiotracer activity near the inferior pole of the left thyroid lobe, which persists on the delayed planar image (B). This finding is suggestive of a parathyroid adenoma (arrow). Please note the relative washout of radiotracer from the normal thyroid gland on the delayed image.

NEUROENDOCRINE TUMOR SCINTIGRAPHY AND TREATMENT

Neuroendocrine tumors arise from tissues originating embryologically from neural crest cells and include pheochromocytomas, paragangliomas, gastric endocrine tumors (eg, carcinoid), and medullary thyroid carcinoma. Small cell lung cancer also falls in this category but is primarily imaged by FDG PET-CT. Both benign and malignant neuroendocrine tumors can be imaged with nuclear medicine studies.

Many neuroendocrine tumors overexpress somatostatin receptors. Somatostatin is a hormone with inhibitory effects on multiple pathways. The radiopharmaceutical indium-111 (In-111) pentetreotide binds to somatostatin receptors 2, 3, and 5, allowing a wide variety of neuroendocrine tumors to be imaged with a high sensitivity. However, some tumors such as insulinomas and medullary thyroid carcinoma are not imaged well with pentreotide. As there is significant physiologic renal, hepatic, and splenic radiotracer uptake, SPECT-CT is routinely performed after whole-body imaging to better evaluate the upper abdomen or lesions of interest seen in planar images (Fig. 2.13). For carcinoid tumors, if the pentreotide study is positive, this is good evidence that the patient will respond to Sandostatin therapy.

Neuroendocrine tumors arising from the adrenergic tissues such as pheochromocytomas and paragangliomas are preferentially imaged with meta-iodobenzylguanidine (MIBG), which concentrates in presynaptic adrenergic nerves. MIBG is also used in the evaluation of neuroblastoma,

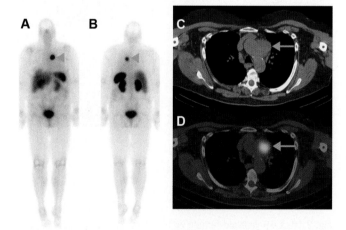

Fig. 2.13 A 54-year-old female with metastatic well-differentiated neuroendocrine carcinoma (carcinoid tumor), referred for restaging. (A) Anterior and (B) posterior whole-body planar images obtained 4 hours after the intravenous administration of 6 mCi of In 111 pentetreotide demonstrating an area of increased radiotracer activity in the mediastinum, compatible with biopsy-proven nodal metastasis (arrowheads). (C) CT and (D) fused SPECT-CT images of the chest demonstrate increased radiotracer activity localizing to a nodal mass in the prevascular region (arrows).

MYOCARDIAL PERFUSION IMAGING

Fundamentally, myocardial perfusion imaging (MPI) detects differences in blood flow to the left ventricle and myocardial extraction of tracers when radiopharmaceuticals are injected during rest and stress conditions caused by a significant coronary artery stenosis. Both SPECT and PET studies are performed. While PET has a higher sensitivity and specificity at 90% and 88% versus 85% and 85% for Tc-99m SPECT, the application of PET is generally limited by cost to patients who are obese and those with an inconclusive MPI SPECT study [1]. Exercise treadmill tests alone have a sensitivity of 75% with many false positives, particularly in women (specificity around 60%) and patients with certain baseline electrocardiography (ECG) abnormalities.

MPI SPECT can be performed with two radiopharmaceuticals, thallium-201 chloride (Tl-201) and Tc-99m agents, in a wide variety of protocols beyond the scope of this text. Tl-201 is a physiologic potassium analogue that is actively transported into myocardial cells with a very high first-pass extraction. Tl-201 is not bound in the cell and redistributes over time into all viable myocardium independent of the blood flow conditions under which it was injected. Due to a long physical half-life of 3 days coupled with a 10-day half-life in the body, the amount of Tl-201 used for imaging is low (up to 4 mCi). Also, the primary imaging photons are x-rays in the range of 69 to 83 keV, which is lower than the optimal range for gamma camera leading to the worst image quality of MPI radiotracers.

The Tc-99m agents, sestamibi and tetrofosmin, have a lower first-pass extraction than Tl-201 but do not redistribute as they are trapped within mitochondria. Tc-99m has a 6-hour half-life allowing for higher dose usage than Tl-201 and is in the optimal range for gamma cameras leading to better image quality than Tl-201 and making ECG-gated images more feasible.

Prior to acquisition of resting images for a baseline, a directed history should be obtained from the patient to ascertain if the stress test would be compromised. Patients need to fast 6 hours prior to the study, refrain from caffeine for 24 hours, and stop beta-blockers, calcium channel blockers, long-acting nitrates, and other drugs based on stress lab instructions. The stress portion of the study may be performed using an exercise treadmill test or pharmacologically. While exercise treadmill provides additional information on functional capacity and ECG changes during exercise, the images obtained do not have a notable sensitivity advantage over pharmacologic stress images. As exercise increases the oxygen demand on the heart, ischemia may be induced and the ECG must be monitored closely. Normal coronary arteries can significantly dilate in response to exercise, while areas with significant stenosis cannot, leading to ischemia and ECG changes. Tl-201 or the Tc-99m agents are injected when the patient reaches

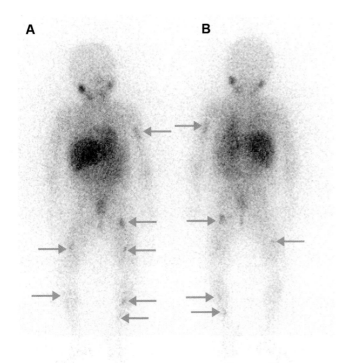

Fig. 2.14 A 3-year-old female with metastatic neuroblastoma. (A) Anterior and (B) posterior I-123 MIBG delayed planar images demonstrate multiple sites of osseous metastases involving the left humerus, femora, and tibiae (arrows).

a malignant neoplasm occurring primarily in children less than 4 years old (Fig. 2.14). The sensitivity for adrenergic tumors is greater than 90% with a similarly high specificity. Many drugs interfere with the uptake of MIBG, so a thorough history must be obtained from the patient prior to imaging.

High-dose I-131 MIBG has been used as a palliative treatment for metastatic neuroendocrine cancers. Due to the high doses used, all patients are admitted to an appropriately shielded hospital room until the level of radiation being emitted from the patient is safe for the public. In addition, MIBG has been used to image the adrenergic innervation of the heart both in congestive heart failure and after heart transplant.

CARDIOVASCULAR SCINTIGRAPHY

Roughly half of the 16 million nuclear medicine procedures performed each year in the United States are cardiac imaging studies. Nuclear medicine studies have the advantage of being noninvasive measurements of several cardiac functions that still provide valuable information in addition to echocardiography, cardiac MRI, and even cardiac catheterization.

85% of the maximum predicted heart rate (MPHR), and the patient exercises for another minute. SPECT imaging is performed within 15 minutes after the exercise stress test. A dobutamine infusion may also be used to pharmacologically stress patients through chronotropic and inotropic effects that increase cardiac oxygen demand and cause ischemia. As with exercise, the radiopharmaceutical is injected once the patient has reached 85% of the MPHR. Many patients cannot tolerate the infusion level of dobutamine need to reach the target heart rate due to side effects. Atropine and low-level exercise such as leg lifts can be used to increase the heart rate when the maximal dobutamine infusion rate does not achieve an adequate heart rate.

The other pharmacologic agents (adenosine, dipyridamole, regadenoson) work by directly dilating the coronary artery and increasing coronary blood flow 3 to 4 times higher than at rest without significantly increasing cardiac demand. Again, arteries with significant stenosis cannot significantly respond to the vasodilatory effects of these drugs, but ischemia is rarely seen unless a steal phenomenon occurs. Thus pharmacologic stress with these agents is an assessment of coronary flow reserve as opposed to true ischemia for exercise stress. Each agent has a set protocol of when to inject the radiopharmaceutical based on infusion time and not heart rate. Up to 50% of patients will have side effects due to vasodilation and, for the nonselective agents adenosine and dipyridamole, bronchoconstriction. The less than 10 second half-life of adenosine leads to side effects resolving quickly after infusion, but side effects of the other two agents may need to be countered by administration of aminophylline. SPECT imaging typically begins 45 minutes after pharmacologic stress to reduce the effect of tracer uptake in the liver. Unlike the pharmacologic agents, exercise decreases the splanchnic circulation in favor of increased peripheral circulation and thus reduces the amount of radiotracer delivered to the liver and allows for earlier imaging.

ECG gating during imaging can be used to create a map of left ventricular wall motion and calculate a left ventricular ejection fraction (LVEF). The ejection fraction is not as robust as those obtained by echocardiography or radionuclide ventriculography. The wall motion and LVEF data play a supporting role in the interpretation of the SPECT images.

The distribution of tracer activity in the rest and stress images is visually assessed. If there are decreased areas of tracer activity on stress images not present on rest, the MPI is positive for a significant flow-limiting lesion in the coronary artery feeding the territory of the observed defect (Figs. 2.15 and 2.16). MPI has a high sensitivity in detecting the most severe lesion but a lower sensitivity for other less severe lesions as the data are scaled to internal counts and do not represent absolute coronary blood flow. Since the MPI has already risk stratified the patient based

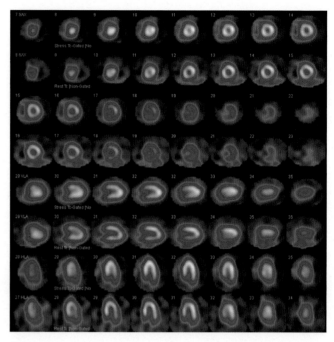

Fig. 2.15 Rest and stress myocardial perfusion study demonstrating normal perfusion throughout the left ventricular myocardium. The stress images are displayed on the top rows and the corresponding rest images are seen on the bottom rows. From top to bottom, the left ventricle is sliced in the short axis (SAX), vertical long axis (VLA), and horizontal long axis (HLA).

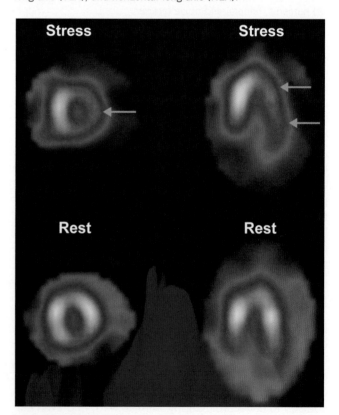

Fig. 2.16 Stress (top row) and rest (bottom row) Tc-99m tetrofosmin myocardial perfusion SPECT images demonstrate a reversible myocardial perfusion defect (arrows on stress images) in the lateral wall, compatible with myocardial ischemia.

on presence of one ischemic area, the lower sensitivity for other lesions is acceptable. In the case of balanced severe reduction in left ventricular coronary flow due to triple vessel disease, stress images may have a visually normal distribution of tracer activity. However, in balanced triple vessel disease, the size of the ventricular cavity may appear larger on stress than rest. While this is termed transient ischemic dilatation (TID), the left ventricle is rarely truly dilated at the time of imaging, but the apparent change is most likely due to inadequate tracer distribution to the subendocardial tissue. When the TID is elevated above a protocol-based threshold, triple vessel disease should be considered.

When perfusion defects are present on both rest and stress images, the defect may represent scar tissue from a prior infarct, hibernating myocardium, or artifact. Artifacts may be caused by attenuation from the patient's body (eg, diaphragm in men, breast in women) and by extracardiac tracer activity in the liver or bowel. The region and appearance of a defect can point to attenuation as the culprit. Diaphragmatic attenuation affects the inferior wall and will demonstrate normal wall motion. If there is a clinical concern, prone imaging can be used to better image the inferior wall. Attenuation correction using additional images from a transmission source such as CT is also used to mitigate tissue attenuation. Wall motion abnormalities support the diagnosis of myocardial infarction. If hibernating myocardium is a clinical concern, viability imaging may be indicated.

PET-CT MPI follows the same basic rest and stress protocol and interpretation of SPECT MPI, with the caveat that all PET studies are performed with attenuation correction to allow for proper reconstruction. Two radiopharmaceuticals are used for PET: N-13 ammonia and rubidium-82. The higher energy of the positron emissions, high target-to-background ratio, and attenuation correction lead to a higher spatial resolution than SPECT and elimination of tissue-based attenuation defects. N-13 ammonia has a short half-life essentially requiring an on-site cyclotron for production. Rubidium-82 (Rb-82) is obtained from a strontium-82 generator placed next to the PET-CT machine. Due to the short half-lives of both tracers, clinical stress studies are almost exclusively pharmacologic. In the near future, PET MPI also may be clinically validated for quantitation of regional coronary blood flow reserve, improving detection of multivessel disease.

VIABILITY IMAGING

Chronically ischemic cardiac tissue reduces its cellular metabolic rate as a survival mechanism and is termed hibernating myocardium. When revascularized, this tissue may return to normal function or show significant functional improvement that scarred tissue cannot. On MPI, this tissue has low uptake of radiotracer on stress and rest,

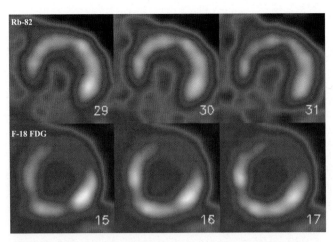

Fig. 2.17 Short axis myocardial perfusion images obtained with Rb-82 PET (top row) demonstrate a large perfusion defect in the inferoseptal wall. Corresponding short axis F-18 FDG PET images (bottom row) demonstrate radiotracer uptake in the inferoseptal wall, compatible with viable myocardium.

making it difficult to distinguish from prior infarct. Two radiopharmaceuticals are used: thallium-201 for SPECT imaging and F-18 fluorodeoxyglucose (FDG) for PET-CT.

Thallium is a potassium analogue that redistributes over time, including into chronically ischemic areas. After injection, images are obtained at 15 minutes and then at 4 or 24 hours. On initial images, the area of questionable viability will have minimal to no tracer accumulation. On delayed images, if the questioned area has increased the tracer accumulation to at least 50% of the known viable walls, this is consistent with viable myocardium and revascularization may be warranted.

FDG is a glucose analogue used by hibernating myocardium, which relies on glycolysis to make ATP in comparison to normal heart musculature, which preferentially uses fatty acids as an energy source. Unlike thallium, tracer uptake in the heart is dependent on the glucose metabolic state of the body. To achieve a euglycemic state, particularly in diabetic and prediabetic patients, glucose loading balanced by insulin administration is used prior to FDG injection. FDG preferentially accumulates in hibernating myocardium, while normal tissue may have no significant tracer uptake. In comparison to rest PET imaging with N-13 ammonia or Rb-82, which demonstrate no significant uptake in hibernating myocardium, FDG accumulation mismatched from the rest images confirms viable tissue (Fig. 2.17).

MUGA

While 2-D echocardiography is the mainstay of left ventricular ejection fraction (LVEF) evaluation, the test is operator and reader dependent, leading to variation in the estimated ejection fraction. In patients undergoing treatment with cardiotoxic chemotherapy requiring serial evaluation of left ventricular ejection fraction, such variability on 2-D echo is undesirable. Radionuclide ventriculography (MUGA, multigated acquisition) solves the variability problem by summing the data from multiple cardiac cycles and not necessitating mathematical models of ventricular shape. 3-D echocardiography and cardiac MRI have similarly low levels of variability to MUGA. When adequate echo windows cannot be obtained, for example in patients who are obese, MUGA can almost always be performed. Right ventricular function can also be assessed using a first-pass technique. Regional wall motion analysis of MUGA is an emerging technique to evaluate wall dyssynchrony prior to cardiac resynchronization and implantable defibrillator placement.

In vivo, modified in vivo, and in vitro methods can be used to tag the red blood cells (RBCs) of the patient, with the in vitro method having the highest binding efficiency at 98%. Using electrocardiographic gating, the radiolabeled RBCs in the left ventricular blood pool are imaged for 300 to 500 cardiac cycles. The cardiac cycle is broken into 8 or 16 parts, and count data from the time period of each cycle are assigned to a bin. The data from the bins are used to create a single summed cardiac cycle. Semiautomated computer analytic software draws regions of interest around the left ventricle at systole and diastole and over a background region of interest to correct for extracardiac blood pool activity (Fig. 2.18). The computer software analysis

has been shown to be highly reproducible in both normal patients and those with cardiac disease.

Ejection fractions greater than 50% are typically considered normal. For patients undergoing cardiotoxic chemotherapy, both the LVEF and the change in LVEF over time are taken into account. Therapy is usually stopped when the LVEF reaches 40% or there has been a drop in LVEF of greater than 20%. Cardiac function can recover after therapy cessation, but the damage may be irreversible.

HEPATOBILIARY AND GASTROINTESTINAL IMAGING

HEPATIC AND SPLENIC IMAGING

Despite the introduction of modern imaging methods such as computed tomography, ultrasound, and magnetic resonance imaging, there are still few specific indications for radionuclide liver and spleen imaging. Following intravenous administration, Tc-99m sulfur colloid is sequestered in the reticuloendothelial (RE) system, and therefore the liver, spleen, and bone marrow can be imaged. Tc-99m sulfur colloid imaging has a role in the evaluation of focal nodular hyperplasia and in the management of patients with portal hypertension to establish the presence of a colloid shift and to differentiate between portal hypertension due to cirrhosis of the liver and noncirrhotic portal fibrosis [2]. Tc-99m sulfur colloid particles are variable in size, ranging from 0.3 to 1.0 μm, depending on the preparation technique. After the intravenous administration, Tc-99m sulfur colloid is rapidly cleared from the blood by the RE system with a half-life of approximately 2½ minutes. The uptake and distribution of Tc-99m sulfur colloid by the organs of the RE system is dependent upon their relative blood flow and the functional capacity of the phagocytic cells. The size of the particles determines the biodistribution of the colloid and the location of radiotracer uptake by the RE system. For example, larger particles are preferentially sequestered by the spleen. Medium-sized particles are phagocytized by the Kupffer cells of the liver, and the smallest particles are taken up by the bone marrow. Under normal circumstances, 80% to 90% of the injected particles are taken up by the liver, 5% to 10% are sequestered by the spleen, and the remainder localize in the bone marrow and other RE sites.

In normal patients, there is homogenous radiotracer activity throughout the liver. The normal spleen exhibits homogeneous radiotracer uptake equal to or less than that of the liver. In the liver, the gallbladder fossa, the region of the falciform ligament, and the porta hepatis can usually be identified on planar images. In cases where there is colloid shift secondary to portal hypertension, the splenic uptake exceeds that of the liver.

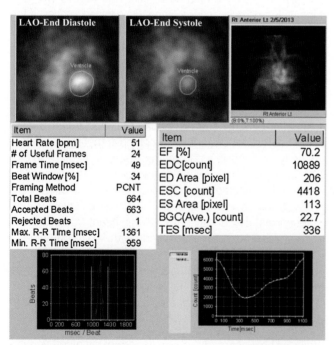

Fig. 2.18 MUGA scan in a 43-year-old male with lymphoma, referred for initial evaluation of left ventricular function prior to chemotherapy. Planar images of the heart are obtained in the anterior and left anterior oblique views for analysis of left ventricular wall motion. Regions of interest are then placed around the left ventricle in end-systole and end-diastole for calculation of the left ventricular ejection fraction. The computer software also displays several values related to gated imaging acquisition.

Focal nodular hyperplasia (FNH) of the liver is a benign tumor seen predominantly in women and thought to represent a hyperplastic (regenerative) response to hyperperfusion by anomalous arteries found in the center of these nodules. On histology, these lesions contain abnormal vessels, bile ductules, and Kupffer cells in an abnormal hyperplastic arrangement. There is normal radiotracer uptake in approximately one-third of the lesions, increased radiotracer uptake in one-third, and decreased activity in the remaining one-third. When the lesions demonstrate normal or increased radiotracer uptake on sulfur colloid images, FNH can be presumed in the correct clinical setting. In the event that there is decreased activity in comparison to the liver parenchyma, the study is inconclusive, and further evaluation with cross-sectional imaging is required.

Splenic imaging with Tc-99m sulfur colloid or Tc-99m labeled heat-denatured red blood cells is widely used to identify suspected residual functioning splenic tissue status post splenectomy in patients with idiopathic thrombocytopenic purpura and to differentiate splenules from other intra-abdominal masses [3]. Tc-99m labeled red blood cells are typically damaged by heating for 20 minutes in a water bath at 49°C to 50°C before they are reinjected in the patient. During imaging, residual splenic tissue can be easily identified by increased radiotracer activity.

GASTROINTESTINAL BLEEDING SCINTIGRAPHY

Acute lower gastrointestinal bleeding (LGIB) refers to blood loss of recent onset originating from a site distant to the ligament of Treitz [4]. Frequent causes of LGIB in adults include diverticulosis, ischemia, hemorrhoids, rectal ulcers, polyps, malignancy, angiodysplasia, inflammatory bowel disease, and other causes [5]. Gastrointestinal bleeding scintigraphy is performed in patients with suspected active LGIB using Tc-99m labeled autologous red blood cells (Tc-99m RBC). The objectives of Tc-99m RBC scans are to locate the bleeding site and to guide further intervention by angiography, when clinically applicable. In general, nuclear scintigraphy is more sensitive to detect active LGIB than conventional angiography. For instance, the minimal detectable bleeding rate of a Tc-99m RBC scan is approximately 0.1 mL/min. In comparison, conventional angiography is able to detect bleeding rates of approximately 1.0 mL/min. The in vitro method for labeling the patient's red blood cells is favored due to its higher labeling efficiency. After the radiotracer is injected intravenously, dynamic images of the abdomen are obtained in the anterior view for 60 to 90 minutes. In case a source of LGIB cannot be identified during this time, delayed images can be performed.

A positive Tc-99m RBC scan requires that the signal generated by the extravasated radiolabeled RBC within the bowel lumen increase in intensity over time and move anterograde or retrograde through the bowel (Fig. 2.19). Small bowel bleeding can be differentiated from colonic bleeding due to its rapid serpiginous movement. An area of activity that remains fixed in location over the duration of the study should raise suspicion of other causes.

HEPATOBILIARY IMAGING

Tc-99m labeled iminodiacetic acids (IDA) such as disofenin or mebrofenin are widely used in hepatobiliary imaging. By far, the major indication for hepatobiliary imaging is to evaluate for acute cholecystitis. IDA labeled radiotracers are removed from the circulation by active transport into the hepatocytes and then secreted into the bile canaliculi. After the intravenous administration of the radiopharmaceutical, dynamic images of the abdomen are obtained in the anterior view for 60 minutes. In normal patients, there is rapid blood clearance with maximum activity in the liver at 10 to 15 minutes, followed subsequently by activity in the intrahepatic and extrahepatic biliary tree and gallbladder (GB). Approximately two-thirds of the biliary excretion bypasses the gallbladder and enters the duodenum, progressing through the small bowel. Normally, all these structures should be seen at 60 minutes (Fig. 2.20). Persistent visualization of blood-pool activity after 5 to 10 minutes is a sign of significant hepatic dysfunction. Normal GB filling within the period of the study implies a patent cystic duct and virtually excludes acute cholecystitis due to obstruction of the cystic duct by a stone, edema, or inflammation. Delayed imaging up to 4 hours can be obtained to detect late filling of the GB in cases of chronic cholecystitis. Morphine sulfate augmentation, 0.04 mg/kg, injected intravenously over 2 to 3 minutes, may be used in lieu of delayed images. Morphine causes temporary spasm of the sphincter of Oddi, raising the intraductal pressure and facilitating the filling of the GB in patients with chronic cholecystitis. Dynamic imaging is usually performed for an additional 30 minutes after the intravenous administration of morphine. If the GB is visualized after delayed imaging or morphine augmentation, acute cholecystitis is considered unlikely (Fig. 2.21).

A gallbladder ejection fraction can be performed in patients with normal imaging studies and persistent right upper quadrant symptoms and suspected biliary dyskinesia. At the completion of a normal hepatobiliary scan, regions of interest are drawn around the GB before and after the slow intravenous administration of sincalide (synthetic cholecystokinin). Subsequently, a GB ejection fraction is calculated according to an algorithm. A patient with an abnormally low ejection fraction may benefit from surgical intervention.

In case of suspected biliary leak after trauma or surgery, delayed images may be necessary depending on the rate of the leak.

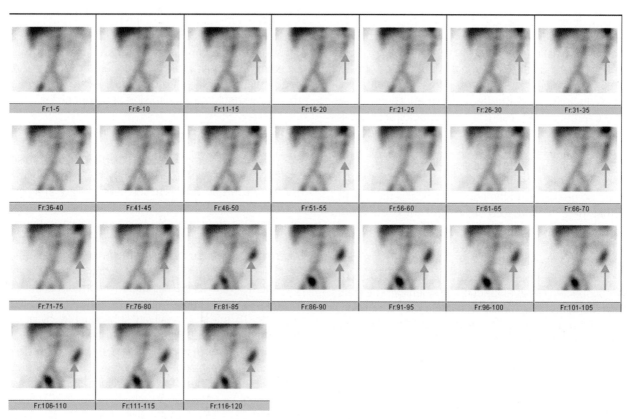

Fr:1-5	Fr:6-10	Fr:11-15	Fr:16-20	Fr:21-25	Fr:26-30	Fr:31-35
Fr:36-40	Fr:41-45	Fr:46-50	Fr:51-55	Fr:56-60	Fr:61-65	Fr:66-70
Fr:71-75	Fr:76-80	Fr:81-85	Fr:86-90	Fr:91-95	Fr:96-100	Fr:101-105
Fr:106-110	Fr:111-115	Fr:116-120				

Fig. 2.19 A 71-year-old male with mantle cell lymphoma presenting with bright red blood per rectum. Dynamic images of the abdomen and pelvis were obtained in the anterior view for 60 minutes after the intravenous administration of 25 mCi of Tc-99m labeled red blood cells. There is linear radiotracer activity in the descending colon, consistent with acute lower gastrointestinal bleeding (arrows).

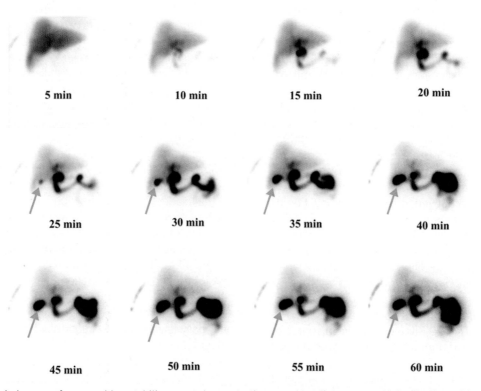

5 min	10 min	15 min	20 min
25 min	30 min	35 min	40 min
45 min	50 min	55 min	60 min

Fig. 2.20 Dynamic images of a normal hepatobiliary scan demonstrating prompt radiotracer uptake by the liver with subsequent excretion into the biliary tree. Activity in the gallbladder (arrows) and small bowel is noted at the expected time points.

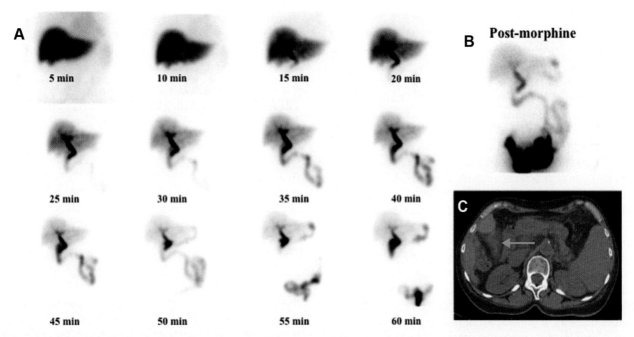

Fig. 2.21 (A) Dynamic images of a hepatobiliary scan obtained for 60 minutes in the anterior view fail to demonstrate radiotracer accumulation in the gallbladder. The patient was administered 4 mg of morphine sulfate intravenously and dynamic imaging was continued for an additional 30 minutes. (B) Postmorphine images at 30 minutes again fail to demonstrate radiotracer activity in the gallbladder. (C) Axial image of the CT component of a SPECT-CT image demonstrates prominent inflammatory changes in the gallbladder fossa (arrow), compatible with acute cholecystitis.

SKELETAL SYSTEM

Nuclear medicine studies are frequently used to evaluate the skeletal system for metastatic and primary bone tumors, trauma, infection, metabolic disorders, infarctions, and bone density as well as to assess the distribution of bone marrow. For patients with painful sclerotic bone metastases, other radiopharmaceuticals are used for pain palliation.

Bone scintigraphy uses a radiopharmaceutical that chemoadsorbs to hydroxyapatite crystals in the osseous matrix and thus localizes avidly to areas of bone turnover. These radiopharmaceuticals are similar in structure to the bisphosphonates used to treat osteoporosis. Bone scintigraphy is very sensitive for areas with increased bone turnover such as tumors, fractures, and acute infection but has a low specificity due to the similarity of their appearance on the study. Thus, clinical history, additional imaging such as SPECT or SPECT-CT, and even examination of the patient can be valuable tools in interpreting the images. More recently, PET-CT bone imaging with sodium fluoride (NaF) has been shown to have a greater sensitivity and specificity than bone scintigraphy, though the higher cost has led to relatively low utilization (Fig. 2.22).

BONE TUMORS

Whole-body bone scintigraphy obtained in the anterior and posterior planar projections has been used for many years as a sensitive and inexpensive survey for sclerotic metastases,

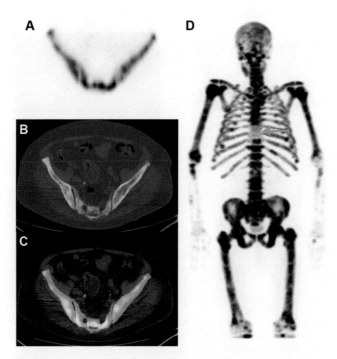

Fig. 2.22 (A) Axial PET, (B) CT, (C) fused PET-CT, and (D) MIP images of a 68-year-old male with metastatic prostate cancer demonstrating diffuse sodium fluoride uptake corresponding to sclerotic lesions throughout the axial and appendicular skeleton. An area of decreased radiotracer activity in the vertebral bodies of T8 and T9 is consistent with prior radiation therapy (arrow).

particularly from prostate and breast cancer. For these cancers, bone scans have roughly a 95% sensitivity, detecting as low as a 5% bone mineral loss as opposed to the 50% loss needed for plain radiographs to detect a lesion. Lytic metastases have a lower sensitivity, especially from multiple myeloma, due to the smaller amount of bone turnover. FDG PET-CT has a higher sensitivity for lytic lesions and lesions involving primarily the bone marrow, as detection relies on the tumor itself and not the bone turnover. Thus PET-CT can play an important role in the evaluation of multiple myeloma. When compared to bone scintigraphy, FDG PET-CT typically detects more lesions per patient, but the number of patients in whom metastatic disease is detected is similar [6].

Sclerotic metastatic lesions demonstrate increased tracer activity. Trauma such as a rib fracture or degenerative changes will also avidly take up radiotracer. Differentiation between benign and malignant processes can be made by the appearance, distribution, and additional imaging such as SPECT-CT. In patients with diffuse metastatic osseous disease, a superscan appearance may be seen, which consists of a relatively uniform increased uptake in the bones and faint to no activity in the kidneys. The superscan reflects the diffuse nature of the metastases (Fig. 2.23).

MRI is the modality of choice for malignant primary bone tumors. Bone scintigraphy has been used as an inexpensive screen for metastases. For benign bone tumors such

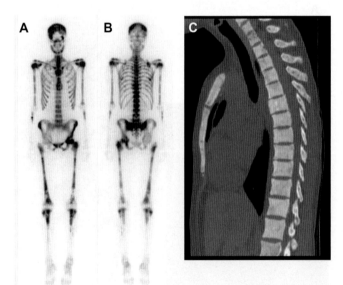

Fig. 2.23 A 23-year-old male with metastatic osteosarcoma. (A) Anterior and (B) posterior whole-body planar images of a bone scan demonstrating diffuse increased radiotracer uptake in the axial and appendicular skeleton, compatible with widespread bone metastases. The kidneys and the urinary bladder are not visualized, consistent with a superscan. (C) Sagittal CT image of the same patient demonstrates diffuse sclerosis of the spine and sternum, compatible with bone metastases.

as osteoid osteomas, bone scintigraphy has largely been supplanted by CT, though it still has a role in occult lesions or in further characterizing atypical bone islands as benign if there is no significant uptake.

TREATMENT OF PAIN RELATED TO OSSEOUS METASTASES

Pain from osseous metastases can be difficult to ameliorate with narcotic medicines, significantly affecting quality of life. Radiation therapy is very useful for treating a small number of metastatic lesions but cannot address widespread metastases. Thus, when widespread metastases are present on bone scintigraphy, radiopharmaceuticals that target areas of bone turnover, samarium-153 EDTMP and strontium-89, can decrease bone pain in up to 70% of patients leading to decreased narcotic use and improved quality of life. The treatment is solely palliative and, while the mechanism of action is not fully understood, the beta radiation most likely damages small nerves in the bone surrounding the tumor with resultant pain reduction for an average of 4 to 6 months. The primary side effect is mild marrow suppression, necessitating weekly blood counts for approximately 8 weeks. Severe neutropenia or thrombocytopenia is rare in properly screened patients. Patients can be treated multiple times as their pain recurs.

Recently, the alpha emitting radiotherapy agent radium-223 dichloride was approved for the treatment of patients with painful osseous metastases from castrate-resistant prostate cancer and without significant soft tissue metastases. As with strontium, radium resides in the same group as calcium on the periodic table and is incorporated into bone. Unlike the beta agents, radium-223 demonstrated a survival benefit in a phase III trial. The relative biologic effectiveness of alpha particles is 20 times that of a particle, but the shorter path length in tissue may limit the damage to surrounding normal tissue. The treatment consists of up to 6 radium-223 injections spaced 4 weeks apart. As with the beta agents, marrow suppression with recovery before 6 to 8 weeks is expected with more severe marrow toxicity occurring occasionally. Further study is needed to confirm the survival benefit and evaluate the treatment in other cancer types.

METABOLIC BONE DISEASE

Whole-body bone scintigraphy is very sensitive to changes in bone turnover from a variety of metabolic abnormalities including hyperparathyroidism, hyperthyroidism, and metal toxicities, though there is rarely an indication for bone scintigraphy to evaluate these processes. In Paget's disease, bone scintigraphy is useful in establishing the extent of the disease, whereas radiographs can establish the diagnosis and CT or MRI can assess possible local

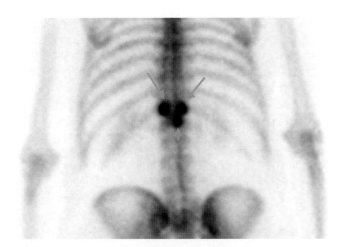

Fig. 2.24 Spot image of a bone scan obtained in the posterior view demonstrating increased radiotracer activity in the vertebral body (arrows) and spinous process (short arrow) of T12 vertebra in a pattern previously described as the "Mickey Mouse" or "champagne glass" sign, associated with Paget's disease.

complications. Active Paget's lesions have increased tracer activity, while older "burned out" lesions have reduced uptake (Fig. 2.24).

OSTEOMYELITIS

While MRI is now the modality of choice for acute osteomyelitis, three-phase bone scintigraphy is very sensitive in distinguishing cellulitis from osteomyelitis. The three phases include an arterial flow phase, a blood pool phase that represents tracer retained in the intracellular spaces, and a delayed phase taken several hours after injection (the same delay that a whole-body bone scan would have). Osteomyelitis will be positive on all three phases, while cellulitis will not have notably increased bone uptake on delayed images (Fig. 2.25). Specificity of three-phase bone scintigraphy is poor at roughly 50% due to increased uptake in all three phases by fractures, neuropathic joint changes, tumors, and many other conditions.

White blood cell scintigraphy, discussed later, can improve the specificity significantly to greater than 70%. In diabetic foot osteomyelitis and infected joint prostheses, dual isotope imaging with indium labeled white blood cells and Tc-99m sulfur colloid for marrow imaging have shown a high accuracy (about 90%) [7]. For spinal osteomyelitis or fungal osteomyelitis, gallium-67 can be used when an MRI is not possible or inconclusive. The sensitivity of white blood cell scintigraphy for spinal osteomyelitis is only 50% and thus too low to be useful. The role of FDG PET in the evaluation of osteomyelitis, including of the spine, is promising based on the current literature, but further studies are needed.

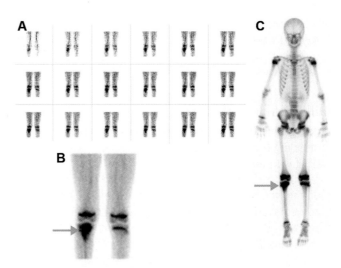

Fig. 2.25 (A) Flow images performed in the anterior view for 60 seconds demonstrate asymmetry with relatively increased blood flow to the region of the right proximal tibia. (B) Blood pool image of the knees obtained in the anterior view demonstrates increased radiotracer activity in the right proximal tibia (arrow). (C) Delayed whole-body planar image shows radiotracer uptake in the right proximal tibia (arrow), confirming the clinical suspicion of osteomyelitis.

BONE TRAUMA

Bone scintigraphy has a very high sensitivity for the bone turnover associated with skeletal trauma, becoming positive several weeks before a subtle fracture becomes apparent radiographically. While MRI has supplanted bone scintigraphy in the evaluation of occult fractures, stress fractures, and shin splints, bone scintigraphy with SPECT is sometimes the only modality by which a lesion is detected. Prosthetic loosening, particularly for knee and hip replacements, can be detected easily with bone scintigraphy due to the increased bone turnover at the bone-prosthesis interface.

Three-phase bone imaging is useful in the evaluation of heterotopic bone that can form in the soft tissue after trauma, particularly in patients with paraplegia. If blood flow and pool images are positive, the heterotopic bone formation is ongoing, and surgery at that time can worsen the disease. Three-phase bone scintigraphy can detect abnormal tracer accumulation in the musculature before radiographic changes are evident.

Complex regional pain syndrome, a nerve disorder typically seen after trauma that results in pain, improper blood flow control, and autonomic dysfunction usually in a limb, has a variety of appearances on three-phase bone scintigraphy based on the stage of disease. Early disease is characterized by increased flow and blood pooling in the affected limb and periarticular uptake on delayed images in every joint below the first joint affected. As the disease progresses, the blood flow and pool imaging normalizes and can become less than the contralateral limb as the nerve damage leads to muscle wasting and contractures. Delayed images will remain positive longer than the first two phases but may normalize or have decreased uptake in later stages of the disease.

BONE MINERAL DENSITY

Osteoporosis is a silent disease of bone loss that increases in incidence with age and costs billions of dollars a year. Half of women and a quarter of men over 50 suffer a fracture due to osteoporosis. Early detection is important in reducing the rate of fracture. Bone mineral density measurements principally of the spine and hips are best to diagnosis osteoporosis and follow a patient over time.

Years ago, dual-photon absorptiometry using gadolinium-153 with 41 and 102 keV gamma ray photopeaks was used, but currently x-ray based dual energy x-ray absorptiometry (DXA) machines are primarily used to assess bone mineral density. The World Health Organization (WHO) bone mass classification system uses a comparison to a young control population (the T-score) to determine if the patient has normal bone mineral density ($\leq$ 1 standard deviation [SD] below the control), osteopenia (1-2.5 SD below the control), or osteoporosis (>2.5 SD below the control). Z scores are matched to age, sex, and race and are important in the evaluation of premenopausal women, children, and men under age 50 (Fig. 2.26).

INFECTION IMAGING

Infection is a significant cause of morbidity and mortality, requiring prompt diagnosis and initiation of therapy. While conventional imaging is the mainstay of infection imaging, nuclear medicine studies remain important in the workup of occult infections and when surgery or trauma alters the normal anatomy.

Prior to CT and MRI, gallium-67 was a key imaging agent for noninvasive evaluation of both infection/inflammation and malignancy. Gallium has a biologic behavior similar to iron and thus is bound by siderophores of bacteria and lactoferrin released by white bloods cells at sites of infection and inflammation. As gallium is not specific and has suboptimal imaging characteristics, the radiotracer is rarely used, though it still has a role to play in vertebral osteomyelitis

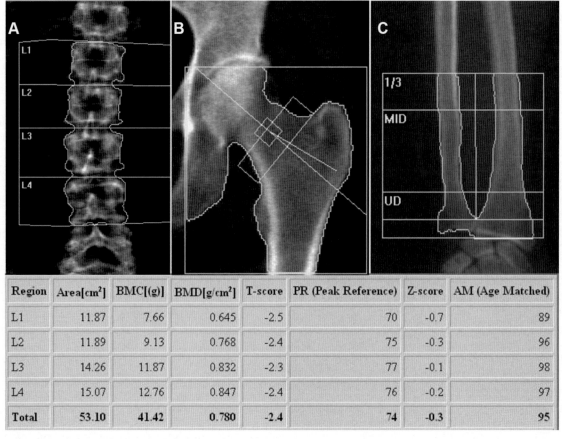

Region	Area[cm²]	BMC[(g)]	BMD[g/cm²]	T-score	PR (Peak Reference)	Z-score	AM (Age Matched)
L1	11.87	7.66	0.645	-2.5	70	-0.7	89
L2	11.89	9.13	0.768	-2.4	75	-0.3	96
L3	14.26	11.87	0.832	-2.3	77	-0.1	98
L4	15.07	12.76	0.847	-2.4	76	-0.2	97
Total	53.10	41.42	0.780	-2.4	74	-0.3	95

Fig. 2.26 Images of the (A) lumbar spine (L1-L4), (B) left hip, and (C) left forearm obtained on dual x-ray absorptiometry equipment. Bone mineral density measurements of the lumbar spine demonstrate a total T-score in the range of osteopenia.

and possibly immunocompromised patients in whom white blood cell activity is inadequate for other studies.

The white blood cells (WBCs) of a patient can be labeled with Tc-99m or In-111 in vitro and readministered to the patient with handling control precautions similar to that of blood transfusions. Approximately 50 mL of blood are taken from the patient and centrifuged to separate the white and red cells, the separated WBCS are labeled with the radioisotope, and quality control measures are performed prior to reinjection. The radiolabeled WBCs will accumulate in areas of infection and, to a lesser extent, inflammation with a high degree of sensitivity for many disease processes. For Tc-99m labeled WBCs, physiologic gut activity can obscure intra-abdominal processes, and thus early imaging prior to 2 hours can be used as opposed to a 4-hour delay for imaging extremities. For In-111 WBCs, imaging is typically performed at 24 hours, though early detection of acute process can be made with 4-hour imaging.

In comparison to a three-phase bone scan, WBC imaging has reported specificities ranging up to 70% to 80% as opposed to 50% or less. To further improve specificity, marrow imaging using Tc-99m sulfur colloid, which is concentrated by the reticuloendothelial system, in conjunction with WBC imaging has been used in both diabetic foot and joint prosthesis infection imaging. If an infection is present, the marrow does not function correctly, resulting in decreased Tc-99m sulfur colloid uptake while the In-111 WBC activity will be present. As the two radioisotopes have different specific energies, the gamma camera can discriminate between the two, allowing the patient to undergo only one imaging session. For joint prosthesis infections, the accuracy of WBC-marrow imaging is greater than 90%. Both WBC and gallium scintigraphy have been used to monitor treatment of osseous infections.

While CT is the modality of choice for intra-abdominal infections, WBC scintigraphy has reported accuracies greater than 90% for several disease processes, but it would be appropriately used only for occult infections after conventional workup. In patients with inflammatory bowel disease, WBC scans have been used to diagnose, determine the extent of bowel involvement, detect recurrence, and discover abscesses. Tc-99m WBCs imaging at 1 hour has been found to be better than In-111 WBCs due to more favorable imaging characteristics.

In patients undergoing PET-CT studies to evaluate cancers, accumulation of FDG in areas of infection and inflammation are potential false positives, but the literature supporting FDG for the diagnosis of infections has been building over the past decade. FDG PET-CT imaging has been demonstrated to have a high sensitivity for aortic graft infections, infectious etiologies of fevers of unknown origin, vertebral osteomyelitis, and prosthesis infections as well as

a high negative predictive value. Currently, FDG PET-CT studies for infection are not reimbursed by most insurance companies including Medicare as the scientific literature is still in development. Prior attempts to label WBCs with FDG have been unsuccessful due to rapid washout of FDG from the cell.

PULMONARY SCINTIGRAPHY

Ventilation and perfusion scintigraphy (VQ) is primarily directed at the detection of pulmonary embolism (PE) through regional quantitation of both ventilation and perfusion, and it is clinically valuable for select indications. Pulmonary embolism has an incidence estimated up to 900,000 people per year in the United States with fatality estimates ranging from 100,000 to 200,000 people per year, with less than half diagnosed prior to death. As the signs and symptom of pulmonary embolism are nonspecific, clinical examination alone does not adequately exclude pulmonary embolism. Criteria such as the Wells score and D-dimer testing have been used to identify low-risk patients, but this typically excludes less than half of patients with suspected PE [8]. Therefore, imaging is the mainstay of PE evaluation. With the advent of multidetector CT, CT pulmonary arteriography (CTPA) is the primary modality used for PE workup, allowing for detection of pulmonary embolism and other etiologies for the patient's symptoms (such as pneumonia, aortic disease, etc). VQ still has a role to play in patients with contraindications to intravenous CT contrast or uninterpretable CTPAs. Additionally, the radiation dose to the breast of young women is high with CTPA, and VQ should be considered as an alternative. In pregnant patients with a normal chest radiograph, a perfusion-only study with roughly one-quarter of the CTPA dose can be employed to reduce the dose to the fetus.

As the name implies, VQ scintigraphy is comprised of two separate studies. The ventilation portion may be performed by inhalation of one of two radiotracers—Tc-99m DTPA or xenon-133. Tc-99m DTPA is a particle that can be aerosolized using a nebulizer. The small particles are deposited by deep breathing into the alveoli. Larger particles and turbulent flow due to diseases such as COPD deposit the DTPA into the central airway leading to reduced tracer distribution in the periphery. Planar images can be obtained in multiple projections or SPECT imaging can be performed. On the other hand, xenon-133 (Xe-133) is a gas allowing for dynamic imaging over time but only in two projections, with the anterior and posterior images being obtained most frequently. Patients are imaged during the initial phase of breathing in the Xe-133 and air mixture, while Xe-133 equilibrates, and during washout of Xe-133. Both delayed tracer wash-in and washout point to ventilatory deficiencies that will lead to shunting of blood away from these regions. SPECT imaging with Xe-133 has been described in the literature but has not been notably translated to the clinic. For both radiopharmaceuticals, ventilation images are typically obtained prior to perfusion images.

Perfusion imaging is performed by intravenous administration of Tc-99m macroaggregated albumin (MAA). MAA is a particle sized primarily in the 10 to 30 μm range. For comparison, the pulmonary capillaries are 7 to 10 μm in size and precapillary arterioles are 35 μm. Thus the MAA lodges in between the precapillary arterioles and capillaries in the lung and breaks down with a 4- to 6-hour biological half-life. As with DTPA, both multiplanar and SPECT imaging can be performed.

VQ studies are interpreted in conjunction with a recent chest radiograph. Segmental areas without MAA tracer activity that follow the triangular prism branching pattern of the pulmonary arteries (colloquially the "wedge to the edge") without similar or greater matching ventilator defects are concerning for pulmonary embolism. Matched or nonsegmental perfusion defects are not consistent with pulmonary embolism. Matched and nonsegmental defects may be due to poor ventilation to a region leading to arterial shunting, pulmonary lesions such as bullae or masses, and attenuation from an enlarged heart, aortic disease, or hiatal hernia. Various interpretation criteria have been used for planar VQ with PIOPED and its subsequent revisions the most widely used. Revised PIOPED criteria break interpretation down into 6 categories based on the defect size, appearance, and matching to estimate the probability of PE: normal (<2%), very low (<10%), low (<20%), intermediate (20%-80%), high (>80%), or nondiagnostic (Fig. 2.27). The actual incidence of PE on intermediate probability studies is 30% to 35%. Clinical pretest probability for PE using risk factor scores can be used to modify the post-test probability of the VQ for PE but require cooperation between the referring and interpreting physician. SPECT VQ is interpreted using not consistent (<10%), consistent, or nondiagnostic for pulmonary embolus. SPECT VQ has a higher sensitivity and specificity than planar VQ, though the literature is still in development.

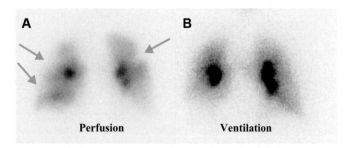

Fig. 2.27 (A) Perfusion image of the lungs obtained in the anterior view demonstrates large segmental defects bilaterally (arrows), which are not matched by similar ventilation abnormalities (B). This pattern on a ventilation-perfusion scan carries a high probability for pulmonary thromboembolism.

If right to left intracardiac or intrapulmonary shunts are present, a portion of the Tc-99m MAA will be delivered to the rest of the body. The shunt is demonstrated on imaging by tracer activity in the brain and the kidneys due to the high percentage of cardiac output directed to these organs. The quantity of the shunt can be calculated, and shunt fraction calculations have been used clinically. Of note, DTPA crosses from the alveoli to the capillaries and is excreted by the kidneys, and thus very mild renal activity on MAA imaging may be related to this physiologic excretion. Activity in the brain is not physiologic.

Quantitation of the ventilation and/or perfusion studies is used in the preoperative evaluation of patients undergoing lung surgery for malignancies with low lung functional capacity and of lung transplant patients. Perfusion quantitation has been used to evaluate the change in blood flow seen after surgical correction of pulmonary artery stenosis. Regions of interest are placed over the lungs in two projections, often the anterior and posterior images, and analysis is performed allowing comparison between the two lungs and within regions of the lung. For lung surgery, the pulmonary function test data can be related to the ventilatory data to decide whether the planned lung resection would leave the patient unable to perform activities of daily living due to inadequate pulmonary reserve.

NUCLEAR ONCOLOGY
LYMPHOSCINTIGRAPHY

Sentinel lymph node biopsy (SLNB) is a minimally invasive procedure employed in the accurate determination of nodal status. It has been studied in the management of patients with breast cancer, melanoma, head and neck tumors, Merkel cell carcinoma, penile carcinoma, and gynecological malignancies [9-12].

The basic principle for SLNB was observed in 1907 when Jamieson described the significance of neoplastic cells spreading to the so-called primary gland, by which he meant the draining lymph node [13]. The term *sentinel node*—the first lymph node in a regional lymphatic basin that receives flow from a primary tumor—was proposed by Gould et al in 1960 when studying cancers of the parotid gland. If the sentinel lymph node is negative on pathology, there is a low likelihood that the cancer has spread to the lymph nodes draining the location of the primary tumor.

Tc-99m sulfur colloid is approved for imaging of the liver and spleen by the United States Food and Drug Administration (FDA) and is widely used for lymphoscintigraphy in the filtered and unfiltered forms. The smaller filtered particles are microfiltered (pore size 0.22 μm—Millipore, Bedford, MA). Unfiltered sulfur colloid has variable range of sizes due to aggregation and can range from 0.3 to 1.0 μm depending on the preparation technique [14]. Particle size determines the kinetics of the radiotracer transit through the lymphatics, and filtered particles move faster [15]. Worldwide, additional radiotracers are utilized. For example, Tc-99m antimony trisulfide (particle size, 0.015-0.3 µm) is commercially available in Australia and Canada and Tc-99m-HSA nanocolloid (particle size, 0.05-0.8 µm) is used in Europe [16].

Radiotracer dose, injection techniques, and imaging protocols vary extensively according to the type of tumor being investigated. For example, in patients with melanoma, dynamic or sequential images are usually performed immediately after the intradermal injection of radiotracer around the primary tumor and continued for 30 to 60 minutes [17]. After images are obtained, the patient is taken directly to the operating room.

In breast cancer, the most popular approaches are to perform an intradermal injection in the skin overlying the primary tumor or subdermal injections in the periareolar area of the ipsilateral breast [18]. Other services have utilized peritumoral injections with similar success rates [19]. Dynamic or sequential images are not routinely performed. Images can be obtained on the same day or the day before surgery [20]. Proponents of the 2-day protocol claim greater efficiency in scheduling with less operating room time wasted in waiting for patients to arrive from the nuclear medicine department [20].

Using the preoperative images as a guide, the surgeon uses a small handheld probe to detect gamma-ray emissions from the radiotracer by means of auditory signals and meter readout of counts. By placing the probe over the region of highest counts, an incision can be made directly over the sentinel lymph node. A SLN is not necessarily the hottest node, although that is often the case. A SLN usually has at least 10 times the background counts, taken at a location remote from the injection site [17]. After the SLN is removed, the probe can be used to detect residual activity and the presence of additional lymph nodes (Fig. 2.28).

The main disadvantage of lymphoscintigraphy is the poor spatial resolution and the lack of detailed anatomy to guide surgeons during excision. Recently, the introduction of new imaging instrumentation such as SPECT-CT promises more accurate depiction of lymphatic channels and draining lymph nodes [21]. SPECT-CT will probably have its highest impact for problem solving and in tumors located in body parts with ambiguous lymph node drainage (Fig. 2.29).

ONCOLOGIC POSITRON EMISSION TOMOGRAPHY

Positron emission tomography (PET) imaging with F-18 fluorodeoxyglucose (FDG) is widely employed in staging, restaging, and evaluation of response to treatment in a variety of cancers. FDG is a glucose analogue and as such can

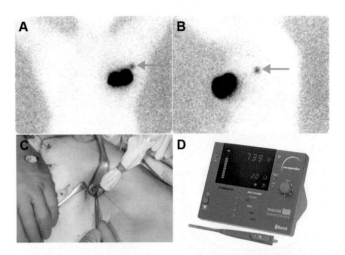

Fig. 2.28 (A) Anterior and (B) posterior images of a 45-year-old female with left breast cancer undergoing lymphatic mapping demonstrate intense radiotracer activity at the injection site in the left breast. A smaller focus of increased uptake in the left axilla (arrow) is compatible with a sentinel lymph node. The patient was subsequently taken to the operating room, where the sentinel lymph node was dissected (C) with the help of a handheld gamma probe (D).

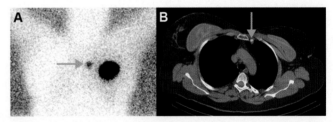

Fig. 2.29 A 61-year-old female with left breast cancer referred for lymphoscintigraphy. (A) Anterior spot view of the chest demonstrates intense radiotracer activity at the injection site in the left breast. In addition, there is a focus of increased radiotracer activity medial to the injection site, compatible with a draining lymph node (arrow). (B) On SPECT-CT imaging, this activity localizes to a normal-sized lymph node in the left internal mammary region (arrow). Due to the abnormal pattern of drainage and absence of activity in the left axilla, the sentinel lymph node biopsy was cancelled.

be used as a surrogate for tissue glucose utilization (metabolism). As increased glucose metabolism is a common feature of many malignancies, F-18 FDG PET imaging has proven valuable in the management of patients with cancer. The basic principle of F-18 FDG imaging is based on Warburg's observation that the increased metabolic demands of rapidly dividing tumor cells required adenosine triphosphate (ATP) generated by glycolysis [22]. FDG is actively transported into cells and converted into FDG-6-phosphate by hexokinase. FDG-6-phosphate, because it is not a substrate for the enzyme responsible for the next step in glycolysis, is then trapped in the cell. The F-18 label allows the location of FDG to be tracked in space and time by

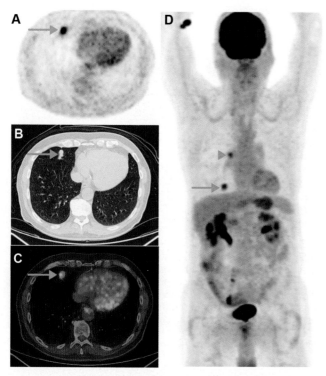

Fig. 2.30 A 75-year-old male with newly diagnosed lung adenocarcinoma, referred for initial staging. (A) Axial PET, (B) CT, (C) fused PET-CT, and (D) MIP images demonstrate increased F-18 FDG activity (SUV max 5.2) localizing to a 2.6 × 1.5 cm right middle lobe nodule, compatible with the primary tumor (arrows). MIP image (D) depicts a second focus of increased radiotracer activity (SUV max 5.0) in the right hilar region (arrowhead), consistent with nodal metastasis.

PET imaging, resulting in an approximation of tissue glucose utilization [23]. In the United States, the Center for Medicare and Medicaid Services has approved reimbursement for FDG PET imaging for several indications, and recent data collected by the National Oncological PET Registry is being used to substantiate the request to expand coverage to other types of cancers [24] (Fig. 2.30).

In addition to F-18 FDG, several other promising radiotracers for PET imaging are currently under investigation for future clinical applications. Table 2.4 contains a listing of novel radiotracers used for PET imaging and their targets in vivo. For more information regarding new agents for PET imaging, the reader is encouraged to visit the Molecular Imaging and Contrast Agent Database (MICAD) [25].

MONOCLONAL ANTIBODY IMAGING

Currently, only one monoclonal antibody (moAb) is routinely used for imaging. In-111 capromab, a murine moAb, is directed at the transmembrane protein prostate membrane specific antigen (PMSA) that is upregulated in prostate cancer and used primarily in patients with occult recurrence after prostatectomy. After bone scintigraphy confirms the absence of osseous metastases, capromab

Table 2.4 Radiolabeled Compounds Used for PET Targeting Specific Processes

Molecular Target/Process	Imaging Probes
Proliferation	[18F]FLT
Apoptosis	[18F]Annexin V
Angiogenesis	[18F]RGD
Hypoxia	[18F]MISO
Choline kinase	[11C]Choline, [18F]Choline
Glucose metabolism	[18F]FDG
Cytoplasmic lipid synthesis	[18F]Acetate, [11C]Acetate
Amino acid transport	[11C]MET [18F]FACBC [18F]FDOPA [11C]Tyrosine (TYR)
Somatostatin receptors	[68Ga]DOTA-TOC [68Ga]DOTA-NOC [68Ga]DOTA-TATE
Androgen receptor	[18F]Dihydrotestosterone (FDHT)
Blood flow	[15O]Water, [13N]Ammonia, [82Rb]Chloride

can be imaged 96 hours after injection as the relatively large moAb has a long residence time in the blood. Due to the persistent blood pool activity and nontarget binding, Tc-99m sulfur colloid and labeled RBCs can be used to delineate the marrow and vascular activity distribution respectively. Capromab has a higher sensitivity for pelvic lymph node metastases than CT or MRI and for detecting small recurrences in the prostatectomy bed.

As the antibody is murine based, the body may develop an elevated level of antibodies direct against the murine component (HAMA or human anti-mouse antibody). Thus, if a capromab study is repeated the HAMA levels must be checked. Elevated HAMA would result in altered biodistribution of the radiotracer, making the study uninterpretable.

MONOCLONAL ANTIBODY THERAPY

Numerous efforts are underway to radiolabel clinically relevant antibodies in order to take advantage of the specificity of the antibody-receptor binding mechanism for radioimmunotherapy. While there are many challenges involved (eg, maintaining immunoreactivity, limiting nontarget cross reactivity, ensuring clearance of these large molecules from the bloodstream to reduce background activity, etc), the potential benefits are substantial.

There are two therapeutic radiolabeled antibodies approved by the Food and Drug Administration (FDA) for clinical use: Y-90 ibritumomab tiuxetan (Zevalin) and I-131 tositumomab (Bexxar). Both of these agents target the CD20 antigen expressed in 90% of B-cell non-Hodgkin's lymphoma (NHL).

Both have shown to benefit patients with low-grade or follicular B-cell NHL who relapse or are refractory to other therapies. Y-90 Zevalin is also approved for previously untreated follicular NHL in patients who achieve a partial or complete response to first-line chemotherapy [26].

Several other radiolabeled monoclonal antibodies are currently under development. Of particular interest are the monoclonal antibodies conjugated to alpha particles. Alpha particles offer key advantages over beta minus particles. They possess a high linear energy transfer (LET) and a limited range in tissue. The high alpha particle LET can produce significant more damage to cancer cells than beta minus particles, with less toxicity to remaining normal tissues [27].

SELECTIVE INTERNAL RADIOTHERAPY

Both primary and metastatic liver tumors receive the majority of their blood supply from the hepatic arteries (up to 95%), while normal hepatic parenchyma receives less than 30%. Several interventional radiology procedures take advantage of the flow differential to treat liver tumors. Selective internal radiotherapy (SIRT) uses tiny spheres that contain the beta emitter yttrium-90 injected into the hepatic arterial system. The Y-90 microspheres flow preferentially into the hypervascular tumors, embolize the precapillary beds, and deliver a high local dose to the tumor and a much lower dose to the surrounding hepatic parenchyma.

Nuclear medicine physicians partner with the interventional radiologists by overseeing the radiation safety aspects of dose delivery, treatment planning, and interpretation of pretherapy and posttherapy nuclear scans. Prior to therapy, Tc-99m MAA is injected into the hepatic artery or a branch to map the tracer distribution of activity in the liver, assess for extrahepatic tracer delivery, and calculate the amount of tracer shunted to the lungs. Extrahepatic radioembolization can cause significant morbidity and possible mortality due to pancreatitis, gastritis, gastric ulceration, radiation pneumonitis, and cholecystitis. Extrahepatic abdominal tracer deposition is assessed with planar, SPECT, and SPECT-CT imaging, with SPECT-CT possessing the greatest sensitivity. A lung shunt fraction is calculated from the planar images, with a fraction greater than 20% precluding treatment due to excessive dose to the lungs. Posttherapy SPECT-CT is also useful in documenting the distribution of the therapy dose in the liver and extrahepatic activity that would alert clinicians to monitor for a specific complication.

RENAL AND UROGRAPHIC SCINTIGRAPHY

Renal scintigraphic studies can assess the movement of substances from the blood to the urine, the movement of urine from the kidney through the urinary tract, renal blood flow, and the presence of normal renal cortex.

DYNAMIC RENOGRAPHIC SCAN

Dynamic renographic scans are comprised of two parts: the blood flow to the kidney in the first minute and the uptake and excretion of the radiotracer over the next 24 to 29 minutes. Two radiopharmaceuticals are used: the tubular excretion agent Tc-99m MAG-3 and glomerularly filtered Tc-99m DTPA. The relative uptake of the kidneys is obtained from the 1- to 3-minute images and can be used in surgical planning. The uptake and excretion from both the renal cortex and whole kidney are calculated from regions of interest and can be displayed graphically (Fig. 2.31). In a normal kidney, tracer uptake peaks prior to 5 minutes and the clearance half-time is ≤ 10 minutes. In obstructed kidneys, adequate clearance is not present and tracer activity can increase over the length of the study (Fig. 2.32). As dilated renal collecting systems can pool the tracer when an obstruction is not present, intravenous furosemide to increase the production of urine and overcome the pooling effect followed by an additional 20 minutes of imaging can distinguish between the two.

Renography can be used to confirm the diagnosis of renovascular hypertension, in which reduced blood flow to the kidney upregulates the renin-angiotensin system (RAS) leading to angiotensin-II mediated vasoconstriction. This potent vasoconstriction on the efferent arteriole from the glomerulus preserves glomerular pressure at the cost of systemic hypertension. Renovascular hypertension accounts for roughly 1% of patients with hypertension, and the mere presence of atherosclerotic renal artery stenosis on conventional imaging is not contributory as the vast majority of those lesions are not functionally significant. After baseline renography, the patient receives an angiotensin converting enzyme (ACE) inhibitor and a repeat renogram is performed. The ACE inhibitor disrupts the RAS causing a drop in glomerular pressure and thus filtration rate. In patients with renovascular hypertension, the renogram significantly changes from baseline to post-ACE in the affected kidney.

In renal transplant patients, renography can be used to assess for rejection, disorders of the vasculature, acute tubular necrosis, urine leak, and obstruction.

RENAL CORTICAL IMAGING

Tc-99m DMSA binds to the renal cortex, allowing planar or SPECT imaging after a 2- to 3-hour delay. As with MAG-3 and DTPA, relative renal uptake calculations can be useful in the presurgical setting. In the pediatric population, DMSA cortical scintigraphy is more sensitive than ultrasound and similar to CT in the detection of acute pyelonephritis. Pyelonephritis appears as one or more wedge-shaped cortical defects on scintigraphy. DMSA is also more sensitive for scarring after pyelonephritis (Fig. 2.33). DMSA can also be used to distinguish a prominent column of Bertin from a renal tumor.

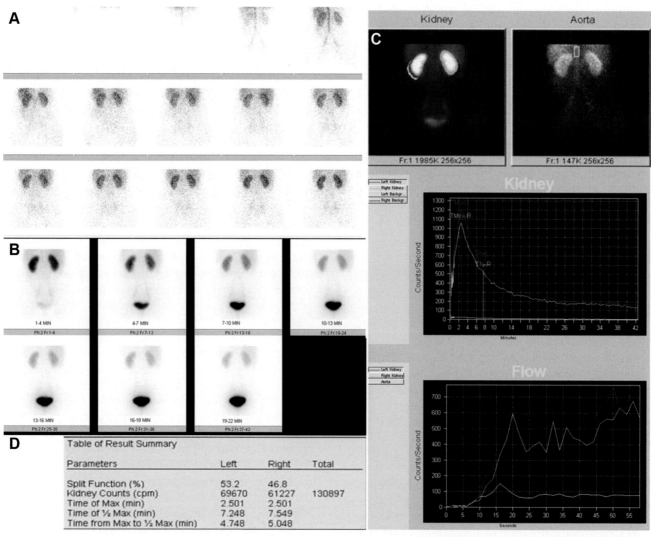

Fig. 2.31 Normal Tc-99m MAG-3 renal scintigraphy. (A) Flow images demonstrate normal and symmetric flow to the kidneys bilaterally. (B) Dynamic images demonstrate prompt and symmetric radiotracer uptake by the kidneys and normal washout over the period of the study. (C) Regions of interest are then drawn around the kidneys and renogram curves are generated. Background subtraction regions of interest are placed around the inferior portions of the kidneys. An aortic region of interest is used to assess the injected bolus, as well as relative perfusion. The renogram curves labeled "Kidney" demonstrate normal time-activity curves with a steep uptake slope (representing the vascular and concentration phases), a distinct peak, and rapid radiotracer excretion.

VOIDING CYSTOGRAPHY

Epidemiologic data suggest a prevalence of vesicoureteral reflux of up to 1.8% of the population, but this may be higher based on imaging studies. Fluoroscopic voiding cystourethrography (VCUG) is typically used for initial evaluation of suspected reflux, providing anatomic detail and grading that nuclear VCUG cannot. However, nuclear VCUG is more sensitive than fluoroscopy. Due to the much lower radiation dose for nuclear VCUG, it is used for following reflux over time and after treatment and for screening asymptomatic siblings of a child with reflux.

CENTRAL NERVOUS SYSTEM SCINTIGRAPHY

Prior to the development of CT and MRI, brain scintigraphy was the only noninvasive method to diagnose a wide variety of diseases of the brain. While many of the vascular and tumor indications are gone, brain scans still provide valuable information by detecting physiologic change prior to anatomic change. In the research arena, radiopharmaceuticals target a myriad of neuroreceptors in addition to blood flow, metabolism, beta-amyloid, and many other processes, leading to advances in our understanding of numerous neurologic and psychiatric diseases.

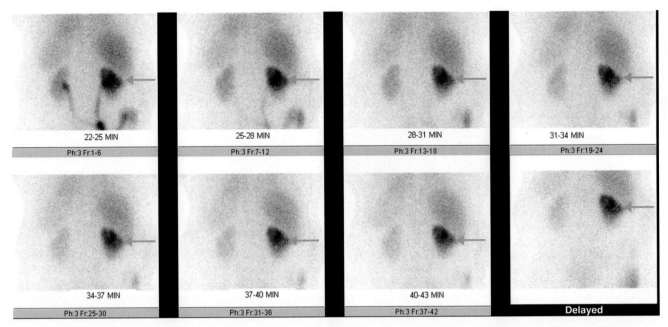

Fig. 2.32 A 60-year-old male with history of bladder cancer, status post radical cystoprostatectomy and ileal conduit urinary diversion. Dynamic images of the kidneys obtained in the posterior view after the administration of 40 mg of Lasix intravenously demonstrate persistent radiotracer activity in the right kidney, compatible with obstruction (arrows). Delayed image obtained after the post-Lasix dynamic imaging demonstrates that significant radiotracer activity persists in the right kidney (arrow), confirming obstruction.

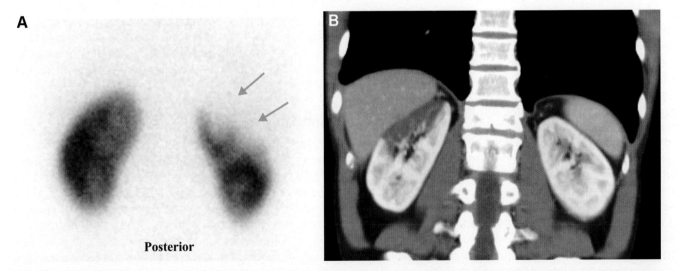

Fig. 2.33 A 63-year-old female with remote history of pyelonephritis. (A) Planar image of the kidneys obtained in the posterior view at 2 hours after the intravenous administration of Tc-99m DMSA demonstrates an area of decreased counts involving the upper and mid poles of the right kidney (arrows). (B) Coronal reformat of a CT image of the abdomen demonstrates a corresponding cortical defect in the upper and mid poles of the right kidney, compatible with scarring (arrow). Used with permission of Aaron C. Jessop, MD.

SEIZURE

In patients whose seizures are refractory to medical therapy when resection of the seizure locus is being considered, multiple tests are used to pinpoint the location of the seizure focus including electroencephalogram, MRI, and scintigraphy. The anatomic abnormalities on MRI do not typically match the full extent of the seizure locus that can be detected on physiologic imaging. Two types of radiopharmaceuticals are used—SPECT Tc-99m cerebral blood flow agents and the PET metabolic agent FDG. The Tc-99m agents, HMPAO and ECD, both cross the blood-brain barrier, enter cells, and become trapped allowing imaging to be delayed up to 2 or 3 hours. Glucose is the fundamental energy source for the brain, and FDG becomes trapped in the cells relative to the regional cerebral glucose metabolism.

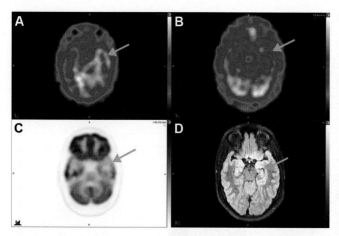

Fig. 2.34 Four imaging studies obtained in the same patient with seizure disorder. (A) Ictal axial SPECT image obtained after the intravenous administration of Tc-99m ECD demonstrates an area of hyperperfusion in the left temporal lobe (arrow). (B) Interictal axial SPECT image with Tc-99m ECD demonstrates hypoperfusion in the left temporal lobe (arrow). (C) Interictal axial F-18 FDG PET image demonstrates asymmetry, with relatively decreased glucose metabolism in the left temporal lobe (arrow) in comparison to the right temporal lobe. (D) Axial MRI image demonstrates reduced volume in the left hippocampus (arrow).

SPECT agents can be used in both ictal and interictal (between seizures) studies. Ictal SPECT has the highest sensitivity at greater than 80% for temporal lobe epileptic loci but requires a specialized setting, as the radiotracer must be injected at the onset of a seizure prior to generalization. Increased blood flow due to the seizure leads to increased tracer deposition in the seizure locus in relation to the rest of the cerebrum. Interictal SPECT has a sensitivity of greater than 60%, and the lower blood flow to the disordered neurons of the locus leads to reduced tracer activity when compared other gray matter. Due to the short half-life of F-18, ictal PET is not feasible. Interictal PET has a sensitivity greater than 70%, and disordered neurons have a lower metabolic rate than normal gray matter, leading to lower tracer activity. In short, the seizure locus will be hot (high tracer activity) on ictal imaging and photopenic (low tracer activity) on interictal imaging (Fig. 2.34).

BRAIN DEATH

Brain death is a clinical diagnosis, but ancillary tests can be useful to clinicians in the establishment of the diagnosis in the setting of equivocal findings, especially when there is concomitant hypothermia or barbiturate intoxication [28]. Using the gamma cerebral perfusion agents, blood flow above the circle of Willis can be assessed very sensitively using planar imaging alone. A positive study is characterized by no activity in the cerebrum signifying absence of blood flow leading to rapid death of cerebral cells. The absence of tracer in the cerebrum does not mean the

patient is brain dead as the flow to the respiratory center in the brain stem is not assessed. However, a positive study can be used to speed the diagnosis of brain death and facilitate more rapid organ donation (Fig. 2.35).

DEMENTIA

Dementia is a rapidly growing problem for the aging population in the United States and is the sixth leading cause of death. Dementias such as Alzheimer's cannot be definitively diagnosed without a brain biopsy, but clinicians use neuropsychiatric testing and judgment to determine the type of dementia. Both FDG PET and the SPECT cerebral blood flow agents have been used to characterize dementias when the type of dementia is unclear. Alzheimer's dementia (AD) demonstrates reduced tracer activity in the temporoparietal cortex early, progressing to have frontal lobe decrease as the disease progresses. Late-stage AD has near global decrease in cortical activity. Frontotemporal dementias are characterized by decreased tracer activity on the frontal and temporal lobes. Other processes such as depression, ALS, and cocaine abuse can have a similar pattern.

F-18 florbetapir and the recently approved F-18 flutemetamol bind to beta-amyloid in the brain, providing information on the density of the plaques. These plaques are a defining feature of AD but are also seen in other diseases and in normal patients. Beta-amyloid binding agents have been used to noninvasively monitor the effect of therapies directed at the plaques. The literature on appropriate use is still in development.

DOPAMINE TRANSPORTER IMAGING

Parkinsonian syndromes can be difficult to distinguish from essential tremor with up to 20% of patients incorrectly diagnosed with Parkinson's disease if not evaluated by a movement disorder specialist. I-123 ioflupane binds to the dopamine transporters on the synapse of striatal neurons and can detect the loss of striatal dopaminergic neuron density. In parkisonian syndromes (Parkinson's, supranuclear palsy, multiple system atrophy) this neuron loss will manifest as decrease and then absence of activity in the putamen and eventually decreased activity in the caudate nuclei as the disease progresses. Essential tremor does not arise from the death of dopaminergic neurons and striatal activity is normal.

CEREBROSPINAL FLUID STUDIES

Radiopharmaceuticals can be placed into the cerebrospinal fluid (CSF) via lumbar puncture or surgical shunt reservoir to trace CSF movement. CT and MRI flow studies are typically first line in the evaluation of hydrocephalus, but scintigraphy can aid when the results are nondiagnostic. In the normal pressure hydrocephalus (NPH), a type of communicating hydrocephalus, In-111 DTPA injected

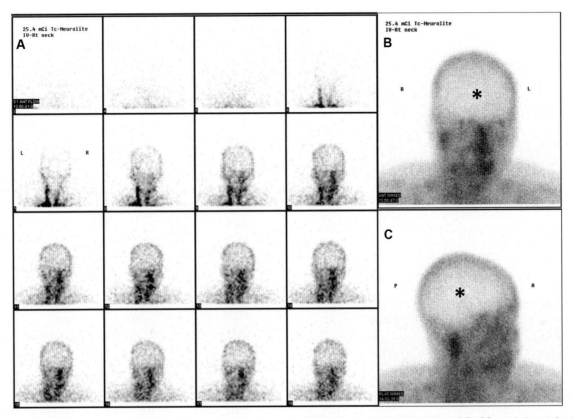

Fig. 2.35 (A) Flow images of the brain obtained in the anterior view after the intravenous administration of Tc-99m ethyl cysteinate dimer (ECD) demonstrate no evidence of brain perfusion. Delayed planar images of the brain obtained in the (B) anterior and (C) right lateral views demonstrate no radiotracer uptake in the brain (asterisk), compatible with the clinical diagnosis of brain death. Used with permission of Aaron C. Jessop, MD.

via lumbar puncture can be followed for 24 hours to see if the flow is normal or slowed with or without abnormal ventricular uptake pointing to NPH as a cause for the patient's symptoms. The classic triad of NPH is dementia, gait disturbance, and urinary incontinence. CSF leaks from the base of skull through the nose and ears after trauma can be detected with a high specificity. Radiotracers can be injected into the shunt reservoirs or intraspinal pump reservoirs to assess for patency of the tubing.

REFERENCES

1. Mc Ardle BA, et al. Does rubidium-82 PET have superior accuracy to SPECT perfusion imaging for the diagnosis of obstructive coronary disease?: a systematic review and meta-analysis. *J Am Coll Cardiol*. 2012;60(18):1828-1837.

2. Chakraborty D, et al. Role of Tc99m sulfur colloid scintigraphy in differentiating non-cirrhotic portal fibrosis from cirrhosis liver. *Indian J Nucl Med*. 2010;25(4):139-142.

3. Pinson AG, et al. Technetium-99m-RBC venography in the diagnosis of deep venous thrombosis of the lower extremity: a systematic review of the literature. *J Nucl Med*. 1991;32(12):2324-2328.

4. Zuccaro G Jr. Management of the adult patient with acute lower gastrointestinal bleeding. American College of Gastroenterology. Practice Parameters Committee. *Am J Gastroenterol*. 1998;93(8):1202-1208.

5. Strate LL. Lower GI bleeding: epidemiology and diagnosis. *Gastroenterol Clin North Am*. 2005;34(4):643-664.

6. Shie P, et al. Meta-analysis: comparison of F-18 fluorodeoxy-glucose-positron emission tomography and bone scintigraphy in the detection of bone metastases in patients with breast cancer. *Clin Nucl Med*. 2008;33(2):97-101.

7. Palestro CJ, et al. Combined labeled leukocyte and technetium 99m sulfur colloid bone marrow imaging for diagnosing musculoskeletal infection. *Radiographics*. 2006;26(3): 859-870.

8. Geersing GJ, et al. Safe exclusion of pulmonary embolism using the Wells rule and qualitative D-dimer testing in primary care: prospective cohort study. *BMJ*. 2012;345:e6564.

9. Paleri V, et al. Sentinel node biopsy in squamous cell cancer of the oral cavity and oral pharynx: a diagnostic meta-analysis. *Head & Neck*. 2005;27(9):739-747.

10. Gupta SG, et al. Sentinel lymph node biopsy for evaluation and treatment of patients with Merkel cell carcinoma: the Dana-Farber experience and meta-analysis of the literature. *Arch Dermatol*. 2006;142(6):685-690.

11. Perdona S, et al. Role of dynamic sentinel node biopsy in penile cancer: our experience. *J Surg Oncol*. 2006;93(3): 181-185.

12. Schneider A. The sentinel concept in patients with cervical cancer. *J Surg Oncol*. 2007;96(4):337-341.

13. JK J, JF D. Lectures on the lymphatic system of the stomach. *Lancet*. 1907;1:1061-1062.

14. Larson SM, Nelp WB. Radiopharmacology of a simplifield technetium-99m-colloid preparation for photoscanning. *J Nucl Med*. 1966;7(11):817-826.

15. Bergqvist L, Strand SE, Persson BR. Particle sizing and biokinetics of interstitial lymphoscintigraphic agents. *Semin Nucl Med*. 1983;13(1):9-19.

16. Tsopelas C. Understanding the radiolabelling mechanism of 99mTc-antimony sulphide colloid. *Appl Radiat Isot*. 2003;59(5-6):321-328.

17. Alazraki N, et al. Procedure guideline for lymphoscintigraphy and the use of intraoperative gamma probe for sentinel lymph node localization in melanoma of intermediate thickness 1.0. *J Nucl Med*. 2002;43:1414-1418.

18. Maza S, et al. Peritumoural versus subareolar administration of technetium-99m nanocolloid for sentinel lymph node detection in breast cancer: preliminary results of a prospective intra-individual comparative study. *Eur J Nucl Med Mol Imaging*. 2003;30(5):651-656.

19. Babiera GV, et al. Lymphatic drainage patterns on early versus delayed breast lymphoscintigraphy performed after injection of filtered Tc-99m sulfur colloid in breast cancer patients undergoing sentinel lymph node biopsy. *Clin Nucl Med*. 2005;30(1):11-15.

20. Yeung HW, et al. Lymphoscintigraphy and sentinel node localization in breast cancer patients: a comparison between 1-day and 2-day protocols. *J Nucl Med*. 2001;42(3):420-423.

21. Mar MV, et al. Evaluation and localization of lymphatic drainage and sentinel lymph nodes in patients with head and neck melanomas by hybrid SPECT/CT lymphoscintigraphic imaging. *J Nucl Med Technol*. 2007;35(1):10-16; quiz 17-20.

22. Warburg O. On the origin of cancer cells. *Science*. 1956; 123(3191):309-314.

23. Sokoloff L, et al. The [14C]deoxyglucose method for the measurement of local cerebral glucose utilization: theory, procedure, and normal values in the conscious and anesthetized albino rat. *J Neurochem*. 1977;28(5):897-916.

24. Hillner BE, et al. The impact of positron emission tomography (PET) on expected management during cancer treatment: findings of the National Oncologic PET Registry. *Cancer*. 2009;115(2):410-418.

25. Molecular Imaging and Contrast Agent Database (MICAD). National Center for Biotechnology Information (US). http://www.ncbi.nlm.nih.gov/books/NBK5330/, 2004-2013.

26. Jacene HA, et al. Comparison of 90Y-ibritumomab tiuxetan and 131I-tositumomab in clinical practice. *J Nucl Med*. 2007;48(11):1767-1776.

27. Scheinberg DA, McDevitt MR. Actinium-225 in targeted alpha-particle therapeutic applications. *Curr Radiopharm*. 2011;4(4):306-320.

28. Wijdicks EF, et al. Evidence-based guideline update: determining brain death in adults: report of the Quality Standards Subcommittee of the American Academy of Neurology. *Neurology*. 2010;74(23):1911-1918.

Chapter 3

Diagnostic Neuroradiology

*By Santosh Shah, Tara Hagopian, Robert Klinglesmith,
and Eliana Bonfante*

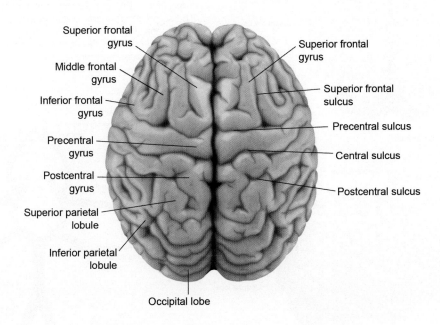

Superior frontal
gyrus

Middle frontal
gyrus

Inferior frontal
gyrus

Precentral
gyrus

Postcentral
gyrus

Superior parietal
lobule

Inferior parietal
lobule

Superior frontal
gyrus

Superior frontal
sulcus

Precentral sulcus

Central sulcus

Postcentral sulcus

Occipital lobe

ANATOMY

This section serves as an introduction to the basic anatomy of the brain, head, neck, and spine. Brain anatomy is complex, and a complete discussion is beyond the scope of this text.

The human brain can be roughly divided into the cerebrum, thalamus, brain stem, and cerebellum. The cerebrum is comprised of the cerebral cortex, basal ganglia, and limbic system. The brain stem includes the midbrain, pons, and medulla. The cerebellum is composed of the cerebellar hemispheres and vermis.

Figures 3.1 to 3.10 illustrate the structures and blood vessels of the brain, head, neck, and spine.

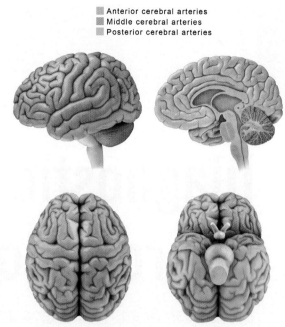

Anterior cerebral arteries
Middle cerebral arteries
Posterior cerebral arteries

Fig. 3.2 Vascular distribution of the brain parenchyma. An understanding of the territories of the major intracranial vessels is important in the diagnosis of stroke and other vascular lesions. The anterior cerebral arteries (blue) supply the anterior parasagittal regions. The middle cerebral arteries (pink) supply most of the lateral cortex of the frontal and superior temporal lobes. The posterior cerebral arteries (green) supply the inferior temporal and occipital lobes.

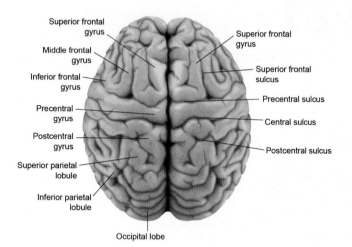

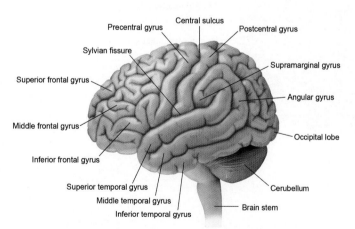

Fig. 3.1 Surface anatomy of the brain. The cerebral cortex is composed of gyri (ridges) and sulci (intervening depressions) divided into 4 lobes: frontal, parietal, temporal, and occipital. The frontal lobe is separated from the parietal lobe by the central sulcus. The sylvian fissure separates the temporal lobe from the more superiorly located frontal and parietal lobes. The occipital lobe is separated from the parietal lobe by the parieto-occipital sulcus.

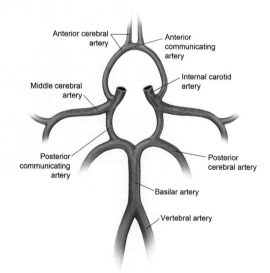

Fig. 3.3 Circle of Willis. The circle of Willis describes a loop of arteries that supply most of the brain. The posterior circulation consists of the 2 vertebral arteries that join to form the midline basilar artery. The basilar artery terminates into paired posterior cerebral arteries. The anterior circulation is predominantly supplied by the internal carotid arteries that terminate into the anterior and middle cerebral arteries. The anterior communicating artery connects both the anterior cerebral arteries, while the posterior communicating arteries connect the anterior and posterior circulation. The circle of Willis plays an important role in providing collateral supply in the setting of arterial occlusions and strokes.

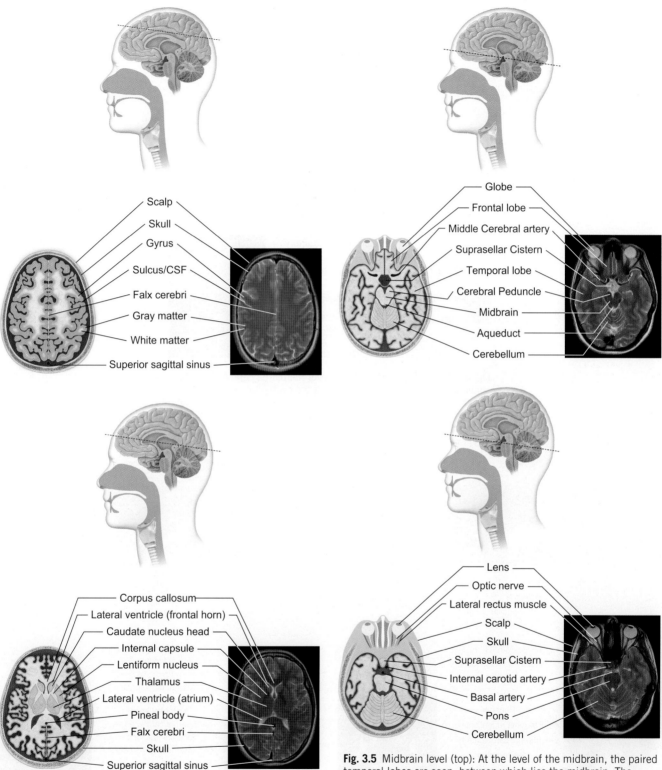

Fig. 3.4 Supraventricular level (top): At the supraventricular level, the frontal and parietal lobes are seen in cross section. The falx cerebri is a dural reflection that separates the 2 hemispheres. The superior sagittal sinus is seen posteriorly.

Lateral ventricular level (bottom): The lateral ventricles are seen on this level as paired frontal horns anteriorly and the atria more posteriorly. The basal ganglia are seen, as are the thalami.

Fig. 3.5 Midbrain level (top): At the level of the midbrain, the paired temporal lobes are seen, between which lies the midbrain. The suprasellar cistern (a cerebrospinal fluid [CSF]–filled space at the base of the brain) is seen in the midline. The midbrain is composed of the tectum, tegmentum, and cerebral penducles. The cerebral aqueduct connects the third ventricle with the fourth ventricle.

Pons level (bottom): At this level the pons is seen, along with inferior temporal lobes and the upper cerebellum. The pons contains several white matter bundles that connect the cerebrum to the cerebellum and medulla and also contains several cranial nerve nuclei.

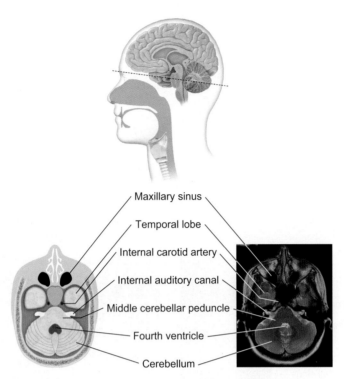

Fig. 3.6 Cerebellum level: At this level the paired cerebellar hemispheres are seen, between which lies the cerebellar vermis. At the cerebellopontine angle, the paired internal auditory canals are seen. Within the internal auditory canals lie the facial, vestibular, and cochlear nerves.

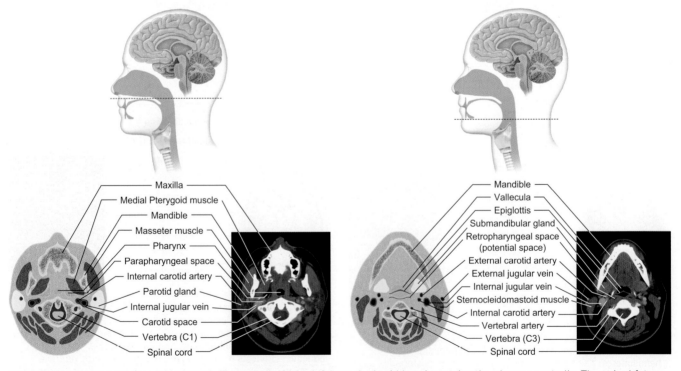

Fig. 3.7 Suprahyoid neck (top and bottom): The suprahyoid neck (above the hyoid bone) contains the pharynx centrally. The paired fat-containing parapharyngeal spaces are seen adjacent to the pharynx. Anterolateral to the parapharyngeal space lies the masticator space, while posterolaterally lies the carotid space. The retropharyngeal and prevertebral spaces lie posterior to the pharynx.

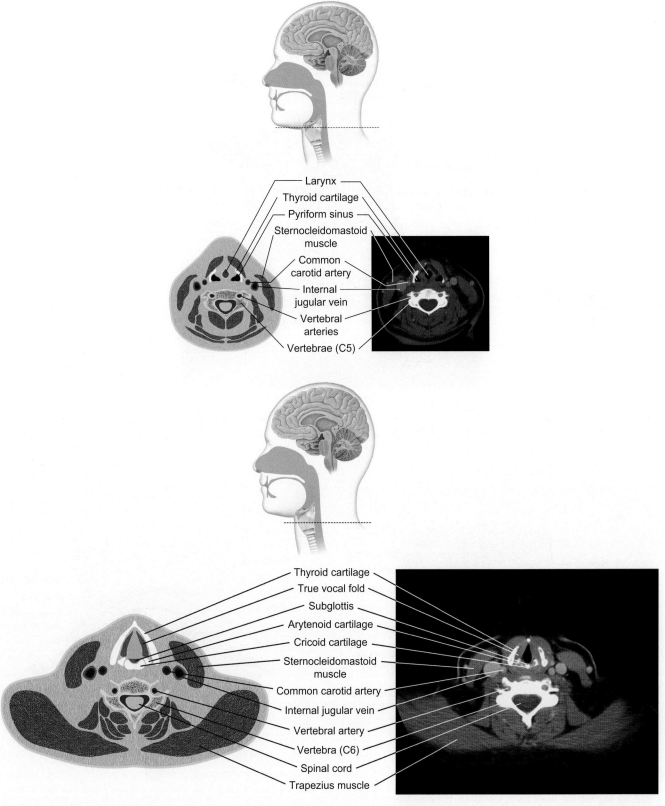

Fig. 3.8 Infrahyoid neck (top and bottom): Below the hyoid bone lie the larynx and hypopharynx. The larynx is surrounded by several cartilaginous structures: thyroid cartilage, cricoid cartilage, arytenoid cartilage, and cricoid cartilage. The vocal cords are situated within the central larynx and divide the larynx into the supraglottic and subglottic spaces. The hypopharynx consists of the piriform sinuses, postcricoid region, and posterior pharyngeal wall.

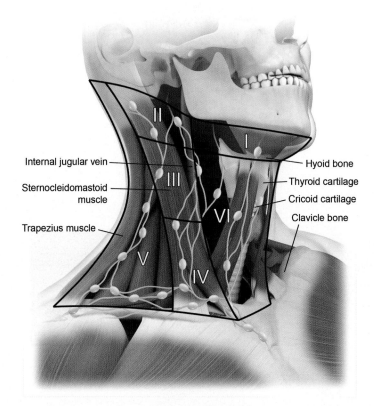

Fig. 3.9 The cervical lymph nodes can be divided into several groups based on anatomical landmarks: Level 1 (submandibular and submental), Level II, III, IV (upper, mid, low internal jugular nodes), V (posterior cervical), VI (visceral).

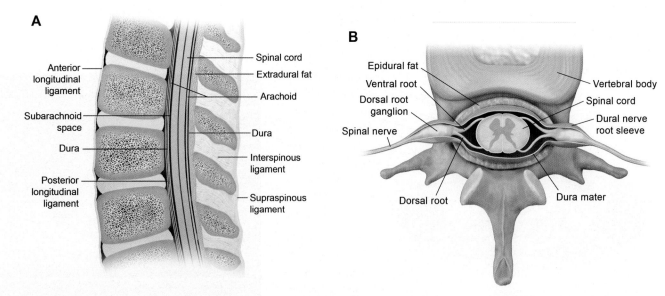

Fig. 3.10 (A) Sagittal diagram of the spine, (B) axial diagram of the spine. The vertebral column contains vertebral bodies, intervertebral disks, and posterior elements. The spinal canal bounded by posterior elements contains the spinal cord, exiting nerve roots, surrounding cerebrospinal fluid, dura, and epidural fat/vessels.

INTRODUCTION TO BRAIN MR SEQUENCES

MR (magnetic resonance) is the cornerstone of modern imaging of the brain and spinal cord. Images are obtained by taking advantage of resonance properties of nuclei under the influence of an external magnetic field. Some basic sequences that the reader should become familiar with are shown in Figs. 3.11 to 3.13.

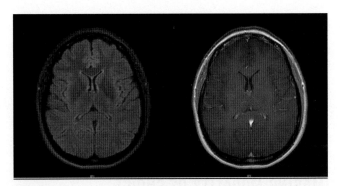

Fig. 3.12 FLAIR imaging (left) is very similar to T2-weighted imaging in which white matter is relatively hypointense; however, the signal from CSF is suppressed. This sequence is helpful as any pathological process resulting in vasogenic or cytotoxic edema is hyperintense. Postcontrast images (right) are T1-weighted sequences obtained after the administration of gadolinium-based contrast agents. The vessels appear bright due to the presence of contrast. Postcontrast images are useful in detection of infectious, inflammatory, and neoplastic processes.

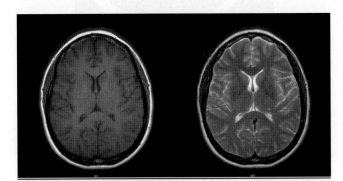

Fig. 3.11 On T1-weighted imaging (left), white matter is bright due to the presence of myelin and gray matter structures including the cortical gray matter appear darker. Note that simple fluid such as CSF is black. Fat, subacute hemorrhage, melanin, and mineralization can appear bright on T1-weighted images. On T2-weighted imaging (right), CSF is bright, and white matter is dark. On both pulse sequences, there is loss of signal from flowing blood referred to as a flow void.

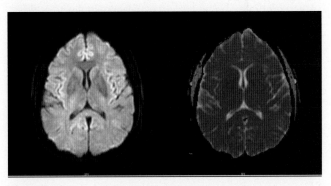

Fig. 3.13 Diffusion weighted imaging (DWI) is a very important tool in neuroimaging. During acute ischemia/infarct and other pathological processes, the diffusion of water molecules is restricted. These regions are hyperintense on diffusion weighted images (left) and dark on ADC images (right).

CASE 1

PATIENT PRESENTATION

A 72-year-old male presents to the emergency department with acute onset of focal sensory loss and right arm weakness.

CLINICAL SUSPICION

Acute ischemic stroke

IMAGING MODALITY OF CHOICE

Noncontrast CT of the head to evaluate for hemorrhage and early ischemic changes. Advantages: fast and readily available, high sensitivity for presence of hemorrhage.

FINDINGS

Cerebral infarcts are the leading cause of disability and fourth leading cause of death in the United States. Patients with acute cerebral ischemia/infarct usually present with sudden-onset neurologic deficit (weakness, sensory loss, aphasia). Risk factors include diabetes, hypertension, smoking, and hyperlipidemia. It is important to realize that the value in CT is not to diagnose an acute ischemic infarct. The role of CT is to exclude hemorrhage, exclude nonischemic pathologies (masses, infections, vascular malformations), and evaluate the volume of infarcted territory. In the setting of cerebral infarcts, the infarcted territory results in contralateral symptomatology.

CT

- Usually normal in the hyperacute phase
- Hyperdense vessel representing acute thrombus (low sensitivity, high specificity) (Fig. C1.1)
- Loss of gray matter–white matter differentiation
  - "Insular ribbon" sign: swelling and blurring of normal gray-white differentiation within the insular cortex
  - Obscured lentiform nucleus
- Parenchymal hypodensity resulting from early cytotoxic edema (Fig. C1.2)
- Gyral swelling with sulcal effacement

  Additional CT examinations that may be performed:

- CT angiography: useful in localizing area of arterial stenosis or occlusion
- CT perfusion: useful in identification of penumbra (brain at risk), which may help stratify patients for therapeutic intervention

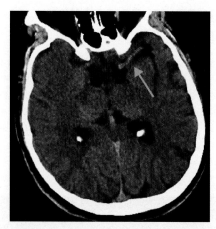

Fig. C1.1 Axial noncontrast CT demonstrating a dense MCA sign (arrow) representing an acutely thrombosed MCA in the setting of acute ischemic infarct.

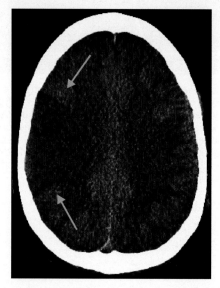

Fig. C1.2 Axial noncontrast CT in a different patient with acute infarct shows a wedge-shaped hypodensity (arrows) with gyral swelling and sulcal effacement.

MRI

- Highly sensitive to diagnose acute infarcts within minutes of onset.
- Areas of acute ischemia restrict free diffusion of water, resulting in elevated signal on DWI images and decreased ADC values (Fig. C1.3).
- Limitations of MRI in the emergency setting include difficulty to transport and monitor unstable patients, longer scan times, limited availability, and contraindications in certain patients (pacemakers, intraocular metallic foreign bodies).

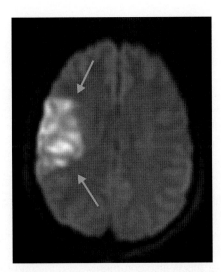

Fig. C1.3 Axial DWI shows a wedge-shaped area of bright signal (arrows) signifying an acute infarct. Corresponding ADC map (not shown) demonstrated decreased signal in this area.

Intravenous treatment of acute ischemic stroke with r-TPA can be considered if it is less than 4.5 hours since symptom onset, there is no CT evidence of hemorrhage, and the infarct does not involve more than one-third of the MCA distribution. Intra-arterial treatment with r-TPA can be considered up to 6 hours after symptom onset.

DIFFERENTIAL DIAGNOSIS
Clinical Differential

- Acute hemorrhagic infarct
- Neoplasm
- Encephalitis
- Todd's paralysis

Imaging Differential

- Hyperdense vessel: high hematocrit, atherosclerosis.
- Parenchymal hypodensity: infiltrating neoplasm, encephalitis/cerebritis, encephalomalacia, dural venous thrombosis with venous congestion and edema.

REFERENCES AND SUGGESTED READING

1. Hand PJ, Wardlaw JM, Rowat AM, et al. Magnetic resonance brain imaging in patients with acute stroke: feasibility and patient related difficulties. *J Neurol Neurosurg Psychiatry.* 2005;76:1525-1527.

2. Jeffrey RB, Manaster BJ, Gurney JW, et al. *Diagnostic Imaging: Emergency.* 3rd ed. Salt Lake City, UT: Amirsys; 2007:32-343. Yousem DM, Grossman RI. *Neuroradiology: The Requisites.* Philadelphia, PA: Mosby; 2010:117-127.

CASE 2

PATIENT PRESENTATION

A 59-year-old hypertensive male presents to the emergency department with headache and acute sensory deficit.

CLINICAL SUSPICION

Hypertensive hemorrhagic stroke

IMAGING MODALITY OF CHOICE

CT head without contrast to evaluate for presence of hemorrhage (Fig. C2.1). Advantages: fast and readily available, high sensitivity for presence of hemorrhage.

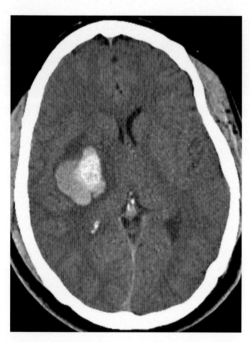

Fig. C2.1 Noncontrast CT shows an oval hyperdense acute bleed centered in the right basal ganglia.

FINDINGS

Chronic hypertension results in damage to small perforating arteries leading to fibrinoid necrosis and vessel fragility. Hemorrhagic strokes account for only 10% of all strokes (the majority are ischemic) and are associated with a higher mortality rate. Patients with hypertension have a fourfold increased risk of intracranial hemorrhage. The most common locations include the basal ganglia/external capsule, thalamus, brain stem, and cerebellum; however, approximately 10% are lobar. Initially, there may be little mass effect or surrounding edema; however, this often develops in the first couple of days leading to patient deterioration. As treatment differs markedly from ischemic stroke, prompt diagnosis is essential.

CT

- Round or oval hyperdense lesion in the brain parenchyma on noncontrast CT with predilection for certain locations as described earlier.
- Other evidence of hypertensive cerebrovascular disease including chronic lacunar infarcts, multiple subacute/chronic microbleeds, and microvascular white matter changes.

MR

Hemorrhage on MR has varied imaging characteristics (Table C2.1, Figs. C2.2 and C2.3):

- Gradient echo sequences may show several hypointense foci secondary to microbleeds. It is important to note that this is also commonly seen in cerebral amyloid angiopathy (disorder of vascular amyloid deposition leading to multiple bleeds).
- No/mild peripheral contrast enhancement.

Table C2.1 Characteristics of Hemorrhage on MR

Age of Hemorrhage	Component	T1	T2
Hyperacute	Oxyhemoglobin	Isointense/hypointense	Hyperintense
Acute	Deoxyhemoglobin	Isointense/hypointense	Hypointense
Subacute	Methemoglobin	Hyperintense	Hyperintense
Chronic	Hemosiderin/ferritin	Hypointense	Hypointense

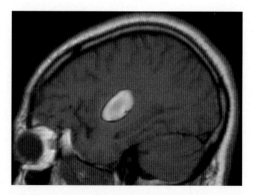

Fig. C2.2 Corresponding sagittal follow-up MRI with bright T1 and T2 FLAIR signal consistent with a late subacute hemorrhage.

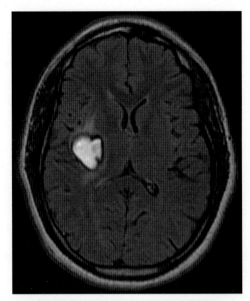

Fig. C2.3 Corresponding axial follow-up MRI with bright T1 and T2 FLAIR signal consistent with a late subacute hemorrhage.

DIFFERENTIAL DIAGNOSIS

Clinical Differential

- Ischemic stroke
- Neoplasm
- Encephalitis/meningitis

Imaging Differential

- Hemorrhagic transformation of an ischemic infarct
- Cerebral amyloid angiopathy
- Underlying neoplasm or vascular lesion
- Cocaine abuse
- Coagulopathy
- Venous thrombosis

REFERENCES AND SUGGESTED READING

1. Jeffrey RB, Manaster BJ, Gurney JW, et al. *Diagnostic Imaging: Emergency.* Salt Lake City, UT: Amirsys 2007:24-26.

2. Yousem DM, Grossman RI. *Neuroradiology: The Requisites.* 3rd ed. Philadelphia, PA: Mosby; 2010:149-153.

CASE 3

PATIENT PRESENTATION

Patient presents to the emergency department after hitting his head in a car accident.

CLINICAL SUSPICION

Traumatic intracranial extra-axial hemorrhage

IMAGING MODALITY OF CHOICE

CT head without contrast. Advantages: fast and readily available, high sensitivity for presence of hemorrhage.

FINDINGS

Injuries involving the central nervous system are the leading cause of death in trauma patients. Intracranial hemorrhage is often seen in patients with moderate to severe head trauma. Acute hemorrhage is usually hyperdense on noncontrast CT images. In some instances the hemorrhage may have low density due to severe anemia, DIC, and hyperacute active bleeding, making its detection more difficult. There are several types of extra-axial hemorrhage based on location, as shown in Fig. C3.1.

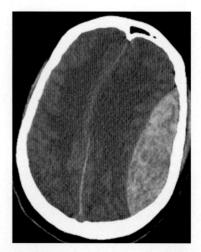

Fig. C3.2 Lens-shaped left frontoparietal epidural hematoma with an overlying skull fracture.

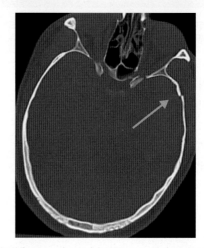

Fig. C3.3 Skull fracture (arrow) in the same injury shown in Fig. C3.2.

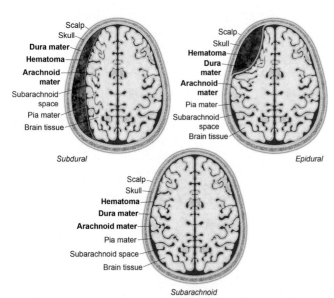

Fig. C3.1 Types of extra-axial hemorrhage.

Epidural Hematoma (EDH)

The epidural space is a potential space between the inner table of the skull and the dura mater. CT shows a hyperdense biconvex extra-axial collection (Figs. C3.2 and C3.3). It does not cross suture lines due to firm attachment of the dura to the suture but may cross the midline. Bleeding most commonly results from tearing of the middle meningeal artery from calvarial fracture, secondary to trauma. Most epidural hematomas are found in the temporal and parietal regions. They may also be found in the posterior fossa secondary to a venous sinus tear. Approximately half of patients will have a lucid interval after the insult.

Subdural Hematoma (SDH)

Collection of blood in the space between the dura mater and the arachnoid layer. CT shows a hyperdense crescentic extra-axial collection (Fig. C3.4). It can cross suture lines but does not cross the midline. Bleeding results from tearing of bridging cortical veins as a result of rotational motion of the brain with respect to the fixed venous structures. This most commonly occurs over the cerebral convexities. Subdural hematomas are often secondary to trauma but can occur secondary to minor trauma in elderly patients and patients on anticoagulation.

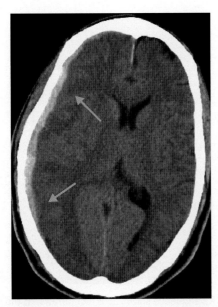

Fig. C3.4 Noncontrast CT (NECT) shows a cresent-shaped hyperdensity (arrow) overlying the right cerebral convexity consistent with acute subdural hematoma.

Subarachnoid Hemorrhage (SAH)

CT shows hyperdensity in the subarachnoid space (Fig. C3.5); 4 different patterns may be seen.

- Adjacent to intraparenchymal or extraparenchymal hematomas: common in severe head trauma.

- Overlying the cerebral hemispheres in isolation: common in mild and moderate head trauma.

- Extensive hemorrhage within the basal cisterns and subarachnoid space: often seen in the setting of nontraumatic subarachnoid hemorrhage from ruptured aneurysm or arteriovenous malformation (AVM). It can also occur from traumatic arterial dissection, sometimes with concomitant skull base fracture.

- Nontraumatic perimesencephalic hemorrhage: focal small hemorrhage in the interpeduncular cistern can be seen in patients presenting with headache without aneurysm. It usually results in no long-term clinical sequelae.

  It is critical to evaluate patients with SAH for an intracranial aneurysm, regardless of a history of head trauma. A ruptured aneurysm may have been the precipitating event prior to the incident leading to the head trauma.

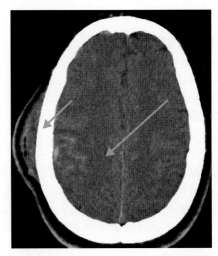

Fig. C3.5 Noncontrast CT shows hyperdensity from subarachnoid hemorrhage in the parietal sulci (long arrow) with overlying soft tissue swelling (short arrow).

DIFFERENTIAL DIAGNOSIS

Clinical Differential

Epidural hemorrhage, subdural hemorrhage, subarachnoid hemorrhage, diffuse axonal injury (DAI), and concussion.

Imaging Differential

- Epidural hemorrhage: subdural hemorrhage, abscess, tumor, inflammatory lesion, extramedullary hematopoiesis.

- Subdural hemorrhage: EDH, subdural hygroma, pachymeningitis (thickened dura), tumor.

- Subarachnoid hemorrhage: exudates in the subarachnoid space, serpentine calcifications from cortical laminar necrosis, arteriovenous malformation, Sturge-Weber syndrome, racemous neurocysticercosis.

REFERENCES AND SUGGESTED READING

1. Jeffrey RB, Manaster BJ, Gurney JW, et al. *Diagnostic Imaging: Emergency*. Salt Lake City, UT: Amirsys; 2007:2-10,16-18.

2. Yousem DM, Grossman RI. *Neuroradiology: The Requisites*. 3rd ed. Philadelphia, PA: Mosby; 2010:159-160,170-174.

CASE 4

PATIENT PRESENTATION

An unconscious trauma patient presents to the emergency department and has a normal noncontrast head CT.

CLINICAL SUSPICION

Diffuse axonal injury (traumatic brain injury)

IMAGING MODALITY OF CHOICE

MRI brain without contrast. Advantages: excellent contrast between normal and edematous brain parenchyma, highly sensitive for small hemorrhages due to susceptibility of blood products.

FINDINGS

Diffuse axonal injury (DAI) is a shearing/stress injury caused by rotational acceleration/deceleration movements of the head. Brain tissues of different densities accelerate/ decelerate at varying speeds, and particularly in regions where these tissues intersect the axons get stretched, resulting in damage. Small white matter vessels may also tear, resulting in petechial hemorrhages. Injuries are most commonly nonhemorrhagic, but hemorrhagic lesions also occur. Initial noncontrast CT is usually normal.

MRI

Multiple bilateral punctate to 1.5 cm round or ovoid foci with the long axis parallel to fiber bundles.

- Nonhemorrhagic foci: bright on T2-weighted and FLAIR sequences.
- Hemorrhagic foci: bright on T1, dark on T2, bright on FLAIR, and very dark on gradient echo images (due to susceptibility from blood products). GRE is the most sensitive sequence.
- DWI may show areas of restricted diffusion (bright signal).

Lesions are found in characteristic locations with increasing order of injury severity:

1. Gray-white matter junction, typically in the frontal and temporal lobes, and cerebral white matter (Figs. C4.1 and C4.2).
2. Corpus callosum, most common in the splenium.
3. Dorsal upper brain stem and cerebellum.
4. Additional less common locations: deep gray matter, internal/external capsule, tegmentum, and fornix. Lesion burden on MRI may predict the degree of potential neurological recovery.

Additional MRI sequences can be performed such as diffusion tensor imaging and MR spectroscopy, which can

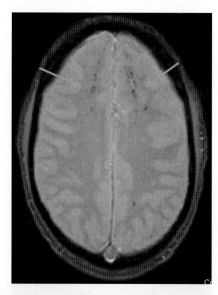

Fig. C4.1 GRE sequence shows dark foci (arrows) at the gray-white junctions indicative of blood products from shearing injuries.

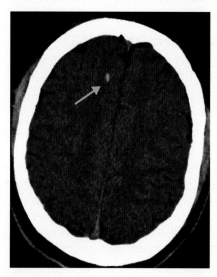

Fig. C4.2 NECT shows an oval hyperdense hemorrhagic lesion (arrow) at the gray-white interface.

be helpful in cases in which conventional MR imaging is inconclusive.

CT

- May show punctate areas of high density (hemorrhage) surrounded by a collar of low-density edema.
- Usually underestimates the extent of the disease.

DAI should be considered if the patient's symptoms are disproportionate to the imaging findings. DAI carries a poor prognosis, and patients may remain in a persistent vegetative state.

DIFFERENTIAL DIAGNOSIS

Clinical Differential

EDH, SDH, SAH

Imaging Differential

- Multifocal nonhemorrhagic lesions: age-related lesions (leukoaraiosis and lacunes), demyelinating disease, Marchiafava-Bignami syndrome (corpus callosum lesions).

- Multifocal hemorrhagic lesions: cerebral amyloid angiopathy, chronic hypertension, cavernous malformations, hemorrhagic metastases.

REFERENCES AND SUGGESTED READING

1. American College of Radiology. ACR Appropriateness Criteria. Head trauma. http://www.acr.org/SecondaryMain MenuCategories/quality_safety/app_criteria/pdf/ ExpertPanelonNeurologicImaging/HeadTraumaDoc5.aspx. Accessed November 19, 2011.

2. Jeffrey RB, Manaster BJ, Gurney JW, et al. *Diagnostic Imaging: Emergency*. Salt Lake City, UT: Amirsys; 2007:1-24.

3. Yousem DM, Grossman RI. *Neuroradiology: The Requisites*. 3rd ed. Philadelphia, PA: Mosby; 2010:180-181.

CASE 5

PATIENT PRESENTATION

A 24-year-old pregnant female presents to her physician with elevated blood pressure and sudden onset of headache and visual disturbance.

CLINICAL SUSPICION

Posterior reversible encephalopathy syndrome (PRES)

IMAGING MODALITY OF CHOICE

MRI head with and without contrast (include DWI). Advantages: T2/FLAIR images are sensitive for edema.

FINDINGS

Bilateral, symmetric, patchy abnormalities classically involving the subcortical white matter of the occipital and parietal lobes. It may also extend to the cortex and involve the temporal and frontal lobes, pons, and cerebellum.

CT

Hypodensity in the subcortical white matter of the occipital and parietal lobes (Figs. C5.1 and C5.2).

MRI

- T2-weighted image/FLAIR: high signal intensity in the affected areas.
- T1-weighted image: corresponding low signal intensity.
- DWI-ADC map: areas of DWI abnormality without ADC correlation are more common, but irreversible ischemia (high DWI signal with decreased ADC signal) may occur.
- Enhancement can be seen but is not a common finding.
- MR perfusion: may show decreased relative cerebral blood volume, decreased cerebral blood flow, and increased mean transit time.
- Areas of hemorrhage are seen in approximately 15% of patients.

Angiography (MRA or Conventional)

May demonstrate a vasculopathy type pattern with areas of vessel irregularity, consistent with vasoconstriction/vasodilation.

The underlying etiology of PRES is thought to be the inability of the posterior circulation to autoregulate in response to acute changes in blood pressure. This results in vascular damage and breakdown of the blood-brain barrier leading to vasogenic edema. Symptoms include headache,

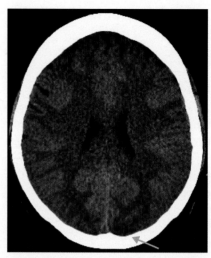

Fig. C5.1 Hypodensity in the left posterior parieto-occipital area in a patient with severe hypertension (arrow).

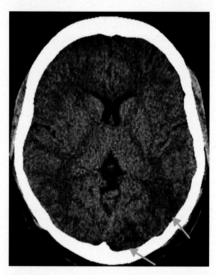

Fig. C5.2 Hypodensity in the left posterior parieto-occipital area in a patient with severe hypertension (arrows).

confusion, seizures, and loss of vision. Interestingly, hypertension is absent in approximately 25% of patients with PRES, alluding to alternative underlying mechanisms of the disease. With prompt diagnosis and treatment of the underlying cause, PRES is usually reversible; in some instances it may progress to infarction.

PRES may be caused by hypertension, preeclampsia/eclampsia, immunosuppressive drugs, chemotherapy (tacrolimus and cyclosporine), sepsis, renal disease, autoimmune diseases, cryoglobulinemia, and hemolytic-uremic syndrome.

DIFFERENTIAL DIAGNOSIS

Clinical Differential

- Primary headache/migraine
- Preeclampsia/eclampsia not associated with PRES
- Venous sinus thrombosis
- Intraparenchymal hemorrhage

Imaging Differential

- Acute ischemic infarct
- Status epilepticus
- Metabolic abnormalities
- Gliomatosis cerebr

REFERENCES AND SUGGESTED READING

1. Bartynski WS. Posterior reversible encephalopathy syndrome, part 1: fundamental imaging and clinical features. *AJNR*. 2008;29:1036-1042.
2. Jeffrey RB, Manaster BJ, Gurney JW, et al. *Diagnostic Imaging: Emergency*. Salt Lake City, UT: Amirsys; 2007;28-30.

CASE 6

PATIENT PRESENTATION

A 28-year-old female presents with sudden onset of severe headache, confusion, and right extremity weakness.

CLINICAL SUSPICION

Intracranial hemorrhage, possibly from vascular malformation

IMAGING MODALITY OF CHOICE

CT head without contrast in the acute setting followed by CTA or MRA. Definitive diagnosis/characterization performed with catheter angiography. Advantages: fast and readily available, high sensitivity for presence of hemorrhage.

FINDINGS

Arteriovenous malformations are abnormal connections/ networks of blood vessels that result in arteriovenous shunting of blood, bypassing blood supply to the brain tissue (Fig. C6.1A,B). They are characterized by an enlarged feeding artery/arteries leading to a nidus of entangled abnormal vessels (no true capillary bed) and early drainage into enlarged draining veins (Fig. C6.2). In the acute setting, noncontrast head CT is the imaging modality of choice.

CT

- Intraparenchymal hematoma if ruptured. Can also result in intraventricular or subarachnoid hemorrhage.
- If unruptured, hyperdense serpentine mass lesion.
- Curvilinear or speckled calcifications may be seen.
- Surrounding hypodensity of gliosis (chronic ischemia or previous hemorrhage).

CTA/MRA

- Intensely enhancing curvilinear structures on CTA, curvilinear flow voids on MRI.
- Dilated feeding arteries and draining veins; veins typically larger than arteries.
- Intranidal aneurysms (found more than 50% of the time).

Catheter angiography provides dynamic information showing the arterial supply and venous drainage of the lesion.

Pitfalls in diagnosis can occur with small lesions, location near a major dural venous sinus, and due to compression from acute hematoma (repeat angiogram is warranted if initial study is normal).

AVMs can be classified using the Spetzler-Martin grading system in order to predict operative outcomes as shown in Table C6.1 (graded 1 to 5 by adding the points in each category).

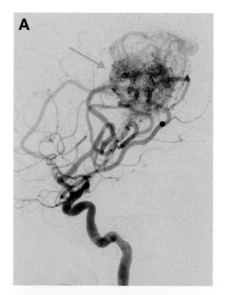

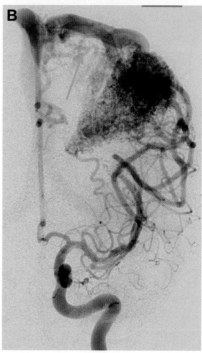

Fig. C6.1 Of left ICA injection shows an AVM nidus (A, arrow) with enlarged early draining cortical veins (B, arrow).

Grades 1 and 2 are treated with surgical resection; Grade 3 lesions receive multimodality treatment (microsurgery/endovascular/radiosurgery); Grades 4 and 5 are not treated, with the exception of recurrent hemorrhages, progressive neurological deficits, steal-related symptoms, and AVM-related aneurysms. Imaging features that are associated with a risk of future hemorrhage include prior hemorrhage (low signal intensity on gradient echo sequence), intranidal aneurysms, venous stasis or ectasia, deep venous drainage, single venous drainage,

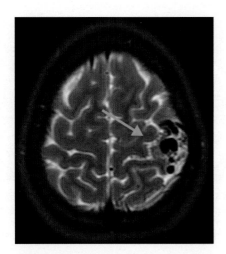

Fig. C6.2 T2-weighted image shows dark serpiginous flow voids (arrow) classic of an AVM.

and deep or posterior fossa locations. Imaging features associated with risk of nonhemorrhagic neurological deficits include high-flow shunt, venous congestion or outflow obstruction, long pial course of draining vein, perifocal or perinidal gliosis, mass effect or hydrocephalus, and arterial steal.

Table C6.1 Spetzler-Martin Grading System

Size of Nidus	Venous Drainage	Adjacent Eloquent Brain
Small (<3cm) = 1	Superficial only = 0	No = 0
Medium (3-6 cm) = 2	Deep = 1	Yes = 1
Large (>6 cm) = 3		

The term *eloquent brain* is defined as regions of the brain that control speech, motor, or sensory function.

DIFFERENTIAL DIAGNOSIS

Clinical Differential

CVA, underlying neoplasm, amyloid angiopathy

Imaging Differential

Hypertensive bleed, other vascular lesions (cavernous hemangioma), intratumoral hemorrhage, dural sinus thrombosis with hemorrhagic infarct, mycotic aneurysm, drug abuse.

REFERENCES AND SUGGESTED READING

1. Geibprasert S, Pongpech S, Fiarakongmun P, et al. Radiologic assessment of brain arteriovenous malformations: what clinicians need to know. *Radiographics.* 2010;30(2):483-501.

2. Jeffrey RB, Manaster BJ, Gurney JW, et al. *Diagnostic Imaging: Emergency.* Salt Lake City, UT: Amirsys; 2007:65.

3. Spetzler RF, Martin NA. A proposed grading system for arteriovenous malformations. *J Neurosurg.* 1986;65(4):476-483.

4. Spetzler RF, Ponce FA. A 3-tier classification of cerebral arteriovenous malformations. *J Neurosurg.* 2011;114(3):842-849.

5. Yousem DM, Grossman RI. *Neuroradiology: The Requisites.* 3rd ed. Philadelphia, PA: Mosby; 2010:165-167.

CASE 7

PATIENT PRESENTATION

A 53-year-old female with history of hypertension present-ing with complaints of intermittent headache. Patient recalls having been diagnosed with benign tumor many years ago.

CLINICAL SUSPICION

Meningioma

IMAGING MODALITY OF CHOICE

In the acute setting, noncontrast CT is obtained to exclude intracranial hemorrhage. MRI is preferred for evaluation of intracranial neoplasms as it provides greater sensitivity, su-perior parenchymal detail, and better tissue contrast.

FINDINGS

Meningiomas are tumors that arise from the meninges and as a result are extra-axial. While most meningiomas are benign (WHO Grade 1), atypical (WHO Grade 2) and ma-lignant meningiomas (WHO Grade 3) can rarely be seen.

CT

- Hyperdense extra-axial mass on noncontrast CT (Fig. C7.1)
- 20% to 25% are calcified
- Hyperostosis (thickening) of the adjacent calvarium
- Avidly enhance, with enhancement of a dural tail

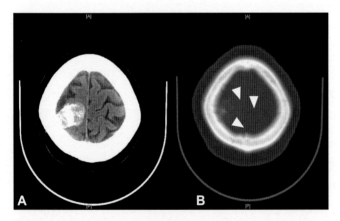

Fig. C7.1 (A) Axial noncontrast CT images at the convexities in brain windows demonstre a hyperattenuating extra-axial mass without significant edema. (B) Bone algorithm reveals minimal calcific content (arrowheads).

MRI

- T1: isointense to hypointense to cerebral cortex; may be heterogeneous due to cystic degeneration and/or hemorrhage (Fig. C7.2).

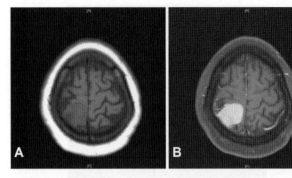

Fig. C7.2 (A) Axial T1 precontrast MRI and (B) postcontrast fat-saturated images demonstrate an enhancing, dural-based mass that measures almost 4 cm in greatest dimension. The mass is nearly isointense to the brain parenchyma on precontrast imaging.

- T2: variable, large lesions can be associated with edema within the subjacent brain parenchyma; visualization of a CSF cleft between mass and adjacent brain paren-chyma is helpful in diagnosis of an extra-axial mass.
- T1+C: avid enhancement with enhancement of a dural tail (Fig. C7.3).

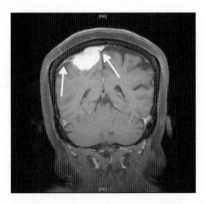

Fig. C7.3 Coronal postcontrast T1 fat-saturated image demon-strating large, extra-axial enhancing mass displacing brain tissue inferiorly. The dural tails are better apparent (arrows).

DIFFERENTIAL DIAGNOSIS

Clinical Differential

While most patients with typical meningioma are asymp-tomatic, patients with larger lesions may present with varied symptoms based upon the location of the lesion. Parasagit-tal lesions may present with seizures and weakness; basi-sphenoid/diaphragm sella lesions with visual defects, and cavernous sinus lesions with cranial nerve palsies.

Imaging Differential

- Metastasis: Dural-based metastasis can mimic meningi-omas; however, patients usually have a known primary tumor and may have other sites of metastatic disease.

- Granuloma: Meningeal involvement from sarcoid or TB can mimic meningioma; however, these patients often have signs/symptoms of disease elsewhere in the body.
- Lymphoma: Extra-axial areas of lymphomatous involvement are usually multifocal and present in patients with known history of lymphoma. Lesions demonstrate hypointensity on T2 images due to hypercellularity.
- Hemangiopericytoma: Can mimic meningioma; however, calcification and hyperostosis are usually absent. Enhancement is usually more heterogeneous.

REFERENCES AND SUGGESTED READING

1. Beutow MP, Beutow PC, Smirniotopoulos JG. From the archives of the AFIP: typical, atypical and misleading features of meningioma. *Radiographics*. 1991;11:1087-1106.
2. Shaman MA, Zak IT, Kupskey WJ. Best cases from the AFIP: involuted sclerotic meningioma. *Radiographics*. 2003;23: 785-780.

CASE 8

PATIENT PRESENTATION

A 48-year-old male presents to his physician with new-onset seizures.

CLINICAL SUSPICION

High-grade glioma / glioblastoma multiforme (GBM)

IMAGING MODALITY OF CHOICE

MRI brain with and without contrast. Advantages: MRI is preferred for evaluation of intracranial neoplasms as it provides greater sensitivity, superior parenchymal detail, and better tissue contrast. Diffusion weighted imaging, perfusion imaging, and MR spectroscopy may be helpful in evaluation of intracranial neoplasms.

FINDINGS

While most intra-axial neoplasms are metastatic, glioblastoma multiforme (WHO grade 4 tumor) accounts for approximately 25% of all intra-axial neoplasms. It is a highly malignant infiltrating astrocytoma with a poor prognosis (10%-15% two-year survival). These tumors can occur anywhere but most commonly arise, in decreasing order of frequency, in the temporal, parietal, and frontal lobes. GBMs can either be a primary tumor (arising de novo) or a secondary tumor (resulting from dedifferentiation of a lower grade astrocytoma).

MRI

- T1: usually heterogeneously isointense to hypointense. Heterogeneity results from internal necrosis; some cases present with hemorrhage.
- T2/FLAIR: heterogneously hyperintense with surrounding edema/infiltrative tumor (Fig. C8.1).

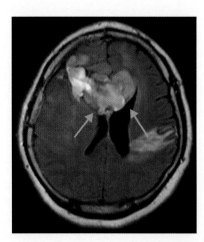

Fig. C8.1 T2 FLAIR shows a slightly heterogenous hyperintense mass crossing the corpus callosum (arrows) giving the classic appearance of a "butterfly" tumor.

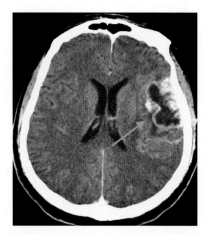

Fig. C8.2 Contrast-enhanced CT reveals a ring-enhancing lesion (arrow) in a different patient with thick peripheral nodularity, biopsy-proven GBM.

- T1+C: variable. Typically there is an irregular rind of enhancement surrounding a central area of necrosis (Fig. C8.2).

The tumor frequently crosses the midline to the contralateral hemisphere by direct extension through the corpus callosum, anterior commisure, or posterior commisure ("butterfly" tumor). It is important to realize that microscopic infiltration of tumor beyond the borders of imaging abnormality. Increased relative cerebral blood volume (rCBV) can be seen on perfusion studies and has been shown to correlate with the histological grade (higher rCBV = higher histological grade). The presence of lactic acid on MR spectroscopy and the presence of intratumoral hemorrhage have also been linked to higher-grade tumors.

DIFFERENTIAL DIAGNOSIS

Clinical Differential

- Medication/drug related seizures, CVA, metabolic disorder, meningitis/encephalitis, posttraumatic, autoimmune/degenerative diseases, neoplasm.

Imaging Differential

- Metastasis.
- Ring-enhancing lesions: abscess, demyelinating disease, resolving hematoma, subacute cerebral infarction, radiation necrosis.
- Corpus callosum lesions: lymphoma, multiple sclerosis.

REFERENCE AND SUGGESTED READING

1. Yousem DM, Grossman RI. *Neuroradiology: The Requisites.* 3rd ed. Philadelphia, PA: Mosby; 2010:72,76-78.

CASE 9

PATIENT PRESENTATION

Patient presents to the emergency department with seizure and has a history of AIDS.

CLINICAL SUSPICION

Opportunistic infection versus neoplasm

IMAGING MODALITY OF CHOICE

MRI brain with and without contrast. Advantages: MRI is preferred for evaluation of intracranial infections or neoplasms as it provides greater sensitivity, superior parenchymal detail, and better tissue contrast.

FINDINGS

The vast majority of primary CNS lymphoma is non-Hodgkins lymphoma and usually occurs in immunocompromised individuals. These lesions are mostly supratentorial in location (above the tentorium cerebelli) and commonly involve the periventricular white matter and deep gray matter. CNS lymphoma may spread along the ventricular lining (subependymal) and cross the midline. It usually presents with multiple lesions that are less than 2 cm in size. Primary CNS lymphoma in immunocompetent patients is less often seen and usually has a later onset.

CT

- High-density mass/masses typically periventricular in location on noncontrast exam with variable enhancement.
- Central necrosis may be present; hemorrhage rarely present.

MR

- T1: isointense or hypointense lesions (Fig. C9.1).
- T2/FLAIR: variable; approximately half will be isointense or slightly hypointense owing to tumor cellularity. Increased T2/FLAIR signal surrounding lesions representing edema.
- T1+C: variable, usually solid or ring enhancement (Fig. C9.2).
- DWI: mildly restricted diffusion due to high cellularity.

An alternative diagnosis found in AIDS patients that must be differentiated from lymphoma (due to similar imaging characteristics) is toxoplasmosis (Table C9.1). Toxoplasmosis is the most common cause of focal lesions in AIDS patients.

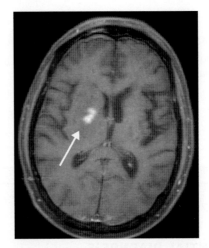

Fig. C9.1 T1 postcontrast image shows a lobulated diffusely enhancing mass in the right basal ganglia in an AIDS patient.

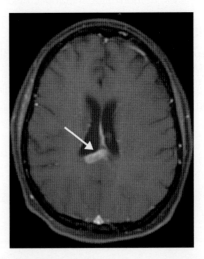

Fig. C9.2 Another AIDS patient with an oval enhancing lesion in the right splenium, crossing midline.

Table C9.1 Lymphoma Versus Toxoplasmosis in AIDS

Characteristic	Lymphoma	Toxoplasmosis
Present with solitary lesion	19%	39%
Lesion size	53% 1-3 cm	52% <1 cm
Solid enhancement	76% if <1 cm, 50% if >1 cm	77% if <1 cm, 23% if >1 cm
Ring enhancement	24% if <1 cm, 50% if >1 cm	23% if <1 cm, 77% if >1 cm
Dense on noncontrast CT	33% of lesions	None
T2-weighted image	55% isointense	Usually hyperintense or mixed
Periventricular/subependymal/ corpus callosum location	25% of pts/38%/3%	3% of pts/none/none
Basal ganglia location	7% of pts	17% of pts
Thallium-201 SPECT scan	Avid uptake (>2cm lesions)	No uptake
MR perfusion	Increased rCBV	Decreased rCBV
MRS	Increased choline and lipid, low NAA	Increased lactate
Steroid/radiation therapy	Very sensitive	No response

From Dina [1] and Yousem and Grossman [4] (see references).

DIFFERENTIAL DIAGNOSIS

Clinical Differential

HIV encephalitis, other CNS infections (toxoplasmosis, CMV, PML, aspergillosis, cryptococcus, TB), alcohol withdrawal, drug toxicity, CVA, hemorrhage, metabolic disorders.

Imaging Differential

- Diffuse/patchy WM abnormalities in AIDS: HIV encephalitis, PML, CMV.
- Focal/multifocal brain lesions in AIDS: toxoplasmosis, lymphoma, tuberculoma, fungal, abscess.

REFERENCES AND SUGGESTED READING

1. Dina TS. Primary central nervous system lymphoma versus toxoplasmosis in AIDS. *Radiology.* 1991;179(3):823-828.
2. Jeffrey RB, Manaster BJ, Gurney JW, et al. *Diagnostic Imaging: Emergency.* Salt Lake City, UT: Amirsys; 2007:60-61.
3. Lee GT, Antelo F, Mlikotic AA. Best cases from the AFIP: cerebral toxoplasmosis. *Radiographics.* 2009;29(4):1200-1205.
4. Yousem DM, Grossman RI. *Neuroradiology: The Requisites.* 3rd ed. Philadelphia, PA: Mosby; 2010:93-94,208-209.

CASE 10

PATIENT PRESENTATION

A 5-year-old female presents to the clinic with several-week history of increasing ataxia and 3-day history of nausea/vomiting.

CLINICAL SUSPICION

Brain tumor

IMAGING MODALITY OF CHOICE

Contrast-enhanced MRI examination. Advantages: provides excellent soft tissue contrast without any radiation exposure.

FINDINGS

Most primary intracranial neoplasms in children occur within the posterior fossa. Patients with posterior fossa tumors can present with symptoms of increased intracranial pressure and cerebellar signs/ataxia. The 3 most common histological lesions are pilocytic astrocytoma, medulloblastoma, and ependymoma in order of decreasing frequency. There are imaging features that may help differentiate these lesions (Figs. C10.1-C10.3).

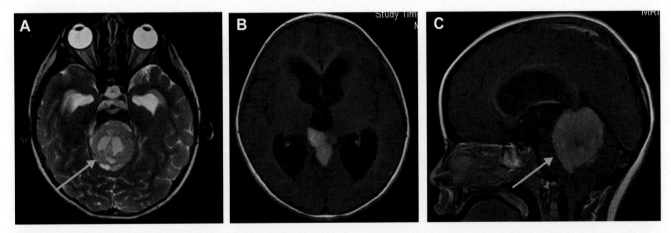

Fig. C10.1 Axial T2 (left) and axial post-contrast (middle) and sagittal post-contrast (right) images demonstrate a heterogeneous mass within the posterior fossa (arrows). Note the presence of obstructive hydrocephalus. Pathology revealed pilocytic astrocytoma.

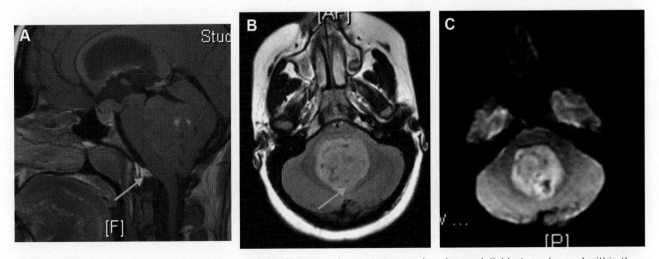

Fig. C10.2 Sagittal postcontrast (A), Axial T2 (B), and DWI (C) images demonstrate an enhancing medulloblastoma (arrows) within the posterior fossa. Tumor demonstrated mildly restricted diffusion.

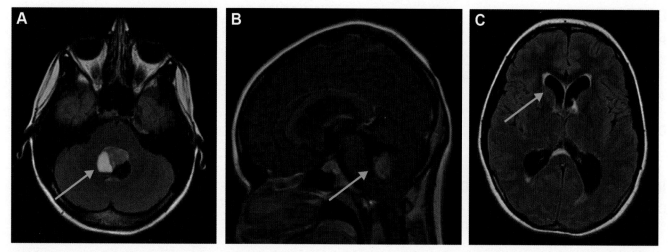

Fig. C10.3 (A) Axial FLAIR image at the level of the posterior fossa ependymoma (arrow) demonstrates a heterogenous mass centered within the fourth ventricle. (B) Sagittal postcontrast image. (C) Axial FLAIR image demonstrates the presence of hydrocephalus (arrow).

Pilocytic Astrocytoma

- WHO Grade 1 astrocytoma
- Peak age of incidence between 5 and 15 years
- 60% of cases occur in the cerebellum, 25% to 30% involve optic pathway
- Usually presents as a cyst with a mural nodule
- CT
  - Cystic lesion with solid mural nodule
  - Calcifications seen in 20%; hemorrhage rarely seen
  - Can cause obstructive hydrocephalus
- MR
  - Cyst contents similar in signal to CSF, but hyperintense on FLAIR images
  - Solid mural nodule that demonstrates intense but heterogeneous contrast enhancement

Medulloblastoma

- Highly malignant WHO Grade 4 primitive neuroectodermal tumor (PNET)
- Arises from the roof of the fourth ventricle, although it may arise from the cerebellar hemispheres in older patients
- CT
  - Hyperdense on NECT
  - Calcifications can be seen in 20% of cases
  - Intratumoral cysts/necrosis in 40% to 50% of cases
  - Often result in hydrocephalus due to obstruction of the fourth ventricle

- MRI
  - T1 isointense, T2 isointense to hyperintense
  - Avidly enhances with contrast
  - Restrict diffusion
- As up to one-third of patients have subarachnoid dissemination, it is critical to image the entire neuraxis.

Ependymoma

- WHO grade 2/3
- Peak age of 1 to 5 years
- Two-thirds are infratentorial, most within fourth ventricle
- Extend from fourth ventricles in to the cisterns
- Can contain hemorrhage, cysts, and calcifications
- CT
  - Fourth ventricular mass with extension through foramen magnum, or extending into the CPA
  - Calcifications, cysts, hemorrhage commonly seen
- MR
  - Heterogenous on T1- and T2-weighted imaging due to cystic foci, hemorrhage, and calcifications
  - Mild to moderate heterogenous enhancement

DIFFERENTIAL DIAGNOSIS

Clinical Differential

Signs and symptoms associated with posterior fossa brain tumors can also be seen in a variety of nonneoplastic conditions, some of which include:

- Seizure disorder
- Pediatric stroke
- CNS infection or postinfectious syndromes

Imaging Differential

The 3 most common pediatric posterior fossa tumors discussed can have overlapping imaging findings; however, the majority of cases can be reliably distinguished based on imaging.

REFERENCES AND SUGGESTED READING

1. Poretti A, Meoded A, Huisman TA. Neuroimaging of pediatric posterior fossa tumors including review of the literature. *J Magn Reson Imaging*. January 2012;35(1):32-47.
2. Yousem DM, Grossman RI. *Neuroradiology: The Requisites*. 3rd ed. Philadelphia, PA: Mosby; 2010:93-94,208-209.

CASE 11

PATIENT PRESENTATION

A 45-year-old female presents to the ED with visual field loss and a cranial nerve palsy.

CLINICAL SUSPICION

Pituitary adenoma

IMAGING MODALITY OF CHOICE

MRI with and without contrast with thin sagittal and coronal sectional imaging. Dynamic postcontrast coronal T1-weighted imaging is very sensitive for detecting small pituitary abnormalities (Figs. C11.1 and C11.2).

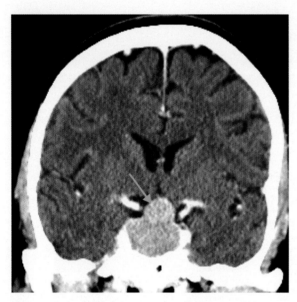

Fig. C11.1 Large enhancing mass (arrow) growing superiorly from the sella turcica with a "snowman" appearance; classic for a pituitary macroadenoma.

FINDINGS

Pituitary adenomas can be described as microadenomas (<10 mm) or macroadenomas (>10 mm). Approximately 75% of pituitary adenomas are hormonally active and are thus found when they are small (microadenomas). When they are not hormonally active, they grow to large sizes (macroadenomas) until patients become symptomatic secondary to mass effect/invasion of adjacent structures. When adenomas grow superiorly, they can compress the optic chiasm producing the classic bitemporal homonymous hemianopsia. At the level of the diaphragma sellae, the tumor gets a waistlike constriction, giving it a "snowman" appearance (soft tumor). Adenomas may also grow laterally and invade the cavernous sinus, producing cranial nerve palsies (CN III, IV, V$_1$, V$_2$, and VI).

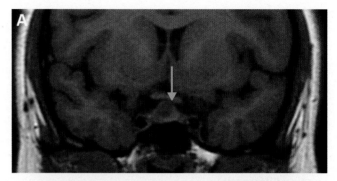

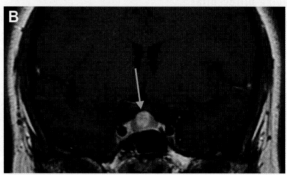

Fig. C11.2 T1 pre contrast (A) shows a subcentimeter hypointense lesion (arrow) in the pituitary gland that is diffusely enhancing on T1 postcontrast images (B) consistent with a microadenoma (arrow).

CT

- Adenomas are usually isodense to gray matter; however, they are often heterogeneous due to cystic formation, necrosis, and hemorrhage.
- With macroadenomas there may be widening and remodeling of the sella turcica. Calcifications are rare.
- Moderate heterogeneous enhancement.

MR

- T1: isointense to gray matter, but can be heterogenous.
- T2: variable signal intensity.
- T1 dynamic postcontrast images: most macroadenomas avidly enhance. Microadenomas enhance, but less than the background pituitary gland.

Determining whether cavernous sinus invasion is present is important, as there is increased morbidity and mortality associated with surgical intervention.

Detection of Cavernous Sinus Invasion

Indications that cavernous sinus invasion is *not* present:
- Tumor remains medial to a line drawn through the midline of the cavernous carotid artery.
- Tumor encases less than 25% of the intracavernous carotid artery.

- Normal pituitary tissue is present between the adenoma and the cavernous sinus.

Indications that cavernous sinus invasion is present:

- Tumor extends lateral to a line drawn along the lateral edge of the cavernous carotid artery.
- Tumor encases less than 50% of the intracavernous carotid artery.

DIFFERENTIAL DIAGNOSIS
Clinical Differential

- Any other mass lesion that can occur in the sellar/suprasellar space (listed under Imaging Differential).
- Multiple sclerosis.
- Inflammatory/infectious process.

Imaging Differential

Suprasellar mass lesions:

- Craniopharyngioma: calcifications and cystic areas are common.
- Rathke cleft cyst.

- Granulomatous hypophysitis.
- Meningioma: homogeneous enhancement, dural tail, and carotid artery narrowing.
- Hypothalamic or optic pathway glioma.
- Metastasis: finding additional lesions helps to suggest this diagnosis.

REFERENCES AND SUGGESTED READING

1. Cottier JP, Destrieux C, Brunereau L, et al. Cavernous sinus invasion by pituitary adenoma: MR imaging. *Radiology.* 2000;215(2):463-469.
2. Yousem DM, Grossman RI. *Neuroradiology: The Requisites.* 3rd ed. Philadelphia, PA: Mosby, 2010:364-367.

CASE 12

PATIENT PRESENTATION

A 17-year-old female presents to the ED complaining of headache and stiff neck.

CLINICAL SUSPICION

Meningitis

IMAGING MODALITY OF CHOICE

MRI brain with and without contrast (Figs. C12.1 and C12.2). Advantages: MRI is preferred for evaluation of intracranial infections as it provides greater sensitivity, superior parenchymal detail, and better tissue contrast.

FINDINGS

Meningitis, or leptomeningitis, is an inflammatory process involving the pia and arachnoid layers of the meninges. Although it is a clinical diagnosis, imaging plays an important role in looking for alternate diagnoses, evaluation prior to lumbar puncture, and to delineate complications of meningitis. Early in the disease process imaging findings are nonspecific and may be normal.

MR

- T2/FLAIR: hyperintense signal following the gyri/sulci or cisternal surface. Subdural collections, which may represent sterile effusions or empyemas.
- T1+C: linear enhancement along the gyri/sulci or cisterns (breakdown of the blood-brain barrier results in contrast leakage into the leptomeninges).
- DWI: increased signal with ADC correlation in areas of infarction.
- MRA: absent venous sinus flow voids if there is thrombosis.

Noncontrast CT of the head can also be performed during the initial workup to exclude subarachnoid hemorrhage or signs of increased intracranial pressure. This can be especially important prior to performing a lumbar puncture for cerebrospinal fluid analysis.

Contraindications to LP

- Impacted cerebellar tonsils in the foramen magnum
- Cerebellar herniation syndromes
- Obliterated or trapped fourth ventricle (expanded ventricle due to obstructed aqueduct and outlet foramina)
- Cerebellar mass or stroke
- Completely effaced basal cisterns/sulci
- Significant subfalcine herniation

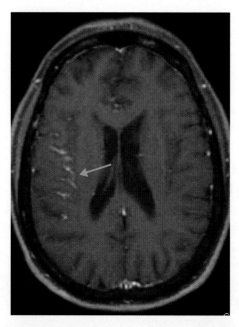

Fig. C12.1 T1 postcontrast image shows linear enhancement in the right sylvian sulci (arrow).

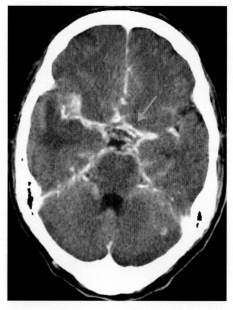

Fig. C12.2 Postcontrast CT, diffuse enhancement along the basal cisterns (arrow).

Complications of Meningitis

- Communicating hydrocephalus is the most common complication. Hydrocephalus implies increased CSF within the ventricular system. This may be due to obstruction within the ventricular system (noncommunicating) or at the level of the arachnoid granulations (communicating).

- Cerebritis/abscess, ventriculitis, subdural empyema.
- Arterial spasm, infectious vasculitis, or dural sinus thrombosis may lead to arterial or venous infarcts (bright signal on DWI).
- Labyrinthitis ossificans: infiltration of the cochlear channels by infected CSF that can result in bilateral hearing loss.

DIFFERENTIAL DIAGNOSIS
Clinical Differential

Migraine, tension headache, subarachnoid hemorrhage

Imaging Differential

Leptomeningeal carcinomatosis, sarcoidosis, subarachnoid hemorrhage, acute stroke. Increased CSF FLAIR signal can be seen with high inspired oxygen, artifact related, or with retained gadolinium in dialysis patients.

REFERENCES AND SUGGESTED READING

1. Hughes DC, Raghavan A, Mordekar SR, et al. Role of imaging in the diagnosis of acute bacterial meningitis and its complications. *Postgrad Med J.* 2010;86:478-485.
2. Jeffrey RB, Manaster BJ, Gurney JW, et al. *Diagnostic Imaging: Emergency.* Salt Lake City, UT: Amirsys; 2007:44-46.
3. Yousem DM, Grossman RI. *Neuroradiology: The Requisites.* 3rd ed. Philadelphia, PA: Mosby; 2010:193-196,253.

CASE 13

PATIENT PRESENTATION

A 37-year-old woman presents to her physician with monocular vision loss.

CLINICAL SUSPICION

Multiple sclerosis (MS)

IMAGING MODALITY OF CHOICE

MRI brain with and without contrast (including sagittal FLAIR sequence) (Figs. C13.1 and C13.2).

FINDINGS

MS is the most common demyelinating disorder in adults. It is thought to be an autoimmune disease with chronic inflammatory process resulting in loss of myelin. There is a female predominance, and it usually occurs between 20 and 40 years of age. MS is the leading cause of nontraumatic neurologic disability in young adults. The diagnosis of MS is based on clinical criteria, cerebrospinal fluid analysis, and MRI findings. MR imaging can be used to support the diagnosis, find alternative diagnoses, and monitor the effects of therapy.

MS lesions can occur anywhere in the brain or spinal cord but have a predilection for certain areas: the periventricular region (known as Dawson's fingers), corpus callosum, subcortical white matter, optic nerves and visual pathway, brain stem, cerebellar peduncles, and cervical spinal cord. Involvement of the callosal-septal interface on sagittal FLAIR images is classic.

MR

- T1: isointense to hypointense lesions with predilection of the above-mentioned locations.

- T2/FLAIR: Lesions are usually hyperintense in signal and ovoid in shape. "Dawson's fingers" is the classic description of perivenular extension along the deep medullary veins that run perpendicular to the long axis of the lateral ventricles (seen on sagittal sequence).

- T1+C: Not all lesions will enhance; enhancement implies active lesions (breakdown of the BBB secondary to inflammation). Nodular/ovoid uniform enhancement (new lesions) that can evolve to ring or arc shaped enhancement (reactivation of older lesions). Occasionally, a lesion may be large and exhibit mass effect simulating a neoplasm (tumefactive MS). These lesions have a leading edge of enhancement that incompletely surrounds the affected area.

- Atrophy of the brain and spinal cord may also be seen.

- Spinal cord lesions are typically peripheral, cross gray-white matter boundaries, and are less than 2 vertebral body segments in length.

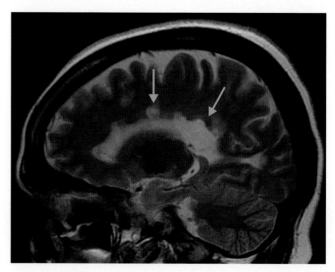

Fig. C13.1 Sagittal T2 shows the classic hyperintense ovoid lesions (arrows) oriented perpendicular to the long axis of the ventricles, "Dawson's fingers."

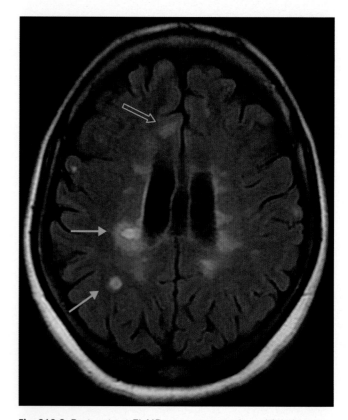

Fig. C13.2 Postcontrast FLAIR sequence reveals multiple hyperintense periventricular and subcortical (open arrow) white matter lesions, some enhancing (arrows).

DIFFERENTIAL DIAGNOSIS
Clinical Differential
- Transverse myelitis
- Lyme disease
- Sarcoidosis
- Vasculitides

Imaging Differential
- Small vessel ischemic disease
- Vasculopathy

- Migraine headaches
- Lyme disease
- Acute disseminated encephalomyelitis

REFERENCES AND SUGGESTED READING
1. Lovblad KO, Anzalone N, Dorfler A, et al. MR imaging in multiple sclerosis: review and recommendations for current practice. *AJNR*. 2010;31:983-989.
2. Yousem DM, Grossman RI. *Neuroradiology: The Requisites*. 3rd ed. Philadelphia, PA: Mosby; 2010:227-232.

CASE 14

PATIENT PRESENTATION

A 19-year-old male presents to his physician with a history of epilepsy.

CLINICAL SUSPICION

Mesial temporal sclerosis (MTS)

IMAGING MODALITY OF CHOICE

MRI brain with and without contrast (including thin coronal T2 images) (Figs. C14.1 and C14.2). Advantages: MR allows for assessment of hippocampal size and signal intensity. CT is insensitive for diagnosing MTS.

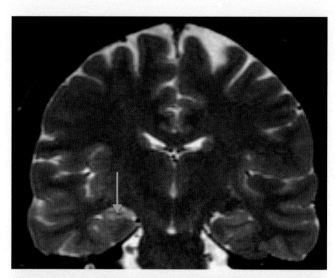

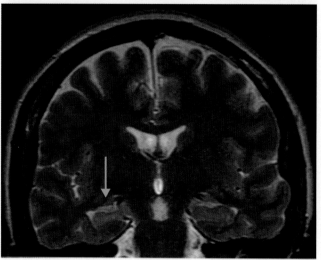

Fig. C14.1 Two different patients with atrophy and increased T2 signal in the right hippocampus (arrows).

FINDINGS

Mesial temporal sclerosis is the most common cause of temporal lobe epilepsy and is a common source of seizures in adolescents and young adults. Temporal lobe epilepsy usually presents with complex partial seizures (complex: altered consciousness; partial: arises from a single focus). MTS has been linked to febrile seizures in infancy, and there is also speculation that perinatal ischemic events may be a cause. The imaging features of MTS reflect neuronal loss and gliosis within the hippocampus and parahippocampal structures.

MRI

- Atrophy of the hippocampus with architectural distortion. Loss of the normal cortical interdigitations of the hippocampal head (90% sensitive).
- T2/FLAIR: hyperintense signal in the hippocampus.
- Decreased size of the ipsilateral fornix, mammillary body, and enlarged temporal horn are secondary signs.
- 20% of cases have bilateral involvement.

It is not uncommon for structural abnormalities to be absent on standard MR imaging. In these cases, advanced MR techniques can be utilized to better evaluate the temporal lobes including hippocampal volume measurements, MR spectroscopy, T2 relaxometry, and diffusion tensor imaging. Positron emission tomography and single photon emission computed tomography (SPECT) may also be helpful in diagnosis.

DIFFERENTIAL DIAGNOSIS

Clinical Differential

Neoplasm, vascular malformation, gliotic abnormalities, cortical developmental abnormalities

Imaging Differential

Herpes encephalitis, cortical dysplasia

REFERENCES AND SUGGESTED READING

1. Deblaere K, Achten E. Structural magnetic resonance imaging in epilepsy. *Eur Radiol.* 2008;18:119-129.
2. Yousem DM, Grossman RI. *Neuroradiology: The Requisites.* 3rd ed. Philadelphia, PA: Mosby; 2010:304-306.

CASE 15

PATIENT PRESENTATION

A 22 month old male with developmental and motor delays, including feeding problems and spastic myoclonus.

CLINICAL SUSPICION

Metabolic disorder, mitochondrial encephalopathy

IMAGING MODALITY OF CHOICE

MRI is the imaging modality of choice (Figs. C15.1 and C15.2). Advantages include high resolution to demonstrate the anatomic structures and the myelination, as well as its lack of ionizing radiation. Due to greater sensitivity to motion, most examinations are performed with sedation/anesthesia.

FINDINGS

Mitochondrial encephalopathies encompass several disorders that arise from defects in genes encoding important enzymes in oxidative phosphorylation. Leigh's disease is the most common mitochondrial disorder in young children. Common findings of Leigh's disease include:

- Delays in myelination patterns
- Symmetric areas of increased T2/FLAIR signal from gliosis within in the deep gray nuclei
  - Cerebral and cerebellar atrophy

MR spectroscopy in mitochondrial disorders may reveal decreased N-acetylaspartic acid (NAA) and elevated

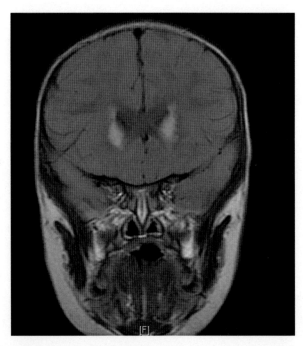

Fig. C15.2 Coronal T2/FLAIR MRI image accentuates the signal changes in the caudate heads.

lactate, owing to the cellular damage that results from defects in the metabolic chain.

Leigh's disease frequently affects motor development and results in poor muscle tone and spasticity. Brain stem findings and abnormal eye movements are also seen. Patients often have multiorgan involvement.

DIFFERENTIAL DIAGNOSIS

Mitochondrial disorders share many anatomical, biochemical and imaging similarities. Differentiation is best made clinically, once a full assessment is complete. The evaluation is complemented with laboratory analysis and in many cases genetic studies. The derangements are progressive and severe. Prognosis is poor in most cases, with most patients dying in infancy or childhood.

Clinical Differential

- MELAS (myelopathy, encephalopathy, lactic acidosis, and strokelike episodes) is frequently asymptomatic at birth. Subsequent episodes of seizures, headache, vomiting, and strokelike events portend progressive dementia.
- Alper's disease is characterized by severe, intractable seizures, motor regression, and liver dysfunction. Eventual ophthalmoplegia and ataxia may develop.
- Kearnes-Sayre: External ophthalmoplegia with retinal pigment abnormality is a clinical hallmark of this disease. Other significant organ involvement includes heart block, sensorineural hearing loss, and mental retardation.

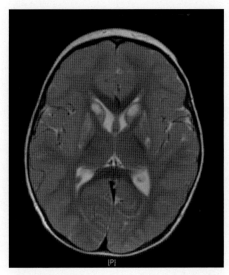

Fig. C15.1 Axial T2-weighted MRI at the level of the foramen of Monro demonstrates abnormally intense signal in the bilateral putamina, globus pallidi, and caudate nuclei. Caudate signal intensity is likely due to acute ischemia. The myelination pattern is normal.

Imaging Differential

- MELAS: At imaging, strokelike lesions are transient and do not necessarily related to a vascular territory.

- Alper's disease: On MRI, there is typically increased T2/FLAIR signal in the basal ganglia, thalamus, and occipital regions.

- Kearnes-Sayre: On MRI, cerebral and cerebellar atrophy can be seen. There is also involvement of the subcortical white matter. Abnormal T2/FLAIR signal intensity can be seen in the basal ganglia and brain stem. Subcortical U fibers may partially demonstrate increased T1 signal.

- The differential diagnosis of signal abnormalities in the basal ganglia includes repeated hypoxic or toxic exposure such as to carbon monoxide.

REFERENCES AND SUGGESTED READING

1. Cheon J, Kim IO, Hwang YS, et al. Leukodystophy in children: a pictorial review of MR imaging features. *Radiographics*. 2002;22:461-476.
2. Geldorf K, Ramboer K, Goethals JM, Verhaeghe L. CT and MRI appearance of mitochondrial encephalopathy. *JBR-BTR*; 2007:90:288-289.
3. Saneto RP, Friedman SD, Shaw DWW. Neuroimaging of mitochondrial disease. *Mitochondrion*. 2008;8:396-413.
4. Valanne L, Ketonen L, Majander AS, Pihko H. Neuroradiologic findings in children with mitochondrial disorders. *AJNR*. 1998;19:369-377.

CASE 16

PATIENT PRESENTATION

Newborn with elevated alpha-fetoprotein levels during pre-natal screening presents with a red lesion on the midline lower back.

CLINICAL SUSPICION

Chiari II malformation

IMAGING MODALITY OF CHOICE

MRI brain and spine without contrast (Figs. C16.1 and C16.2).

FINDINGS

Chiari II malformation is characterized by a number of congenital abnormalities of the brain and spine. This disorder is broadly understood as hindbrain anomalies associated with a spinal myelomeningocele. One proposed mechanism for Chiari II is that leakage of CSF through the open spinal defect leads to the underdevelopment of the posterior fossa, which in turn leads to overcrowding and displacement of the posterior fossa structures. A number of radiologic abnormalities can be seen, but not all in every patient:

Supratentorial Brain

- Hydrocephalus
- Colpocephaly (asymmetric dilation of the occipital horns of the lateral ventricles)
- Agenesis of the corpus callosum, partial or complete, predominately affecting the splenium
- Fenestration of the falx cerebri allowing gyral herniation across midline (interdigitation)
- Enlargement of the massa intermedia (interthalamic band of gray matter)
- Dysplasia of the posterior cingulate gyrus

Infratentorial (Hindbrain)

- Underdeveloped posterior fossa.
- Cerebellar displacement: tonsillar herniation—downward displacement of the cerebellar tonsils greater than 5 mm below the foramen magnum with pointed, rather than the normal rounded, shape of the inferior tonsils. Anterior wrapping around the brain stem. Towering superior cerebellum.
- Vermis, fourth ventricle (elongated), and brain stem displaced inferiorly through the foramen magnum.
- Cervicomedullary kink (due to fixed attachment of the upper cervical cord).

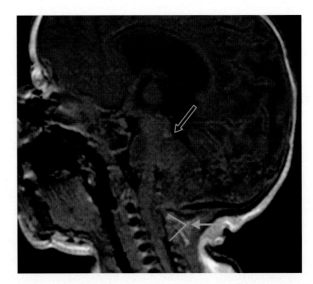

Fig. C16.1 Sagittal T1: small posterior fossa with inferior hernation of the cerebellar tonsils (arrow) and tectal beaking (open arrow).

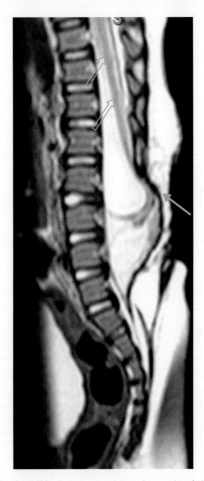

Fig. C16.2 Sagittal T2 shows a myelomeningocele of the lower spine (arrow) as well as a syrinx in the lower cord (open arrows).

- Tectal beaking (dorsal part of the midbrain).
- Dysplastic tentorium.
- Low-lying torcula with a low transverse sinus.

Spine

- Myelomeningocele: failure of the neural tube to close; usually lumbar
- Tethered cord
- Syrinx

Screening with prenatal ultrasound is important as early diagnosis and treatment can potentially decrease the severity of the disease. Myelomeningoceles can be identified as early as 10 weeks gestation and intracranial abnormalities as early as 12 weeks. Prenatal ultrasonography can reveal the "lemon" sign (concavity of the frontal bones on axial image) or the "banana" sign (anterior curvature of the cerebellum). Pregnant mothers should take folate supplements to significantly decrease the risk of the fetus developing a neural tube defect. Some centers perform fetal surgery to correct spinal myelomengioceles.

DIFFERENTIAL DIAGNOSIS

Clinical Differential

Isolated meningocele, closed spinal dysraphism

Imaging Differential

- Posterior fossa abnormalities: other Chiari malformations (I, III), intracranial CSF hypotension, multisutural craniosynostosis syndromes
- Spinal abnormalities: meningocele, closed spinal dysraphism

REFERENCES AND SUGGESTED READING

1. Brant WE, Helms CA. *Fundamentals of Diagnostic Radiology*. Vol 1. 3rd ed. Philadelphia, PA: LWW; 2007:231-232.
2. Cai C, Oakes JW. Hindbrain herniation syndromes: the Chiari malformations (I and II). *Semin Pediatric Neurol*. 1997;4(3):179-191.
3. Yousem DM, Grossman RI. *Neuroradiology: The Requisites*. 3rd ed. Philadelphia, PA: Mosby; 2010:297-298.

CASE 17

PATIENT PRESENTATION

A 25-year-old female presents to the emergency room with 1 day history of painful left eye and fever for the past 2 days. In addition, she reports having purulent nasal drainage. Physical examination reveals erythema with gaze restriction. Visual field is normal. Laboratory examination reveals leukocyotosis with left shift.

CLINICAL SUSPICION

Orbital cellulitis

IMAGING MODALITY OF CHOICE

Contrast-enhanced CT of the orbits (Figs. C17.1-C17.3). Advantages:

- Can be performed quickly in the ER setting
- Excellent sensitivity in detecting orbital cellulitis
- Less susceptible to motion artifacts than MR
- Allows assessment of adjacent paranasal sinuses

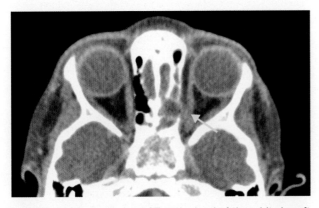

Fig. C17.1 Contrast-enhanced CT at the level of the orbits in soft tissue window demonstrating opacification of the left ethmoid air cells with extension of inflammatory changes through the lamina papyracea into the extraconal orbit. A small periosteal abscess buckles the left medial rectus muscle (arrow).

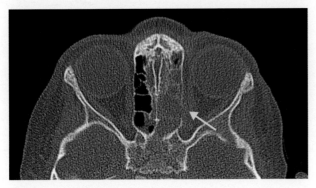

Fig. C17.2 Bone windows demonstrate erosion of the lamina papyracea (arrow).

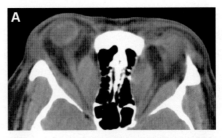

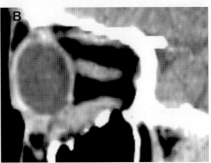

Fig. C17.3 (A) Graves' orbitopathy with bilateral enlargement of the extraoccular muscles sparing the tendinous portion. (B) Inflammatory pseudotumor involving the inferior rectus. Note involvement of the musculotendinous junction.

FINDINGS

Preseptal cellulitis is defined as inflammation confined to orbital soft tissues anterior to the orbital septum. The orbital septum is a membrane that extends from the orbital rims to the eyelids which seprates the orbit into the anterior preseptal and posterior postseptal spaces. Postseptal cellulitis (also termed orbital cellulitis) extends posterior to the orbital septum. Inflammatory changes of orbital cellulitis are usually due to an adjacent sinusitis which involves the extraconal orbit.

CT

- Thickening and edema of soft tissues within the orbit posterior to the orbital septum. Inflammatory changes may result in proptosis of the eye.
- Low attenuation rim enhancing subperiosteal abscess may be seen in more advanced cases.
- Thickening of adjacent extroocular muscles suggests myositis.
- Potential complications of orbital sinusitis include ophthalmic vein thrombosis possibly with extension to the cavernous sinus. Intracranial extension may result in epidural and subdural empyemas, meningitis, and/ or cerebritis.

DIFFERENTIAL DIAGNOSIS
Clinical Differential

- Inflammatory pseudotumor: most common cause of painful proptosis, which results from infiltration of inflammatory cells without known cause anywhere in the orbit.

- Graves' orbitopathy: usually bilateral enlargement of the extraocular muscles in the setting of Graves' disease. It spares the musculotendinous junctions.

Imaging Differential

- Inflammatory pseudotumor: usually no adjacent sinus inflammation.

- Graves' orbitopathy: usually bilateral enlargement of the extraocular muscles in the setting of Graves' disease. It spares the musculotendinous junctions.

- Orbital mass: usually no adjacent sinus inflammation seen.

REFERENCES AND SUGGESTED READING

1. Jain A. Orbital cellulitis in children. *Int Ophthalmol Clin.* 2001;41:71.

2. Givner LB: Perioribtal versus orbital cellultis. *Pediatric Infect Dis J.* 2002;21(12):1157-1158.

3. Sobol SE, Marchand J, Tewfik TL, et al. Orbital complications of sinusitis in children. *J Otolaryngol.* 2002; 31(3):131-136.

CASE 18

PATIENT PRESENTATION

A 55-year-old woman with complaints of painless proptosis of the left eye developing over the past 6 months. Patient reports no other symptomatology and has an unremarkable past medical history. Physical examination reveals proptosis without gaze restriction or visual field defect.

CLINICAL SUSPICION

Orbital mass

IMAGING MODALITY OF CHOICE

CT imaging of the orbits with contrast (Figs. C18.1 and C18.2). Advantages: readily available and rapidly acquired.

FINDINGS

The most common adult orbital mass is a cavernous hemangioma. Orbital hemangiomas are nonneoplastic masses composed of dilated vascular channels. Patients usually present with slowly progressive painless proptosis.

CT

- Well-defined mass usually within the intraconal compartment of the orbit.
- Heterogenous enhancement that progressively fills in on delayed imaging.
- Calcifications can be seen in a minority of cases.

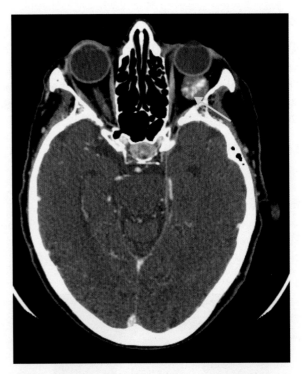

Fig. C18.2 Left-sided intraconal mass representing hemangioma. Note the presence of calcifications (arrow).

DIFFERENTIAL DIAGNOSIS

Clinical Differential

- Thyroid orbitopathy
- Sinonasal mucocele
- Lacrimal gland tumor
- Orbital metastasis

Imaging Differential

- Optic nerve sheath meningioma
- Schwannoma
- Hemangiopericytoma

REFERENCES AND SUGGESTED READING

1. Koeller KK, Smirniotopoulos JG. Orbital masses. *Semin Ultrasound CT MR*. June 1998;19(3):272-291.
2. Bilaniuk LT. Orbital vascular lesions: role of imaging. *Radiol Clin North Am*. January 1999;37(1):169-183, xi.

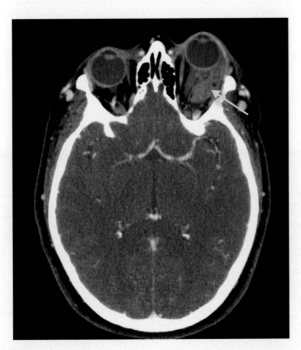

Fig. C18.1 Contrast-enhanced CT reveals a left-sided enhancing intraconal hemangioma (arrow) resulting in proptosis.

CASE 19

PATIENT PRESENTATION

A 45-year-old female presents with a 2-month history of facial asymmetry overlying the left angle of the mandible. Patient reports no pain. Physical examination reveals slight asymmetry of the left parotid region.

CLINICAL SUSPICION

Parotid mass

IMAGING MODALITY OF CHOICE

Contrast-enhanced CT or MR examination (Figs. C19.1 and C19.2). Advantages:

● CT: relatively easy to obtain, less cost than MRI

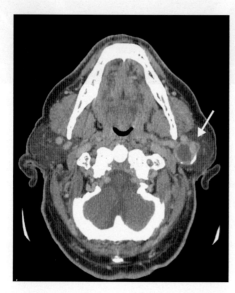

Fig. C19.1 Contrast-enhanced axial CT image demonstrates a well-circumscribed centrally necrotic lesion (arrow) within the deep lobe of the left parotid gland. Note the presence of dystrophic calcifications in the periphery of the lesion.

● MR: no ionizing radiation, less incidence of contrast allergy

FINDINGS

Parotid masses encompass a wide array of different pathologies. The vast majority of parotid masses are benign, with benign mixed tumor (pleomorphic adenoma) constituting about 80% of cases. Metastatic lymphadenopathy and salivary gland tumors constitute the majority of malignant parotid masses. The following are characteristic imaging findings of pleomorphic adenoma:

CT

● Homogenously (small) to heterogeneously (large) enhancing ovoid mass with gentle lobulations

● May have dystrophic calcifications

MR

● T1: hypointense

● T2: hyperintense; T2 hypointense rim can be seen representing a pseudocapsule

● T1+C: mild to moderate enhancement

DIFFERENTIAL DIAGNOSES

● Warthin tumor: heterogeneous mass usually seen within the parotid tail.

● Metastatic lymphadenopathy: usually seen as unilateral or bilateral enlarged nodes within the parotid glands in the setting of skin squamous cell carcinoma or melanoma.

● Salivary gland malignancy: may demonstrate ill-defined margins with local extension.

● Lymphoma: may present in lymph nodes or as a primary parotid mass.

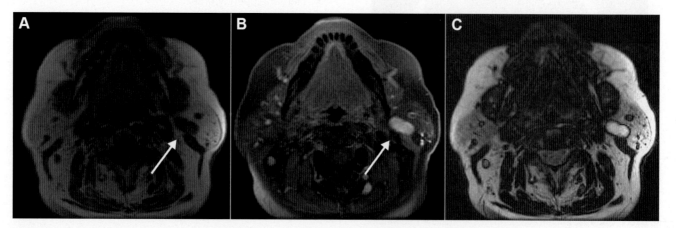

Fig. C19.2 (A) Axial T1 and (B) postcontrast image demonstrate a homogenously hypointense enhancing lobulated mass (arrow) in the left parotid gland. (C) T2 images demonstrate homogenous hyperintense lesion with a hypointense pseudocapsule.

REFERENCES AND SUGGESTED READING

1. Shah GV. MR imaging of the slaviary glands. *Magn Reson Imaging Clinc N Am*. 2002;10:631.

2. Kakimoto N, Gamoh S, Tamaki J, Kishino M, Murakami S, Furukawa S. CT and MR images of pleomorphic adenoma in major and minor salivary glands. *Eur J Radiol*. Mar 2009;69(3):464-472.

3. Howlett DC, Kesse KW, Hughes DV, Sallomi DF. The role of imaging in the evaluation of parotid disease. *Clin Radiol*. August 2002;57(8):692-701.

CASE 20

PATIENT PRESENTATION

A 46-year-old female presents to the clinic with unilateral sensorineural hearing loss and tinnitus.

CLINICAL SUSPICION

Vestibular schwannoma (VS)

IMAGING MODALITY OF CHOICE

MRI brain and internal auditory canal (thin sections) with and without contrast (Fig. C20.1). Advantages: no skull base artifact as seen with CT, better soft tissue contrast.

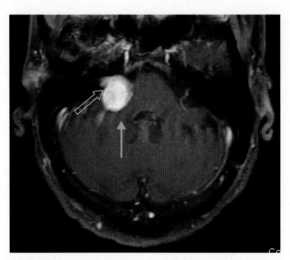

Fig. C20.1 T1 postcontrast image shows an enhancing "ice cream on cone" shaped mass in the right CPA extending into the internal auditory canal (open arrow).

FINDINGS

MR

- Globular/cylindrical shaped tumor in the cerebellopontine angle (CPA).
- Extension of tumor into the internal auditory canal with expansion of the canal.
- Tumor border makes an acute angle with the petrous temporal bone.
- All pulse sequences: isointense to hypointense to pontine tissue.
- T1+C: avid homogenous contrast enhancement.
- T2/FLAIR: cystic changes can be seen but are less common; peritumoral edema may be present.
- GRE: calcification, hemorrhage.

VS are benign tumors that arise from the Schwann cells that surround the superior vestibular branch of cranial nerve VIII (most commonly; less commonly involving the inferior vestibular branch). They are found in the cerebellopontine angle and account for 80% to 90% of CPA tumors. It is important to try to differentiate vestibular schwannomas from meningiomas, which account for 10% to 15% of CPA tumors, for presurgical planning and counseling. Some clues to the diagnosis of a meningioma include sessile tumor with a broad base against the tentorium, obtuse angle with the petrous temporal bone, homogeneous enhancement, dural tail, calcification, and hyperostosis of the overlying bone. Bilateral vestibular schwannomas is virtually pathognomonic for neurofibromatosis type 2.

DIFFERENTIAL DIAGNOSIS

Clinical Differential

- Viral vestibulitis
- Vascular occlusive disease
- Perilymphatic fistula

Imaging Differential

Cerebellopontine angle masses:

- Meningioma
- Epidermoid cyst, arachnoid cyst
- Facial nerve schwannoma
- Aneurysm
- Paraganglioma, ependymoma
- Metastasis
- Lipoma

REFERENCES AND SUGGESTED READING

1. American College of Radiology. ACR Appropriateness Criteria. Vertigo and hearing loss. http://www.acr.org/SecondaryMainMenuCategories/quality_safety/app_criteria/pdf/ExpertPanelonNeurologicImaging/VertigoandHearingLossDoc14.aspx. Accessed November 26, 2011.

2. Thamburaj K, Radhakrishnan VV, Thomas B, et al. Intratumoral microhemorrhages on T2* weighted gradient-echo imaging helps differentiate vestibular schwannoma from meningioma. *AJNR*. 2008;29:552-557.

3. Yousem DM, Grossman RI. *Neuroradiology: The Requisites*. 3rd ed. Philadelphia, PA: Mosby; 2010:63.

CASE 21
PATIENT PRESENTATION

A 34-year-old female who presents to her primary care physician for an enlarging neck mass over the past few years. Clinical examination reveals a thyroid nodule within the right thyroid gland with palpable adjacent jugular chain lymphadenopathy. Laboratory examination reveals normal TSH.

CLINICAL SUSPICION

Thyroid nodule, concern for malignant thyroid nodule

IMAGING MODALITY OF CHOICE

Ultrasound (Figs. C21.1 and C21.2). Advantages: readily available, no ionizing radiation, low cost.

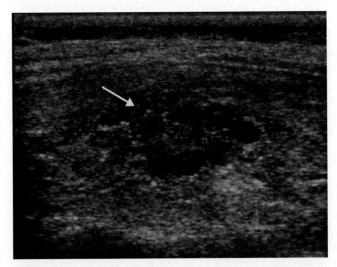

Fig. C21.1 Gray-scale ultrasound demonstrates an irregular, solid hypoechoic nodule within the right thyroid gland (arrow). Note the presence of microcalcifications.

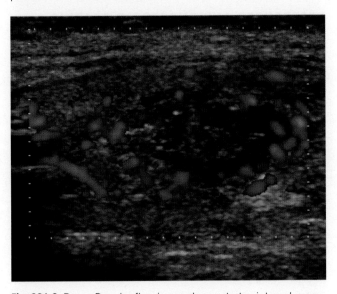

Fig. C21.2 Power Doppler flow image demonstrates internal vascularity within the nodule.

FINDINGS

Although benign thyroid nodules are much more common than malignant thyroid nodules, there are several ultrasound imaging features that may help identify nodules that are at increased risk for malignancy:

- Microcalcifications
- Hypoechogenicity
- Irregular margins or no halo
- Solid
- Intranodal vascularity

Thyroid nodules that are felt to be at increased risk for malignancy are biopsied by fine needle aspiration.

DIFFERENTIAL DIAGNOSIS
Clinical Differential

- Benign thyroid nodule: Most thyroid nodules are benign thyroid adenomas.
- Parathryoid adenoma: Usually parathyroid adenomas are outside the thyroid gland and are seen in patients with hypercalcemia.
- Thyroid cyst: no associated features.

Imaging Differential

- Benign thyroid nodule: Although imaging appearances overlap, benign thyroid nodules lack suspicious imaging features.
- Parathryoid adenoma: Usually parathyroid adenomas are outside the thyroid gland and are seen in patients with hypercalcemia.
- Thyroid cyst: cystic structure on imaging.

REFERENCES/SUGGESTED READING

1. Moon W. Benign and malignant thyroid nodules: US differentiation—multicenter retrospective study. *Radiology*. June 2008;247:762-770.
2. Frates MC, Benson CB, Charboneau JW, et al. Management of thyroid nodules detected at US: Society of Radiologists in Ultrasound consensus conference statement. *Radiology*. December 2005;237:794-800. doi:10.1148/radiol.2373050220.

CASE 22
PATIENT PRESENTATION

A 45-year-old female presents with 6-month history of weight loss, heat intolerance, and tremor. Physical examination reveals a diffusely enlarged thyroid gland. TSH values are below the reference range with elevated free T4 levels.

CLINICAL SUSPICION

Hyperthyroidism, Graves' disease

IMAGING MODALITY OF CHOICE

Initial imaging evaluation of suspected hyperthyroidism consists of a nuclear medicine thyroid scan using either Tc-99m pertechnetate or I-123 (Fig. C22.1). Imaging can be performed 20 minutes after injection of 3 to 5 mCi Tc99m pertechnetate or 4 hours after injection of 0.1 to 0.4 mCi I-123. Advantages: thyroid scintigraphy is the best way to evaluate if hyperthyroidism is due to increased endogenous production of thyroid hormone.

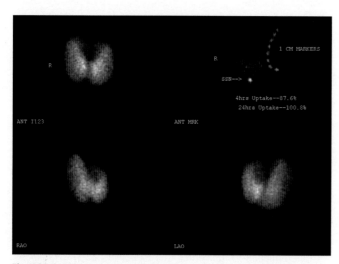

Fig. C22.1 Planar images obtained 4 hours after administration of I-123. There is diffusely increased radiotracer uptake within both lobes of the thyroid. Radioactive iodine uptake is markedly increased.

FINDINGS

Graves' disease is an autoimmune disorder that results in endogenous overproduction of thyroid hormone due to the presence of thyroid-stimulating autoantibodies. The stimulated thyroid gland utilizes iodide at a faster rate than a normal gland, resulting in the following imaging findings:

- Homogenous increased radiotracer uptake with increased target-to-background ratio
- Elevated radioactive iodine uptake (>15% at 4 hours, >35% at 24 hours)

DIFFERENTIAL DIAGNOSIS
Clinical Differential

- Subacute thyroiditis: Postinfectious thyroiditis that results in hyperthyroidism from release of preformed thyroid hormone.
- Toxic multinodular goiter: Hyperthyroidism results from one or several nodules that demonstrate increased uptake.
- Exogenous thyroid hormone: Exogenous thyroid hormone can result in symptoms of hyperthyroidism.

Imaging Differential

- Subacute thyroiditis: Radioactive iodine uptake is decreased in subacute thyroiditis.
- Toxic multinodular goiter: The remainder of the thyroid gland is usually suppressed and only faintly visible. These cases of hyperthyroidism require higher doses of I-131 for treatment.
- Exogenous thyroid hormone: In these cases, TSH suppression results in decreased thyroid uptake.

REFERENCES AND SUGGESTED READING

1. Floyd JL, Rosen PR, Borchert RD, et al. Thyroid uptake and imaging with iodine-123 at 4-5 hours: replacement of the 24-hour iodine-131 standard. *J Nucl Med.* August 1985;26(8):884-887.
2. Cappelli C. The role of imaging in Graves' disease: a cost effectiveness analysis. *Eur J Radiol.* January 2008;65(1):99-103.

CASE 23

PATIENT PRESENTATION

A 60-year-old female presents to her primary care physician with a 2-month history of memory loss and insomnia. Basic metabolic profile reveals calcium of 11.2. The serum creatinine, BUN, and calculated GFR are normal. PTH levels are elevated.

CLINICAL SUSPICION

Hypercalcemia possibly from primary hyperparathyroidism

IMAGING MODALITY OF CHOICE

Dual phase Tc-99m sestamibi nuclear parathyroid planar images followed by SPECT/CT (Figs. C23.1-C23.3).

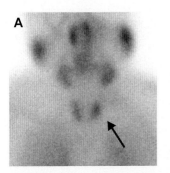
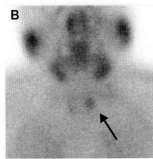

Fig. C23.1 (A) Immediate anterior planar image demonstrates uptake within the thyroid gland as well as within the left inferior parathyroid adenoma (arrow). (B) Delayed anterior planar images reveals washout of the thyroid gland with increased conspicuity of the parathyroid adenoma (arrow).

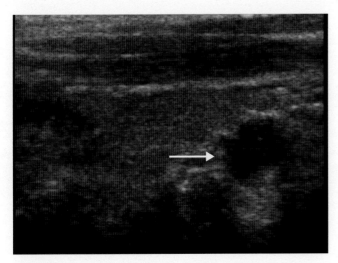

Fig. C23.2 Longitudinal gray-scale ultrasound image through the left thyroid lobe demonstrates an extrathyroidal hypoechoic lesion (arrow) representing a left inferior parathyroid adenoma.

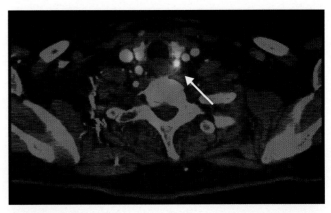

Fig. C23.3 SPECT/CT axial fused image demonstrates marked increased uptake within a left inferior parathyroid adenoma (arrow).

FINDINGS

Parathyroid adenoma (75%-85%) is the most common cause of primary hyperparathyroidism followed by parathyroid hyperplasia (10%-15%) and carcinoma (0.5%-5%). Usually there are 4 parathyroid glands, 2 superior and 2 inferior, located posterior to the thyroid gland; however, they can vary in number and location. The purpose of imaging is to confirm the presence of parathyroid pathology and to localize the parathyroid adenoma in order to guide surgical planning. 10 to 20 minutes after injection of Tc-99m sestamibi, anterior planar images are obtained. Delayed images are obtained 90 minutes postinjection.

Tc-99m Sestamibi

- Early images demonstrate uptake by both thyroid and parathyroid tissue. Since most parathyroid adenomas retain the radiotracer longer than the thyroid gland, delayed images demonstrate relatively increased uptake within the parathyroid adenoma.

- SPECT/CT: useful for more accurate localization and when planar images are equivocal.

DIFFERENTIAL DIAGNOSIS

Clinical Differential

- Secondary hyperparathyroidism (HPT): end organ resistance to PTH, usually from renal failure, resulting in hyperparathyroidism without hypercalcemia.

- Teritiary hyperparathyroidism: long-standing secondary HPT resulting in autonomous production of PTH.

- Malignancy: Several different malignancies can result in hypercalcemia either due to metastatic disease or from paraneoplastic effects.

Imaging Differential

- Thyroid adenoma: Benign thyroid adenomas can demonstrate decreased washout on delayed images in comparison with normal thyroid tissue, which may be confused for a parathyroid adenoma.
- Ectopic thyroid tissue: Ectopic thyroid tissue may simulate parathyroid adenoma on scintigraphy.
- Parathyroid carcinoma: Similar scintigraphic appearance, however, may present with regional lymph nodal metastasis.

REFERENCES AND SUGGESTED READING

1. Eslamy HK, Ziessman HA. Parathyroid scintigraphy in patients with primary hyperparathyroidism: 99mTc sestamibi SPECT and SPECT/CT. *Radiographics*. September-October 2008;28(5):1461-1476.
2. Tublin ME, Pryma DA, Yim JH, et al. Localization of parathyroid adenomas by sonography and technetium tc-99m sestamibi single-photon emission computed tomography before minimally invasive parathyroidectomy: are both studies really needed? *J Ultrasound Med*. February 2009;28(2):183-189.

CASE 24

PATIENT PRESENTATION

A 75-year-old male presents to the emergency room with an episode of right lower extremity weakness lasting for a few hours. Physical examination reveals no residual weakness. Both CT and MR examinations of the brain reveal no acute abnormalities. A left carotid bruit is auscultated.

CLINICAL SUSPICION

Carotid stenosis with transient ischemic attack (TIA)

IMAGING MODALITY OF CHOICE

US with Doppler evaluation of the carotid arteries (Figs. C24.1 and C24.2). Advantages: readily available, low cost, real-time, evaluation of flow dynamics.

FINDINGS

Ultrasound evaluation of carotid stenosis mainly consists of gray-scale and Doppler evaluation. The main objective of imaging is to quantify the level of stenosis or obstruction: mild, moderate, severe, near or complete occlusion as the severity of stenosis, along with clinical symptomatology, guides treatment. Gray-scale ultrasound (US) allows visualization of the atherosclerotic plaque, which can vary in echogenicity from hypoechoic (soft, noncalcified) to echogenic (calcified). Calcified plaques are considered more stable and less likely to embolize than hypoechoic soft plaques. Doppler evaluation allows for hemodynamic assessment of blood flow within the artery allowing estimation of the level of stenosis.

Gray Scale

- Atherosclerotic plaque: may vary from hypoechoic (soft plaque) to highly echnogenic calcified plaque
- Luminal narrowing: varying from minimal decrease in lumen caliber to complete occlusion

Doppler

- Mild (< 50%) stenosis:
  - Peak systolic velocity (PSV) < 125 cm/s
  - Internal carotid/common carotid artery ratio (ICA/CCA) ratio < 2
- Moderate (50%-69%) stenosis
  - PSV: 125 to 230 cm/s
  - ICA/CCA: 2 to 4
- Severe (> 70%) stenosis:
  - PSV: > 230 cm/s
  - ICA/CCA > 4
  - Poststenotic turbulence with damped waveforms

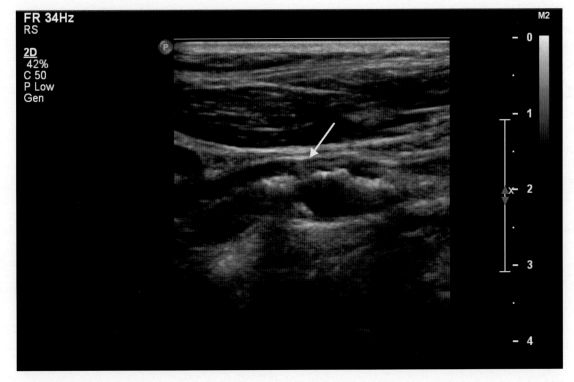

Fig. C24.1 Gray-scale ultrasound reveals the presence of atheroslerotic calcifications involving the carotid bulb and proximal internal carotid artery (arrow).

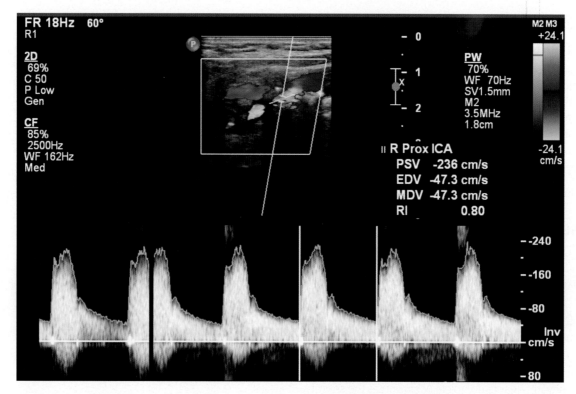

Fig. C24.2 Color and spectral Doppler reveals increased peak systolic velocity at the level of stenosis.

- Near complete occlusion (90%-99%):
  - Variable PSV
- Complete occlusion:
  - Undetectable PSV

DIFFERENTIAL DIAGNOSIS

- Carotid dissection: usually involves the ICA distal to the carotid bifurcation.
- Fibromuscular dysplasia: often affects both internal carotid and external carotid arteries and appears as alternating beading and stenosis.

REFERENCES AND SUGGESTED READING

1. Grant EG, Benson CB, Moneta GL, et al. Carotid artery stenosis: gray-scale and Doppler US diagnosis—Society of Radiologists in Ultrasound Consensus Conference. *Radiology.* November 2003;229(2):340-346. Epub September 18, 2003. Review.

2. Screening for carotid artery stenosis: U.S. Preventive Services Task Force recommendation statement. *Ann Intern Med.* December 18, 2007;147(12):854-859.

CASE 25

PRESENTATION

A 58-year-old man with chronic back pain and prior history of lumbar spine surgery presents with persistent back pain and fever.

CLINICAL SUSPICION

Discitis/osteomyelitis

IMAGING MODALITY OF CHOICE

Contrast-enhanced MRI (Figs. C25.1 and C25.2). Advantages: MR imaging is sensitive to findings of osteomyelitis, with positive findings in as few as 3 days. It shows the extraosseous involvement and the compromise of the cord/nerve roots. Disadvantages: the presence of metallic devices introduces artifacts that degrade image quality.

FINDINGS

Discitis/osteomyelitis refers to infection involving the intervertebral disc and adjacent vertebral bodies. Pathogens enter the disc space through trauma or surgery or are spread hematogenously. The intervertebral discs lack vascularity, and thus are unable to mount sufficient immune responses to infection.

MRI

- Decreased bone marrow signal intensity on unenhanced T1-weighted imaging with postcontrast enhancement of involved vertebral bodies.

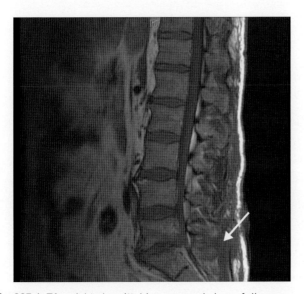

Fig. C25.1 T1-weighted sagittal image reveals loss of disc space height, with decreased signal in the endplates of L5 and S1 adjacent to the affected disc. Granulation tissue (arrow) from the prior laminectomy at this level can be appreciated posteriorly.

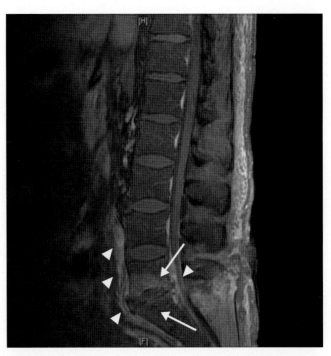

Fig. C25.2 T1-weighted postcontrast image shows enhancement in the vertebral body endplates (arrows) surrounding the infected disc at L5-S1. Disc space height loss is again demonstrated. Increased epidural space enhancement denotes extension of infection to tissues surrounding the spinal cord. Paraspinal soft tissues are inflamed anteriorly and posteriorly (arrowheads).

- Decreased disc space/disc height with or without destruction of adjacent vertebral body endplates.
- Increased T2 signal intensity and enhancement of involved discs compared to adjacent normal discs.
- Paravertebral soft tissue inflammatory changes and/or paravertebral/epidural abscess.

DIFFERENTIAL DIAGNOSIS

Clinical Differential

- Postoperative pain: a symptom not uncommon after surgical procedures intended to correct or alleviate chronic back pain. However, pain and fever are worrisome for infectious etiology, as surgery itself is a risk factor for spinal infection.
- Rheumatoid spondylitis: most commonly in cervical spine
- Spinal tumor: also may present with chronic back pain, may also present with paralysis or loss of bowel or bladder function.

Imaging Differential

- Postoperative pain/failed back surgery syndrome: usually do not present with endplate destruction. Failed back surgery syndrome comprises various different entities including spinal stenosis, instability, recurrent herniation, fibrosis, and arachnoiditis.

- Postoperative granulation tissue: enhancement in the surgical tract is an expected postoperative finding.

REFERENCES AND SUGGESTED READING

1. Berquist TH, Fenton DS. Spine. In: Berquist TH, ed. *Musculoskeletal Imaging Companion*. 2nd ed. Philadelphia, PA: Lippincott Williams & Wilkins; 2007:32-124.

2. Ledermann HP, Schweitzer ME, Morrison WB, Carrino JA. MR imaging findings in spinal infections: rules or myths? *Radiology*. 2003;228:506-514.

3. Pineda C, Espinosa R, Pena A. Radiographic imaging in osteomyelitis: the role of plain radiography, computed tomography, ultrasonography, magnetic resonance imaging and schintigraphy. *Semin Plast Surg*. 2009;23:80-89.

4. Witte RJ, Lane JI, Miller GM, Krecke KN. Spine. In: Berquist TH, ed. *MRI of the Musculoskeletal System*. Philadelphia, PA: Lippincott Williams & Wilkins; 2006:121-202.

CASE 26

PATIENT PRESENTATION

A 57-year-old female presents with back pain after a fall. No neurological deficits were revealed on examination.

CLINICAL SUSPICION

Compression fracture in the setting of osteoporosis

IMAGING MODALITY OF CHOICE

Noncontrast CT provides superior demonstration of osseous structures, as plain films may underestimate the extent of spinal canal narrowing or miss posterior element fractures. Coronal and sagittal reformatted images are recommended for identification of fractures that are in the axial plane of imaging (Figs. C26.1 and C26.2).

FINDINGS

Noncontrast CT allows evaluation of all cortical margins of each vertebral body level, including articular pillars, lamina, and spinous processes.

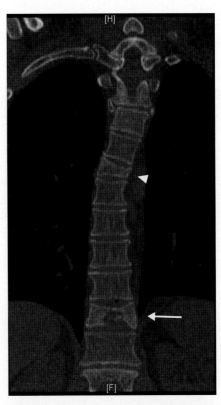

Fig. C26.2 Coronal noncontrast CT image shows dextroscoliosis centered around chronic, lateral compression deformity of T6 (arrowhead). An acute compression fracture of the T11 vertebral body results in vacuum phenonomenon in the T10-11 disc space and approximately 50% vertebral body height loss (arrow).

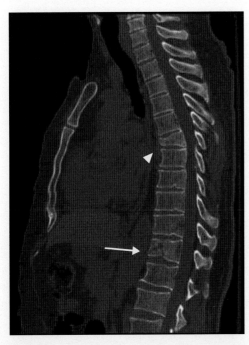

Fig. C26.1 Sagittal reformatted noncontrast CT image of the thoracic spine demonstrates anterior compression deformity of the T6 vertebral body (arrowhead). An additional deformity is seen along the inferior endplate of T11, with approximately 50% anterior height loss (arrow).

CT

- Diffuse, decreased bone mineral density seen in the setting of osteopenia
- Change in the contour of vertebral body cortical bone
- Wedge-shaped vertebral body in the area of compression
- Displaced fragments (of particular importance if found in the canal)
- Paraspinal soft tissue hematoma (occasionally)

Physical examination should include neurological assessment. Deficits will identify and localize cord injury, inferring areas of focus for radiologic assessment of fragment retropulsion/canal narrowing. MRI evaluation is recommended in the case of clinical neurological deficits.

DIFFERENTIAL DIAGNOSIS
Clinical Differential
Traumatic fracture, muscle spasm, cancer-related fracture

Imaging Differential

- Burst fracture: subset of unstable compression fractures usually seen in the setting of trauma. Retropulsion of fracture fragments into the spinal canal is frequently seen.
- Pathological fracture: fractures due to infection or tumor. Fracture lines will be visible, just as in any fracture. Osseous tumor is usually apparent. Aggressive-appearing bony changes include trabecular destruction and distortion of eroded cortical bone.

REFERENCES AND SUGGESTED READING
1. Eastlack RK, Bono CM. Fractures and dislocations of the thoracolumbar spine. In: Bucholz RW, Heckman JD, Court-Brown CM, eds. *Rockwood and Green's Fractures in Adults*. 6th ed. Philadelphia, PA: Lippincott, Williams & Wilkins; 2006:1544-1581.
2. Hsu JM, Joseph T, Ellis AM. Thoracolumbar fracture in blunt trauma patients: guidelines for diagnosis and imaging. *Injury*. 2003;34:426-433.
3. Sheridan R, Peralta R, Rhea J, Ptak T, Novelline R. Reformatted visceral protocol helical computed tomographic scanning allows conventional radiographs of the thoracic and lumbar spine to be eliminated in the evaluation of blunt trauma patients. *J Trauma*. 2003;55:665-669.

CASE 27

PATIENT PRESENTATION

A 25-year-old female with recurrent intractable postural headaches, relieved with supine positioning. There has been no history of trauma or surgery. The patient had no significant prior illnesses or infections. Prior CT and MRI imaging were negative.

CLINICAL SUSPICION

Cerebrospinal fluid leak

IMAGING MODALITY OF CHOICE

For suspected CSF leak, initial imaging with CT or MRI is obtained to evaluate for signs of intracranial hypotension. When the results of these exams are negative, radionuclide cisternograms with delayed imaging are indicated, including evaluation of the entire neuraxis (Figs. C27.1 and C27.2).

FINDINGS

CT/MRI

- MRI or CT examination may show secondary signs of intracranial hypotension such as low-lying tonsils, sagging midbrain, or subdural collections in the convexities. Meningoceles or fistula within the auditory canals or

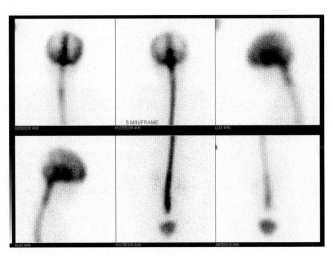

Fig. C27.1 Normal CSF radionuclide cisternogram demonstrates expected distribution of radiotracer in the cranium and along the spinal dural space.

sinuses are also possible, and correlate with CSF otorhinorrhea. These were not present in the current case.

Radionuclide Cisternography (RNC)

- Nuclear medicine technique in which radiotracer is injected intrathecally, after which imaging is performed under a gamma camera.

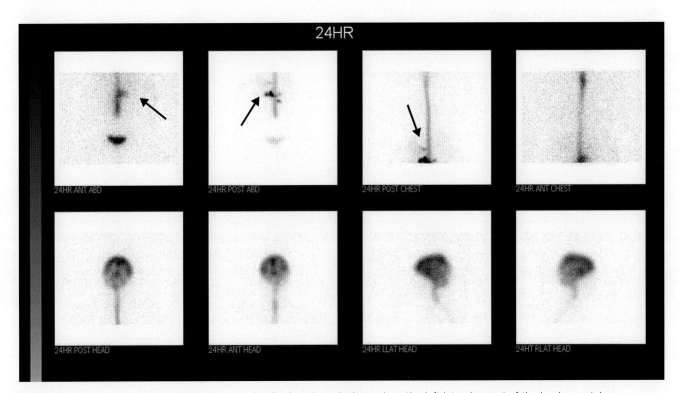

Fig. C27.2 24-hour delayed imaging of radiotracer distribution shows leakage along the left lateral aspect of the lumbar vertebrae, consistent with a CSF leak (arrows).

- Direct findings of CSF leak on radionuclide imaging include collections of tracer uptake outside anatomic location of CSF, such as in the paranasal sinuses or adjacent to the spinal cord. Delayed imaging increases the sensitivity of these findings.

- Indirect findings on radionuclide imaging include early bladder filling, lack of radiotracer detection along the intracranial cerebral convexities, early washout of tracer around the spinal cord, and abnormal outlining of spinal root sleeves.

- Treatment options include rest as necessary, epidural blood patch, and intrathecal saline infusion. Surgery is reserved for cases of dural injury or refractory/persistent leaks.

DIFFERENTIAL DIAGNOSIS
Clinical Differential

- Subarachnoid/intracranial hemorrhage: Such hemorrhage classically presents as acute, debilitating headache.

- Migraine headache: These headaches tend to be more common in female patients. Clinical symptoms include unilateral, pulsatile cephalgia with associated photophobia and/or nausea. Classic migraine headaches are preceded by prodromal symptoms such as scotoma or paresthesias.

- Factitious disorder: Although physicians must always be alert to the risk of psychological/psychiatric and addiction etiologies for chronic pain presentation, this should not be the initial differential consideration.

Imaging Differential

- Subarachnoid/intracranial hemorrhage: Noncontrast CT examination will reveal even small amounts of high-attenuation fluid in subarachnoid spaces. After initial stabilization, additional etiologies such as hypertension, vasculitis, or primary renal syndromes should be sought.

- Migraine headache: Deep white matter signal abnormalities are seen in T2/FLAIR imaging. These were absent in this case.

REFERENCES AND SUGGESTED READING

1. Stone JA, Castillo M, Neelon B, Mukherji SK. Evaluation of CSF leaks: high-resolution CT compared with contrast-enhanced CT and radionuclide cisternography. *AJNR.* 1999; 20:706-712.

2. Morioka T, Aoki T, Tomoda Y, et al. Cerebrospinal fluid leakage in intracranial hypotension syndrome: usefulness of indirect findings in radionuclide cisternography for detection and treatment monitoring. *Clin Nucl Med.* 2008;33:181-185.

3. Yoo HM, Kim SJ, Choi CG, et al. Detection of CSF leak in spinal CSF leak syndrome using MR myelography: correlation with radioisotope cisternography. *AJNR.* 2008;29:649-654.

CASE 28

PATIENT PRESENTATION

A 28-year-old male with neck pain following a motor vehicle collision. Articular column fracture was diagnosed on trauma CT evaluation.

CLINICAL SUSPICION

Discoligamentous injury

IMAGING MODALITY OF CHOICE

CT of the cervical spine without contrast is the preferred initial imaging modality of cervical spine trauma in a high-risk patient (Figs. C28.1 and C28.2). Advantages include superior resolution of fractures, especially with the use of coronal and sagittal reformatted images. Disadvantages include poor resolution of subtle ligamentous or cord injury. Lateral mass fractures are frequently associated with discoligamentous injury and multiplane instability. If there is clinical or imaging suspicion of soft tissue, neural, or ligamentous injury, noncontrast MRI imaging is indicated (Fig. C28.3).

FINDINGS

CT

Evaluation of imaging in acute cervical spine trauma begins with an assessment of alignment and fractures. Any finding of malalignment or fracture raises the suspicion for ligamentous and neural injury. Compromise of spinal column patency is a potential surgical emergency and is also likely clinically apparent.

Fractures are typically seen as disruption of the cortical margins of bone. This is best demonstrated by CT. Evaluation of occult, nondisplaced fractures and soft tissue and ligamentous injury is better made with MRI.

The current case demonstrates unilateral articular pillar fracture—a stable injury. There is no suspicion of canal narrowing. Only mild anterolisthesis is seen on the sagittal images. However, physical examination findings motivated the ER team to request MRI evaluation.

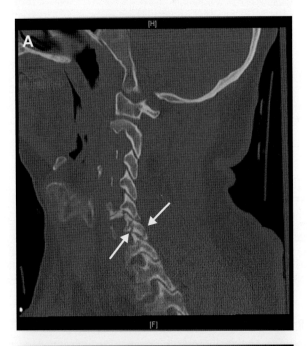

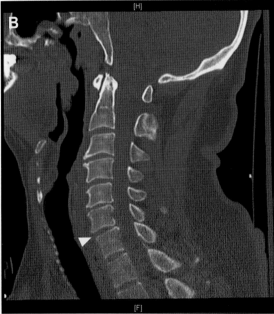

Fig. C28.2 (A) Noncontrast CT of the cervical spine in sagittal plane again demonstrating fracture lines in the left articular pillar of C6 (arrows). (B) More medially, slight anterolisthesis of C6 on C7 can be appreciated (arrowhead).

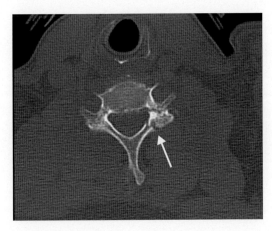

Fig. C28.1 Initial noncontrast cervical spine CT examination in the axial plane reveals fracture of the left articular pillar at C6 (arrow). The fracture fragment is minimally displaced.

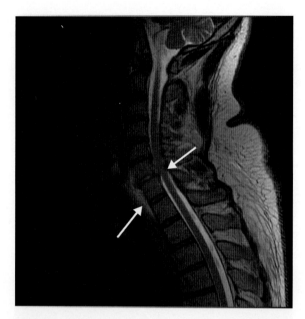

Fig. C28.3 T2-weighted MRI in sagittal plane demonstrates disruption of the anterior and posterior longitudinal ligaments over the C6-C7 disc space (arrows). Increased T2 signal anterior to the vertebral bodies signifies acute soft tissue edema. Mild anterolisthesis at this level is again visible. Spinal cord signal is normal.

MR

Findings of ligamentous injury include disruption of the ligamentous contour and increased soft tissue and disc T2 signal (edema).

DIFFERENTIAL DIAGNOSIS

Clinical Differential

Whiplash/strain, hyperextension injury, flexion injury, herniated disk, carotid dissection.

Imaging Differential

- Whiplash/strain: Primarily a soft-tissue injury, there will be no associated fractures or significant findings on CT. Muscle strain may be evident as decreased attenuation and/or swelling on CT.

- Hyperextension injury: Precise mechanism of cervical spine injury is frequently unknown at the time of initial evaluation. Some authors argue that mechanism is less prognostically useful than thorough injury description. In a hyperextension injury there is usually widening of the anterior disc space and posterior element fractures. Spinous process fractures can also be seen.

- Flexion injury: At most spinal levels, flexion injury results in anterior compression deformity. Sagitally oriented fractures through the vertebral body are also common.

REFERENCES AND SUGGESTED READING

1. Jansson KA, Gill K. Management of spine fractures. In: Pape HC, Sanders R, Borrelli J, eds. *The Poly-traumatized Patient with Fractures: A Multidisciplinary Approach.* New York: Springer; 2011:151-165.

2. Kotani Y, Abumi K, Ito M, Minami A. Cervical spine injuries associated with lateral mass and facet joint fractures: new classification and surgical treatment with pedicle screw fixation. *Eur Spine J.* 2005;14:69-77.

3. Mirvis, SE. Imaging of cervical spine trauma. In: Mirvis SE, Shanmuganathan K, eds. *Imaging in Trauma and Critical Care.* 2nd ed. Philadelphia, PA: Elselvier; 2003:185-296.

4. Vaccaro AR, Hulbert RJ, Fischer C, et al. The sub-axial cervical spine injury classification system (SLIC): a novel approach to recognize the importance of morphology, neurology and integrity of the discoligamentous complex. *Spine.* 2007;21:2365-2374.

CASE 29

PRESENTATION

A 47-year-old female with chronic lower back pain.

CLINICAL SUSPICION

Lumbar disc herniation with radiculopathy

IMAGING MODALITY OF CHOICE

MRI is the imaging modality of choice in patients suspected of having intervertebral disc pathology (Figs. C29.1-C29.3). CT myelography involves injection of contrast into the intrathecal space, and it usually is reserved for patients who cannot undergo MRI examination, especially in those patients with metallic implants such as non-MR-compatible pacemakers or pain pumps.

FINDINGS

MRI

- Extension of disc material beyond the confines of the normal disc space. The damaged disc material will be isointense to the normal disc on T1, but may be hypointense on T2 depending on the level of desiccation.
- Bulge: refers to extension of disc tissue beyond the normal ring size, and involves greater than 50% of the disc circumference.
- Herniation involves less than 50% of the disc circumference. Focal herniation involves less than 25% of the disc circumference. Broad-based herniation involves greater than 25% of the disc circumference.
- Protrusion: a form of focal herniation in which the base of the protuberance is broader than its body.

- Extrusion: a form of focal herniation in which the base of the protuberance is narrower than its body.
- Sequestered disc fragment can only result from extrusion and involves the migration of separated disc material from the disc of origin.

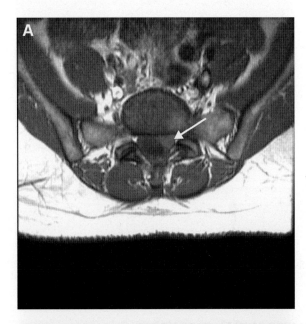

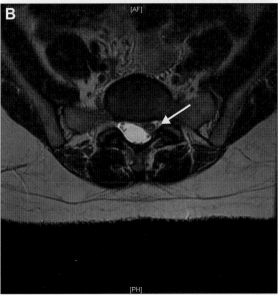

Fig. C29.2 (A) Axial T1-weighted image at S1 showing extruded disc material occupying the left lateral recess, narrowing the canal at this level (arrow). (B) Axial T2-weighted image at S1 showing extruded disc material occupying the left lateral recess (arrow). A nerve root of the cauda equina is displaced posteriorly (arrowhead).

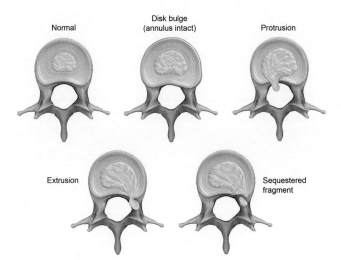

Fig. C29.1 Disc herniation nomencature.

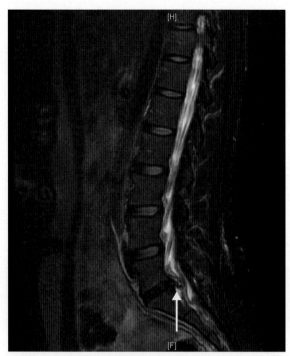

Fig. C29.3 Sagittal T2-weighted image shows extruded disc material projecting inferiorly and impinging upon the S1 nerve root (arrow).

DIFFERENTIAL DIAGNOSIS

Clinical Differential

Lumbar strain, pathologic fracture, multiple myeloma, dural fibrosis, facet synovial cyst, drop metastasis

Imaging Differential

- Dural fibrosis: degenerative fibrosis may have the appearance of a mass causing thecal impingment. The use of postcontrast sequences will demonstrate prompt enhancement; a protruded/extruded disc will not. Additionally, fibrosis is less likely to be focal and more frequently causes circumferential involvement.

- Facet synovial cyst: secondary to facet degeneration. A cyst with heterogeneous signal intensity, extending from the facet joint into the spinal canal, usually the lateral recess, may have similar appearance to an extruded disk. Images in multiple planes help to establish its relationship with the facet joint.

- Drop metastases: It would be unusual for drop metastases in the spine—such as from medulloblastoma or ependymoma—to present first as low back pain. Postcontrast sequences would be helpful in unclear cases, as metastases frequently enhance. Other metastases may involve the vertebral bodies or posterior elements, places the disc material cannot migrate.

REFERENCES AND SUGGESTED READING

1. Fardon DF, Milette PC. Nomenclature and classification of lumbar disc pathology: recommendations of the combined task forces of the North American Spine Society, American Society of Spine Radiology, and American Society of Neuroradiology. *Spine.* 2001;26(5):E93-E113.

2. Haughton V. Imaging intervertebral disc degeneration. *J Bone Joint Surg Am.* April 2006;88 Suppl 2:15-20.

3. Modic MT, Ross JS. Lumbar degenerative disc disease. *Radiology.* 2007;245:43-61.

CASE 30

PATIENT PRESENTATION

A 57-year-old female presents with gradual onset of bilateral upper and lower extremity weakness and numbness. Imaging of the brain is normal.

CLINICAL SUSPICION

Spinal cord neoplasm, possibly spinal cord astrocytoma

IMAGING MODALITY OF CHOICE

Precontrast and postcontrast MRI with fat saturation in axial and sagittal planes provides demonstration of tumor location, extent, and involvement or effect on canal and assists with surgical planning in the case of myelopathy (Figs. C30.1-C30.3).

FINDINGS OF SPINAL CORD ASTROCYTOMA
MRI

- Usually isointense to the normal cord on T1-weighted images.
- Cystic component to the mass appears isointense to CSF on T1- and T2-weighted imaging.

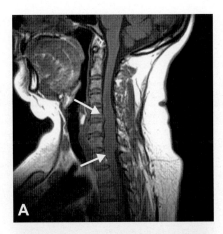

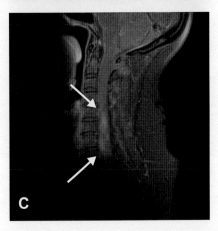

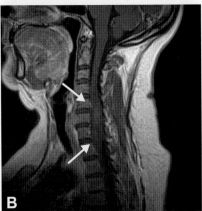

Fig. C30.2 Sagittal T1-weighted precontrast (A) and postcontrast (B), as well as postcontrast fat-saturated (C) images of the cervical spine showing enhancing intramedullary mass extending from C5 to T1 (arrows). No cystic component is present. The cord appears expanded along the extent of the tumor.

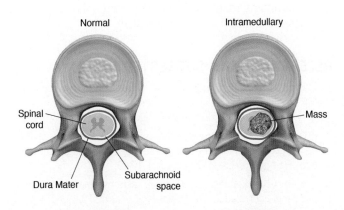

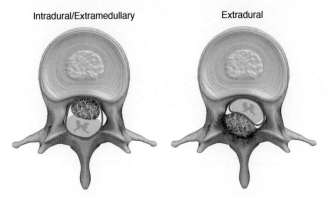

Fig. C30.1 Axial diagram demonstrating different locations of spinal neoplasms.

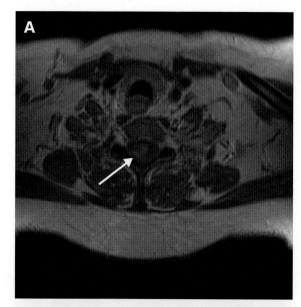

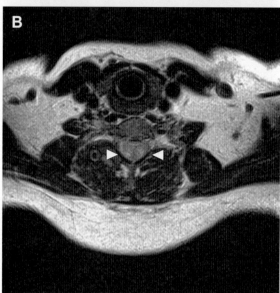

Fig. C30.3 Axial postcontrast (A) and T2-weighted images (B) through the cervical spine at the level of C6 showing enhancing intramedullary mass (arrow). The spinal cord has expanded, leaving virtually no CSF space (arrowheads).

- The mass usually causes cord expansion.
- Postcontrast imaging will demonstrate enhancement of the tumor, distinguishing it from normal cord. Fat-saturated sequences help differentiate abnormal enhancement from the presence of fatty elements. Leptomeningeal enhancement, corresponding to spread of tumor, is also common.

- These tumors tend to be located eccentrically in the canal as opposed to ependymoma, which arise from the ependymal lining.
- Calcification occurs occasionally.

DIFFERENTIAL DIAGNOSIS
Clinical Differential

Ependymoma, arteriovenous malformation, syringohydromyelia, schwannoma, neurofibroma, and meningioma can all cause symptoms similar to the presentation discussed in this case.

Imaging Differential

- Ependymoma: more commonly have a cystic or necrotic component. These tumors tend to be more centrally located. Hemorrhagic foci are common. T2-weighted signal is hyperintense to spinal parenchyma.
- Arteriovenous malformation: will contain serpiginous flow voids on T2-weighted imaging. Enhancement is avid, with rapid washout. These lesions more commonly occur in the lower cord and rarely affect the caliber of the cord or canal.
- Syringohydromyelia: will be fluid signal and cystic on all sequences. These lesions do not enhance.
- Schwannoma/meningioma/neurofibroma: these masses are intradural extramedullary.

REFERENCES AND SUGGESTED READING

1. Horger M, Ritz R, Beschorner R, et al. Spinal astrocytoma: MR imaging findings at first presentation and following surgery. *Eur J Radiol.* 2011;79:389-399.
2. Koeller KK, Rosenblum RS, Morrison AL. Neoplasms of the spinal cord and filum terminale: radiologic-pathologic correlation. *Radiographics.* 2000;20:1721-1749.
3. Koeller KK, Rushing EJ. Pilocytic astrocytoma: radiologic-pathologic correlation. *Radiographics.* 2004;24:1693-1708.

CASE 31

PATIENT PRESENTATION

A 12-year-old male presenting with gradual onset of gait disturbance over past several weeks. No history of trauma. Physical examination demonstrates reduced pain and temperature sensation involving the lower extremities.

CLINICAL SUSPICION

Focal spinal cord lesion, possibly syrinx

IMAGING MODALITY OF CHOICE

MRI is the imaging modality of choice to assess the spinal cord (Figs. C31.1 and C31.2). It also permits the evaluation of the spinal canal and the surrounding osseous and ligamentous structures.

FINDINGS

- Liquid content of the cyst cavity will be hypointense on T1-weighted images and fluid signal (hyperintense) on T2-weighted images.
- Frequently associated with Chiari I malformation (constellation of findings include tonsillar herniation, small posterior fossa, and posterior angling of the odontoid process).

DIFFERENTIAL DIAGNOSIS

Clinical Differential

Spinal cord tumor, posttraumatic cyst, central cord dilation

Imaging Differential

- Spinal cord tumor, cystic: typically heterogeneous on T1-weighted images, hyperintense on T2, variable contrast enhancement.
- Posttraumatic cyst: should be considered when there is a history of trauma. The cystic area results from myelomalacia and degeneration.
- Central cord dilation (ventriculus terminalis): These cystic structures are seen near the conus and are infrequently associated with other findings, whereas low-lying syringomyelia is associated with spina bifida occulta, syndactyly, and pes cavus.

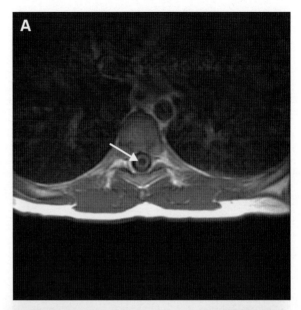

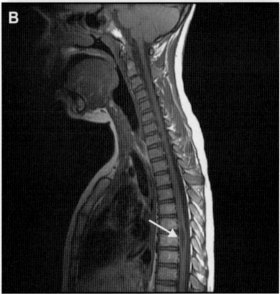

Fig. C31.1 Axial (A) and sagittal (B) T1-weighted MRI images of the upper thoracic spine demonstrating a focal, fusiform area of low signal intensity extending from T7 to T9 (arrows).

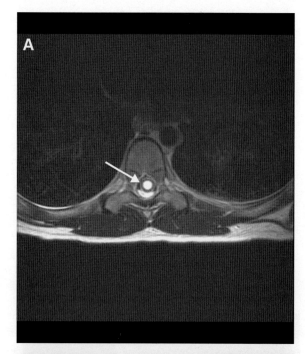

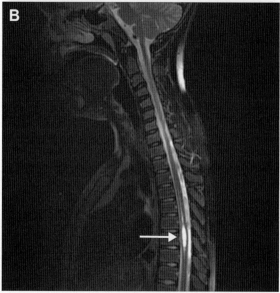

Fig. C31.2 Axial (A) and sagittal (B) T2-weighted images through the thoracic spine revealing fluid-intensity signal within the widened central canal at T7 through T9 (arrows).

REFERENCES AND SUGGESTED READING

1. Coleman LT, Zimmerman RA, Rorke LB. Ventriculus terminalis of the conus medullaris: MR findings in children. *AJNR.* 1995;16:1421-1426.

2. Elster AD, Chen MY. Chiari I malformations: clinical and radiologic reappraisal. *Radiology.* 1992;183:347-353.

3. Guinto G, Abdo M, Arechiga N, Zepeda E. Different types of syringomyelia and their management: part I. *Contemp Neurosurg.* 2009;31:1-8.

CASE 32

PATIENT PRESENTATION

A 30-year-old female with history of chronic ear infections presents with several-month history of hearing loss. Physical examination reveals a pearly white tumor at the pars flaccida.

CLINICAL SUSPICION

Cholesteatoma

IMAGING MODALITY OF CHOICE

Temporal bone CT without contrast. Advantages: high-resolution images of the temporal bone allow evaluation of small structures that may be eroded in the setting of cholesteatoma (Figs. C32.1 and C32.2).

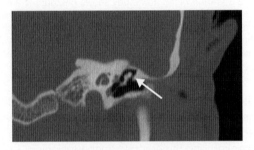

Fig. C32.1 Normal middle ear. Note the normal scutum (arrow) and the tympanic membrane with intact ossicles.

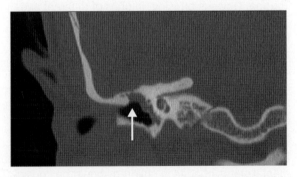

Fig C32.2 The presence of a soft tissue density mass (arrow) in Prussak's space erodes the scutum as well as the ossicles.

FINDINGS

An acquired cholesteatoma results from ingrowth of squamous epithelium through the tympanic membrane into the middle ear. The most common type of acquired cholesteatoma is the pars flaccida type (80%) with the following imaging charactersitics on temporal bone CT:

- Soft tissue mass in Prussak's space (lateral to the head of the malleus).
- Commonly erodes the scutum (bony plate from the lower edge of which the tympanic membrane is attached).
- Often results in ossicular erosion (usually the long process of the incus).
- Although contrast-enhanced imaging is usually not performed in the evaluation of cholesteatoma, there is usually no contrast enhancement if contrast is used.

Complications of cholesteatoma include intracranial extension, which may cause meningitis, venous thrombosis, CSF leak, erosion of labyrinth with creation of perilympatic fistula, and facial nerve palsy.

DIFFERENTIAL DIAGNOSIS

- Congenital middle ear cholesteatoma: congenital ectodermal rest in the middle ear cavity that is far less common than acquired cholesteatomas. Bone and ossicular erosion can be seen but is less common than in acquired cholesteatoma.
- Middle ear cholesterol granuloma: usually occurs in patients with multiple ear infections resulting in repeated episodes of hemorrhage into the middle ear cavity. Can result in bone and ossicular erosion similar to cholesteatoma.
- Glomus tympanicum paraganglioma: usually presents as a pulsatile red mass behind the eardrum on clinical examination. On imaging, this lesion does not cause bone or ossicular erosions.

REFERENCES AND SUGGESTED READING

1. Mafee MF. MRI and CT in the evaluation of acquired and congenital cholesteatomas of the temporal bone. *J Otolaryngol.* August 1993;22(4):239-248.
2. Alexander AE. Clinical and surgical application of reformatted high-resolution CT of the temporal bone. *Neuroimaging Clin N Am.* 1998;8:631.

CASE 33

PATIENT PRESENTATION

A 2-year-old female arrives to the emergency room non-responsive with a Glasgow Coma Scale of 3 and no brain stem signs. No external injuries are noted. The parents report the child has been behaviorally challenging, requiring "extra discipline."

CLINICAL SUSPICION

Nonaccidental trauma resulting in brain death

IMAGING MODALITY OF CHOICE

The initial study to evaluate a patient with mental status changes is brain CT (Figs. C33.1 and C33.2). In the setting of a patient in whom no cerebral or brain stem activity can be elicited, a nuclear medicine cerebral blood flow study is an adjunct to the clinical diagnosis of brain death; it should never be considered the final diagnostic determination.

FINDINGS

A patient clinically suspected of brain death is administered a radiotracer that reflects brain metabolism, usually technetium-99m-HMPAO or Tc-99m ECD. The radiopharmaceutical crosses the blood-brain barrier and is taken up by the cerebrum, cerebellum, and brain stem. If there is no cerebral perfusion or metabolism, no radiotracer uptake is seen, which supports a clinical diagnosis of brain death. By comparison, the extracranial circulation will be relatively increased, resulting in a "hot" focus in the area

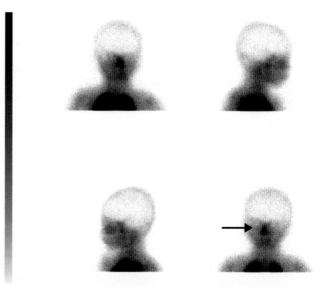

Fig. C33.2 Cerebral blood flow study shows photopenic area (white) in the intracranial cavity representing a lack of intracranial blood flow, consistent with the clinical diagnosis of brain death. The exam demonstrates comparatively intense uptake of radiopharmaceutical in the face/extracranial circulation, referred to as the "hot nose" sign (arrow).

of greatest preserved perfusion—the face. This finding has been termed the "hot nose" sign as a central area of increased uptake over the face is present overlying a photopenic background of cerebral hypoperfusion.

DIFFERENTIAL DIAGNOSIS

- Trauma: Obvious bruising, injuries of different ages, and/or an inconsistent history should raise suspicion for nonaccidental trauma. Most institutions employ a protocol for trauma assessment in children that includes physical examination and survey radiography.

- Cerebral edema: Multiple etiologies for cerebral edema exist, including toxic exposure and seizure. Reversible causes for brain edema are usually assessed during the initial evaluation.

- Encephalitis/meningitis: Infectious etiologies for acute mental status change in children should be considered. However, absent supporting clinical history or signs/symptoms of infection, further investigation and imaging is warranted.

REFERENCES AND SUGGESTED READING

1. Donohue KJ, Frey KA, Gerbaudo VH, Mariani G, Nagel JS, Shulkin B. Procedure guideline for brain death scintigraphy. *J Nucl Med.* 2003;44:846-851.

2. Huang AH. The hot nose sign. *Radiology.* 2005;235:216-217.

3. Mettler FA, Guiberteau MJ. Radionuclide brain imaging. In: *Essentials of Nuclear Medicine.* 4th ed. Philadelphia, PA: Saunders; 1998:82-83.

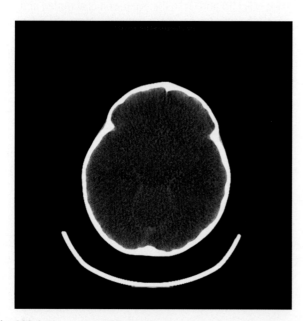

Fig. C33.1 Noncontrast CT examination of the brain demonstrates loss of gray-white matter distinction and complete effacement of the sulci and cisterns, consistent with global cerebral edema.

CASE 34

PATIENT PRESENTATION

A 3-year-old child with history of fever presents to the emergency room with difficulty swallowing. Physical examination reveals erythema of the pharyngeal soft tissues with neck stiffness and bilateral cervical lymphadenopathy.

CLINICAL SUSPICION

Pharyngitis complicated by retropharyngeal abscess

IMAGING MODALITY OF CHOICE

Contrast-enhanced CT examination of the neck (Fig. C34.1). Advantages: CT is a readily available imaging study that defines the extent of the inflammatory process and assists in identifying the presence of a drainable abscess. The use of intravenous contrast is helpful in differentiating between abscess and nonpurulent collections and useful in evaluating vascular complications. The patient is scanned from level of skull base to carina.

FINDINGS

Retropharyngeal abscess represents the spread of infection usually from pharyngitis or tonsillitis to the retropharyngeal space, either from direct extension or from lymphatic drainage. Less common causes include ventral extension from a prevertebral infection or from a penetrating foreign body. Contrast-enhanced CT findings are as follows:

- Thickening of the retropharyngeal soft tissues (inflammation of tissues posterior to the oropharynx).

- A well-defined low-intensity collection usually surrounded by an enhancing rim is consistent with abscess. Early abscesses may not demonstrate rim enhancement.

- Suppurative inflammation without drainable fluid collection is generically termed a phlegmon, which may proceed to an abscess if inadequately treated.

- A large abscess may narrow the airway or extend into the carotid space, resulting in vascular complications such as jugular vein thrombosis and carotid artery pseudoaneurysm.

DIFFERENTIAL DIAGNOSIS

Clinical Differential

Fever with airway symptoms:

- Croup: self-limiting condition caused by parainfluenza virus infection resulting in subglottic edema.

- Exudative tracheitis: subglottic infection involving the tracheal mucosa with presence of inflammatory membranes.

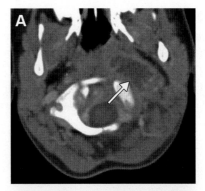

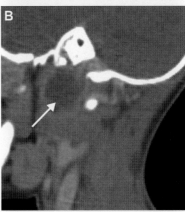

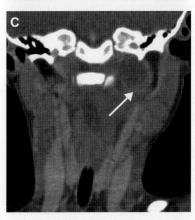

Fig. C34.1 Axial (A) and sagittal (B) oriented contrast-enhanced CT of the neck demonstrates thickening of the retropharyngeal soft tissues with the presence of a low-density fluid collection with peripheral enhancement consistent with an abscess (arrows). (C) Coronal CT imaging demonstrates abscess displacing the left carotid artery and jugular vein. Note the presence of asymmetrically enlarged left cervical lymphadenopathy (arrow).

- Epiglottitis: inflammation of the epiglottis that results in airway compromise. Rarely seen after the routine immunization against *Haemophilus influenzae* type b.

Radiological Differential

- Retrophanyngeal edema: nonpurulent inflammation within the retropharngeal tissues from pharyngitis/tonsillitis.

- Lymphatic malformation, lymphatic obstruction can result in fluid collection in the retropharyngeal space.

REFERENCES/SUGGESTED READING

1. Craig FW. Retropharyngeal abscess in children. *Pediatrics*. June 2003;111(6, pt 1):1394-1398.

2. Dawes. Retropharyngeal abscess in children. *ANZ J Surg*. June 2002;72(6):417-420.

3. Chong VF. Radiology of the retropharyngeal space. *Clin Radiol*. October 2000;55(10):740-748.

CASE 35

PATIENT PRESENTATION

A 65-year-old male with complaints of "fullness in throat" and dysphagia developing over the past few months. He reports a 50-year history of smoking and drinking regularly. A large mass is identified at the base of the tongue and enlarged cervical lymph nodes are palpated bilaterally.

CLINICAL SUSPICION

Head and neck squamous cell carcinoma (SCC)

IMAGING MODALITY OF CHOICE

CT soft tissue neck with contrast (Fig. C35.1). Advantages: rapidly acquired examination that estimates size and extent of local disease and allows for assessment of regional lymph nodes.

FINDINGS

Head and neck squamous cell carcinoma involves patients in the fifth through seventh decades of life and affects men 3 to 5 times more often than women. Risk factors include tobacco use, drinking, and HPV exposure. Contrast-enhanced CT findings include:

- Enhancing mucosal lesion representing primary tumor.
- If nodal disease is present, there is nodal enlargement usually over 1 cm. Involved lymph nodes may demonstrate central necrosis.

DIFFERENTIAL DIAGNOSIS

Clinical Differential

- Lymphoid hyperplasia
- Benign salivary gland tumor
- Lymphoma
- Sarcoma

Diagnostic Differential

- Nonsquamous head/neck cancer
- Metastasis
- Lymphoma

REFERENCES/SUGGESTED READING

1. Weber AL, Romo L, Hashmi S. Malignant tumors of the oral cavity and oropharynx: clinical, pathologic, and radiologic evaluation. *Neuroimaging Clin N Am*. August 2003;13(3):443-464.

2. Sigal R, Zagdanski AM, Schwaab G, et al. CT and MR imaging of squamous cell carcinoma of the tongue and floor of the mouth. *Radiographics*. July 1996;16(4):787-810.

3. Mukherji SK, Castelijns J, Castillo M. Squamous cell carcinoma of the oropharynx and oral cavity: how imaging makes a difference. *Semin Ultrasound CT MR*. December 1998;19(6):463-475. Review.

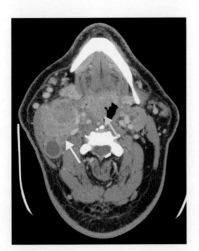

Fig. C35.1 Axial contrast-enhanced CT image demonstrates a large enhancing mass arising from the right base of tongue (yellow arrow). Note the presence of large metastatic lymph nodes (white arrow) bilaterally, right greater than left.

Chapter 4

Cardiothoracic Imaging

By Nakul Gupta, Eduardo J. Matta, and Sandra A. A. Oldham

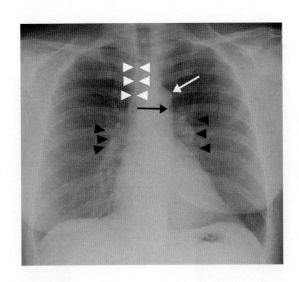

BASIC RADIOLOGIC ANATOMY OF THE CHEST

In order to identify pathologic changes in the chest, it is important to understand the radiologic anatomy. Since chest radiography and CT are the primary modalities for imaging the chest, these will be depicted in Figs. 4.1 to 4.6. While the heart and lungs are the dominant structures in the chest, it is important to remember that many other important structures are depicted on radiographs and CT scans of the chest, such as the great vessels, esophagus, tracheobronchial tree, rib cage, etc. Many of these structures are contained within the mediastinum. For practical purposes, it is useful to compartmentalize the mediastinum as described by Felson [1]. The anterior and middle mediastinum are divided on the lateral chest radiograph by a line extending along the anterior tracheal border and inferiorly along the posterior border of the heart. The middle and posterior mediastinum are separated by a line 1 cm posterior to the anterior margin of the thoracic vertebral bodies. While this differs from traditional anatomic boundaries, it proves useful radiographically.

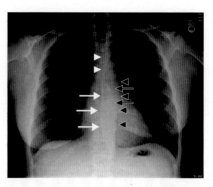

Fig. 4.2 Normal PA view of the chest. This is the same study as Fig. 4.1; however, the window and level settings have been adjusted to allow for improved visualization of the mediastinal borders. Black arrowheads annotate the lateral border of the descending aorta. Black arrows demarcate the left paraspinal stripe. White arrowheads demonstrate the anterior junction line, formed where the pleura of the right and left lungs appose anteriorly. Finally, the azygoesophageal recess is marked by white arrows, formed by the interface of the right lower lobe with the esophagus and azygous vein. Please note the importance of altering window/level settings in order to maximize visualization of normal anatomic structures and therefore pathology as well.

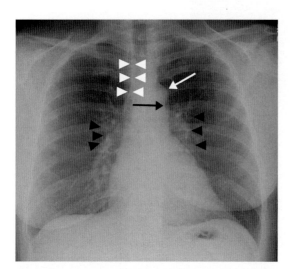

Fig. 4.1 Normal PA view of the chest. This is a female patient (note the breast shadows). White arrowheads denote the right paratracheal stripe. This is normally 4 mm or less in thickness. The white arrow annotates the aortic knob, which is created by the aortic arch being seen somewhat en face, slightly oblique. The black arrow denotes the AP window. The hilar angles are demarcated bilaterally by the black arrowheads, and are normally concave as in this patient. The right heart border (mostly the right atrium) is border forming with the right middle lobe, and the left heart border (mostly the left ventricle) is border forming with the lingula.

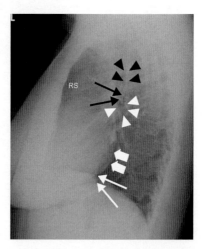

Fig. 4.3 Normal lateral chest radiograph. RS denotes the retrosternal clear space. An opacity in this region would suggest an anterior mediastinal mass. Black arrowheads mark the posterior wall of the trachea. Thin black arrows denote the posterior wall of the bronchus intermedius, and white arrowheads outline the right main bronchus, which is seen en face on the lateral projection. Thick white arrows demonstrate the posterior border of the left atrium, and thin white arrows annotate the posterior border of the IVC. Note how the vertebral bodies become more lucent inferiorly; loss of this lucency is a useful sign when assessing for a retrocardiac opacity.

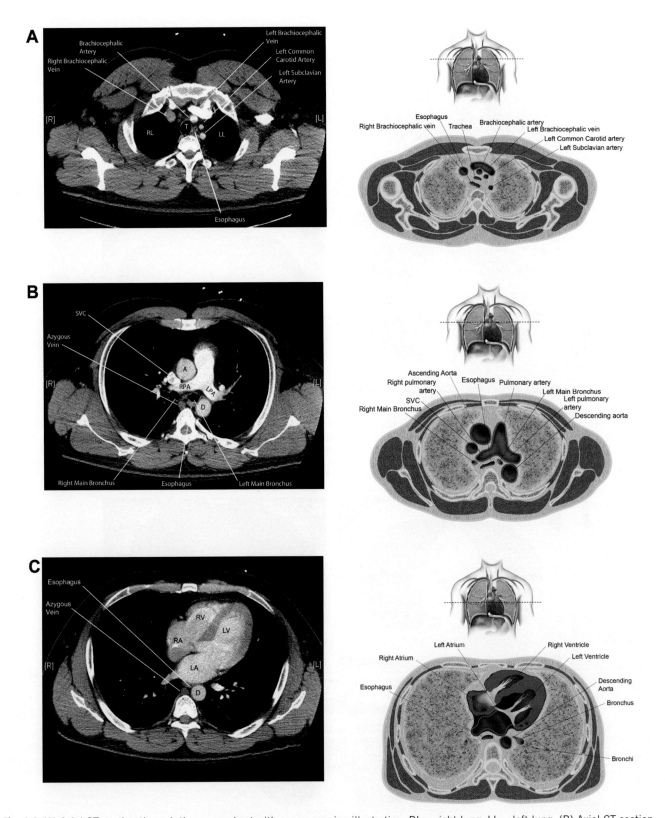

Fig. 4.4 (A) Axial CT section through the upper chest with accompanying illustration. RL = right lung, LL = left lung. (B) Axial CT section through the pulmonary artery with accompanying illustration. A = ascending aorta, D = descending aorta, RPA = right pulmonary artery, LPA = left pulmonary artery. (C) Axial section through the heart with accompanying illustration. LV = left ventricle, RV = right ventricle, RA = right atrium, LA = left atrium, D = descending aorta.

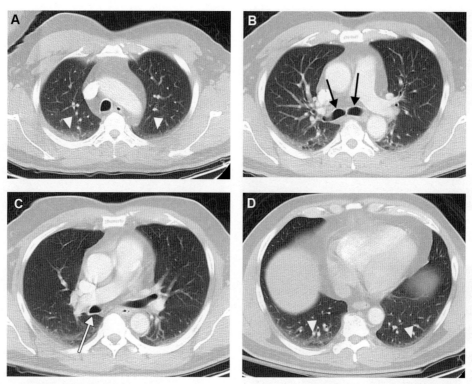

Fig. 4.5 Representative axial CT sections in lung windows, superior to inferior. (A) Axial section through the apices. Note the bilateral dependent hazy opacity (white arrowheads). This is due to areas of subsegmental or discoid atelectasis, and is seen commonly. If the patient were scanned in the prone position rather than supine, then this would be seen in the ventral aspect of the lungs. (B) Axial section just below the carina demonstrates the right and left main bronchi (black arrows). (C) Axial section slightly inferior to (B) demonstrates the posterior wall of the bronchus intermedius (white arrow). (D) Axial section through the lung bases again demonstrates bilateral dependent atelectasis (white arrowheads). This is seen nearly ubiquitously at the lung bases.

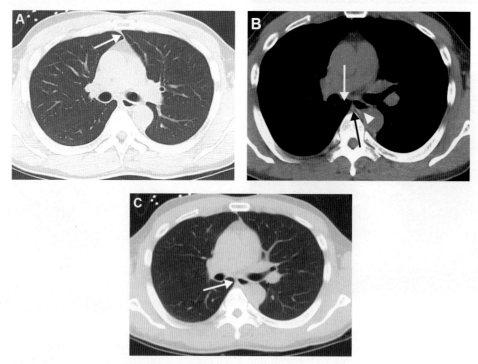

Fig. 4.6 Additional axial CT sections, different patient. (A) Axial section just below the carina demonstrates the anterior junction line (white arrow). (B) Axial section slightly lower than (A) in soft tissue windows demonstrates the azygos vein (black arrow), esophagus (white arrowhead), and the azygoesophageal recess (white arrow). (C) Lung windows better demonstrate the lung–mediastinum interface (white arrow), which creates the azygoesophageal recess on chest x-rays.

The right lung is divided into upper, middle, and lower lobes by pleural reflections known as fissures (Fig. 4.7). The major fissure is obliquely oriented from superior to inferior, and divides the right lower lobe posteroinferiorly from the upper and middle lobes anterosuperiorly. The minor fissure is horizontally oriented and divides the right upper and middle lobes. Each lobe is divided into segments based on bronchovascular supply. The right upper lobe is divided into apical, anterior, and posterior segments. The right middle lobe is divided into medial and lateral segments. The right lower lobe is divided into a superior segment and 4 basal segments (medial, anterior, lateral, and posterior). The left upper lobe is divided into the apicoposterior segment and anterior segment. The lingua is divided into superior and inferior segments. The left lower lobe consists of a superior

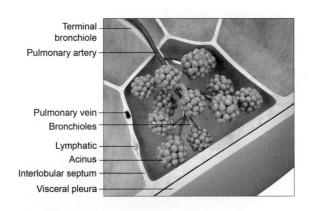

Fig. 4.8 Secondary pulmonary lobule.

segment, but only contains three basal segments instead of four (anterior, lateral, and posterior).

The smallest functional unit of the lung is known as the secondary pulmonary lobule (Fig. 4.8). Each lobule is demarcated by interlobular septae, which contain lymphatics and pulmonary veins. Interlobular septae are not normally visible on radiographs, and only occasionally faintly seen on HRCT. When they become visible, it is usually because they are diseased. The lobule is supplied centrally by a terminal bronchiole and accompanying centrilobular pulmonary artery, which are together known as the bronchovascular bundle. A second set of lymphatics also runs with the bronchovascular bundle.

REFERENCE AND SUGGESTED READING

1. Felson B. *Chest Roentgenology*. WB Saunders, PA; 1973.

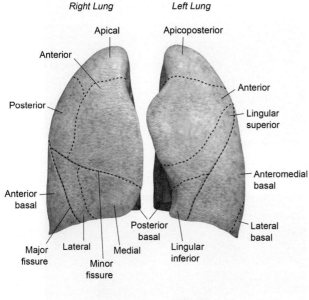

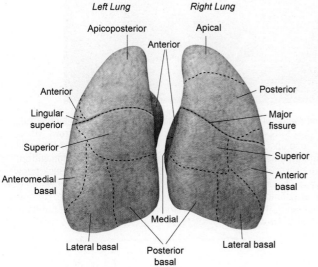

Fig. 4.7 Segmental anatomy of the lungs. Top diagram is an anterior view; bottom diagram is a posterior view.

CASE 1: PNEUMONIA

PATIENT PRESENTATION

A 50-year-old female presents with fever, cough, and chest pain.

CLINICAL SUSPICION

Pneumonia

IMAGING MODALITY OF CHOICE

Chest x-ray, preferably PA and lateral views (Figs. C1.1-C1.5)

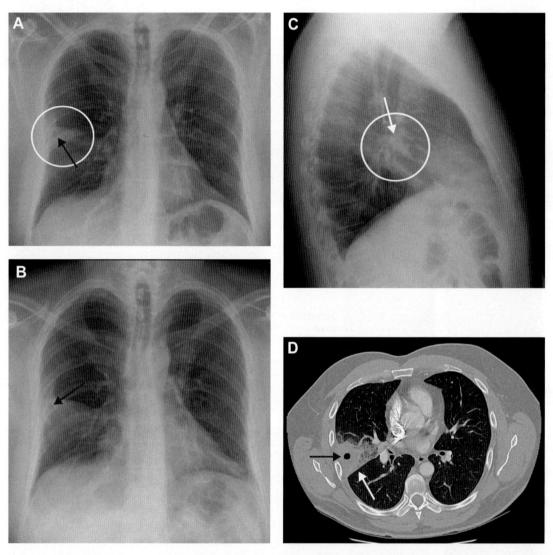

Fig. C1.1 Necrotizing right middle lobe pneumonia. (A) Initial frontal chest radiograph demonstrates a hazy opacity bordered by the minor fissure superiorly, indicating right middle lobe location (white circle). There is a rounded lucency within this opacity (black arrow). (B, C) PA and lateral views obtained 24 hours later show worsening right middle lobe opacity (white circle). The rounded lucency is more well defined (black arrow). (D) Chest CT in lung windows performed at the same time as (B) and (C) demonstrates focal consolidation within the right middle lobe (white arrow) with an area of lucency consistent with necrosis, more apparent than on the chest x-rays (black arrow). Necrotizing pneumonias may be caused by *Staphylococcus aureus*, *Klebsiella pneumoniae*, as well as anaerobic organisms (often when due to aspiration). Fungal organisms should also be considered in the appropriate clinical setting. Occasionally, it may be difficult to differentiate necrotizing pneumonia from a cavitary malignancy. In necrotizing pneumonia, there is typically a larger area of surrounding pulmonary consolidation. Also, cavities resulting from malignancy typically have more nodular walls.

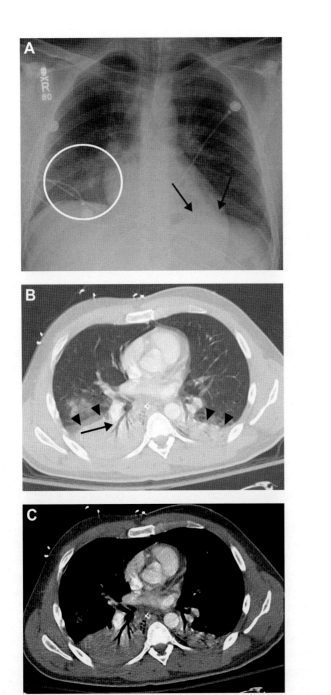

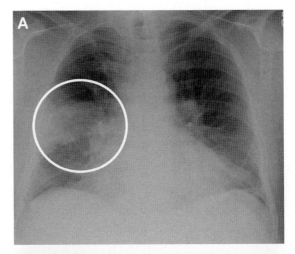

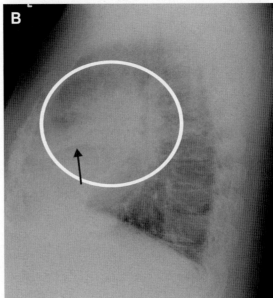

Fig. C1.3 Right upper lobe pneumonia. (A) PA view of the chest demonstrates a large airspace opacity in the right mid lung zone. (B) Lateral view of the chest localizes the opacity to the right upper lobe anterior segment.

Fig. C1.2 Pneumonia. (A) Portable AP chest radiograph demonstrates a hazy right lower lung opacity (white circle) and a retrocardiac opacity that partially obscures the left hemidiaphragm (black arrows). The patient is intubated and there is a nasogastric tube. (B) Axial chest CT in lung windows demonstrates bilateral dependent consolidation, right worse than left (black arrowheads). Note the air bronchograms (black arrow). (C) Same study as B, now in soft tissue windows. Note how the consolidated lung does not enhance. If this were atelectasis, the lung would demonstrate enhancement.

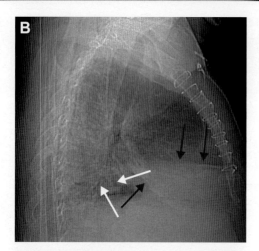

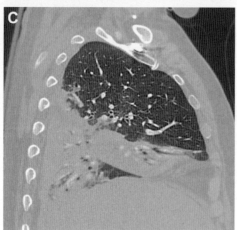

Fig. C1.4 Right upper and lower lobe pneumonia. (A) Initial AP chest radiograph demonstrates airspace opacity in the right lower lung zone (white circle) bordered by the minor fissure superiorly (white arrow), indicating right middle lobe consolidation. (B) Lateral scout from CT scan obtained the same day demonstrates right middle lobe consolidation (black arrows). There are also multiple air bronchograms seen posteriorly (white arrows), suggesting right lower lobe consolidation as well. (C) Sagittal reformatted CT in lung windows demonstrates right middle and lower lobe consolidation. Blood cultures were positive for *Streptococcus pneumoniae.* The patient was HIV positive.

FINDINGS

Classic inhalationally acquired pneumonias follow one of several radiographic patterns: a lobar pattern, lobular or bronchopneumonia pattern, or an interstitial pattern. Lobar pneumonias are due to filling of distal airspaces with a fibrinopurulent exudate. Radiographically, they manifest as airspace opacities that are largely confined to one lobe and often demonstrate "air bronchograms," which are branching patent airways seen against a background of opacified airspaces. These airspace opacities are often described as fluffy, hazy, or consolidative opacities. Lobar pneumonias are most often due to bacterial infections, and *Streptococcus pneumoniae* is a typical organism. There is little, if any, volume loss, and there may even be volume expansion manifest by bulging fissures, especially in *Klebsiella* infections. A lobular or bronchopneumonia pattern is due to patchy consolidation of the lung and is typically caused by bacterial infection, for example *Staphylococcus aureus*. There is considerable overlap between lobar and bronchopneumonia patterns, as the patchy opacities seen in a bronchopneumonia may progress and become confluent, thus resembling a lobar pneumonia. Also, the same organism may cause a bronchopneumonia pattern in one individual, and a lobar pattern in another. The "silhouette sign" is a useful sign to localize an area of consolidation. The premise of the silhouette sign is that when two structures of similar densities are abutting each other, the border between them is not visible on a radiograph. The diaphragmatic and cardiomediastinal borders on a chest x-ray are visible because the mediastinum and diaphragm are of soft tissue density (approximately the same as water), and are outlined by the lungs, which are of primarily air density. When the portion of lung in contact with one of these borders becomes diseased (eg, with pneumonia, edema, hemorrhage, etc, which are all similar to water density), then that border becomes obscured, or "silhouetted." For instance, the right heart border on a frontal view of the chest is mostly bordered by the middle lobe (RML). Therefore, obscuration of the right heart border often signifies disease in the RML. The left heart border is often obscured by disease in the lingula, the right border of the ascending aorta is often obliterated by RUL anterior segment disease, disease silhouetting the diaphragm is in either the right or the left lower lobe, and disease obliterating the left border of the aortic knob localizes to the LUL apicoposterior segment.

Aspiration pneumonitis and pneumonia are distinct clinicopathologic entities that bear discussion as well. Aspiration events will vary in distribution depending on the position of the patient at the time of aspiration. If aspiration occurs in the supine position, the gravity-dependent portions of the lungs are the superior segments of the lower lobes and the posterior segments of the upper lobes. In

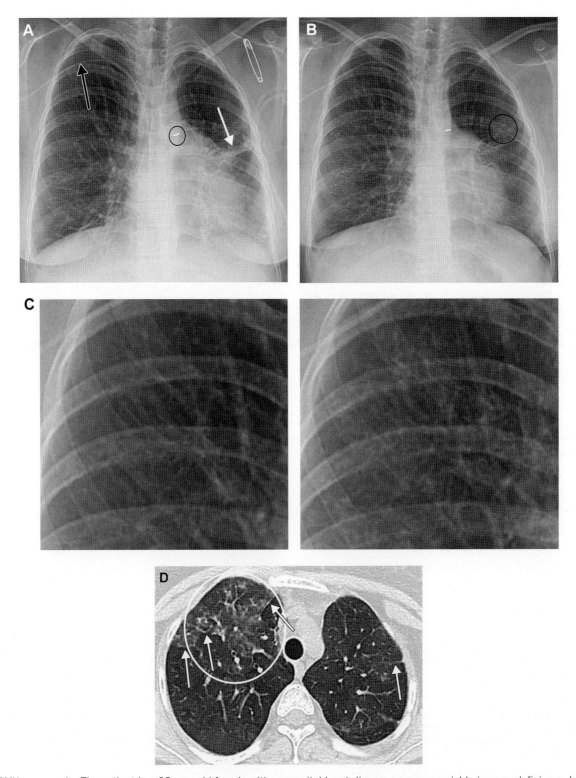

Fig. C1.5 CMV pneumonia. The patient is a 22-year-old female with congenital heart disease, common variable immunodeficiency, being treated for Burkitt's lymphoma. (A) Baseline frontal chest x-ray demonstrates a right upper extremity PICC (black arrow), PDA ligation clip (black circle), and some scarring in the left lung, probably from prior infections in this immunocompromised patient (white arrow). (B) Several months later the patient presented with fever and cough. Chest x-ray demonstrates subtly increased reticular opacities throughout most of the right lung. Faint nodular opacities in the left lung are annotated as well (black circle). (C) Magnified view of a portion of the right upper lung with baseline image on the left and admission chest x-ray on the right. Although subtle, note the increased linear densities in the right image. (D) Axial chest CT demonstrates patchy ground glass opacities in the right upper lobe (white circle). Compare this to the denser consolidation seen in Figs. C1.2 and C1.4. White arrows indicate examples of reticular opacities. Bronchoalveolar lavage was performed, and CMV was isolated.

the upright position, the right middle lobe and basilar segments of the lower lobes are affected. In general, the right lung is affected more due to the more vertical orientation of the right main bronchus. Aspiration pneumonitis is most often the result of aspirating sterile but acidic gastric contents, and is also known as Mendelson's syndrome. Aspiration pneumonia results when oropharyngeal secretions colonized by microorganisms are aspirated. Radiographically, it is not often possible to differentiate the two. Sterile pneumonitis may clear more rapidly and without antibiotic therapy, while aspiration pneumonia may progress to necrosis, cavitation, and abscess formation. Severe acute aspiration events may cause severe lung injury and can lead to ARDS.

Interstitial patterns are usually caused by atypical bacteria (ie, *Mycoplasma pneumoniae*), or viral infections (such as influenza, RSV, adenovirus, HSV, varicella, etc). They are characterized pathologically by an inflammatory infiltrate primarily confined to the interstitium of the lung and the walls of the alveoli, without dense filling of the alveolar airspaces. There may be obstruction of small airways due to the inflammation, resulting in areas of resorptive atelectasis. Radiographically, interstitial opacities are often described as reticular (consisting of predominantly linear densities), nodular (predominantly small rounded opacities), or reticulonodular (a combination of both). At CT, these findings may be easier to appreciate, and subtle cases may only be visible with CT. Additionally, CT often demonstrates "ground glass" opacities, which are not as dense as frank consolidation and have a hazier appearance. Pathologically, these opacities represent partial filling or collapse of alveolar airspaces, as well as infiltration of the interstitium below the resolution of CT.

Clinical Differential

COPD exacerbation, aspiration, myocardial infarction, pulmonary embolism

Imaging Differential

Airspace opacities are most often due to pneumonia, edema, contusion, or hemorrhage. Clinical information is often required to distinguish between these entities. Atelectasis may also mimic airspace opacity, although evidence of volume loss is often present, and can aid in the diagnosis. The differential diagnosis of cavitary pneumonias includes fungal infection, tuberculosis, and malignancy.

REFERENCES AND SUGGESTED READINGS

1. Felson B. *Chest Roentgenology*. WB Saunders, PA; 1973.
2. Marik PE. Aspiration pneumonitis and aspiration pneumonia. *N Engl J Med*. 2001;344:665-671.

CASE 2: PLEURAL EFFUSION

PATIENT PRESENTATION

Progressive shortness of breath over the past several days to weeks. On exam, there are decreased breath sounds at the right lung base.

CLINICAL SUSPICION

Pleural effusion (Figs. C2.1-C2.4)

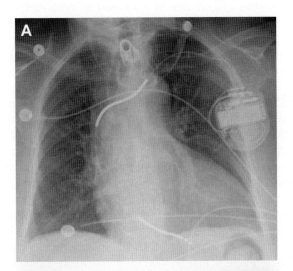

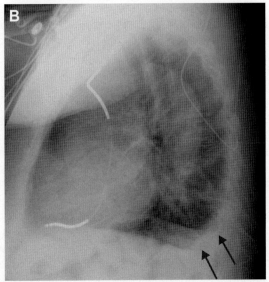

Fig. C2.1 Small pleural effusion. (A) PA view of the chest demonstrates sharp lateral costophrenic angles, no evidence of pleural effusion. The cardiac silhouette is enlarged, and there is an AICD/pacemaker. (B) Lateral view demonstrates blunting of the posterior costophrenic angles, indicating small bilateral pleural effusions (black arrows). On the lateral view, the right hemidiaphragm can be followed anteriorly, while the left hemidiaphragm will be silhouetted by the heart and will be lost anteriorly. Therefore, the lower black arrow indicates the right costophrenic angle in this case, and the upper arrow is the left.

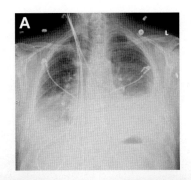

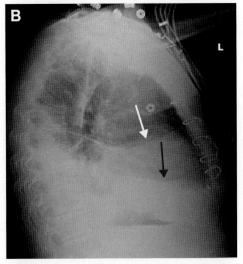

Fig. C2.2 Large bilateral pleural effusions. (A) PA view of the chest demonstrates large bilateral pleural effusions, right worse than left with hazy bibasilar opacities and menisci. (B) Lateral view demonstrates the menisci as well, left (white arrow) and right (black arrow).

IMAGING MODALITY OF CHOICE

Chest x-ray. CT can be a useful adjunct in characterizing empyemas and loculated effusions.

DISCUSSION

Frontal and lateral views should be obtained, and decubitus views are helpful as well to demonstrate mobility/layering of fluid to exclude loculation. Decubitus views are also the most sensitive to small amounts of fluid. CT is helpful in complicated cases (ie, empyema, loculation), as well as to evaluate for underlying lung or pleural masses. Administration of contrast material is helpful whenever possible, especially when looking for underlying masses or if an exudative effusion is suspected (ie, empyema).

The pleural space physiologically contains up to 5 cc of fluid. Mobile pleural effusions will travel to the most dependent portion of the pleura, which will vary depending on the position in which the patient is imaged. When the patient is erect, this is typically the posterior costophrenic recess, and this is why lateral views are more sensitive to detect

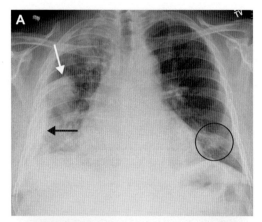

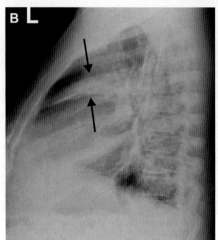

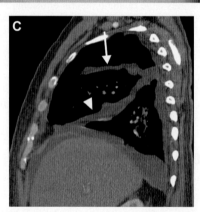

Fig. C2.3 Pseudotumor caused by fluid tracking along the minor fissure. (A) PA view of the chest demonstrates smooth, lentiform right lateral pleural thickening (black arrow) suspicious for pleural effusion. There is a nodular opacity in the right midlung zone (white arrow). An ill-defined hazy opacity is also seen at the left lung base (black circle). (B) Lateral view of the chest fails to demonstrate the nodular lesion seen in the right midlung on the frontal view. However, there is fluid noted to be tracking in the minor fissure (black arrows). This creates an illusion of a nodular or mass lesion on frontal views of the chest, and it is often described as a pseudotumor. This is most often seen in association with congestive heart failure or other transudative effusions. (C) Sagittal reformatted CT scan in soft tissue windows demonstrates fluid tracking along the major (white arrowhead) and minor (white arrow) fissures. There was no mass. Ill-defined opacity at the left lung base was due to scarring, likely from prior infection.

small effusions compared to frontal views. A frontal view may require 200 to 500 cc of fluid to be present before blunting of the lateral costophrenic recesses will become evident, whereas approximately 50 cc may be necessary to see blunting of the posterior costophrenic recess on a lateral view [1]. The lateral decubitus view is actually the most sensitive, and may be able to detect as little as 10 cc of fluid [2]. After filling the posterior and lateral recesses, moderate sized effusions will typically extend superiorly and produce a meniscus, which is easily identified. Very large effusions can result in compressive atelectasis of most of the lung as well as contralateral mediastinal shift due to their space occupying effects, and can result in complete opacification of the hemithorax. These are often due to malignancy. Pleural fluid can accumulate in a variety of locations, including within the fissures, the subpulmonic space, and along the mediastinum. Subpulmonic effusions in particular can be difficult to assess on a frontal view. Some signs to look for include elevation of the hemidiaphragm, lateral displacement of the peak of the hemidiaphragm, and (only on the left side) increased distance between the gastric bubble and the diaphragm. In all of these signs, it is not actually the hemidiaphragm that is displaced, rather it is the subpulmonic collection silhouetted against the diaphragm that you are seeing. On a supine frontal view of the chest, pleural fluid will layer posteriorly, and may reach a very large size before being detectable. A hazy gradient opacity overlying the entire hemithorax may be the only clue. Larger effusions will eventually cause blunting of the lateral costophrenic recess, and a meniscus may be seen as well. Very large effusions will extend to the lung apex, producing an "apical cap."

Many patients with pneumonia develop simple parapneumonic effusions, of which a small percentage will go on to develop into an empyema due to secondary infection of the pleural fluid. While this may not be readily identifiable on plain films (unless it is loculated), contrast-enhanced CT can be helpful and will demonstrate thickening and enhancement of the pleura. Additionally, there will often be a "split-pleura" sign, which is when both the visceral and parietal leaves of the pleura are thickened and enhancing, and are seen to be separated by an empyema or exudative effusion [3]. Loculated effusions can be demonstrated by lack of mobility on decubitus views of the chest. Additionally, they tend to lose their meniscoid shape, and may appear as peripheral lentiform-shaped collections on frontal views, which may be indistinguishable from pleural masses based on x-ray alone. CT is again helpful in this situation, and will demonstrate fluid attenuation within a loculated pleural effusion, as opposed to a pleural mass. Ultrasound may allow direct visualization of the fibrinous septations responsible for the loculation, and may be used to guide thoracentesis. Hemorrhagic pleural effusions can sometimes be distinguished on CT

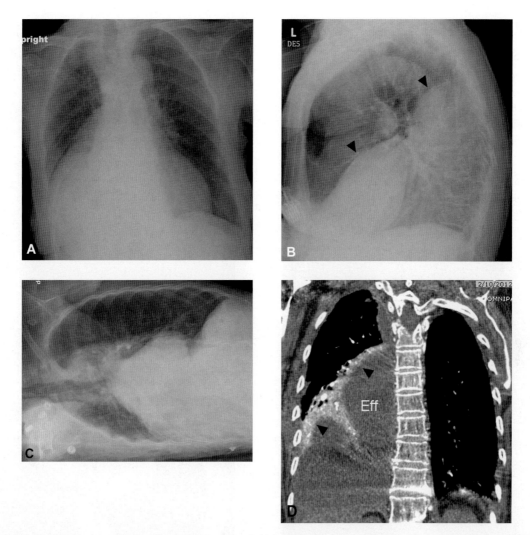

Fig. C2.4 Loculated pleural effusion. (A) There is elevation of the right hemidiaphragm on PA view. (B) Lateral view. The left hemidiaphragm is visible and silhouetted by the heart anteriorly. The right hemidiaphragm appears elevated (black arrowheads) likely due to a large subpulmonic effusion. (C) Right lateral decubitus view does not demonstrate layering of the effusion, indicating that it is loculated and not freely mobile. (D) Coronal reformatted contrast-enhanced CT in soft tissue windows demonstrates a large subpulmonic effusion (Eff) and adjacent enhancing atelectatic lung (black arrowheads).

due to the higher attenuation of blood compared to water. Additionally, a hematocrit effect may be seen, which is manifest by layering high-density material due to clotted blood products.

Drainage of pleural effusions whether for diagnostic or therapeutic purposes can be achieved in a variety of ways, depending largely on institutional or operator preference. Ultrasound, CT, and fluoroscopy are all commonly used. Ultrasound has the advantage of being portable, allowing for bedside drainage, and avoids radiation exposure as well.

Clinical Differential

Pneumonia, atelectasis, and lung cancer may all present with shortness of breath and decreased breath sounds.

Radiologic differential diagnosis

Imaging findings of a simple pleural effusion are fairly typical and pathognomonic. CT may be helpful in differentiating a simple effusion from an empyema as described on the previous page.

REFERENCES AND SUGGESTED READING

1. Blackmore CC, Black WC, Dallas RV, et al. Pleural fluid volume estimation: a chest radiograph prediction rule. *Acad Radiol.* 1996;3:103-109.

2. Moskowitz H, Platt RT, Schachar R, et al. Roentgen visualization of minute pleural effusion: an experimental study to determine the minimum amount of pleural fluid visible on a radiograph. *Radiology.* 1973;109:33-35.

3. Kraus GJ. The split pleura sign. *Radiology.* 2007;243:297-298.

CASE 3: PULMONARY EDEMA

PATIENT PRESENTATION

A 72-year-old male with past medical history of ischemic cardiomyopathy presents with increasing shortness of breath. A third heart sound and pulmonary rales are heard on auscultation, and there is pitting edema of the lower extremities. BNP is elevated.

CLINICAL SUSPICION

Decompensated congestive heart failure (CHF), pulmonary edema (Figs. C3.1-C3.3)

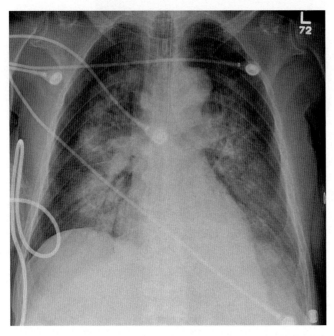

Fig. C3.1 "Batwing" pulmonary edema. Frontal chest radiograph demonstrates bilateral perihilar airspace opacities consistent with batwing pulmonary edema. This tends to be seen with acute or rapid development of heart failure. Also, there is thickening of the minor fissure, which is due to subpleural accumulation of fluid.

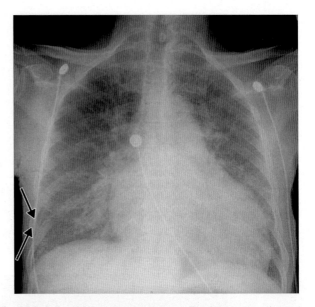

Fig. C3.2 Interstitial pulmonary edema. Frontal chest radiograph demonstrates diffuse bilateral reticular opacity as well as Kerley B lines (two are annotated with black arrows). These represent distended pulmonary lymphatic channels within the interlobular septae due to fluid overload. The cardiac silhouette is grossly enlarged in this patient with CHF.

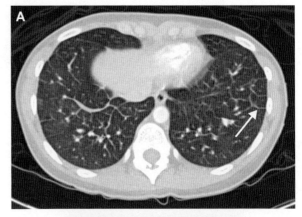

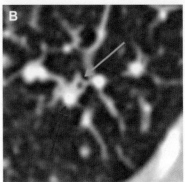

Fig. C3.3 Interstitial pulmonary edema. (A) Axial chest CT demonstrates smooth thickening of interlobular septae (white arrow) in a patient with interstitial pulmonary edema. This is the CT equivalent of Kerley B lines seen on chest x-rays. (B) Magnified view from the RLL in the same patient demonstrates bronchial wall thickening (green arrow), which is the CT equivalent of peribronchial cuffing seen on radiographs. Also, note that the adjacent pulmonary artery branch (red arrow) is slightly larger than the bronchus.

IMAGING MODALITY OF CHOICE

Chest x-ray, preferably upright PA and lateral views. Echocardiography is helpful in assessing cardiac function and chamber size among other things.

FINDINGS

Pulmonary edema can be broadly classified as being due to increased hydrostatic pressure, or due to increased capillary permeability. Hydrostatic edema is primarily due to left heart failure and volume overload states. Radiographically, hydrostatic edema typically progresses through three stages, which have been shown to correlate with a rising pulmonary capillary wedge pressure through each stage. The first stage is pulmonary venous hypertension, which is accompanied by vascular redistribution to the upper lobes, and is demonstrated by cephalization on a frontal radiograph (increased vessel diameter in the upper lobes on an erect film). The second stage is interstitial pulmonary edema, which is due to fluid accumulating in the interstitium of the lung, and due to dilation of lymphatic channels as they begin to drain the excess fluid. This is manifested radiographically by interlobular septal thickening (visible as Kerley "B" lines on a chest x-ray which are thin horizontal lines perpendicular to the pleural surface seen at the lung bases), peribronchial cuffing (thin, circular densities seen due to thickening of bronchial walls secondary to fluid accumulation), and hazy vessel margins. Small pleural effusions may also be seen, which may only manifest as mild pleural thickening. The third phase is frank alveolar edema, due to fluid extravasation into the alveolar space. Radiographically, this is manifest by consolidative opacities, which tend to have ill-defined margins. Classically, they may be in a perihilar or "bat-wing" distribution, although varying patterns are possible, and the pattern may gradually shift depending on patient positioning. The presence of cardiomegaly suggests underlying CHF and can add confidence to the diagnosis, but cardiomegaly can also be seen in patients with renal failure or other causes of volume overload. On an upright and inspiratory PA view of the chest, a rough assessment of cardiomegaly can be made using the cardiothoracic ratio. This is defined as the maximal transverse diameter of the cardiac silhouette divided by the internal diameter of the thorax, measured at the highest point on the right hemidiaphragm. In normal adults, this ratio is less than 0.5. It is important to note that the cardiac silhouette is magnified on AP projections, and this ratio cannot be used. Also, expiratory phase imaging will artificially elevate this ratio. On CT, the main finding in interstitial edema is smooth interlobular septal thickening. Bronchial wall thickening will also be seen, and is the basis

of peribronchial cuffing seen on chest x-rays. Central pulmonary arteries will be enlarged, and may be larger than the adjacent bronchus. As the edema progresses into the alveolar space, lobular ground glass opacities will develop, often in a geographic pattern. Pleural effusions may also be present.

Permeability edema can be due to numerous conditions. Common ones include sepsis, blood transfusion (TRALI), chemical pneumonitis (eg, aspiration), and pancreatitis. Radiographically, it is manifest by nonspecific bilateral air space opacification which is often symmetric, and can be a component of acute respiratory distress syndrome (ARDS) and acute lung injury (ALI), which are clinical diagnoses consisting of multiple criteria. The opacities may initially be patchy and inhomogeneous, but may rapidly coalesce and lead to diffuse opacification. Since permeability edema is primarily an alveolar process, septal lines (ie, Kerley B lines) and peribronchial cuffing are not commonly seen. In patients with ARDS, be on the lookout for complications of barotrauma (such as pneumothorax and pneumomediastinum), as lung compliance is reduced and patients are often on positive pressure ventilation. Superimposed pneumonias are common, and are impossible to distinguish radiographically from the surrounding edema. On CT, the typical pattern is of dense opacification of the dependent portions of the lung, with ground glass opacity layered on top of that, and any normal lung at the very top in the most nondependent regions. The distribution is bilateral, but may be asymmetric and inhomogeneous. The pattern may have a geographic appearance, where uninvolved lobules are seen adjacent to involved lobules. Although septal lines are not often seen on x-rays, interlobular septal thickening is often seen on CT. Pleural effusions may again be present.

Clinical Differential

Pneumonia, myocardial infarction, pulmonary embolism

Imaging Differential

Airspace disease due to hemorrhage or infection may resemble alveolar edema. Interstitial edema may resemble viral or atypical pneumonias.

REFERENCES AND SUGGESTED READING

1. Storto ML, Kee ST, Golden JA, Webb WR. Hydrostatic pulmonary edema: high-resolution CT findings. *AJR*. 1995;165:817-820.
2. Gluecker T, Capasso P, Schnyder P, et al. Clinical and radiologic features of pulmonary edema. *RadioGraphics*. 1999;19(6):1507-1631.

CASE 4: PNEUMOTHORAX

PATIENT PRESENTATION

A 20-year-old male presents with acute onset of left-sided chest pain. On examination he is tall and thin, and breath sounds are absent on the left.

CLINICAL SUSPICION

Pneumothorax

IMAGING MODALITY OF CHOICE

Chest x-ray (Figs. C4.1-C4.4). This should preferably be performed in the upright position initially, although lateral decubitus views offer the greatest sensitivity. Some small pneumothoraces may only be visible on CT.

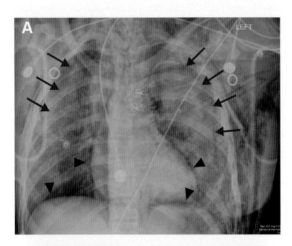

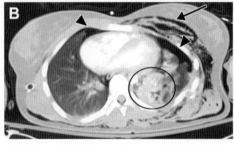

Fig. C4.1 Bilateral posttraumatic pneumothorax. (A) Portable AP chest radiograph obtained in the emergency department demonstrates a faintly visible pleural line bilaterally (black arrows) as well as lucency along the diaphragmatic and cardiac borders (black arrowheads) consistent with bilateral pneumothorax. Also note the extensive subcutaneous emphysema particularly over the left chest and extending into the neck. (B) Axial chest CT again demonstrates bilateral pneumothoraces (black arrowheads). There is extensive pulmonary contusion in the left lung (black circle) as well as subcutaneous chest wall emphysema (black arrow).

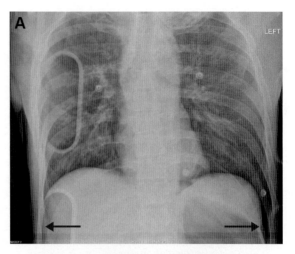

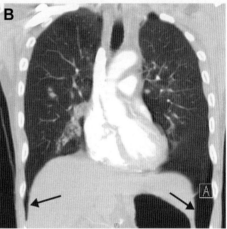

Fig. C4.2 Deep sulcus sign. (A) Portable AP chest x-ray obtained in the emergency department demonstrates air tracking deep within the lateral costophrenic sulci, known as the deep sulcus sign, bilaterally (black arrows). This is indicative of bilateral pneumothorax. (B) Chest CT with coronal reformation demonstrates the basis for this finding (black arrows).

FINDINGS

On an upright frontal view of the chest most pneumothoraces are classically manifest by a visible visceral pleural line. No lung markings will be visible peripheral to the pleural line, and there will often be mediastinal shift toward the side of the pneumothorax due to the associated volume loss (with the exception of a tension pneumothorax). The contralateral lung will then be somewhat hyperexpanded and more lucent, and the collapsed lung will be shrunken and more radiopaque.

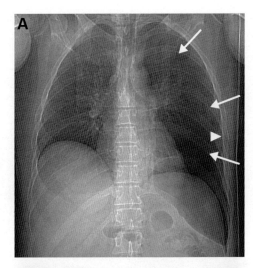

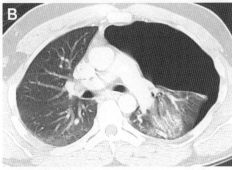

Fig. C4.3 Tension pneumothorax. (A) Scout image from chest CT demonstrates a left rib fracture (white arrowhead) and large left pneumothorax (white arrows). (B) Axial section from the CT scan demonstrates a large left pneumothorax as well as mild rightward mediastinal shift, suspicious for a tension pneumothorax. The patient was hemodynamically stable however. Radiographic evidence of tension physiology does not always correlate with the clinical syndrome, as demonstrated here.

On a supine film, small pneumothoraces may not be readily visible, and sensitivity is greatly reduced. Many signs of pneumothorax on a supine film have been described. One of these is the "deep sulcus sign," which is deepening of the costophrenic angle and increased lucency due to subpulmonic accumulation of air [1]. Other signs of subpulmonic pneumothorax include deepening of the cardiophrenic angle, "double diaphragm sign" (when the inferior extent of the anterior pleural space becomes visible separate from the dome of the diaphragm), and visible well-defined pericardial fat pads [2, 3]. Collections of air

anteromedially can be manifest by increased sharpness or lucency along the ipsilateral cardiomediastinal border [2]. Sometimes, overlying skin folds or the lateral margin of the scapula may simulate a pneumothorax radiographically, and result in a false positive diagnosis. In these cases, pulmonary vascular markings can usually be seen extending beyond the skin fold or scapular margin, excluding a pneumothorax.

In problematic cases, a lateral decubitus view can be helpful. Since the air will rise to a nondependent location, the contralateral decubitus view should be obtained. For example, if a left-sided pneumothorax is suspected, a right lateral decubitus view should be obtained (ie, with the right side down and the left side up). The air should then rise and be visible along the left chest wall. CT can also be performed in questionable cases, and should easily demonstrate air within the pleural space.

Tension pneumothorax is classically described as a large pneumothorax with contralateral mediastinal shift. However, it is important to note that the presence of contralateral mediastinal shift does not always correlate with clinical findings of tension physiology (ie, impaired venous return due to increased intrathoracic pressure resulting in hypotension) [4].

Bronchopleural fistulas are most often seen as a complication of cardiothoracic surgery (ie, pneumonectomy), however, they can also be created due to malignancy, or infection. These can be suspected clinically in the setting of a pneumothorax that is refractory to treatment. CT is the imaging modality of choice, as the fistulous communication can often be directly visualized. Xe-133 ventilation scanning can also be helpful, and will demonstrate accumulation of radiotracer in the pleural space on washout images. This confirms the presence of a bronchopleural fistula, although it does not aid in localization [5].

Clinical Differential

Pulmonary embolism, myocardial infarction, pneumonia, costochondritis.

Imaging Differential

There are several pitfalls in the diagnosis of pneumothorax on plain radiographs including skin folds and the lateral margin of the scapula. Knowledge of these pitfalls will aid in their avoidance. On CT the appearance of a pneumothorax is characteristic.

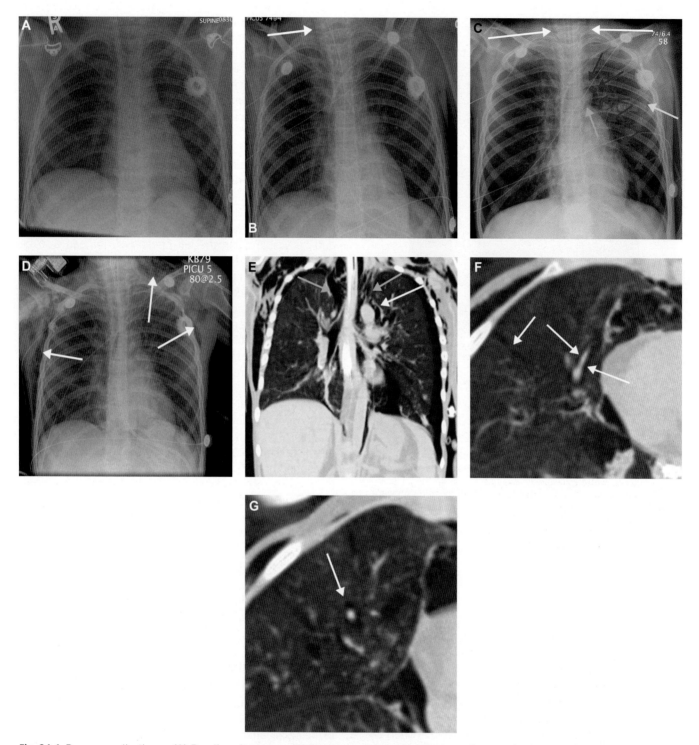

Fig. C4.4 Pneumomediastinum. (A) Baseline chest x-ray. (B) Chest x-ray obtained while the patient was intubated in the intensive care unit demonstrates linear lucency along the right paratracheal region extending into the neck, consistent with pneumomediastinum. (C) Subsequent chest x-ray the next day demonstrates lucency extending into the neck bilaterally (white arrows). Additionally, there is lucency along the aortic knob and left heart border (red arrows). There is lucency along the undersurface of the aortic arch (green arrow). Yellow arrow points to the lateral margin of the left scapula, which may simulate a pneumothorax. (D) By the third day, extensive subcutaneous emphysema has developed. (E) A CT scan was performed at this time, and a coronal reformat demonstrates the lucency surrounding the aortic knob that was seen on the x-ray (white arrow). Additionally, there are bilateral pneumothoraces that were not well seen on x-ray (red arrows). Green arrows demonstrate gas extending from the mediastinum into the neck. (F) Axial CT in lung windows demonstrates branching tubular lucencies in the lung (white arrows) consistent with pulmonary interstitial emphysema. There is also air surrounding a pulmonary artery branch in the RML. (G) Different section again demonstrates gas surrounding a pulmonary artery branch (white arrow). All of these findings were likely the result of barotrauma due to positive pressure ventilation.

REFERENCES AND SUGGESTED READING

1. Gordon R. The deep sulcus sign. *Radiology.* 1980;136:25-27.
2. Tocino IM. Pneumothorax in the supine patient: radiographic anatomy. *RadioGraphics.*1985;5(4):557-586.
3. Ziter FMH Jr, Westcott JL. Supine subpulmonary pneumothorax. *AJR.* 1981;137:699-701.
4. Clark S, Ragg M, Stella J. Is mediastinal shift on chest x-ray of pneumothorax always an emergency? *Emerg Med* (Fremantle) 2003;15:429-433.
5. Qureshi NR, Gleeson FV. Imaging of pleural disease. *Clin Chest Med.* 2006;27(2):193-213.

CASE 5: PULMONARY CONTUSION

PATIENT PRESENTATION

A 45-year-old male status post high-speed MVA involving blunt trauma to the chest complains of chest pain and hemoptysis.

CLINICAL SUSPICION

Pulmonary contusion

IMAGING MODALITY OF CHOICE

While large contusions may be evident on chest radiographs, CT is usually the modality of choice (Figs. C5.1 and C5.2). Although iodinated contrast is not necessary to diagnose a pulmonary contusion, it is very helpful in the setting of chest trauma, particularly to evaluate the aorta.

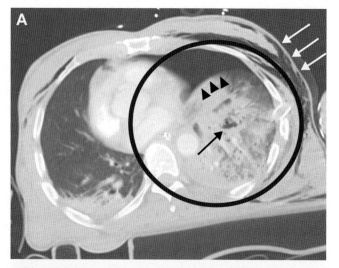

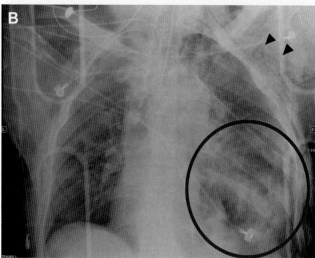

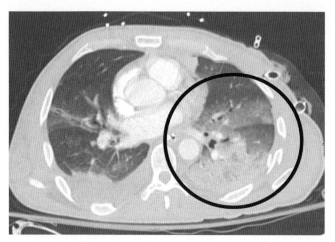

Fig. C5.1 Pulmonary contusion. Axial chest CT in a patient with blunt chest trauma demonstrates a large area of ground glass as well as denser consolidative opacity in the left lower lobe and lingula (black circle) consistent with pulmonary contusion.

Fig. C5.2 Pulmonary contusion and laceration. (A) Axial CT from another patient with blunt chest trauma demonstrates a left pneumothorax (black arrowheads) and subcutaneous emphysema (white arrows). There is extensive ground glass and consolidative opacity within the collapsed left lung (black circle). Also note the several small lucent areas (black arrow) consistent with pulmonary lacerations. (B) Frontal chest x-ray demonstrates consolidative opacity over the left lung base, in the area of the contusion (black circle). Subcutaneous emphysema is evident (black arrowheads). A chest tube has been placed to re-expand the lung.

FINDINGS

Pulmonary contusions are caused by blunt chest trauma, and pathologically they represent blood in the alveoli, which can cause hemoptysis. Radiographically, they typically manifest as a ground glass opacity with ill-defined borders in a geographic distribution. More severe cases may demonstrate frankly consolidative opacities. They stabilize in appearance by 24 hours, and resolve over the course of a week. A pulmonary opacity that appears more than 24 hours after the initial trauma is not therefore due to contusion. Pulmonary lacerations are caused by penetrating trauma usually and are manifest radiographically by rounded lucencies, which may be surrounded or obscured by surrounding contused lung. The lucent areas often contain air-fluid levels secondary to blood within the lesion, and are caused by disruption of the lung parenchyma with resulting recoil of the surrounding lung tissue. A true blood filled cyst is termed a pulmonary hematoma.

Clinical Differential

In the setting of trauma, the complaints of chest pain and hemoptysis are highly suggestive of pulmonary contusion.

Imaging Differential

On imaging alone, contusion may be indifferentiable from air space disease due to infection, edema or aspiration. The history suggests the diagnosis, as do other ancillary findings of trauma, such as concomitant rib fractures.

REFERENCES AND SUGGESTED READING

1. Van Hise ML, Primack SL, Israel RS, et al. CT in blunt chest trauma: indications and limitations. *RadioGraphics.* 1998;18:1071-1084.
2. Kaewlai R, Avery LL, Asrani AV, et al. Multidetector CT of blunt thoracic trauma. *RadioGraphics.* 2008;28:1555-1570.

CASE 6: PULMONARY EMBOLISM

PATIENT PRESENTATION

A 69-year-old female with breast cancer presents with acute onset of shortness of breath and pleuritic chest pain. On examination, the patient is tachycardic and O_2 saturation is 90% on room air.

CLINICAL SUSPICION

Pulmonary embolism (PE)

IMAGING MODALITY OF CHOICE

Pulmonary CT angiography is now the criterion standard (Figs. C6.1-C6.10). This has essentially replaced

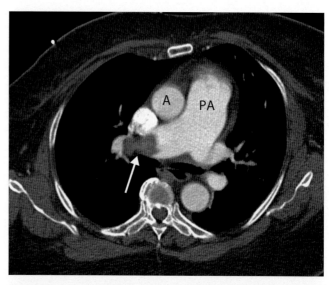

Fig. C6.2 Acute pulmonary embolism with likely pulmonary arterial hypertension. There is an intraluminal filling defect, consistent with an acute pulmonary embolism (white arrow). The pulmonary arterial trunk (PA) is larger than the adjacent ascending aorta (A), suggesting pulmonary arterial hypertension, likely due to the large PE.

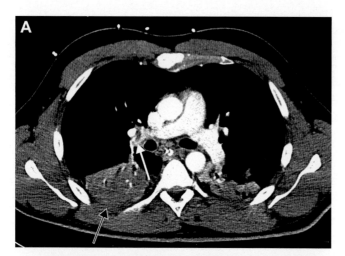

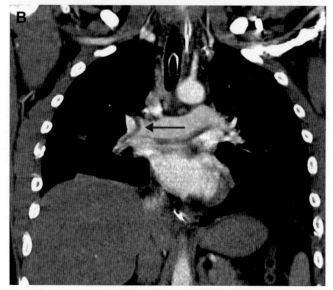

Fig. C6.1 Acute pulmonary embolism. (A) There is an intraluminal filling defect forming a concave border with the contrast material (white arrow). There is also right lower lobe consolidation (black arrow), which could represent a pneumonia or infarction in the appropriate clinical setting. (B) Coronal reformation in the same patient better demonstrates the thrombus (black arrow).

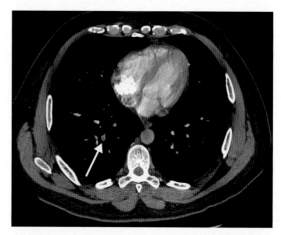

Fig. C6.3 Segmental pulmonary embolus. (A) Filling defect is seen within the right lower lobe posterior segment pulmonary artery (white arrow). It has a rounded configuration with a thin rim of contrast surrounding it, suggesting that it is acute.

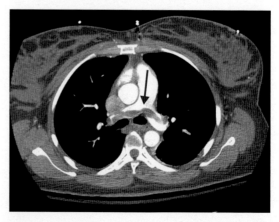

Fig. C6.4 Saddle embolus. There is a rope-shaped filling defect straddling the bifurcation of the main pulmonary artery, extending into the right and left pulmonary arteries (black arrow), consistent with a saddle embolus.

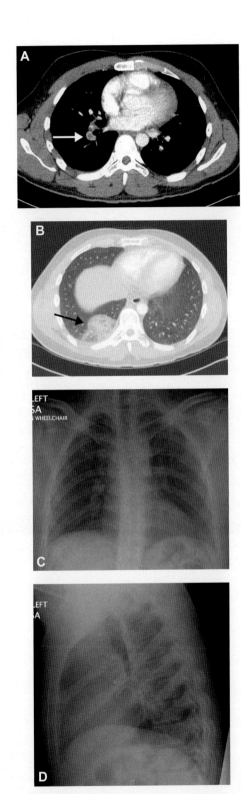

Fig. C6.5 Pulmonary embolism and infarction. (A) CT angiogram of the chest demonstrates a filling defect in the right lower lobe pulmonary artery (white arrow) which was seen straddling the anterior and posterior segments on contiguous sections, consistent with a pulmonary embolism. (B) Axial section in lung windows more inferiorly demonstrates a peripheral wedge shaped opacity in the posterior segment of the right lower lobe, consistent with an infarct (black arrow). (C, D) PA and lateral chest x-ray obtained the same day do not show any abnormality, stressing the insensitivity of chest radiographs for pulmonary embolism.

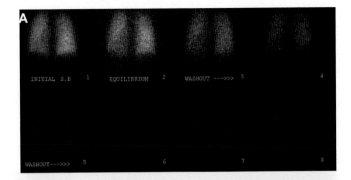

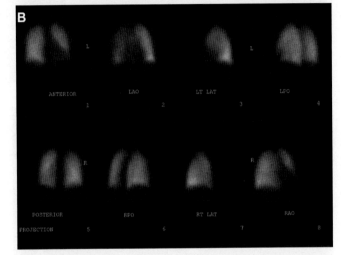

Fig. C6.6 Normal V/Q scan. (A) Ventilation images demonstrate uniform aeration of the lungs with normal washout. (B) Perfusion images in the standard projections demonstrate homogenous perfusion to both lungs, without focal defects.

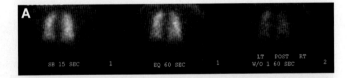

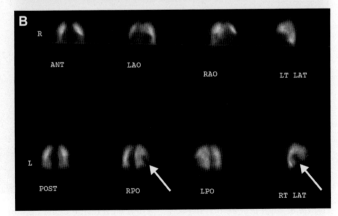

Fig. C6.7 Intermediate probability V/Q scan. (A) Ventilation images demonstrate no focal defects. (B) Perfusion images demonstrate a segmental defect involving the anterior basal segment of the right lower lobe (white arrows), giving an intermediate probability for pulmonary embolism. CT angiogram performed 5 days later did not demonstrate any pulmonary emboli, although the patient received anticoagulation in the interim, and it is conceivable that any potential thrombus may have resolved.

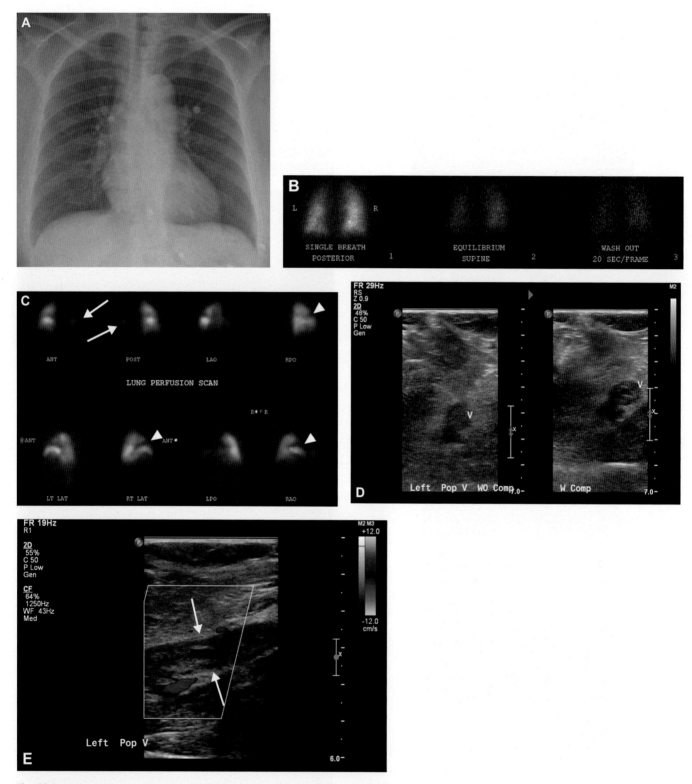

Fig. C6.8 High probability V/Q scan. (A) PA view of the chest demonstrates subtle decrease in vascular markings in the left lung as compared to the right (Westermark sign). (B) Ventilation scan in the same patient is normal. (C) Perfusion scan demonstrates greatly diminished perfusion to the left lung (white arrows) and a moderate sized segmental defect involving the anterior segment of the right upper lobe (white arrowhead), consistent with a high probability of pulmonary embolism. (D) Grayscale Doppler of the left lower extremity in the same patient demonstrates a noncompressible popliteal vein with echogenic thrombus within the lumen. (E) Color Doppler demonstrates lack of flow within the popliteal vein (v), which is completely occluded with echogenic thrombus (white arrows). A few foci of color flow are seen in adjacent collaterals.

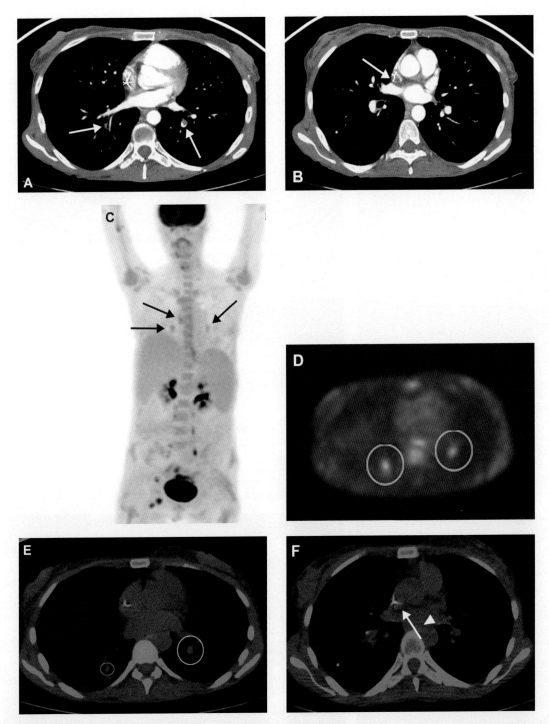

Fig. C6.9 Chronic pulmonary embolism. (A) CT angiogram demonstrates a partially occlusive eccentric filling defect within the posterior basal segment of the left lower lobe as well as an occlusive filling defect in the posterior basal segment of the right lower lobe (white arrows). The morphology of the thrombus in the left lower lobe suggests chronic pulmonary embolism. (B) Different section from the same study demonstrates low attenuation thrombus around the tip of a central catheter (white arrow), which could be a source of emboli. This was a cancer patient with an indwelling port-catheter. (C) Whole body MIP from a PET-CT performed the next day demonstrates foci of low level FDG uptake within the medial lung bases bilaterally as well as slightly higher in the mediastinum (black arrows). Physiologic excretion is seen within the renal pelvises, along the ureters, and in the bladder. Malignant foci are present in the right groin. (D) An axial section from the PET portion of the study localizes the two lower foci to the posterior basal segments bilaterally (white circles). (E) Fused PET-CT image demonstrates that these foci are within the pulmonary arteries, corresponding to the filling defects seen on the prior CTPA (white circles). (F) Another fused PET-CT image demonstrates low-level uptake within the catheter tip thrombus as well (white arrow). Low-level uptake in the esophagus (white arrowhead) is likely physiologic. It is thought that FDG uptake may be secondary to glucose metabolism by the inflammatory cellular infiltrate including activated macrophages, neutrophils, and fibroblasts within an organizing thrombus.

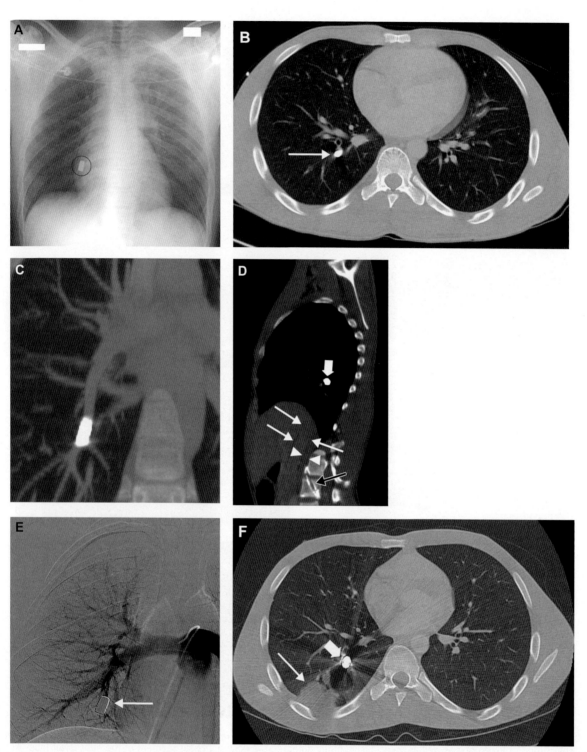

Fig. C6.10 Bullet pulmonary embolus. (A) Portable AP chest x-ray demonstrates a bullet projecting over the medial right lung base (black circle). No evidence of hemothorax, pneumothorax, or other traumatic injury to the chest. Note that since this is only a single view, it could be external to the patient as well. (B) Axial chest CT demonstrates that the bullet is within the right posterior basal segment pulmonary artery branch (white arrow). (C) Coronal MIP nicely demonstrates the intra-arterial location of the bullet. (D) Sagittal CT reconstruction demonstrates the bullet tract through the lumbar spine (black arrow). From there, the bullet entered the IVC (thin white arrows) and then migrated intravascularly into the pulmonary arterial tree via the right heart. There is a retroperitoneal hematoma (white arrowheads). The bullet itself is again seen (thick white arrow). (E) Catheter pulmonary angiogram was performed several days later, also demonstrating the intravascular nature of the bullet (white arrow). The bullet appeared to be stable in position compared to the earlier CT scans, and it was decided to leave the bullet in situ, rather than attempt to retrieve it. (F) Repeat chest CT obtained approximately one week later demonstrates interval development of a peripheral somewhat wedge-shaped opacity consistent with an infarct (thin white arrow) in the territory of the embolized vessel (thick white arrow).

catheter pulmonary angiography and has been demonstrated to be significantly more sensitive, especially for small (ie, segmental and subsegmental) emboli [2]. V/Q scans still have a role in patients who cannot receive iodinated contrast. Some authors advocate perfusion only scans (a V/Q scan without the ventilation component) in pregnant or young women in an effort to reduce radiation dose, although reported doses vary widely and many, if not most, institutions still prefer CT angiography (CTA) [6]. Doppler ultrasound of the lower extremities is also useful in detecting deep venous thrombosis (DVT), the leading cause of pulmonary embolism.

Advantages of Pulmonary CTA

Pulmonary CT angiography is widely available, fast, noninvasive, and very reliable when the study is of good quality. Also, other causes of the patient's symptoms are often identified, even if negative for pulmonary embolism. Excluding inconclusive studies, the sensitivity of CTA for detecting pulmonary embolism was 83% and the specificity was 96% in the PIOPED II study [3].

Disadvantages of Pulmonary CTA

Entails exposure to radiation and iodinated contrast. The exam will be limited if the patient is excessively tachypneic and unable to hold their breath throughout the scan, although scan times are now typically less than 15 seconds on modern multidetector CT scanners. Also, a large bore IV or power injectable central venous catheter is required to withstand the high contrast flow rates needed (typically 4.0-5.0 cc/s).

Radiologic Findings of Pulmonary Embolism

On a pulmonary CTA, the key finding is a filling defect within the pulmonary arterial tree. In an acute pulmonary embolus, this filling defect may occlude the entire vessel, resulting in complete nonopacification and sometimes even mild enlargement of the vessel. Alternatively, it may lie centrally within the vessel and be surrounded by a thin rim of contrast material, producing a target appearance on a transverse section of the vessel or a tram-track appearance on a longitudinal section. The embolus is frequently seen straddling a vascular bifurcation where the embolus gets hung up at the bifurcation, with portions of the embolus going into different segments of a vessel. When imaged longitudinally, the trailing edge (more proximal end) of the thrombus typically has a concave appearance. Finally, it may lie against the wall of the vessel, in which case it will usually form acute angles and maintain a rounded appearance (this is important in differentiating from chronic pulmonary embolus, which will be discussed later) [4]. On a noncontrast CT, large central emboli can rarely be seen as a hyperdense clot within the pulmonary trunk or in the

main pulmonary arteries [1]. If there is an associated pulmonary infarct, this typically appears as a peripheral wedge shaped opacity in the territory of the affected vessel(s), and there may or may not be an associated pleural effusion. An additional benefit to CTA for detection of pulmonary embolism is the ability to detect DVT of the lower extremities concurrently using the same contrast bolus by performing a delayed CT venogram through the pelvis and lower extremities after imaging the chest. The drawback to this approach is increased radiation dose, and this information may be readily obtained by Doppler ultrasound as well (although the IVC and iliac veins are difficult to evaluate sonographically).

Several indirect signs of pulmonary embolism on chest x-rays have been historically described, which lack sensitivity, but deserve mention nonetheless. In fact, the chest x-ray may be entirely normal, and the patient may have a massive PE. Massive acute emboli or extensive chronic emboli may cause pulmonary arterial hypertension, which can manifest as an enlarged pulmonary arterial shadow and/or right heart enlargement on chest x-ray in the setting of cor pulmonale. The Westermark sign is the presence of diminished and/or narrowed vascular markings in the affected vascular territory secondary to regional oligemia. Hampton's hump is a peripheral wedge shaped opacity representing an infarct. While these signs have been reported to have a high specificity, sensitivity and positive predictive value remain low [5].

Ventilation/Perfusion scintigraphy (V/Q scan) has declined in popularity with the advent of CTA; however, it remains a viable option for patients in whom iodinated contrast is contraindicated. The key finding of PE on a V/Q scan is termed a "V/Q mismatch," which is an area of lung that is ventilated, but not perfused. Although specific protocols vary by institution, the premise is similar. For the ventilation portion, the patient inhales a radioactive gas (Xe-133 or Kr-81m) or aerosol (Tc-99m DTPA), and breath hold, equilibrium, and washout images are typically obtained. For the perfusion portion, Tc-99m-MAA is injected intravenously and again images are obtained with a gamma camera in multiple projections. The ventilation and perfusion images are then compared, and assessed for focal defects (areas of photopenia) corresponding to segmental territories. Based on the number and size of matched/mismatched defects and comparison with a recently performed chest x-ray as well as other factors, the likelihood of pulmonary embolism is then assessed based on criteria derived from the PIOPED study [6]. The probability is usually stratified into the following categories: normal, low probability, intermediate probability, and high probability. There have been several proposed modifications to these criteria since the original study, and the latest recommendations can be found in the Society of Nuclear Medicine practice guidelines.

Chronic pulmonary emboli are best imaged with CTA as well, and are more irregular in appearance than acute emboli. When imaged longitudinally, the trailing edge tends to form a concave border with the contrast media as opposed to a convex border typically seen with acute emboli. Chronic thrombus is often eccentric in location within the vessel and is adherent to the vessel wall. This results in intimal irregularities, which often form obtuse angles with the wall when imaged transversely, as compared to the acute angles typically formed by acute emboli. Progressive organization and resorption of the thrombus can lead to the formation of bands and webs within the thrombus as it recanalizes [7]. Often, however, it may not be possible to definitively differentiate acute from chronic thrombi.

Clinical Differential

Pneumonia, myocardial infarction, pleuritis, pericarditis, GERD.

Imaging Differential

The typical appearance of a pulmonary embolism is virtually pathognomonic. Occasionally, artifact from either respiratory or cardiac motion may limit evaluation of certain vessels or mimic a filling defect, leading to either false positive or false negative result. Differentiation of acute and chronic emboli may often be made, as described on page 161. Tumor thrombi and pulmonary artery sarcoma will also present as filling defects, but typically demonstrate enhancement of the thrombus.

REFERENCES AND SUGGESTED READING

1. Kanne JP, Gotway MB, Thoongsuwan N, Stern EJ. Six cases of acute central pulmonary embolism revealed on unenhanced multidetector CT of the chest. *AJR*. 2003;180:1661-1664.

2. Wittram C, Waltman AC, Shepard JA, Halpern E, Goodman LR. Discordance between CT and angiography in the PIOPED II study. *Radiology*. 2007;244(3):883-889.

3. Stein PD, Fowler SE, Goodman LR, et al. Multidetector computed tomography for acute pulmonary embolism. *N Engl J Med*. 2006;354(22):2317-2327.

4. Wittram C, Maher MA, Yoo AJ, et al. CT angiography of pulmonary embolism: diagnostic criteria and causes of misdiagnosis. *RadioGraphics*. 2004;24:1219-1238.

5. Worsley DF, Alavi A, Aronchick JM, et al. Chest radiographic findings in patients with acute pulmonary embolism: observations from the PIOPED study. *Radiology*. 1993;189(1):133-136.

6. Gottschalk A, Sostman HD, Coleman ER, et al. Ventilation-perfusion scintigraphy in the PIOPED study. Part II. Evaluation of the scintigraphic criteria and interpretations. *J Nucl Med*. 1993;34:1119-1126.

7. Wittram C, Kalra MK, Maher MM, et al. Acute and chronic pulmonary emboli: angiography-CT correlation. *AJR*. 2006;186: S421-S429.

8. Wittram C, Scott JA. 18F-FDG PET of pulmonary embolism. *AJR*. 2007;189:171-176.

CASE 7: TUBERCULOSIS

PATIENT PRESENTATION

A 36-year-old male prisoner presents with worsening cough for several weeks, recently with occasional flecks of blood. On review of systems, he also complains of occasional fevers and night sweats.

CLINICAL SUSPICION

Tuberculosis (TB)

IMAGING MODALITY OF CHOICE

Chest x-ray, PA and lateral views (Figs. C7.1-C7.4). Typical chest x-ray findings and positive sputum cultures/smears

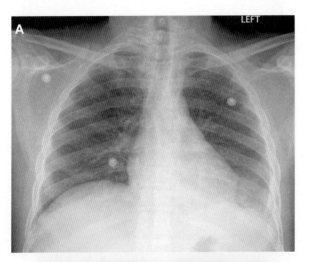

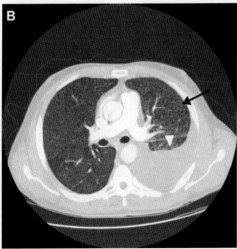

Fig. C7.1 Miliary tuberculosis. (A) Frontal chest radiograph demonstrates innumerable tiny nodules distributed throughout both lungs. There is a hazy opacity at the left lung base with obscuration of the diaphragm, suggesting a pleural effusion. (B) Axial chest CT from the same patient also demonstrates innumerable tiny nodules randomly distributed, which were due to miliary tuberculosis in this HIV positive patient. One of these is annotated (black arrow). There is a large left pleural effusion (white arrowhead).

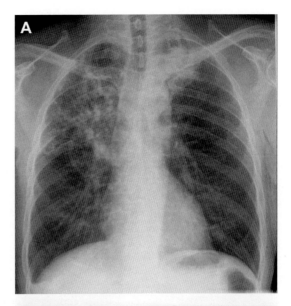

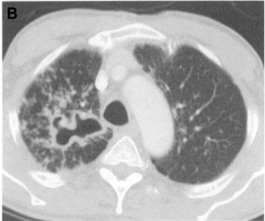

Fig. C7.2 Postprimary (reactivation) tuberculosis. (A) Frontal chest radiograph demonstrates patchy airspace opacities in the right upper lung, and to a much lesser extent in the left apex as well. In the appropriate clinical setting, opacities that demonstrate an apical predominance should raise suspicion for reactivation tuberculosis. (B) Axial chest CT from the same patient demonstrates right upper lobe reticulonodular opacities with a large, irregular, cavity. Note that the cavity is more readily apparent on the CT as compared to the radiograph. The patient was HIV positive, and had a CD4 count of 525.

are all that is typically needed to make the diagnosis. CT can be helpful in adding confidence to the diagnosis, although it is usually not necessary.

FINDINGS

Lymphadenopathy is the hallmark of primary tuberculosis, especially in pediatric age groups. The incidence of lymphadenopathy declines with increasing age, however. The right hilar nodes and right paratracheal nodes are classically the most commonly involved, although any combination of mediastinal and hilar nodes may be affected. This right-sided

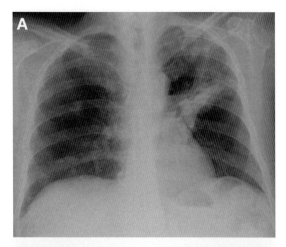

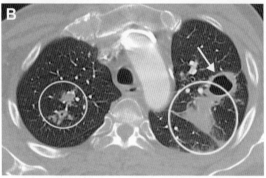

Fig. C7.3 Reactivation tuberculosis. (A) Frontal chest radiograph demonstrates patchy airspace consolidation in both upper lungs, left worse than right. (B) Axial chest CT demonstrates patchy consolidative opacities in the apices (white circles) as well as a cavity (white arrow).

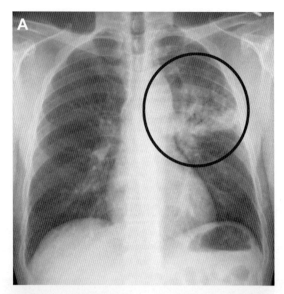

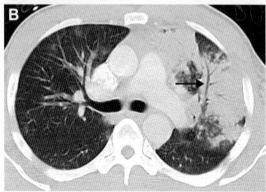

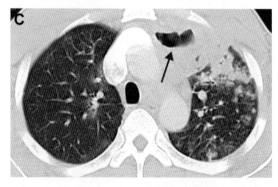

Fig. C7.4 HIV patient with reactivation tuberculosis. (A) Frontal chest x-ray demonstrates left upper lobe consolidation (black circle). (B) Axial chest CT also demonstrates left upper lobe consolidation with an air bronchograms (black arrow). (C) Different section from the same scan demonstrates an area of cavitation that is not apparent on the radiograph (black arrow). Sputum cultures demonstrated *Mycobacterium tuberculosis*. The patient had a CD4 count of 228.

predominance is felt to be due to the higher statistical likelihood of any airborne infection entering the right lung due to the anatomy. In extrapulmonary TB, other nodal groups throughout the body may be affected as well. The classic appearance of tuberculous adenopathy is peripheral enhancement with central hypodensity, which pathologically corresponds to a centrally necrotic but peripherally vascular and inflamed lymph node. In the proper clinical setting this appearance is highly suggestive of TB, although metastatic carcinoma and suppurative adenitis (particularly in the neck) may also have this appearance. In contrast to the incidence of lymphadenopathy in primary TB, the incidence of parenchymal involvement and pleural effusions increase with age. Focal consolidative opacity is the most common parenchymal finding in primary TB, although patchy or multifocal involvement can also occur. Unlike postprimary disease, there is no definite lobar predilection for primary TB. When pleural effusions occur, they are most often unilateral and on the same side as the infection, but can be bilateral. In a few percent of cases, a pleural effusion may be the only finding of primary TB, although it most commonly occurs in conjunction with parenchymal disease.

Postprimary or reactivation TB is classically manifest by apical and posterior opacities and cavitary lesions, although there may also be disease beyond these locations. Particularly, the apical and posterior segments of the upper lobes and the superior segments of the lower lobes are the favored sites. Nodular opacities (ie, tuberculomas) may predominate in a few patients, and some of these may go on to cavitate. On CT, in addition to these findings, there is usually also evidence of bronchogenic spread manifest by centrilobular nodules in a "tree-in-bud" configuration, which represent infectious/necrotic material impacted within respiratory and terminal bronchioles. As their name implies, centrilobular nodules are found in the center of the secondary pulmonary lobules. As such, a centrilobular distribution of nodules will exhibit subpleural sparing as the distal airways do not extend all the way to the pleural surface. This is in contrast to a lymphatic distribution, in which pleural surfaces are involved as well. Pleural effusions can occur in reactivation disease. In contrast to primary TB, hilar and mediastinal adenopathy is uncommon in postprimary disease.

Miliary disease most often occurs in the immunocompromised, and consists of innumerable tiny nodules in a random distribution throughout both lungs, with a basilar predominance consistent with hematologic dissemination. There may be associated consolidative and/or cavitary parenchymal disease with or without lymphadenopathy. Early on, miliary disease may not be seen on chest x-ray, and only seen on CT. The pattern of findings in HIV positive individuals varies with the degree of immune suppression. When immune function is maintained (CD4 > 200), the typical reactivation pattern of disease is seen, similar to immunocompetent hosts. As immune function becomes compromised (CD4 < 200), there is increasing trend toward a primary pattern of disease dominated by lymphadenopathy and noncavitary consolidative opacities.

Nontuberculous mycobacterial infections (NTMB) can cause a spectrum of diseases. In the "classic" form, it consists of apical fibrocavitary disease, which is indistinguishable from postprimary TB, and there is a predilection for older men with underlying COPD or other chronic lung disease. There is a bronchiectatic or "nonclassic" form as well, which has a predilection for older white women, and has been termed "Lady Windermere" syndrome. Radiologic findings include centrilobular nodules (which may be in a tree-in-bud pattern) and bronchiectasis, most commonly affecting the right middle lobe and lingula. NTMB can also be a cause of solitary pulmonary nodules in asymptomatic patients. In those with HIV and CD4 counts of less than 100, NTMB most commonly causes disseminated disease in which the primary finding is lymphadenopathy, which may involve mediastinal and hilar groups as well as abdominal and other extrathoracic groups. More recently, NTMB have been associated with a form of hypersensitivity pneumonitis termed "hot tub lung." This is felt to represent a hypersensitivity reaction to nontuberculous mycobacteria growing in hot tubs, and presents with similar findings to hypersensitivity pneumonitis on imaging. On CT, findings include ground glass nodules and ground glass opacities, as well as air trapping on expiratory scans.

Clinical Differential

Lung cancer, bronchiectasis, fungal infection

Imaging Differential

Nontuberculous necrotizing pneumonia, lung cancer, fungal infection.

REFERENCES AND SUGGESTED READING

1. Leung AN. Pulmonary tuberculosis: the essentials. *Radiology.* 1999;210:307-322.
2. Martinez S, McAdams HP, Batchu CS. The many faces of pulmonary nontuberculous mycobacterial infection. *AJR.* 2007; 189:177-186.

CASE 8: OPPORTUNISTIC INFECTION

PATIENT PRESENTATION

A 35-year-old male with history of HIV and CD4 count of 70 presents with acute onset of shortness of breath and cough for 2 days.

CLINICAL SUSPICION

Pneumocystis pneumonia (PCP)

IMAGING MODALITY OF CHOICE

Initially PA and lateral views of the chest (Figs. C8.1-C8.5). Chest CT may be helpful as well.

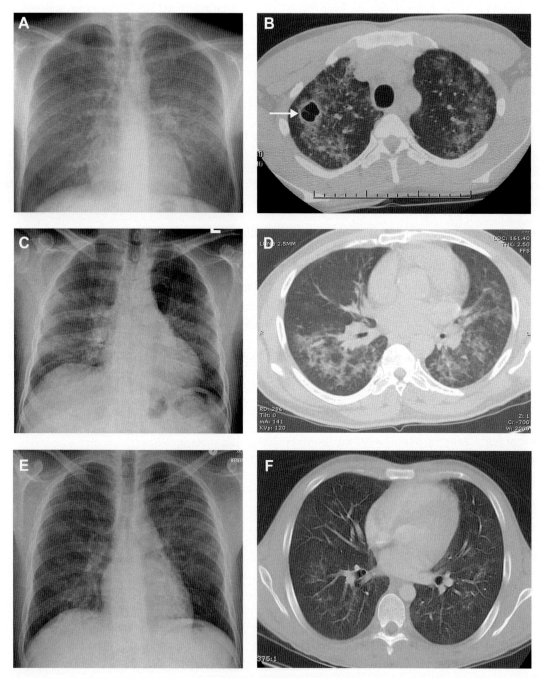

Fig. C8.1 Pneumocystis pneumonia. (A) PA chest x-ray demonstrates diffuse bilateral reticular opacity in a perihilar distribution. The patient had a history of HIV. (B) Axial chest CT in a different patient demonstrates bilateral patchy ground glass opacities with reticular opacities as well. A pneumatocele is demonstrated (white arrow). Rupture of pneumatoceles can cause pneumothorax. (C) A different patient. PA view of the chest demonstrates faint bilateral interstitial opacities in a patient with HIV. (D) Same patient as C, axial chest CT in lung windows demonstrates bilateral patchy ground glass opacity. BAL samples demonstrated *Pneumocystis jiroveci.* (E) PA chest x-ray demonstrates interstitial and patchy faint airspace opacities in another HIV patient. (F) Axial chest CT from the same patient as E demonstrates patchy ground glass opacities, although less impressive than in (D).

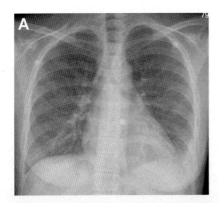

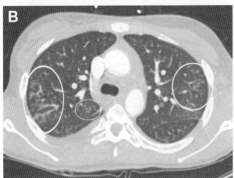

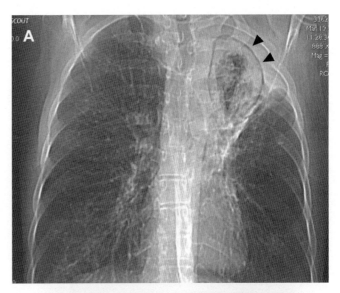

Fig. C8.2 Airway-invasive aspergillosis. (A) Initial chest radiograph from a 25-year-old female with discoid lupus on chronic immune suppression demonstrates bilateral diffuse reticulonodular opacities. (B) Chest CT demonstrates patchy clusters of nodular opacities, predominantly centrilobular in nature, demonstrating a "tree-in-bud" pattern in some places. This pattern is nonspecific and represents impaction of small terminal airways with mucus and/or pus. In this patient, BAL samples eventually grew *Aspergillus terreus*. This appearance is most consistent with an airway invasive pattern of aspergillosis, although not specific. Similar appearance can be seen with mycobacterial, viral or atypical pneumonias, or other fungal pneumonias.

FINDINGS

PCP is typically seen in patients with AIDS who have a CD4 count of less than 200 cells/mm^3 or are otherwise immune suppressed (ie, bone marrow transplant patients). On the frontal chest radiograph, the classic findings are perihilar reticular and ground glass opacities. If sufficiently large, thin-walled cysts (pneumatoceles) may be appreciated. If one of these cysts ruptures, pneumothorax may result. In fact, spontaneous pneumothorax can be the presenting finding in some patients. However, in some patients, the chest x-ray may be interpreted as normal and subtle findings may only be seen at CT. CT findings include fairly symmetric bilateral ground glass opacity with relative sparing of the periphery, and there may be superimposed smooth interlobular septal thickening resulting in a "crazy-paving" pattern. It should be noted that this pattern is not specific for PCP, and may be seen in other entities such as pulmonary alveolar proteinosis, ARDS, and NSIP among others.

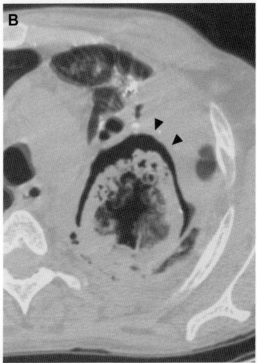

Fig. C8.3 Mycetoma. (A) Scout image from CT scan demonstrates a heterogeneous rounded lesion in the left upper lobe with internal lucencies and surrounding crescent of air (black arrowheads). (B) Chest CT demonstrates a heterogeneous masslike lesion with internal foci of air surrounded by an air crescent nondependently (black arrowheads). The appearance is consistent with a mycetoma. If there was any doubt, the patient could be reimaged in the prone position and the mycetoma would shift position to remain dependent.

Smaller pneumatoceles may be seen that were not apparent on chest x-ray. A nuclear gallium-67 scan will demonstrate bilateral diffuse pulmonary uptake and is highly sensitive for the detection of PCP. However, it lacks specificity, as there

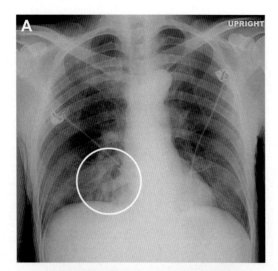

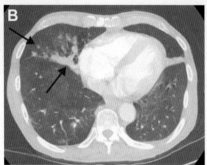

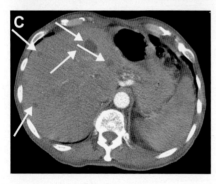

Fig. C8.4 Cryptococcal pneumonia and disseminated crypto-coccosis. (A) Portable AP chest radiograph demonstrates an ill-defined opacity that partially obscures the right heart border, suggesting right middle lobe consolidation. The patient presented with hemoptysis and had a history of HIV. He had been noncompliant with HAART medication for several years, and his CD4 count was 35. (B) Chest CT demonstrates patchy consolidation in the right middle lobe, as well as a few nodular opacities (black arrows). Note how this abuts the right heart border, which was obscured on the x-ray as well. This appearance is suspicious for infection, although bacterial, fungal or mycobacterial etiologies would all be possible in this clinical setting. (C) Axial CT section through the upper abdomen demonstrates numerous nonspecific hypodense lesions in the liver. Differential diagnosis would include cysts, metastases or fungal abscesses. Serum cryptococcal antigen was positive, and disseminated cryptococcosis was diagnosed.

may be pulmonary gallium-67 uptake in a variety of pulmonary infections and inflammatory processes. It is rarely performed nowadays.

Endemic mycoses (histoplasmosis, blastomycosis, and coccidioidomycosis) may affect both immunocompetent and immunocompromised hosts. Radiographically, there are many similarities between these infections. In acute pneumonia due to these organisms, consolidative opacities are commonly seen, and may contain air bronchograms. This pattern is indifferentiable from typical community acquired pneumonias. In more indolent cases, solitary or multifocal nodular opacities may be seen, which can be indifferentiable from malignancy. These nodules may go on to cavitate, in which case they often demonstrate an apical predominance that can mimic postprimary tuberculosis. There may be associated scarring with resultant parenchymal distortion and traction bronchiectasis. In some cases, reticulonodular opacities may be the predominant finding in endemic mycoses. In severe disseminated cases, a miliary pattern may be seen consisting of innumerable tiny nodules diffusely in both lungs. This is typically only seen in immunocompromised patients. Hilar and mediastinal adenopathy are more likely to be seen in cases of histoplasmosis and coccidioidomycosis as compared to blastomycosis. Definitive diagnosis of the various endemic mycoses is usually impossible on the basis of imaging alone, and the diagnosis ultimately rests on clinical and laboratory findings and identification of the causative organism in sputum or lavage samples, or FNA/biopsy specimens.

Aspergillus fumigatus can cause a spectrum of disease in the human host, and may affect either immune competent or immunocompromised hosts in differing capacities. Saprophytic aspergillosis is caused by growth of fungal elements within a preexisting lung cavity (most commonly due to prior tuberculous infection). Radiologically, this is demonstrated by the presence of a rounded mass within an existing cavity, typically with a crescent of air surrounding it (air crescent sign). If there is doubt about whether a lesion represents a cavitating nodule/mass or a mycetoma within a preexisting cavity, the patient can be imaged in different positions (ie, prone and supine). A mycetoma will be mobile and therefore move to the dependent portion of the cavity, whereas a cavitating nodule or mass will appear unchanged. *Aspergillus* can also cause disease due to a hypersensitivity reaction, termed allergic broncho-pulmonary aspergillosis (ABPA). This is typically seen in long-standing asthmatics, and is manifest pathologically by plugs of inspissated mucus within proximal airways containing *Aspergillus* organisms as well as eosinophils. There may be peripheral eosinophilia in the blood as well. Radiologic findings include mucoid impaction and extensive proximal cylindrical bronchiectasis, typically with upper lobe predominance. Mucus plugs may be of high density due to extensive inspissations, and sometimes calcification

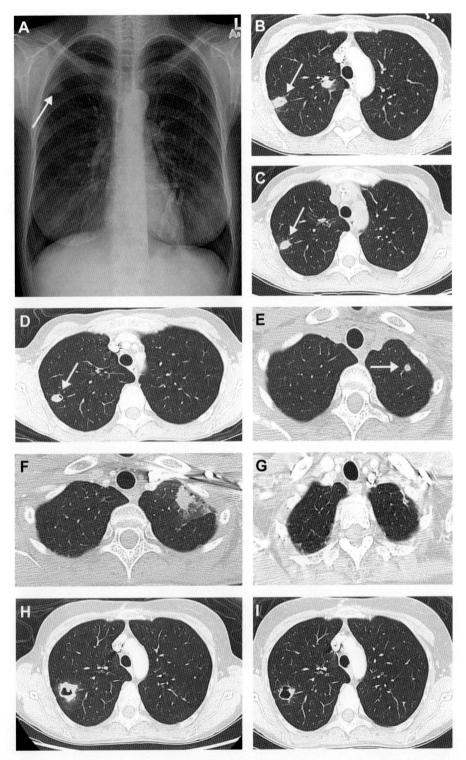

Fig. C8.5 Fungal pneumonia and *Nocardia*. (A) Frontal chest radiograph demonstrates a nodular opacity in the right upper lung zone (white arrow). The patient was recently status post bone marrow transplant and had chest pain. (B) Chest CT demonstrates a spiculated right upper lobe nodule (white arrow). Given the clinical history, fungal infection was favored, although a malignancy would have a similar appearance. Bronchoscopy revealed fungal hyphal elements, although a specific organism was not isolated. Empiric antifungal therapy was initiated. (C, D) Follow-up CT scans demonstrate progressive involution of the nodule. (E) Axial section through the apices from the same exam as (D) demonstrates a new nodule in the left apex (white arrow). This was suspicious for a new infection since the old lesion appeared to be responding to treatment. (F) Short-term follow-up CT demonstrates rapid growth of the new left upper lobe nodule. Repeat bronchoscopy was performed, and cultures this time demonstrated Nocardia. (G) The patient was begun on antibiotics for *Nocardia* as well, and the nodule involuted. (H) Follow-up chest CT demonstrates growth and cavitation of the initial right upper lobe nodule. Upon further questioning, the patient admitted stopping taking antifungal medications secondary to nausea. (I) Antifungal therapy was restarted, and the lesion decreased in size and became more thin-walled.

may be seen. Semi-invasive aspergillosis is characterized by chronic necrotizing granulomatous inflammation, and typically infects chronically debilitated or mildly immunocompromised patients. Radiologic findings include slowly progressive consolidative or nodular opacities which may cavitate and which may progress over months to years. The findings may resemble postprimary tuberculosis. Angioinvasive aspergillosis is typically seen in severely immunocompromised patients and is caused by invasion of small to medium-sized pulmonary arteries leading to hemorrhagic infarcts. At CT, these infarcts classically present as nodular opacities surrounded by a zone of ground glass attenuation (hemorrhage), termed the "halo sign." However, this is nonspecific and may be seen in several other entities such as Kaposi's sarcoma, hemorrhagic metastases, as well as other causes. They may also present as pleural-based wedge shaped opacities, similar to classical lung infarcts.

Cryptococcus neoformans may infect both immune competent and immunocompromised hosts. Infections in immune competent patients are often asymptomatic, while disseminated disease may occur in immunocompromised patients. Typical radiographic patterns are nonspecific as with other fungal infections, and include single or multiple nodules or masslike opacities or consolidative opacities. Nodules or masses may go on to cavitate in immunocompromised hosts. Pleural effusions and hilar and/or mediastinal adenopathy are also more common in immunocompromised hosts.

Clinical Differential

The differential diagnosis for pneumonia in the immunocompromised patient is long, including bacterial, fungal, and viral etiologies.

Imaging Differential

Depends on the radiologic findings. Differential diagnosis for "crazy paving" includes PCP, sarcoidosis, AIP, diffuse hemorrhage, and pulmonary alveolar proteinosis. When fungal pneumonias present with consolidative opacities, bacterial pneumonia is in the differential. When presenting as solitary to multifocal nodules or masses, malignancy and lymphoma may be in the differential diagnosis, and when a miliary pattern is seen, TB, metastases, and viral pneumonia should be in the differential diagnosis.

REFERENCES AND SUGGESTED READING

1. Franquet T, Muller NL, Gimenez A, et al. Spectrum of pulmonary aspergillosis: histologic, clinical, and radiologic findings. *RadioGraphics.* 2001;21:825-837.
2. Fang W, Washington L, Kumar N. Imaging manifestations of blastomycosis: a pulmonary infection with potential dissemination. *RadioGraphics.* 2007;27:641-655.
3. Rossi SE, Erasmus JJ, Volpacchio M. "Crazy-paving" pattern at thin-section CT of the lungs: radiologic-pathologic overview. *RadioGraphics.* 2003;23:1509-1519.
4. McAdams HP, Rosado-de-Christenson ML, Lesar M. Thoracic mycoses from endemic fungi: radiologic-pathologic correlation. *RadioGraphics.* 1995;15:255-270.
5. McAdams HP, Rosado-de-Christenson ML, Templeton PA. Thoracic mycoses from opportunistic fungi: radiologic-pathologic correlation. 1995;15:271-286.

CASE 9: SEPTIC EMBOLI

PATIENT PRESENTATION

A 30-year-old male with history of IV drug abuse presents with fever, cough, and chest pain.

CLINICAL SUSPICION

Septic pulmonary emboli

IMAGING MODALITY OF CHOICE

Initial PA and lateral chest x-ray; CT may be helpful as well (Figs. C9.1 and C9.2).

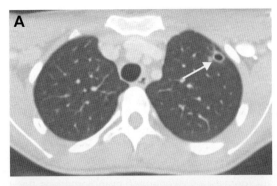

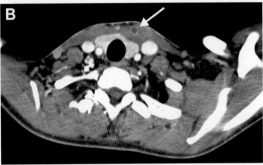

Fig. C9.2 Superficial thrombophlebitis and septic emboli. (A) Axial chest CT demonstrates a small cavitary lesion with mildly thick walls in the left upper lobe (white arrow). (B) CT of the neck demonstrates thrombosis of a superficial neck vein that is nonenhancing, expanded, and peripherally enhancing (white arrow). These findings are indicative of superficial thrombophlebitis, which was felt to be the source of the emboli. The patient had pharyngitis and was admitted for high fever and altered mental status as well as swelling in the neck related to the thrombophlebitis. This is similar to Lemierre's syndrome, in which severe bacterial pharyngitis causes septic thrombophlebitis of the internal jugular vein, which can then cause septic pulmonary emboli as well as showering septic emboli elsewhere in the body. In this case, however, a superficial vein was involved rather than the internal jugular vein. Blood cultures grew alpha-hemolytic streptococcus.

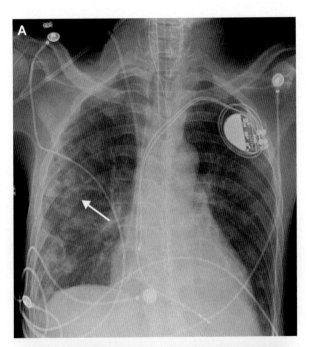

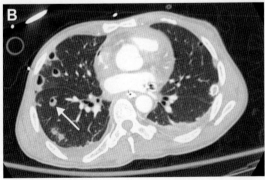

Fig. C9.1 Infected pacemaker lead with septic emboli. (A) Frontal chest x-ray demonstrates numerous cavitary lesions (white arrow). They are present bilaterally, although there are more in the right lung. (B) Axial chest CT from the same patient demonstrates multiple cavitary nodules, as well as some smaller nodules that have not cavitated yet. The patient had an infected pacemaker lead that was the source of the emboli.

FINDINGS

Septic emboli develop when embolic fragments to the lung contain microorganisms. Typical sources include line infections, tricuspid valve endocarditis, and IV drug use. Septic pulmonary emboli represent hematogenous or blood-borne infection to the lungs, different from bronchogenic infections such as pneumonia. Positive blood cultures are frequently found. Bacterial and fungal etiologies are both possible. Radiographically, there will be multiple nodules, which may be of similar sizes if they were the result of a single embolic shower, or of varying sizes if there are multiple embolic events. The nodules are often large and cavitated, containing air-fluid levels. Rupture of one of these cavities into the pleural space results in empyema, pneumothorax, or a combination of both. There is typically a lower lobe predominance due to the increased blood flow to the lung bases. CT findings are essentially the same as at chest x-ray, with the exception that smaller lesions will be more apparent. Also, occasionally a pulmonary artery branch may be seen leading up to some of the lesions, termed the "feeding vessel" sign. In uncomplicated cases, CT may not be necessary, as the diagnosis is often readily made based on the chest x-ray and clinical setting alone.

Clinical Differential

Pneumonia, coronary vasospasm, pulmonary embolism

Imaging Differential

Cavitary metastases, Wegener's granulomatosis, laryngeal papillomatosis. Cavities with a thicker, more irregular, and nodular wall tend to favor malignancy, but this is by no means pathognomonic, and correlation with clinical findings and/or biopsy is necessary.

REFERENCES AND SUGGESTED READING

1. Hagan IG, Burney K. Radiology of recreational drug abuse. *RadioGraphics*. 2007;27:919-940.

2. Han D, Lee KS, Franquet T, et al. Thrombotic and nonthrombotic pulmonary arterial embolism: spectrum of imaging findings. *RadioGraphics*. 2003;23:1521-1539.

CASE 10: ATELECTASIS

PATIENT PRESENTATION

A 76-year-old male with extensive smoking history presents with shortness of breath and decreased breath sounds over the left upper lung.

CLINICAL SUSPICION

Lobar collapse

IMAGING MODALITY OF CHOICE

Chest x-ray, PA and lateral views (Figs. C10.1-C10.7)

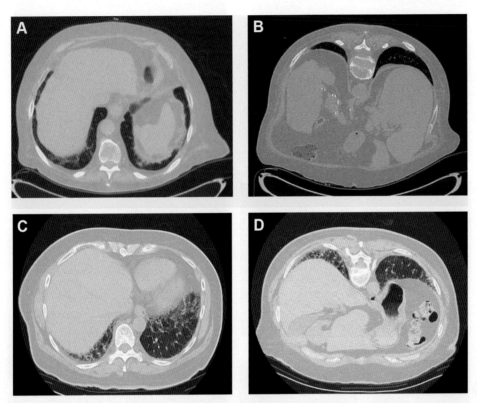

Fig. C10.1 Differentiating subsegmental atelectasis from fibrosis. (A) Supine images from a chest CT demonstrate bilateral linear opacities at the lung bases. (B) Prone images obtained during the same session do not show these same opacities, indicating that they represent subsegmental (or discoid/platelike) atelectasis. This typically occurs in dependent regions of the lung and can be differentiated from early fibrotic changes by imaging in the prone position, as in this case. Atelectatic changes will typically resolve in the prone position, while true fibrotic changes will remain unchanged. (C) Supine and (D) prone images from a different patient than (A) and (B) demonstrate bibasilar reticular opacities that did not change between supine and prone imaging, indicating fibrosis.

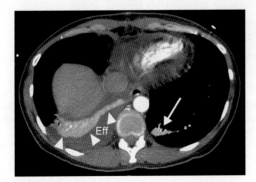

Fig. C10.2 Compressive atelectasis. There is a right pleural effusion (Eff) with compressive atelectasis of the right lower lobe (white arrowheads). Note the uniform enhancement of the atelectatic lung, which helps to differentiate it from consolidated lung, which would not enhance. An area of subsegmental atelectasis is also noted at the left lung base (white arrow).

DISCUSSION

The term atelectasis refers to collapse of alveoli, with resulting volume loss. Mechanistically, atelectasis may be either resorptive, compressive, or cicatricial. Resorptive atelectasis is secondary to an obstructing endobronchial lesion with resorption of air distal to the obstruction and resulting volume loss. Compressive atelectasis is volume loss due to compression from an adjacent space-occupying lesion, often a pleural effusion. Cicatricial atelectasis is volume loss due to parenchymal fibrosis. Morphologically, several types of atelectasis are recognized. Round atelectasis refers to a small round area of nonaerated lung due to overlying pleural adhesions that prevent it from expanding. There is often a "comet tail" representing the feeding bronchovascular bundle. Discoid or "platelike" atelectasis refers to areas of

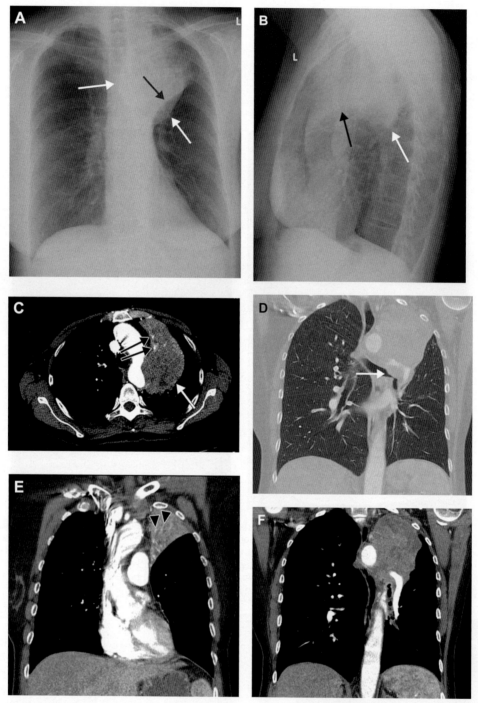

Fig. C10.3 Central mass (squamous cell carcinoma) with left upper lobe collapse. (A) Frontal radiograph demonstrates hazy left upper lung zone opacity with a concave border (black arrow) which is consistent with left upper lobe collapse. There is also a convex border-forming structure projecting over this same area, suggesting an underlying mass, which also results in tracheal compression (white arrows).
(B) Lateral radiograph demonstrates concave border of the collapsed left upper lobe with anterior displacement of the major fissure (black arrow). Convex border of the underlying mass is seen more posteriorly (white arrow). The lateral view is somewhat limited by rotated positioning. (C) Axial contrast-enhanced chest CT at the level of the aortic arch demonstrates a heterogeneous centrally located mass (white arrow) abutting the aorta. There is atelectatic lung anterior to the mass, which contains normal appearing pulmonary vessels (black arrows), although the heterogeneous attenuation of this lung suggests post obstructive pneumonitis or pneumonia. (D) Coronal CT section with lung widows demonstrates high-grade stenosis of the left main bronchus, and the left upper lobe bronchus is not visualized, as it is completely occluded. Note tracheal compression by the medially displaced aortic arch. (E) Coronal CT section in soft tissue windows demonstrates the collapsed left upper lobe responsible for the concave shadow on the frontal chest radiograph. Normal pulmonary vessels are annotated (black arrowheads). Heterogeneous attenuation of this lung again suggests post obstructive pneumonitis or pneumonia.
(F) Another coronal CT section in soft tissue windows more posteriorly than (E) demonstrates the mass responsible for the convex border on the radiographs. Note the lack of normal pulmonary vessels in the mass as compared to the atelectatic lung in (E).

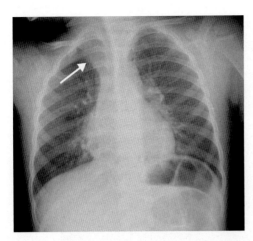

Fig. C10.4 Right upper lobe collapse. Frontal chest radiograph demonstrates streaky perihilar opacities consistent with viral bronchiolitis in this child. There is a hazy concave bordered opacity in the right upper lung zone consistent with right upper lobe collapse. There is subtle elevation of the medial portion of the right hemidiaphragm, as well as rightward mediastinal shift due to volume loss.

subsegmental atelectasis manifest by bandlike linear opacities. These are often seen at the lung bases due to the relatively poorer ventilation in these regions. When the areas of atelectasis involve larger portions of the lung, the terms segmental or lobar collapse are applied, depending on the anatomic extent of involvement. Classic patterns of lobar collapse can typically be diagnosed solely on the basis of chest radiographs, and the clinical scenario will dictate the most likely etiology. For example, collapse of an entire lung in a child is most likely due to an aspirated foreign body (although this more often presents with hyperinflation due to ball-valve effect). In the ambulatory adult patient, lobar collapse is a classic presentation of an obstructing bronchogenic carcinoma, while in the ventilated ICU patient it is most commonly due to a mucus plug.

The upper lobes typically collapse anteriorly and medially. On the right, elevation of the minor fissure may be seen on the frontal view, as well as right paratracheal density, elevation of the right hilum, and compensatory hyperinflation of the middle and lower lobe. On the lateral view, there may be anterior displacement of the major fissure and obliteration of the retrosternal clear space. Left upper lobe collapse may present with similar signs on the left, and classically there is a hazy veil-like opacity over the left hemithorax on the frontal view, with obscuration of the left upper cardiac border and aortic knob.

Right middle lobe collapse is often best demonstrated on the lateral projection, where there will be inferior displacement of the minor fissure and a triangular or band like opacity in the area of the right middle lobe with associated volume loss. On the frontal view, there may be

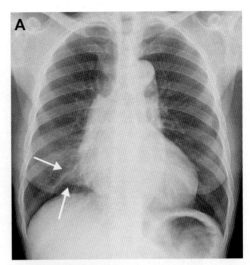
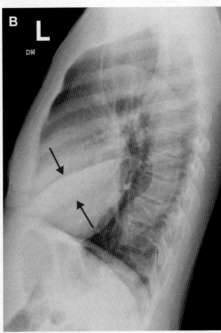

Fig. C10.5 Collapse of the medial basal segment of the right lower lobe. Frontal chest radiograph demonstrates a hazy triangular shaped opacity that does not obliterate the right heart border. Lateral chest radiograph demonstrates a triangular opacity (black arrows) bordered anteriorly by the major fissure. This could easily be confused for RML collapse, but the right heart border would usually be obscured in RML collapse, and more important the RML would be bordered posteriorly by the major fissure on the lateral view instead of anteriorly.

obscuration of the right heart border and hazy opacity over the right lower lung zone which may have a triangular configuration. Of note, right middle lobe collapse is often seen in asthmatics, especially in children.

The lower lobes tend to collapse medially and posteriorly against the spine. On the frontal view, there may be

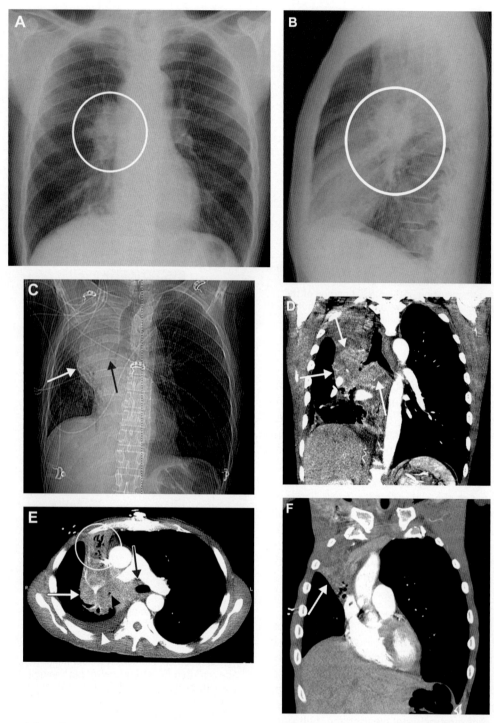

Fig. C10.6 Right upper lobe collapse due to obstructing hilar mass (undifferentiated large cell carcinoma). (A, B) Initial PA and lateral chest radiographs demonstrate lobulated contour and increased opacity of the right hilum suspicious for an underlying mass. Hazy opacity along the right heart border on the PA view may be due to post obstructive pneumonitis and/or atelectasis, however, the patient was lost to follow-up. (C) Scout view from CT scan obtained approximately four months later when the patient re-presented. There is opacification of the right upper lung zone with a centrally convex border (white arrow) which suggests an underlying mass. Note how the combination of a central convex border with a more peripheral convex border forms a reverse S configuration; this is known as the S sign of Golden. There is rightward tracheal and mediastinal shift with elevation of the right hemidiaphragm indicating volume loss. The overall picture is consistent with RUL collapse secondary to an obstructing mass. Additionally, the right main bronchus is cut off (black arrow). (D) Coronal contrast-enhanced chest CT with narrowed window/level settings demonstrates an enhancing right hilar mass (white arrows) invading the mediastinum and occluding the right main bronchus. Compare this to the scout view. (E) Axial contrast-enhanced CT demonstrates enhancing right hilar mass (white arrow) invading the mediastinum (black arrow). Black arrowhead denotes a highly stenotic left upper lobe bronchus. White circle denotes atelectatic lung anteriorly with air bronchograms. Lack of enhancement in this lung suggests post obstructive pneumonitis or pneumonia. Small right pleural effusion is also present (white arrowhead). (F) Coronal section more anterior than D demonstrates atelectatic LUL containing lucent bronchi and pulmonary vessels. Note the smooth, concave border.

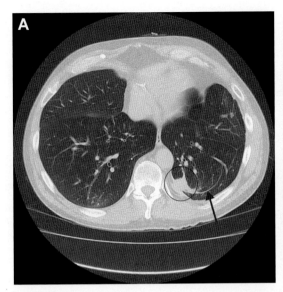 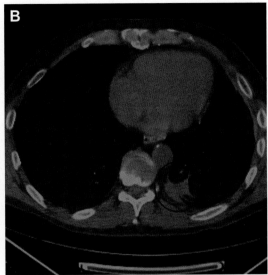

Fig. C10.7 Round atelectasis. (A) There is a nodular opacity at the left lung base (black circle). Note the comet tail (black arrow). The patient had had a pleural effusion earlier, and the opacity developed after the pleural effusion resolved. This is a typical appearance for round atelectasis. (B) PET scan demonstrates lack of FDG uptake in the lesion, consistent with the diagnosis.

a triangular opacity in the lower paravertebral region that obscures the medial portion of the diaphragm. There may be elevation of the diaphragm secondary to volume loss, and there may also be compensatory hyperinflation of the upper lobe. On the lateral view, there will be a triangular opacity posteriorly with posterior displacement of the major fissure and obscuration of the posterior portion of the diaphragm.

Clinical Differential

Differential diagnoses for causes of lobar collapse include foreign body, mucus plug, and bronchogenic carcinoma.

Imaging Differential

Classic findings of lobar and segmental collapse may be confidently diagnosed radiographically. Subsegmental atelectasis may be more difficult to distinguish from early pneumonias, as there may not be an appreciable degree of volume loss.

Round atelectasis may be difficult to distinguish from other causes of solitary pulmonary nodules, particularly malignancy and granulomatous or fungal infection.

REFERENCES AND SUGGESTED READING

1. Robbins LL, Hale CH. The roentgen appearance of lobar and segmental collapse of the lung: a preliminary report. *Radiology*. 1945;44:107-114.

2. Robbins LL, Hale CH. The Roentgen appearance of lobar and segmental collapse of the lung: IV. Collapse of the lower lobes. *Radiology*. 1945;45:120-127.

3. Robbins LL, Hale CH. The roentgen appearance of lobar and segmental collapse of the lung: V. Collapse of the right middle lobe. *Radiology*. 1945;45:260-266.

4. Robbins LL, Hale CH. The roentgen appearance of lobar and segmental collapse of the lung: VI. Collapse of the upper lobes. *Radiology*. 1945;45:347-355.

CASE 11: LUNG CANCER

PATIENT PRESENTATION

A 75-year-old male with 50 pack year smoking history with new onset of cough for the past 3 months, nonproductive. Review of systems also reveals unintentional 20 lb weight loss over that same period.

CLINICAL SUSPICION

Lung cancer

IMAGING MODALITY OF CHOICE

PA and lateral views of the chest for initial workup, followed by contrast-enhanced chest CT (Figs. C11.1-C11.7).

DISCUSSION

Lung cancers are broadly classified as either small cell carcinoma (SCLC) or non–small cell carcinoma (NSCLC). The

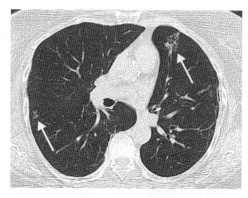

Fig. C11.2 Adenocarcinoma. Axial chest CT demonstrates two areas of fine nodularity (white arrows), one in the lingula, the other in the right lower lobe. Biopsy of the lingular lesion revealed adenocarcinoma of the lung.

non–small cell group consists of three primary entities (ignoring carcinoid tumors for the purposes of this discussion): adenocarcinoma, squamous cell carcinoma, and large cell carcinoma. Many risk factors for lung cancer are recognized, including smoking and radon exposure. While the majority of lung cancers are associated with smoking, radon is thought to account for the bulk of lung cancers in nonsmokers, and approximately 10% of sporadic lung cancers in general. Of the pathologic subtypes, small cell and squamous cell carcinoma show the closest association with smoking. Adenocarcinoma is the most common subtype overall, and its incidence as a whole is rising as well. Lung cancer is staged using the TNM system, with the most recent seventh edition published in 2009 by the International Association for the Study of Lung Cancer (IASLC).

Adenocarcinomas arise from the bronchiolar or alveolar epithelium and thus tend to be more peripheral in

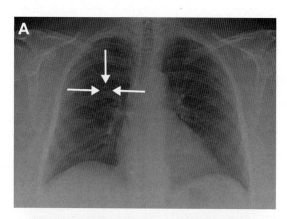

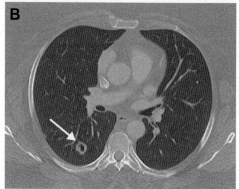

Fig. C11.1 Adenocarcinoma. (A) Frontal chest x-ray demonstrates a faint round cystic lesion in the right upper lung zone. (B) Axial chest CT demonstrates a thick walled cavitary lesion. Biopsy revealed adenocarcinoma of the lung.

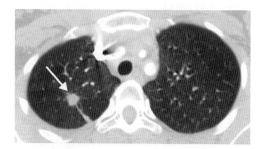

Fig. C11.3 Adenocarcinoma. Axial chest CT demonstrates a right upper lobe nodule (white arrow) which was biopsied and found to be adenocarcinoma of the lung. The patient already had stage IV disease.

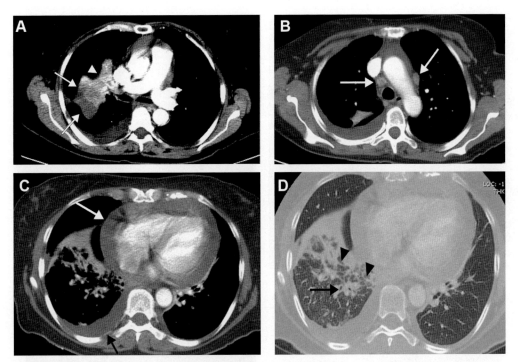

Fig. C11.4 Adenocarcinoma. (A) Axial contrast-enhanced chest CT demonstrates a mass in the right lung (white arrows) which is of relatively low attenuation compared to the enhancing atelectatic lung anteriorly (white arrowhead). (B) The patient had ipsilateral and contralateral mediastinal adenopathy (white arrows). (C) Pleural (black arrow) and pericardial (white arrow) effusions were sampled and found to be malignant. (D) Lung windows demonstrate peribronchial thickening (black arrow) and reticular opacities (few are annotated with black arrowheads) which suggest lymphangitic spread of tumor. Biopsy of the mass demonstrated adenocarcinoma of the lung.

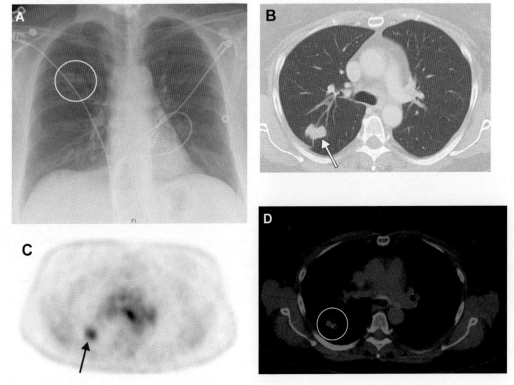

Fig. C11.5 Squamous cell carcinoma. (A) Frontal chest x-ray demonstrates a lobulated opacity in the right upper lung zone. (B) Axial chest CT in lung windows demonstrates a lobulated and spiculated mass, suspicious for malignancy. (C) Corresponding axial PET image from a PET-CT scan demonstrates hypermetabolic FDG uptake in the same area as the mass. (D) Fused PET-CT image confirms this finding. While the focus of increased FDG uptake was easily attributed to the mass in this case even without the fusion images, they are often helpful in equivocal cases. This was squamous cell carcinoma of the lung.

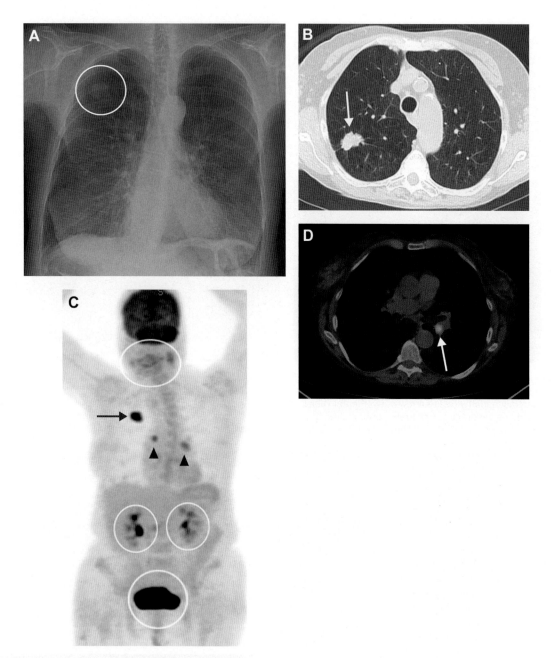

Fig. C11.6 Small cell carcinoma. (A) Frontal chest x-ray demonstrates a nodular opacity in the right upper lung (white circle). (B) Axial chest CT demonstrates a spiculated right upper lung mass suspicious for malignancy (white arrow). (C) Planar whole body PET image demonstrates hypermetabolic FDG uptake in the mass (black arrow) as well as in bilateral hilar lymph nodes (black arrowheads). Physiologic salivary and renal excretion is annotated (white circles). (D) Axial fused PET-CT image from the same examination as (C) demonstrates hypermetabolic FDG uptake within left hilar nodes (white arrow). This was a case of small cell carcinoma.

location. The developmental spectrum of adenocarcinoma is thought to begin with atypical adenomatous hyperplasia (AAH), followed by adenocarcinoma in situ (AIS), minimally invasive adenocarcinoma (MIA) and finally adenocarcinoma. AAH and AIS are considered premalignant lesions. AAH presents as a ground glass nodule without solid component and is typically 5 mm or less in size, although there is no size cutoff. AIS is similar in appearance to AAH, but tends to be slightly larger and more opaque and irregular, although it is still nonsolid. Minimally invasive adenocarcinoma presents as a predominantly nonsolid nodule but with a solid component of 5 mm or less. As the solid

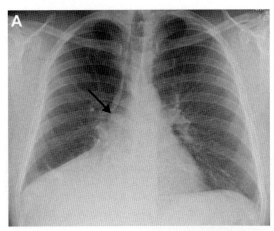
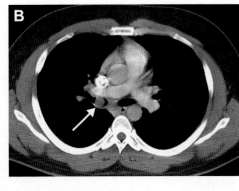
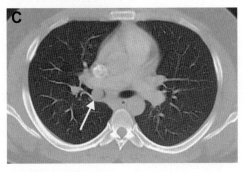

Fig. C11.7 Bronchial carcinoid. (A) Frontal chest x-ray demonstrates a rounded opacity projecting over the bronchus intermedius (black arrow). There is right lower lobe collapse with rightward mediastinal shift and elevation of the right hemidiaphragm. (B) Axial chest CT in soft tissue and (C) lung windows demonstrate the endobronchial nature of the mass. This was a bronchial carcinoid tumor.

component grows beyond 5 mm, they are classified as adenocarcinoma. Adenocarcinomas typically appear as ill-defined spiculated nodules or masses, although the margins may appear to be well defined or lobulated as well. This CT classification is based upon pathologic studies, where ground glass areas on CT have been correlated with areas of "lepidic" growth along the alveolar and bronchial epithelium, but without frank invasion. Areas of solid density have been shown to correlate with areas of invasive tumor, and signify a more aggressive lesion. Not uncommonly, patients may have multifocal lesions.

SCC tends to arise centrally from main, lobar, or segmental bronchi. These lesions often grow into the bronchi, causing cough, hemoptysis, and/or central obstruction. Radiographically, there may be a central mass with collapse or post obstructive pneumonia of the affected pulmonary lobe or segment. This may be demonstrated by the reverse "S" sign of Golden on a chest radiograph, which is manifest by a focal convexity due to an underlying mass within an otherwise concave border of a collapsed lobe. All pneumonias in adults should be followed up for radiographic resolution to exclude the presence of an obstructing

endobronchial mass which may have been obscured by the surrounding consolidation on the initial chest x-ray or CT. SCC often demonstrates central necrosis which may go on to cavitate. Although most SCCs arise centrally, they are a common histologic subtype of the superior sulcus or "Pancoast" tumor.

Large cell carcinoma is an aggressive neoplasm, which is sometimes a diagnosis of exclusion when microscopic features of other subtypes are not seen. Most are reclassified as either SCC or adenocarcinoma when electron microscopy is performed. Radiographically, they appear as large masses that are most commonly peripheral in location, but may be central as well.

Small cell carcinoma arises from neuroendocrine cells lining the main or lobar bronchi. As such, it typically presents as a central mass, which may extrinsically compress bronchi, although it does not typically grow into the bronchial lumen as squamous cell carcinoma often does. Rather, it tends to grow into the bronchial wall and peribronchial connective tissues. The majority of cases have metastasized to mediastinal lymph nodes by the time of imaging diagnosis, and sometimes the primary tumor may not be evident. CT is the examination of choice for evaluating the extent of mediastinal adenopathy. This extensive adenopathy can lead to compression of central bronchi with resulting post obstructive pneumonia or lobar collapse, as well as compression of the SVC with resultant SVC syndrome (although SVC syndrome may occur with any cause of mediastinal mass or adenopathy).

Clinical Differential

Tuberculosis, metastasis

Imaging Differential

Metastasis, tuberculosis, fungal infection, lymphoma, round atelectasis, pulmonary AVM

REFERENCES AND SUGGESTED READING

1. Rosado-de-Christensen ML, Templeton PA, Moran CA. Bronchogenic carcinoma: radiologic-pathologic correlation. *RadioGraphics*. 1994;14:429-446.

2. Lee KS, Jeong YJ, Han J, et al. T1 Non–small cell lung cancer: imaging and histopathologic findings and their prognostic implications. *RadioGraphics*. 2004;24:1617-1636.

3. UyBico SJ, Wu CC, Suh RD, et al. Lung cancer staging essentials: the new TNM staging system and potential imaging pitfalls. *RadioGraphics*. 2010;30:1163-1181.

4. Detterbeck FC, Boffa DJ, Tanoue LT. The new lung cancer staging system. *Chest*. 2009;136:260-271.

5. Austin JHM, Garg K, Aberle D, et al. Radiologic implications of the 2011 classification of adenocarcinoma of the lung. *Radiology*. 2013;266:62-71.

CASE 12: SOLITARY PULMONARY NODULE

PATIENT PRESENTATION

A 50-year-old nonsmoking female with incidental finding of a solitary 5 mm pulmonary nodule on CT angiogram of the chest performed to assess for pulmonary embolism.

CLINICAL SUSPICION

Solitary pulmonary nodule

IMAGING MODALITY OF CHOICE

Chest CT (Figs. C12.1-C12.5)

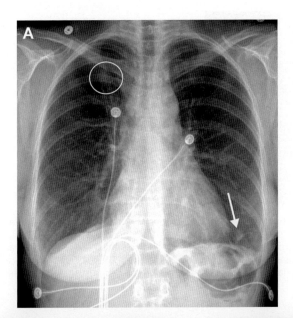

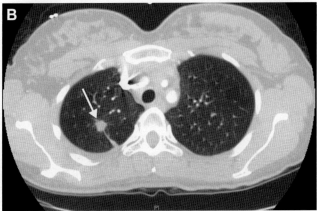

Fig. C12.1 Adenocarcinoma of the lung. (A) Frontal chest radiograph demonstrates a faint nodular opacity at the right lung apex (white circle). This is partially obscured by an overlying rib, making it difficult to discern. Note the nipple shadow at the left lung base (white arrow). (B) Axial chest CT demonstrates a spiculated nodule at the right lung apex, confirming chest radiograph findings (white arrow). This proved to be adenocarcinoma of the lung, and the patient already had stage IV disease.

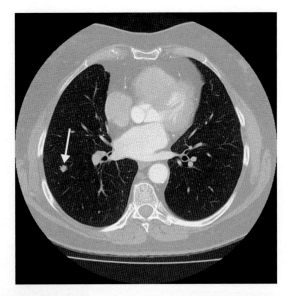

Fig. C12.2 Adenocarcinoma of the lung. Axial chest CT demonstrates a nodule in the right lung with lobulated borders (white arrow). This was adenocarcinoma of the lung.

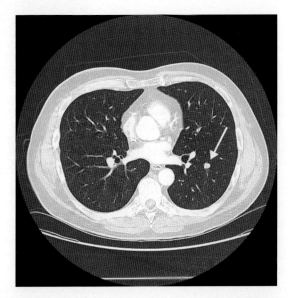

Fig. C12.3 Metastatic melanoma. Axial chest CT demonstrates a lobulated nodule in the left lower lobe (white arrow). This was metastatic melanoma.

DISCUSSION

Nodules are defined as rounded opacities of <3 cm diameter. If the lesion is >3 cm it is called a mass. The differential diagnosis is broad, and includes malignant neoplastic entities such as primary lung carcinoma and metastatic carcinoma, benign neoplastic entities such as hamartoma, infectious entities such as granuloma or round pneumonia, and inflammatory entities such as sarcoidosis, rheumatoid nodule, and Wegener's granulomatosis. There are numerous

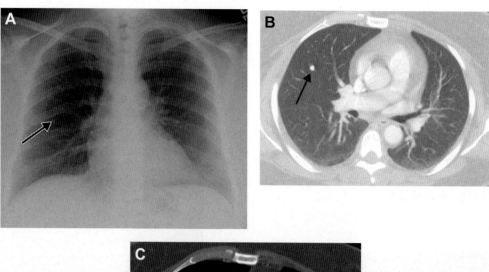

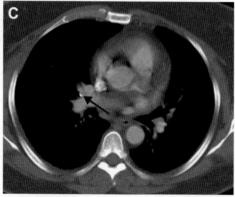

Fig. C12.4 Calcified granuloma. (A) Frontal chest radiograph demonstrates a tiny well-defined nodular opacity in the right mid lung (black arrow). (B) Axial chest CT in lung windows demonstrates a diffusely calcified nodule consistent with a granuloma (black arrow). (C) Soft tissue windows demonstrate a calcified ipsilateral hilar lymph node (black arrow). This constellation of findings most likely represents a Ranke complex from prior TB exposure. There was no evidence of active disease. A Ranke complex consists of a Ghon lesion (which is a calcified pulmonary parenchymal tuberculoma) and an ipsilateral calcified hilar lymph node. This is seen in healed primary tuberculosis.

other more obscure entities as well. In the absence of contributory clinical history, the primary concern when a nodule is found in the lung is typically the exclusion of malignancy.

When assessing risk of malignancy, the first criteria to consider is the size of the lesion. Lesions smaller than 1 cm are more likely to be benign, while those >1 cm in size are more likely malignant. Certain morphologic characteristics are also helpful, such as the presence and morphology of calcifications and the presence of fat in a lesion. Patterns of benign calcification include central, laminated, and diffuse solid calcifications which are indicative of granulomas, and "popcorn" type calcifications which are indicative of hamartomas (although this pattern is very rare). The presence of fat density within a lesion is indicative of a hamartoma, and therefore benignity. Any other patterns of calcification (such as amorphous, eccentric, or punctuate calcifications) are indeterminate. The margin of a lesion is an important factor to consider. Irregular, lobulated or

spiculated nodules tend to be malignant, whereas perfectly smooth nodules tend to be benign. Other characteristics such as the density of the lesion, and the wall thickness of a cavitary lesion are also considered when assessing risk of malignancy, however these criteria are not sufficiently sensitive to allow for confident diagnosis.

In the absence of definitively benign or malignant features, the nodule must be considered indeterminate. There are then two possible management strategies. One is to pursue definitive diagnosis via biopsy, and the other is to follow with serial imaging on the assumption that malignant lesions will demonstrate growth while nonmalignant lesions will largely remain unchanged in appearance. The optimal interval for follow-up is based on the doubling time of lung cancers, which is approximately 6 months for solid appearing nodules, and can be 2 years or longer for ground glass nodules. However, these estimates vary widely from tumor to tumor. Another complicating factor is the fact that small nodules may grow a substantial percentage in terms of

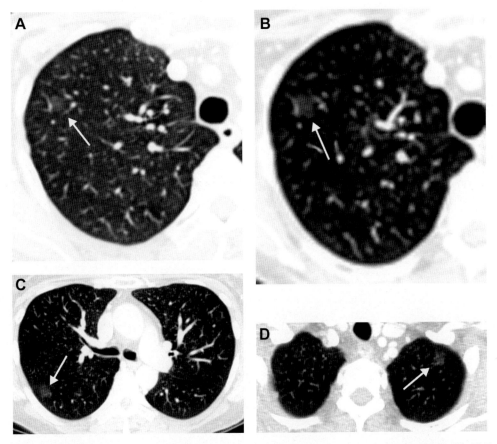

Fig. C12.5 Multifocal adenocarcinoma in situ (AIS), formerly known as bronchioloalveolar cell carcinoma (BAC). (A, B) Two chest CT sections obtained approximately 2 years apart demonstrate a ground glass nodule in the right upper lobe with interval growth between the two studies. (C, D) Axial chest CT sections from the same patient demonstrate additional ground glass nodules bilaterally. Biopsy of one of the lesions demonstrated atypical pneumocyte hyperplasia (more commonly known as atypical adenomatous hyperplasia or AAH) which is thought to be a precursor lesion of adenocarcinoma of the lung. However, multiple nodules had demonstrated interval growth and are most consistent with AIS. Several remained stable in appearance and are most consistent with AAH. The progression of AAH to adenocarcinoma is further discussed elsewhere in this text.

volume without this being readily apparent visually on CT. For example, a spherical 4 mm nodule may double in volume, but will still only be 1 mm larger in diameter.

The Fleischner Society has released guidelines for the management of incidentally detected indeterminate solitary pulmonary nodules in patients 35 years of age or older based on the size of the nodule and presence of patient risk factors for malignancy. High-risk patients are those with a history of smoking or other risk factors for lung cancer, and low-risk patients are defined as those with no or minimal smoking history, and absence of other known risk factors. For nodules 4 mm or less in size in low-risk patients, benignity can be assumed, and no follow-up is needed. In a high-risk patient, a single 12-month follow-up chest CT is sufficient if there is no interval change. For nodules greater than 4 to 6 mm in size in a low-risk patient, a single 12-month follow-up chest CT is sufficient if there

is no interval change. In a high-risk patient, initial follow-up is recommended at 6 to 12 months, followed by a second follow-up study at 18 to 24 months if there is no change. For nodules greater than 6 to 8 mm in size in a low-risk patient, initial follow-up is recommended at 6 to 12 months, followed by a second follow-up study at 18 to 24 months if there is no change. In a high-risk patient, follow-up is recommended at 3 to 6, 9 to 12, and 24 months if there is no interval change. For nodules greater than 8 mm in size in both low and high-risk patients, follow-up can be obtained at around 3, 9, and 24 months if there is no change, or alternatively, definitive assessment for malignancy can be pursued with PET and/or biopsy [1]. Dynamic contrast-enhanced CT can also be performed to assess for malignancy, although this is not commonly done. The specific management strategy in these scenarios also varies by institution, based on locally available equipment and expertise.

Clinical Differential

Hamartoma, granuloma, intrapulmonary lymph node, metastasis, primary lung cancer, scar/fibrosis, septic embolus, sarcoidosis, rheumatoid nodule, Wegener's granulomatosis.

Imaging Differential

Same

REFERENCES AND SUGGESTED READING

1. MacMahon H, Austin JHM, Gamsu G, et al. Guidelines for management of small pulmonary nodules detected on CT scans: a statement from the Fleischner Society. *Radiology*. 2005;237:395-400.

2. Winer-Muram HT. The solitary pulmonary nodule. *Radiology*. 2006;239:34-49.

3. Erasmus JJ, Connolly JE, McAdams HP, et al. Solitary pulmonary nodules: part I. Morphologic evaluation for differentiation of benign and malignant lesions. *RadioGraphics*. 2000;20:43-58.

4. Erasmus JJ, Connolly JE, McAdams HP. Solitary pulmonary nodules: part II. Evaluation of the indeterminate nodule. *RadioGraphics*. 2000;20:59-66.

CASE 13: BRONCHIECTASIS

PATIENT PRESENTATION

A 45-year-old male with history of prior TB presents with chronic cough productive of foul smelling sputum.

CLINICAL SUSPICION

Bronchiectasis

IMAGING MODALITY OF CHOICE

Chest CT (Figs. C13.1 and C13.2)

DISCUSSION

Bronchiectasis refers to abnormal permanent dilation of the bronchi, and is secondary to destruction of the muscular and elastic tissue surrounding these structures. Symptoms include productive cough, foul smelling sputum, and hemoptysis. Initial imaging may often consist of a chest radiograph, in which parallel linear shadows representing the bronchial walls may be seen. CT is the modality of choice in evaluating for the presence and extent of bronchiectasis due its cross sectional nature. There are three types of bronchiectasis recognized morphologically. Cylindrical bronchiectasis consists of diffuse dilation of the bronchus. Varicose bronchiectasis consists of focal areas of narrowing with intervening areas of dilation, giving a "string of pearls" appearance. Cystic bronchiectasis is the most severe form

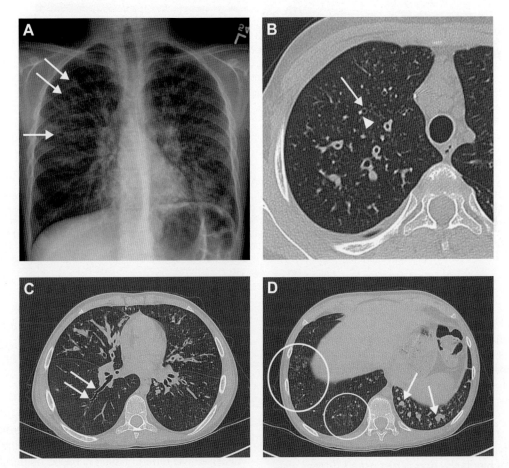

Fig. C13.1 Cystic fibrosis. (A) PA chest radiograph demonstrates innumerable rounded lucencies, several of which are annotated (white arrows). They appear to radiate outward from the hilum, suggesting bronchiectasis rather than cystic lung disease. (B) Axial chest CT from the same patient demonstrates bronchiectasis. As a rule of thumb, the diameter of a bronchus and its adjacent pulmonary artery branch should be approximately equal. In this example, the bronchus (white arrow) is larger in diameter than the adjacent pulmonary artery branch (white arrowhead), suggesting bronchiectasis. Multiple bronchi also demonstrate thickened walls. (C) Same patient. A bronchus seen in longitudinal cross-section (white arrows) demonstrates cylindrical bronchiectasis. (D) Same patient. Cross section through the lung bases demonstrates multiple rounded opacities that actually represent mucus impacted bronchi. Although this is difficult to ascertain on only one image, following these structures on more superior sections would demonstrate their connection to the bronchial tree. Patchy areas of clustered tiny nodular opacities (some in a "tree-in-bud" configuration) are also present (white circles), and in this case are likely due to mucus or pus filled bronchioles.

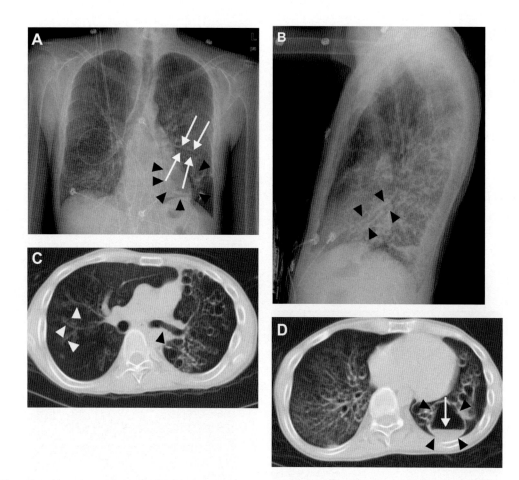

Fig. C13.2 Cystic and varicose bronchiectasis. (A) PA chest radiograph demonstrates bronchiectasis (white arrows). There is also a large cystic lesion in the left lung base (black arrowheads). (B) Lateral view of the same patient also demonstrates bronchiectasis (black arrowheads). (C) Axial CT in lung windows demonstrates a "string of pearls" appearance consistent with varicose bronchiectasis. Black arrowhead denotes a dilated left main bronchus. (D) Axial CT through the lung bases demonstrates the large cystic lesion seen in (A) (black arrowheads). This was proven to communicate with the bronchial tree on contiguous sections, indicating that it is cystic bronchiectasis, rather than some other form of cystic lung disease (ie, lung abscess). There is an air-fluid level (white arrow) due to pooling of secretions.

and is manifest by saclike dilation of bronchi, typically more severe in the periphery.

The most common congenital cause of bronchiectasis is cystic fibrosis. Other congenital causes include Kartagener syndrome (immotile cilia syndrome or primary ciliary dyskinesia), Mounier Kuhn syndrome, and William Campbell syndrome. The most common acquired cause of bronchiectasis is post infectious, typically chronic necrotizing infections. Allergic bronchopulmonary aspergillosis (ABPA) typically causes a predominantly central cylindrical bronchiectasis, and is discussed further elsewhere in this text. Pulmonary fibrosis can also lead to a phenomenon of "traction bronchiectasis" caused by fibrosis that results in retraction of the surrounding lung tissue. Infection with atypical mycobacteria can cause bronchiectasis both in immunocompromised and immune competent hosts.

Clinical Differential

Often, bronchiectasis is asymptomatic. When symptomatic, it may present with cough, foul smelling sputum, and hemoptysis. The differential diagnosis in that case would include pneumonia and tuberculosis.

Imaging Differential

As mentioned in the previous section, the main differential consideration for bronchiectasis on imaging is cystic lung disease. The differentiation is based on demonstrating that the "cysts" are actually dilated airways.

REFERENCES AND SUGGESTED READING

1. Kuhlman JE, Reyes BL, Hruban RH, et al. Abnormal air-filled spaces in the lung. *RadioGraphics*. 1993;13:47-75.
2. Hartman TE, Primack SL, Lee KS, et al. CT of bronchial and bronchiolar diseases. *RadioGraphics*. 1994;14:991-1003.

CASE 14: CHRONIC OBSTRUCTIVE PULMONARY DISEASE

PATIENT PRESENTATION

A 75-year-old male with 50 pack years smoking history presents with chronic cough and production of small amounts of nonpurulent sputum.

CLINICAL SUSPICION

COPD

IMAGING MODALITY OF CHOICE

Chest x-ray (Figs. C14.1-C14.4)

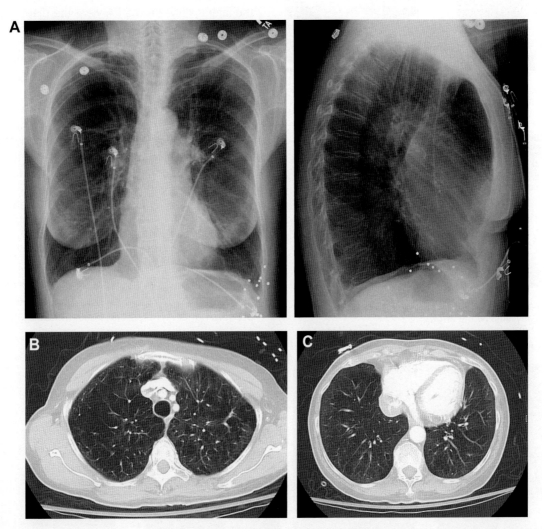

Fig. C14.1 Emphysema. (A) PA and lateral views of the chest demonstrate hyperinflated lungs with flattening of the diaphragm. Shrapnel projects over the left lower chest. (B) Axial chest CT in lung windows through the upper lobes demonstrates severe centrilobular emphysema. (C) Severe but less advanced changes are seen in the lower lobes.

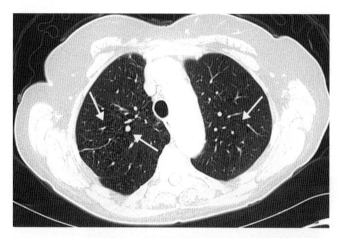

Fig. C14.2 Axial contrast-enhanced CT of the chest demonstrates centrilobular emphysema (white arrows), not as advanced as in Fig. C14.1.

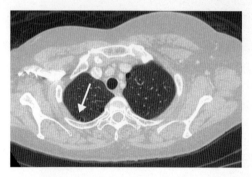

Fig. C14.3 Axial chest CT through the upper lobes demonstrates paraseptal emphysema (white arrow).

DISCUSSION

COPD is a clinical diagnosis based on evidence of pulmonary obstruction which is not fully reversible. Radiologically, obstruction can be suggested by the presence of increased lung volumes. Additionally, there can be evidence of emphysema, which can be the substrate for developing the clinical syndrome of COPD. Increased lung volumes can be inferred by flattening of the diaphragm and increased AP diameter of the chest, which are best appreciated on the lateral view. On the PA view, the diaphragm may also appear flattened and the heart may appear to be smaller relative to the surrounding lungs. However, it is important to note that many of these findings may be mimicked by an exuberant inspiratory effort, and this is a classic pitfall.

Emphysema is an abnormal permanent enlargement of the airspaces distal to the terminal bronchiole accompanied by destruction of their walls and without obvious fibrosis [2]. Several different types of emphysema are generally identified on the basis of their distribution. Centrilobular emphysema is the most common and is manifest by destruction of the central portions of the secondary pulmonary lobule. This form of emphysema is typically more severe in the upper lobes. Paraseptal emphysema is manifest by selective destruction of airspaces along the interlobular septae with centrilobular sparing, and is typically seen in subpleural regions. Panlobular emphysema is uniform destruction of airspaces within the entire secondary pulmonary lobule, and this typically takes a lower lobe predominance. This is classically associated with alpha-1

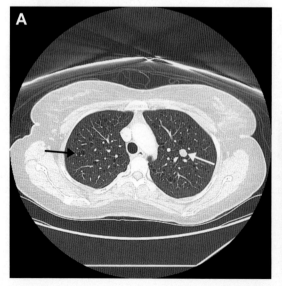

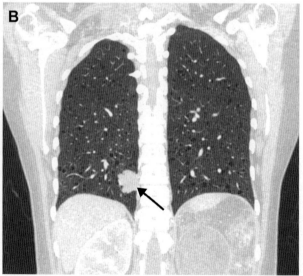

Fig. C14.4 Lymphangioleiomyomatosis (LAM). (A) Axial CT demonstrates numerous bilateral small rounded lucencies, one of which is denoted by a black arrow. Some of these demonstrate thin, barely perceptible walls. Also note the left upper lobe nodule (white arrow). (B) Coronal reformat from the same study demonstrates lower lung zone predominance, which would be atypical for emphysema. Also note the right lower lobe mass (black arrow). The patient had a history of tuberous sclerosis, which is associated with LAM. Additionally, the patient had colon cancer, with pulmonary metastases.

antitrypsin deficiency. Finally, paracicatricial emphysema is destruction and enlargement of airspaces associated with fibrosis of the lung, such as that related to prior infection. While the types of emphysema discussed in this section may be easily appreciated on CT, they cannot be differentiated on chest radiographs alone. Emphysematous changes can be suggested on chest x-ray by areas of lucency, and if severe, bullae may be seen typically in the apical regions. Areas of emphysema may also appear as lucent areas within consolidated lung, in which case they may be misinterpreted as areas of necrosis or abscess formation. When assessing severity of emphysema, it is important to stress that clinical severity often does not correlate with the extent of radiologic findings.

Chest radiography is often performed in the setting of an acute COPD exacerbation, typically to assess for pneumonia as a precipitating factor. Chest CT, while demonstrating emphysematous changes exquisitely, need not be routinely performed since it does not usually alter management. That being said, it does play a role in preoperative evaluation when lung reduction surgery is being considered.

Clinical Differential

Other causes of cough and shortness of breath, including pneumonia, interstitial lung disease, and pulmonary embolism.

Imaging Differential

Differential diagnosis for hyperexpanded lungs would include foreign body aspiration or mucus plug, although these are usually unilateral while COPD will be bilateral. Differential diagnosis for emphysema includes cystic lung diseases (such as lymphangioleiomyomatosis) which may resemble centrilobular emphysema. It is important to recognize differences in distribution (emphysema will have an apical predominance) and to recognize that cysts will have a wall, while emphysema will look more like a "hole."

REFERENCES AND SUGGESTED READING

1. Foster WL Jr, Gimenez EI, Roubidoux MA, et al. The emphysemas: radiologic-pathologic correlations. *RadioGraphics*. 1993;13:311-328.
2. Snider GL, Kleinerman J, Thurlbeck WM, Bengali ZK. The definition of emphysema: report of a National Heart, Lung and Blood Institute, Division of Lung Diseases, workshop. *Am Rev Respir Dis*. 1985;132:182-185.

CASE 15: SARCOIDOSIS

PATIENT PRESENTATION

A 35-year-old black female presents with worsening cough, arthralgias and a nodular erythematous rash over the extensor surface of the lower extremities.

CLINICAL SUSPICION

Sarcoidosis

IMAGING MODALITY OF CHOICE

Chest x-ray should be performed for initial global assessment, with high-resolution chest CT (HRCT) performed subsequently (Figs. C15.1-C15.5).

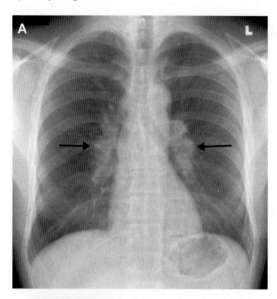

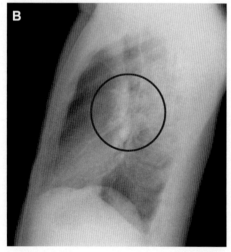

Fig. C15.1 Stage 1 sarcoidosis. (A) PA chest x-ray demonstrates bilateral hilar adenopathy (black arrows). Note the bulging convex border of the hilar angles. (B) Lateral view also demonstrates hilar adenopathy (black circle). Sarcoidosis is often staged as follows: stage 0, normal chest x-ray; stage 1, only lymphadenopathy; stage 2, lymphadenopathy and parenchymal disease; stage 3, only parenchymal disease; stage 4, pulmonary fibrosis.

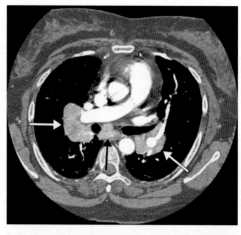

Fig. C15.2 Axial contrast-enhanced chest CT demonstrates bilateral hilar adenopathy (white arrows) as well as subcarinal adenopathy (black arrow) in a patient with sarcoidosis.

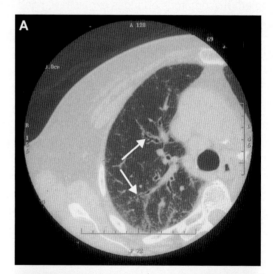

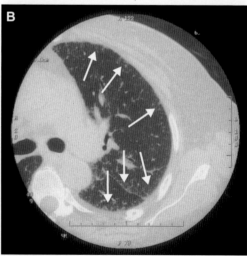

Fig. C15.3 Parenchymal sarcoidosis. Axial high-resolution CT images demonstrate perilymphatic nodules typical for sarcoidosis. White arrows annotate peribronchovascular nodules in (A), and perifissural and subpleural nodules in (B).

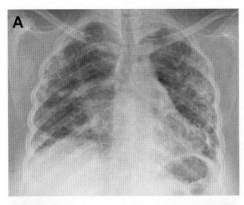

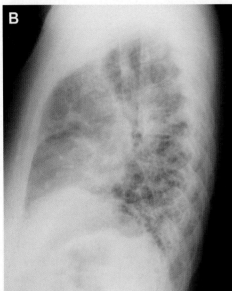

Fig. C15.4 Stage IV sarcoidosis. (A) PA and (B) lateral views of the chest demonstrate end stage sarcoidosis with diffuse coarse reticular opacities, low lung volumes and honeycombing indicative of fibrosis.

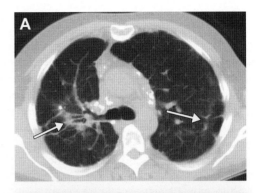

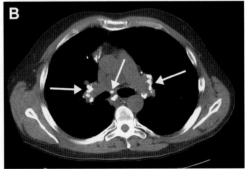

Fig. C15.5 Chronic sarcoidosis. (A) Axial chest CT in lung windows demonstrates bilateral central upper lobe scarring (white arrows) with mild traction bronchiectasis in the right lung. (B) Soft tissue windows demonstrate calcified bilateral hilar and mediastinal lymph nodes (white arrows). The findings were radiographically stable for several years. It is not uncommon for pulmonary sarcoidosis to eventually "burn-out" as is likely in this case.

FINDINGS

Histopathologically, pulmonary sarcoidosis is manifest by noncaseating granulomatous inflammation within the pulmonary interstitium, preferentially along pulmonary lymphatics and bronchovascular bundles. Healing response to this inflammation eventually leads to fibrosis in the late stages of illness. Hilar and mediastinal lymph nodes are typically involved.

Radiographically, the most typical finding is symmetric bilateral hilar adenopathy. Often, there is mediastinal adenopathy as well, most commonly in the right paratracheal group. The combination of right paratracheal, right and left hilar adenopathy has been called the 1-2-3 sign. Unilateral hilar adenopathy is not typical for sarcoidosis and other diagnoses (such as TB or malignancy) should be considered. Isolated mediastinal adenopathy without hilar involvement is also rare. Involved lymph nodes can calcify, often peripherally in an "eggshell" pattern (although this can be seen in other entities as well, such as silicosis).

Approximately half of patients will have evidence of parenchymal disease in addition to nodal disease. Although rare, it is possible to have parenchymal disease without nodal disease. Parenchymal disease is most typically manifest by bilateral symmetric reticulonodular opacities with a preference for the mid to upper lung zones. The nodules are usually tiny (few mm in size) and in a perilymphatic distribution, meaning that they are predominantly seen along bronchovascular bundles and along pleural surfaces. This is best evaluated with HRCT. Small nodules may coalesce to produce larger nodules. Less commonly, a more mass-like pattern may be seen, with multiple scattered larger nodules or masses measuring up to a few centimeters in diameter. These tend to have well-defined borders and may contain air bronchograms as well. Some patients will go on to develop fibrosis, manifest by parenchymal and airway distortion, coarse linear opacities, and cystic changes. These changes predominate in the mid to upper lung zones, and the loss of volume often leads to hilar elevation. Pulmonary air cysts or cavities may rupture and result in spontaneous pneumothorax, or may become secondarily infected with *Aspergillus* and result in mycetoma formation.

Although less commonly performed now, gallium-67 scanning can be of use in diagnosis and monitoring of sarcoidosis as well. Classically, uptake will be seen in bilateral hilar and right paratracheal nodal stations, termed the "lambda" sign (this is the equivalent of the 1-2-3 sign discussed earlier). Another often quoted sign is the "panda" sign, created by uptake in the salivary, parotid, and lacrimal glands. In the proper clinical setting, these are supportive of the diagnosis of sarcoidosis, although Ga-67 uptake is nonspecific, and can be seen in any granulomatous disease and in many malignancies. Ga-67 scanning has also been used to monitor response to treatment, with uptake decreasing in treated or inactive lesions, but persisting in areas of active disease.

Clinical Differential

Connective tissue disease, lymphoma, tuberculosis, Langerhans cell histiocytosis

Imaging Differential

Silicosis, Coal workers' pneumoconiosis, TB, lymphangitic carcinomatosis, hypersensitivity pneumonitis

REFERENCES AND SUGGESTED READING

1. Criado E, Sanchez M, Ramirez J, et al. Pulmonary sarcoidosis: typical and atypical manifestations at high-resolution CT with pathologic correlation. *RadioGraphics*. 2010;30:1567-1586.

CASE 16: INTERSTITIAL LUNG DISEASE

PATIENT PRESENTATION

A 60-year-old female with no prior medical history presents with worsening shortness of breath for 6 months and non-productive cough. On examination, there are fine crackles at the lung bases.

CLINICAL SUSPICION

Idiopathic pulmonary fibrosis

IMAGING MODALITY OF CHOICE

Noncontrast chest CT with high-resolution protocol (HRCT). Chest x-ray should be performed initially; however, HRCT should be performed even if the chest x-ray is normal if there is suspicion for interstitial lung disease (ILD) (Figs. C16.1-C16.4).

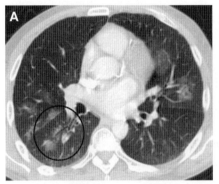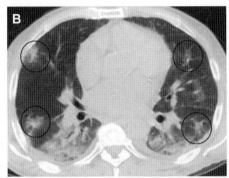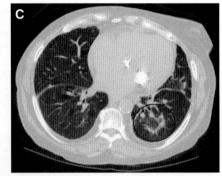

Fig. C16.1 Cryptogenic organizing pneumonia. (A) Axial chest CT demonstrates patchy ground glass opacities, some of which are in a peri-bronchial distribution (black circle). (B) Axial section more inferiorly demonstrates that some of the opacities are more consolidative in appearance and are in a peripheral distribution (black circle). (C) Different patient. There is an "atoll" sign (black circle) manifest by central ground glass opacity with a rim of denser opacity peripherally, which has been likened to the circular coral reef with a central lagoon of an atoll. While this has traditionally been associated with COP, it can be seen in other diseases as well.

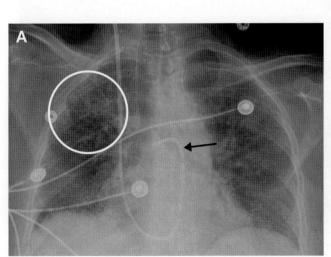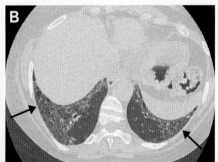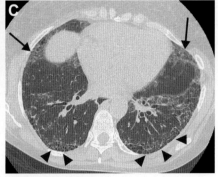

Fig. C16.2 Scleroderma. (A) Portable AP chest radiograph demonstrates bibasilar reticular opacities. Additional reticular opacities are seen in the right upper lung zone (white circle). Note the pulmonary artery catheter. (B) Axial chest CT through the lung bases in lung windows demonstrates bibasilar reticulation and areas of honeycombing (black arrows). There is mild ground glass opacity, but the reticular opacities are the predominant finding. (C) Axial section more superiorly also demonstrates areas of ground glass opacity (black arrows) and areas of honeycombing (black arrowheads). Note the mildly dilated esophagus. The overall picture is most consistent with fibrotic NSIP or UIP. Findings were fairly stable over the course of 5 years favoring NSIP, which has a better prognosis than UIP.

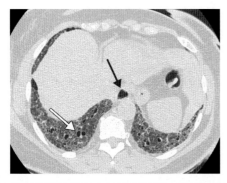

Fig. C16.3 Scleroderma. Axial chest CT at the lung bases demonstrates reticular opacities, traction bronchiectasis (white arrow), and ground glass opacity. Note the dilated esophagus (black arrow). Overall, the findings are consistent with NSIP with features of both fibrotic and cellular forms.

FINDINGS

It is helpful to categorize chronic interstitial pneumonias on the basis of pathologic findings. Six main pathologic entities will be briefly discussed here: usual interstitial pneumonia (UIP), acute interstitial pneumonia (AIP), nonspecific interstitial pneumonia (NSIP), cryptogenic organizing pneumonia (COP), desquamative interstitial pneumonia (DIP) and respiratory bronchiolitis-associated interstitial lung disease (RB-ILD). The latter two (DIP and RB-ILD) are often grouped under the heading of smoking-related interstitial lung diseases, and may represent a spectrum of the same disease process. It is important to note that while many of the above entities may occur idiopathically, they can also have myriad causes including collagen vascular diseases, and pulmonary drug toxicities. While radiographic findings may be diagnostic in UIP, in most other cases the findings are nonspecific, and biopsy may be required for a definitive diagnosis.

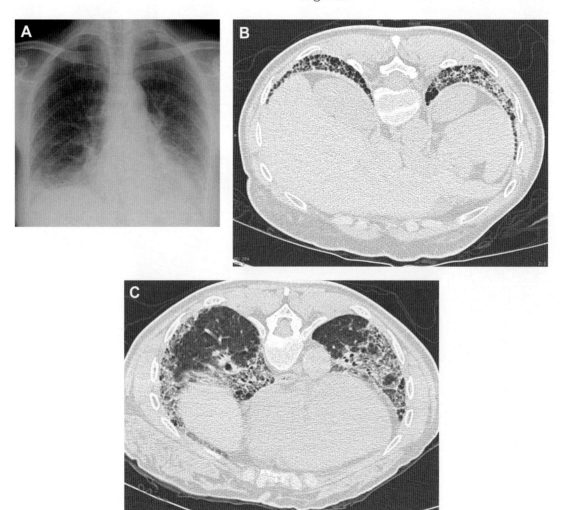

Fig. C16.4 UIP. (A) PA view of the chest demonstrates bilateral fairly symmetric fine peripheral and basilar reticular opacities. (B) Axial high-resolution chest CT section through the lung bases in the same patient demonstrates basilar reticulation and honeycombing, consistent with fibrosis. (C) More superior section from the same patient also demonstrates the largely peripheral nature of the findings. The overall picture is most consistent with UIP. The patient had SLE.

UIP is characterized pathophysiologically by repetitive lung injury with an exuberant fibroblastic healing response. Radiographically, areas of active inflammation are characterized by fine reticular or ground glass opacities, which progress to more coarse appearing reticular opacities and eventually honeycombing as fibrosis progresses. UIP can be idiopathic (idiopathic pulmonary fibrosis or IPF) or the result of many entities, including collagen vascular diseases such as rheumatoid arthritis, scleroderma, SLE, and dermatomyositis/polymyositis, asbestosis, chronic hypersensitivity pneumonitis and chemotherapeutic drugs.

AIP is a rapidly progressive disease characterized pathologically by diffuse alveolar damage, and it can be thought of as being an idiopathic form of ARDS. Radiographic findings are therefore identical to ARDS, and consist of diffuse ground glass opacity and consolidation, often in a gradient of increasing density from nondependent to more dependent regions. There is a very high mortality.

COP is a disorder of unknown etiology characterized by plugs of organizing granulation tissue within alveoli and distal airways. It has been associated with a number of disorders including viral infections, toxic inhalation, collagen vascular disease, drug reaction, and organ transplantation. Radiographically, it is characterized by patchy peribronchial and peripheral consolidative or ground glass opacities. There is often associated bronchiectasis and bronchial wall thickening.

NSIP is something of a waste basket diagnosis for cases which do not fit neatly into other categories. Pathologically, a cellular form and a fibrotic form are recognized. In the cellular pattern of NSIP, fibrosis is absent and the salient CT findings are ground glass and consolidative opacities in a symmetric, peripheral, and basilar distribution. The fibrotic form may demonstrate linear and reticular opacities in a similar distribution, and eventual honeycombing. NSIP may be idiopathic or associated with drug reactions or collagen vascular disease.

DIP is seen almost exclusively in cigarette smokers and is characterized pathologically by intra-alveolar collections of macrophages. Radiographically, it is characterized by bibasilar reticular opacities, with ground glass opacities also seen in a minority of cases as well. Thus, it is difficult to differentiate radiographically from early UIP, although UIP inexorably progresses to fibrotic honeycombing, while DIP does not.

RB-ILD is characterized by the presence of intraluminal macrophages within respiratory bronchioles, and is seen exclusively and commonly in smokers. Radiographically, it is characterized by ground glass centrilobular nodules, and there may be areas of air trapping due to involvement of small airways. Fibrotic changes such as reticular opacities and honeycombing are not seen.

Clinical Differential

Many of these entities present with progressive dyspnea and cough, and the clinical differential may include chronic infection, malignancy, and airway disease (such as COPD or asthma) in addition to interstitial lung diseases.

Imaging Differential

Varies with the radiographic findings. The differential diagnosis for honeycombing includes UIP and fibrotic NSIP, and may be a late finding in sarcoidosis as well as pneumoconioses. Differential diagnosis for AIP (idiopathic ARDS) includes infection, pulmonary edema, and alveolar proteinosis as well as a myriad of other causes of diffuse alveolar damage (DAD). Differential diagnosis for COP includes chronic infection, lymphoma, metastatic, or primary malignancy and sarcoidosis. Clinical information and sometimes biopsy are needed to narrow the above differential diagnoses.

REFERENCES AND SUGGESTED READING

1. Mueller-Mang C, Grosse C, Schmid K, et al. What every radiologist should know about idiopathic interstitial pneumonias. *RadioGraphics.* 2007;27:595-615.

2. Kligerman SJ, Groshong S, Brown KK, et al. Nonspecific interstitial pneumonia: radiologic, clinical, and pathologic considerations. *RadioGraphics.* 2009;29:73-87.

3. Kim EA, Lee KS, Johkoh T, et al. Interstitial lung diseases associated with collagen vascular diseases: radiologic and histopathologic findings. *RadioGraphics.* 2002;22:S151-S165.

CASE 17: ASBESTOS-RELATED DISEASES

PATIENT PRESENTATION

A 70-year-old retired shipyard worker presents with shortness of breath and chest pain. He also notes 20 lb. weight
loss over the last 6 months.

CLINICAL SUSPICION

Asbestosis, mesothelioma

IMAGING MODALITY OF CHOICE

Chest x-ray for initial work up, followed by chest CT with
contrast (Figs. C17.1 and C17.2). High-resolution protocols are helpful to evaluate for early fibrotic changes associated with asbestosis.

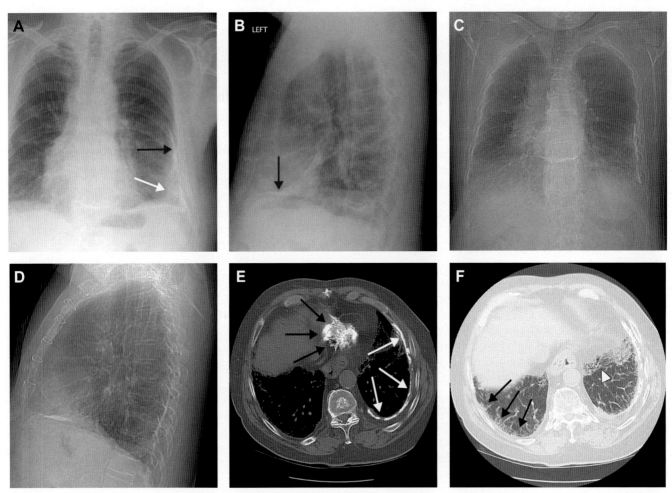

Fig. C17.1 Pleural plaques and lung asbestosis. (A) PA view of the chest demonstrates a high-density linear opacity peripherally near the
lung base consistent with a calcified pleural plaque (black arrow). There is a hazy peripheral basilar opacity, which is poorly defined on this
radiograph. (B) Lateral view again demonstrates a dense linear opacity projecting along the diaphragm, consistent with calcified plaque
(black arrow). (C,D) Calcified nature of these opacities is better demonstrated on these frontal and lateral scout views from a CT scan.
Ill-defined bibasilar reticular opacities are also seen. (E) Axial chest CT in bone window demonstrates calcified plaque along the inferior
pericardium (black arrows). This was seen on the lateral view of the chest in (B). Calcified pleural plaque (white arrows) was responsible
for the peripheral linear opacity on the frontal view of the chest in (A). (F) Axial chest CT in lung windows demonstrates bibasilar peripheral reticular opacities (black arrows). Early honeycombing is also present (white arrowhead). This pattern would be indistinguishable from
UIP, but the presence of calcified pleural plaques in characteristic locations is more consistent with parenchymal asbestosis and asbestos-
related pleural disease.

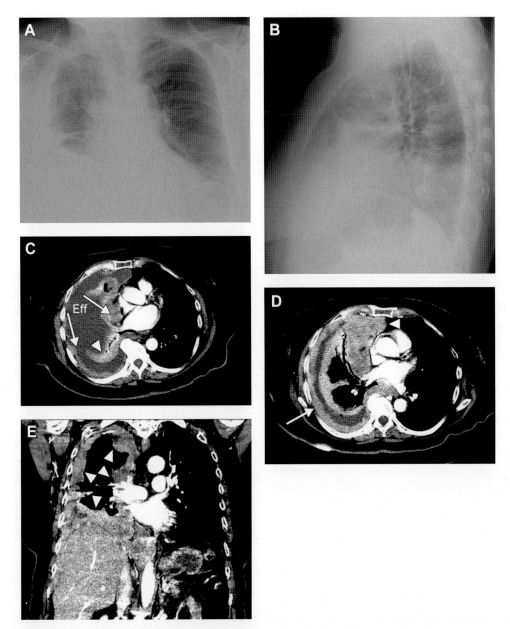

Fig. C17.2 Mesothelioma. (A, B) PA and lateral views of the chest at initial presentation demonstrate a large right pleural effusion, with fluid tracking in the minor fissure. Bulging of the right mediastinal border on the frontal view suggests that there is thickening or fluid tracking along the mediastinal pleura as well. (C) Axial contrast-enhanced CT demonstrates a large right pleural effusion (Eff) with compressive atelectasis (white arrowhead); however, it also reveals irregular pleural thickening which enhances, suspicious for malignancy (white arrows). There is also involvement of the mediastinal pleura. The patient was lost to follow-up. (D) Axial contrast-enhanced CT two months later when the patient re-presented demonstrates progression of pleural thickening, now with circumferential involvement (white arrow). There is a small pleural effusion as well, with associated atelectasis. There is extensive masslike involvement of the mediastinal pleura, and mediastinal invasion (white arrowhead). (E) Coronal reformation from the same study demonstrates the circumferential nature of the pleural thickening as well (white arrowheads). Percutaneous pleural biopsy demonstrated mesothelioma. The patient had a history of household asbestos exposure in Mexico.

DISCUSSION

Asbestos-related thoracic disease encompasses both lung disease (asbestosis) and pleural disease (asbestos-related pleural diseases) which may have benign and malignant etiologies. Lung disease results from inhalation and retention of asbestos fibers in the lungs, and there is a long latency period (20-40 years or more) between the exposure and the onset of disease. Pleural involvement is the most common manifestation of asbestos-related disease. Benign pleural disease includes pleural effusions, diffuse pleural thickening, and pleural plaques. Pleural effusions usually occur within 10 years of exposure, are usually unilateral, and are exudative and hemorrhagic in character. They usually resolve over a period of months, although they can persist or recur. Upon resolution of the pleural effusion, diffuse pleural thickening (DPT) may develop. DPT has been defined as a continuous sheet of pleural thickening more than 5 cm wide, more than 8 cm in craniocaudal extent, and more than 3 mm thick [1]. The margins tend to be ill-defined and irregular, and calcification is rare. DPT often involves the apex and costophrenic angle, and therefore can cause blunting of the costophrenic angle on chest x-ray.

Pleural plaques are the most common manifestation of asbestos exposure, and are typically seen 20 to 30 years after exposure. Pathologically, they are discrete areas of fibrosis. They are typically bilateral, and tend to involve the mid-portion of the posterolateral chest wall as well as the dome of the diaphragm (which is very characteristic). The mediastinal pleura may also be involved. The apices and costophrenic angles are not usually involved, which can help to differentiate from pleural plaques due to TB exposure and prior trauma or empyema, respectively. Calcification can be seen. These pleural plaques are not premalignant. Radiographically, pleural plaques are seen as well-defined focal areas of pleural thickening. They may be difficult to detect with chest radiography due to lack of calcification, and especially if involving the anterior chest wall or paravertebral region. CT is therefore far superior for detection of pleural plaques due to its cross sectional nature. Pleural plaques may be associated with fibrotic changes in the underlying lung, manifest by short linear interstitial opacities radiating from the plaque. Areas of pleural thickening and fibrosis may lead to "round atelectasis," which is manifest by a round subpleural opacity produced by the pleural fluid buoying up the lung base resulting in infolding of the lung upon itself, with overlying pleural thickening. A "comet tail" is often seen, which is thought to represent bronchovascular structures entering the area of atelectatic lung.

Malignant mesothelioma is strongly associated with asbestos exposure, and can occur with short exposures, although there is a dose-response relationship. It is manifest by progressive pleural thickening, with eventual encasement of the lung. There is often an associated pleural effusion. It metastasizes via lymphatic and hematogenous dissemination. Chest radiograph may demonstrate a pleural effusion with associated lobulated pleural thickening and volume loss in the affected hemithorax. It may advance along interlobular fissures, and extend into the chest wall. Asbestos exposure is also a risk factor for bronchogenic carcinoma, particularly with concomitant smoking history. Radiographically and clinically, the presentation is similar to other bronchogenic carcinomas.

Parenchymal asbestosis is manifest by interstitial pulmonary fibrosis secondary to intrapulmonary asbestos fibers. Radiographically, it can be manifest by subpleural reticular opacities with a basilar predominance. This may be more apparent on CT. There may also be associated ground glass opacities and small nodular opacities. Advanced cases may result in honeycombing. There is often associated asbestos-related pleural disease as discussed in this section. Overall, the findings may be difficult to distinguish from other interstitial lung disease, especially UIP/IPF.

REFERENCES AND SUGGESTED READING

1. Lynch DA, Gamsu G, Aberle DR. Conventional and high-resolution tomography in the diagnosis of asbestos-related diseases. *RadioGraphics*. 1989;9:523-551.

2. Roach HD, Davies GJ, Attanoos R, et al. Asbestos: when the dust settles—an imaging review of asbestos related disease. *RadioGraphics*. 2002;22:S167-S184.

3. Kim KI, Kim CW, Lee MK, et al. Imaging of occupational lung disease. *RadioGraphics*. 2001;21:1371-1391.

4. Tyszko SM, Marano GD, Tallaksen RJ, et al. Best cases from the AFIP—malignant mesothelioma. *RadioGraphics*. 2007;27:259-264.

CASE 18: PNEUMOCONIOSIS

PATIENT PRESENTATION

A 65-year-old retired male who spent his entire career working as a sandblaster presents with chronic shortness of breath.

CLINICAL SUSPICION

Silicosis

IMAGING MODALITY OF CHOICE

Initial PA and lateral views of the chest. CT of the chest (typically using a high-resolution protocol, which may vary by institution) is the most sensitive exam (Figs. C18.1 and C18.2).

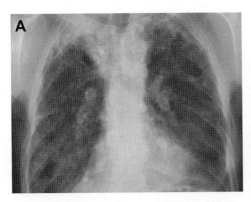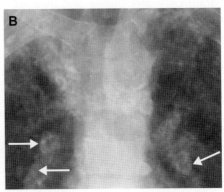

Fig. C18.1 Silicosis. (A) Frontal chest x-ray demonstrates innumerable tiny pulmonary nodules bilaterally. (B) Cropped and zoomed view of the hila demonstrates numerous hilar lymph nodes that are peripherally calcified in an "eggshell" pattern. A few are marked with white arrows. This pattern of calcification, while nonspecific, is classically associated with silicosis. It can also be seen in coal workers' pneumoconiosis, sarcoidosis, as well as other entities.

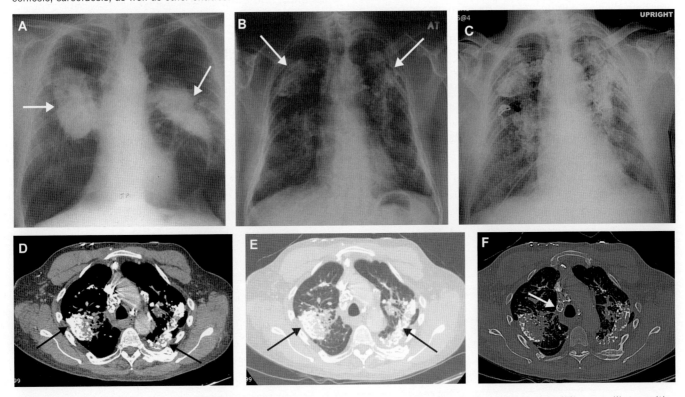

Fig. C18.2 Silicosis with progressive massive fibrosis (PMF). (A) Frontal chest x-ray demonstrates large bilateral perihilar masslike opacities (white arrows). There is retraction of the peripheral lung parenchyma, resulting in relative lucency of the lung apices and bases. Note the peaking or tenting of the left hemidiaphragm as well, due to retraction. (B) Frontal chest x-ray in a different patient demonstrates bilateral upper lobe masslike opacities (white arrows) as well as scattered nodules bilaterally which appear to be calcified. (C) Frontal chest x-ray from the same patient 4 years later is largely unchanged accounting for differences in technique. (D) Axial CT performed at the same time demonstrates bilateral upper lobe conglomerate opacities with extensive coarse calcification (black arrows). (E) Similar section in lung windows. (F) On bone windows, calcified mediastinal adenopathy is present, some of which demonstrates an eggshell pattern (white arrow). The patient had been a sandblaster in the past, consistent with the diagnosis of silicosis. PMF can also be seen in end-stage sarcoidosis and CWP, and can be confused for malignancy if the history is not known and if the findings are not as striking as they are in these cases.

DISCUSSION

Pneumoconioses are a group of diseases caused by an inflammatory reaction to inhaled mineral dusts. Silicosis and anthracosis (coal worker's pneumoconiosis, or CWP) will be discussed further here, although other inorganic dusts such as beryllium and tin are known to cause lung disease as well. Although silicosis and CWP differ in pathophysiology, they are radiographically very similar, and may not be possible to differentiate in individual cases. Silicosis is the most common occupational lung disease, and is most often seen in sandblasters and miners, as it is most often caused by inhaled quartz dust. The quartz is ingested by macrophages, which release inflammatory mediators such as TNF. The earliest manifestations are tiny nodules typically ranging from 1 to 10 mm with a posterior upper lung predilection (as these areas have the poorest lymphatic drainage) which may go on to calcify. The nodules are in a perilymphatic distribution, meaning they are seen both along bronchovascular bundles as well as along fissural and pleural surfaces. Aggregates of subpleural nodules may resemble pleural plaques. Hilar adenopathy may be seen as well, which may calcify. An eggshell pattern of hilar calcification can be very suggestive of silicosis in the appropriate clinical setting, and is much more common in silicosis than in CWP. Advanced silicosis leads to an entity known as progressive massive fibrosis (PMF), which develops by coalescence of individual silicotic nodules into a large masslike lesion, which may have areas of central necrosis. They are typically bilaterally symmetric, and although they begin in the upper peripheral lung zone, they migrate toward the hilum over time, leaving behind areas of emphysematous lung. Notably, patients with silicosis are at higher risk of developing tuberculosis as well as lung cancer. Coal worker's pneumoconiosis appears very similar to silicosis radiographically. Early disease is manifest by "coal macules," which are similar to the tiny nodules with a posterior upper lung predilection seen in silicosis. Advanced disease leads to PMF, just as in silicosis as well. At biopsy, birefringent silicate crystals can usually be identified in cases of silicosis, whereas CWP is characterized by anthracotic pigmentation and coal-laden macrophages.

Clinical Differential

Interstitial lung disease, COPD, CHF

Imaging Differential

Sarcoidosis, silicosis, CWP can all present with small nodules in a perilymphatic distribution. Hypersensitivity pneumonitis also present with perilymphatic nodules, however, this entity typically also includes ground glass opacity and areas of air trapping. When there is cavitation, TB should enter the differential, and may be superimposed upon a pneumoconiosis. PMF may be the common end result of silicosis, sarcoidosis, and CWP. PMF may resemble malignancy, and a high index of suspicion is required since these patients are predisposed to lung cancer as well.

REFERENCES AND SUGGESTED READING

1. Chong S, Lee KS, Chung MJ, et al. Pneumoconiosis: comparison of imaging and pathologic findings. *RadioGraphics*. 2006;26:59-77.
2. Kim KI, Kim CW, Lee MK, et al. Imaging of occupational lung disease. *RadioGraphics*. 2001;21:1371-1391.

CASE 19: ANTERIOR MEDIASTINAL MASS

PATIENT PRESENTATION

A 50-year-old female with fatigue, weakness, double vision, worse at the end of the day.

CLINICAL SUSPICION

Myasthenia gravis, rule out thymoma.

IMAGING MODALITY OF CHOICE

Contrast-enhanced chest CT (Figs. C19.1-C19.5).

FINDINGS

The most common anterior mediastinal masses (in no particular order) are substernal extension of thyroid goiter, lymphoma and other diseases associated with enlarged lymph nodes such as sarcoidosis and metastatic disease, thymoma, and germ cell tumors (including teratoma). These are commonly known as the 4 Ts, (thyroid, thymus/thymoma, teratoma, and terrible lymphoma). Many mediastinal masses may initially come to attention as an incidental finding on a chest x-ray performed for another indication, and there can be many clues to determine the location of such a mass (ie, anterior, middle, or posterior mediastinum) based

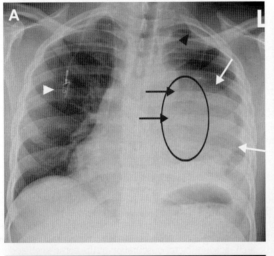
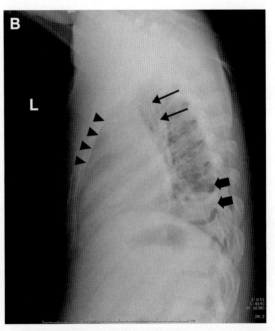
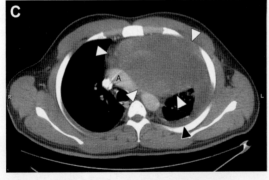

Fig. C19.1 A 34-year-old male with mediastinal germ cell tumor. (A) Frontal view of the chest demonstrates large leftward bulge of the mediastinal contour obscuring the left heart border (white arrows). Pulmonary vascular markings are visible through the lesion, confirming that it is outside the lung parenchyma. The left hilus is visible through the lesion as well (black oval), indicating that it is either anterior or posterior mediastinal (this is known as the *hilum overlay sign*). The descending aorta is visible through the mass as well (black arrows) indicating that it is not posterior mediastinal, so must therefore be anterior mediastinal. There is a left pleural effusion as well (black arrowhead). A CT injectable port-catheter is present over the right hemithorax with a Huber needle attached (white arrowhead). (B) Lateral view demonstrates opacification of the retrosternal clear space (black arrowheads) confirming anterior mediastinal mass. Left pleural effusion (thick black arrows) is demonstrated by obscuration of the left hemidiaphragm and increasing opacity of the lower thoracic vertebral bodies, which normally decrease in opacity inferiorly on the lateral view. Only one hemidiaphragm is visible here, and it can be inferred to be the right hemidiaphragm since it is not silhouetted out by the heart anteriorly. Thin black arrows indicate the posterior wall of the trachea. (C) Axial contrast-enhanced CT of the chest slightly inferior to the level of the aortic arch demonstrates a large, heterogeneously enhancing anterior mediastinal mass (white arrowheads) abutting the aortic arch and anterior chest wall. Ascending aorta is denoted by the letter (A). Black arrowhead indicates left pleural effusion. Serum AFP was massively elevated, consistent with an endodermal sinus (yolk sac) tumor. No testicular primary was identified on ultrasound, and this was therefore felt to be a primary mediastinal germ cell tumor.

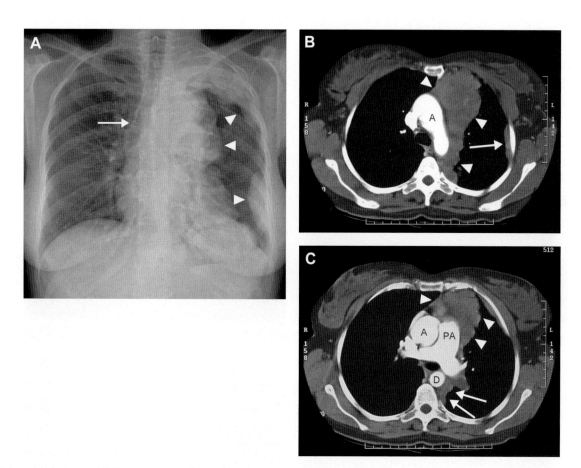

Fig. C19.2 Invasive thymoma. (A) Frontal chest radiograph demonstrates bulky lobulated pleural-based opacities along the lateral, mediastinal and apical pleural surfaces (white arrowheads). There is rightward deviation of the trachea (white arrow) suggesting a mediastinal mass. The aortic knob is obliterated, suggesting anterior mediastinal location. The descending aorta is not visible either, suggesting involvement of the posterior mediastinum or mediastinal pleura. (B) Axial contrast-enhanced CT of the chest at the level of the aortic arch (A) demonstrates a lobulated heterogeneously enhancing anterior mediastinal mass (white arrowheads) that abuts the aortic arch, accounting for obscuration of the aortic knob and rightward tracheal shift on the frontal radiograph. White arrow denotes pleural thickening, due to metastatic disease in this case. (C) Axial slice more inferiorly than B demonstrates the anterior mediastinal mass (white arrowheads), and mediastinal pleural involvement (white arrows) abutting the descending aorta, accounting for loss of the descending aortic shadow on frontal radiograph. PA = pulmonary trunk, D = descending aorta, A = ascending aorta.

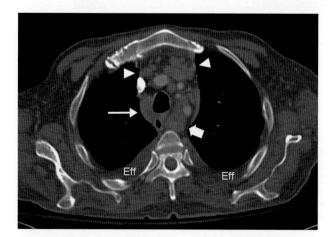

Fig. C19.3 Hodgkin's lymphoma. Axial contrast-enhanced CT superior to the aortic arch demonstrates numerous enlarged anterior mediastinal prevascular lymph nodes (white arrowheads). Right paratracheal adenopathy (thin white arrow) and paraesophageal adenopathy (thick white arrow) are also annotated. Eff = pleural effusion (bilateral). The patient also had bilateral hilar adenopathy (not shown).

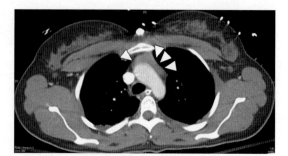

Fig. C19.4 Normal residual thymus, 18-year-old female trauma patient. Note the smoothly contoured bilobed homogeneously enhancing appearance in the expected location of the thymus (white arrowheads). As in this case, the normal thymus frequently has concave borders. This should not be confused for mediastinal hematoma or anterior mediastinal mass in this age group.

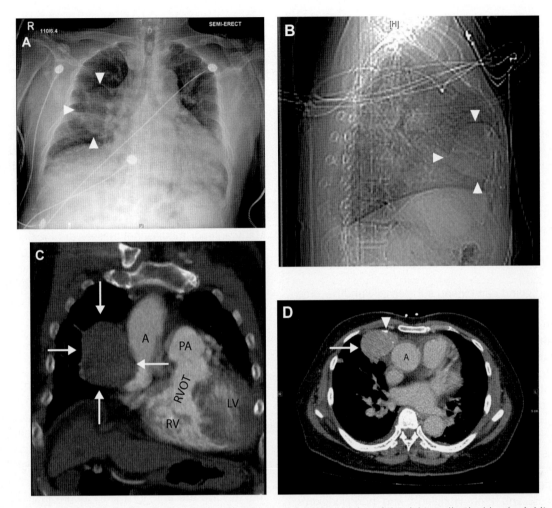

Fig. C19.5 Thymoma. (A) Frontal chest radiograph demonstrates rounded convex bulging of the right mediastinal border (white arrowheads). Pulmonary vascular markings are visible through the lesion, confirming mediastinal location, as opposed to a pulmonary mass. The right hilus is also seen through the lesion, localizing it to the anterior or posterior mediastinum (*hilum overlay sign*). The right heart border is obscured, suggesting anterior mediastinal location. (B) Lateral scout image from CT scan confirms anterior mediastinal location (white arrowheads). (C) Coronal contrast-enhanced CT demonstrates a round homogeneous anterior mediastinal mass abutting the ascending aorta A (white arrows). Compare to frontal chest radiograph. RV = right ventricle, LV = left ventricle, RVOT = right ventricular outflow tract, PA = pulmonary artery. (D) Axial contrast-enhanced chest CT shows the same mass (white arrow) with few calcifications (white arrowhead). A = ascending aorta.

solely on the chest x-ray. There are many clues on the standard PA and lateral chest radiographs that can suggest an anterior mediastinal location. These include retrosternal opacity on the lateral view, obliteration of the anterior junction line, bony destruction or erosion of the sternum (very rare), and a widened right paratracheal stripe (although this can also be seen in middle mediastinal masses). If the hilum is visible through the lesion, then that suggests that the lesion is either anterior or posterior to the hilum. If the lesion is anterior to the hilum, then it could be anterior mediastinal in location. Some anterior mediastinal lesions may silhouette and obscure a portion of the heart border, although middle mediastinal masses may

also do this. Preservation of posterior structures such as the descending aortic shadow excludes a posterior location. Although radiographs may suggest the presence of an anterior mediastinal mass, they are not typically useful in narrowing the differential diagnosis.

The thymus gland is proportionally largest during infancy, although it reaches its absolute maximum mass during adolescence. Afterward, it begins to involute, although a small amount of remnant tissue may remain. The normal thymus gland appears as a bilobed homogeneous soft tissue structure in the anterior mediastinum draped over the ascending aorta anteriorly on CT scans. Thymomas are neoplasms composed of thymic epithelial cells and intermixed lymphocytes, and are typically broadly classified as invasive or noninvasive. They can be graded histologically using the WHO classification scheme, although this does not always predict invasiveness. The Masaoka-Koga system stages thymomas based on invasiveness, and is clinically more useful. On CT, thymic neoplasms appear as an oval or lobulated soft tissue mass in the anterior mediastinum. Small lesions may demonstrate homogeneous enhancement, while larger lesions tend to be more heterogeneous and may demonstrate areas of necrosis or cystic degeneration. Calcifications may be present. Invasive thymomas have a tendency for pleural metastasis, which is often unilateral. Thymic carcinomas are the highest WHO grade thymic epithelial neoplasm, and are typically invasive. Thymic tumors are often associated with myasthenia gravis, although many other paraneoplastic syndromes have been described.

The thyroid gland can extend substernally and become quite large, extending into the anterior mediastinum. It may come to attention incidentally on a chest x-ray, or may produce symptoms from mass effect upon the trachea. The appearance on chest radiographs is nonspecific, but suggestive due to the location of the mass. Typically, there is a mass in the region of the thoracic inlet, with widening of the right paratracheal stripe. On CT, the thyroid gland is seen extending into the anterior mediastinum from the neck. It is usually high in attenuation due to accumulated iodine, and is heterogeneous in appearance due to a multinodular goiter.

Lymphomas are a common etiology for an anterior mediastinal mass, and both Hodgkin's and non-Hodgkin's (NHL) types may involve this location, although other sites are typically involved as well. Hodgkin's disease will often involve the anterior mediastinum as well as hilar nodes, although the anterior mediastinum may rarely be the only site of disease. Lymphoma may appear as enlarged isolated lymph nodes, or as a mass of conglomerate lymph nodes. Thymic enlargement can also be seen in lymphoma, and may be indifferentiable from thymoma. Calcifications are rare in untreated lymphoma, and should suggest a different diagnosis.

Many types of germ cell tumors may arise from germ cell rests in the anterior mediastinum. The most common is mature cystic teratoma. Other lesions include seminoma, immature teratoma, choriocarcinoma, embryonal cell

carcinoma, and endodermal sinus tumor. Only mature cystic teratomas will be further discussed here, since they often have a typical appearance that is pathognomonic. Mature teratomas are benign lesions, although they may demonstrate slow growth. They contain cells derived from all three germ cell layers. They are often cystic and multiloculated, although some may be unilocular. The presence of calcification, fat, fluid, and soft tissue elements is pathognomonic for a teratoma. A fat-fluid level is sometimes seen, and is also diagnostic. Solid portions may demonstrate enhancement on postcontrast images.

Clinical Differential

Many anterior mediastinal masses are incidentally discovered. When symptomatic, it is usually due to airway compression resulting in nonspecific symptoms of chest pain, shortness of breath, and/or coughing. The clinical differential in such cases would include pneumonia and bronchogenic carcinoma.

Imaging Differential

The 4 Ts, (thyroid, thymus/thymoma, teratoma, and terrible lymphoma). "Thyroid" refers to a large substernal goiter. Thymic lesions may include cysts, thymic lymphoma, thymoma, and thymic carcinoma. In addition to teratomas, both seminomatous and nonseminomatous germ cell tumors may arise in the anterior mediastinum from embryonic germ cell rests. Finally, in addition to "terrible lymphoma," other processes involving the lymph nodes may involve the anterior mediastinum including TB, sarcoidosis, and metastasis.

REFERENCES AND SUGGESTED READING

1. Whitten CR, Khan S, Munneke GJ, et al. A diagnostic approach to mediastinal abnormalities. *RadioGraphics*. 2007;27:657-671.

2. Tecce PM, Fishman EK, Kuhlman JE. CT evaluation of the anterior mediastinum: spectrum of disease. *RadioGraphics*. 1994;14:973-990.

3. Gibbs JM, Chandrasekhar CA, Ferguson EC, et al. Lines and stripes: where did they go? from conventional radiography to CT. *RadioGraphics*. 2007;27:33-48.

4. Benveniste MFK, Rosado-de-Christenson ML, Sabloff BS, et al. Role of imaging in the diagnosis, staging, and treatment of thymoma. *RadioGraphics*. 2011;31:1847-1861.

CASE 20: MIDDLE MEDIASTINAL MASS

PATIENT PRESENTATION

A 45-year-old female with intermittent low grade fevers and night sweats.

CLINICAL SUSPICION

Non-Hodgkin's lymphoma (NHL)

IMAGING MODALITY OF CHOICE

CT with intravenous contrast (Fig. C20.1)

DISCUSSION

Both Hodgkin's and NHL may involve mediastinal and hilar nodal groups. While Hodgkin's disease is more likely to involve the anterior mediastinal group, NHL is more likely to involve middle mediastinal and hilar node groups. While CT is the examination of choice and readily demonstrates hilar and mediastinal adenopathy, detection of mediastinal masses and the ability to localize masses to the anterior, middle or posterior mediastinum on plain radiographs are necessary since a chest x-ray will often be the initial imaging modality. Structures within the middle mediastinum include the great vessels, trachea, heart and pericardium, lymph nodes, and the vagus, phrenic, and left recurrent

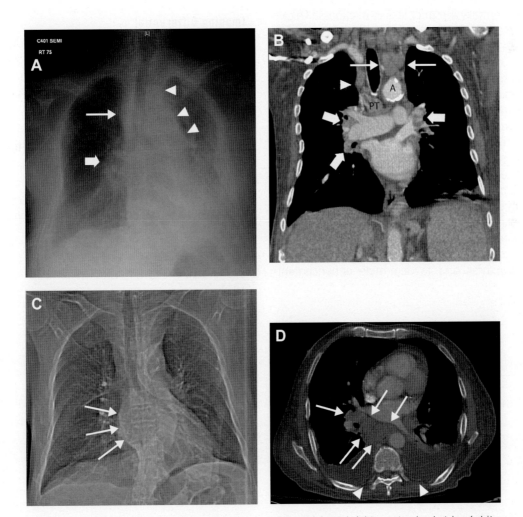

Fig. C20.1 Hodgkin's lymphoma. (A) Frontal chest radiograph demonstrates a thickened right paratracheal stripe (white arrow). There is also thickening of the left paratracheal stripe with a bulging contour and obscuration of the aortic arch and convex bulging of the AP window (white arrowheads). Convex right hilar bulge is also seen (thick white arrow). (B) Coronal contrast-enhanced chest CT demonstrates extensive mediastinal and hilar adenopathy responsible for chest x-ray findings. Right paratracheal adenopathy (white arrowhead), left paratracheal adenopathy (thin white arrows), and bilateral hilar adenopathy are seen (thick white arrows). A denotes aortic arch, which was obscured on chest x-ray by the surrounding adenopathy. PT denotes pretracheal adenopathy. (C) CT scout image from the same patient demonstrates an irregular bulging of the right paraspinal stripe (white arrows). (D) Axial chest CT demonstrates extensive mediastinal adenopathy (white arrows). Bilateral pleural effusions are present (white arrowheads).

laryngeal nerves. Middle mediastinal masses can therefore involve any of these structures, and the differential diagnosis is broad. Lymph node enlargement is the most common source of a middle mediastinal mass, and may be due to infection (ie, tuberculosis, histoplasmosis), malignancy (ie, metastatic disease, lymphoma), as well as other conditions (ie, sarcoidosis, Castleman's disease). Lymph nodes that are greater than 1 cm in size in short axis are considered to be enlarged, although it is quite possible to have malignant lymph nodes that are smaller than this. Other middle mediastinal masses include vascular lesions as well as duplication cysts of foregut and mesothelial origin.

Detection of mediastinal masses on plain radiographs is dependent upon identification of abnormal mediastinal contour. One of these contours is the right paratracheal stripe, which is normally 4 mm or less in thickness. Thickening or bulging of this border should raise suspicion for an underlying mass or adenopathy. While normally seen only on a minority of chest radiographs, widening or bulging of the left paratracheal stripe is also suspicious for underlying mass or adenopathy. The AP window normally has a concave border with the adjacent lung, and convexity of this border is abnormal and should suggest underlying mass, often adenopathy. It is important to differentiate mediastinal masses from masses arising in the adjacent lung. A smooth interface with obtuse angles at the superior and inferior borders of the mass suggests mediastinal origin. If air bronchograms are seen, this confirms pulmonary origin. Once a mediastinal mass is suspected on x-rays, CT scan should be performed for confirmation. Intravenous contrast is helpful to provide contrast between vascular and nonvascular structures and to determine enhancement characteristics of the lesion. CT can be helpful in differentiating the etiology of middle mediastinal masses in addition to localizing them. For example, duplication cysts will be of roughly water density, while adenopathy will be of a higher soft tissue density. Centrally necrotic, rim-enhancing lymph nodes can also be demonstrated, which may suggest tuberculosis. Vascular lesions such as aneurysms can be easily identified with the administration of intravenous contrast.

Clinical Differential

In this case with low grade fever and night sweats, the clinical differential would include indolent infection, such as TB or atypical pneumonia as well as lymphoma.

Imaging Differential

The differential for mediastinal masses due to adenopathy includes lymphoma, TB, histoplasmosis, sarcoidosis, metastatic disease and Castleman's disease. Other middle mediastinal masses include bronchogenic cysts, tracheal tumors, and aortic aneurysms.

REFERENCES AND SUGGESTED READING

1. Whitten CR, Khan S, Munneke GJ, et al. A diagnostic approach to mediastinal abnormalities. *RadioGraphics*. 2007;27:657-671.

2. Gibbs JM, Chandrasekhar CA, Ferguson EC, et al. Lines and stripes: where did they go? from conventional radiography to CT. *RadioGraphics*. 2007;27:33-48.

CASE 21: POSTERIOR MEDIASTINAL MASS

PATIENT PRESENTATION

A 65-year-old male with history of alcoholism presents with dysphagia.

CLINICAL SUSPICION

Esophageal cancer

IMAGING MODALITY OF CHOICE

Endoscopy. Chest CT with contrast is helpful in staging (Figs. C21.1-C21.3).

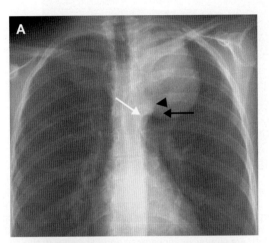

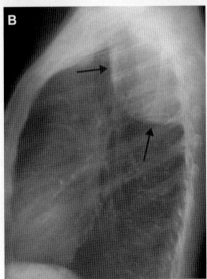

Fig. C21.1 Posterior mediastinal mass. (A) PA chest radiograph demonstrates a smooth bordered opacity projecting over the left apex. The aortic knob is preserved (black arrowhead), indicating that the mass is not likely anterior mediastinal. Pulmonary vessels are visible through the mass (black arrow), suggesting that this is not a primary lung mass. The left paraspinal stripe is border forming (white arrow), suggesting posterior mediastinal location. (B) This is confirmed on the lateral view (black arrows).

FINDINGS

The esophagus resides in the posterior mediastinum. The posterior mediastinum is bordered anteriorly by the posterior wall of the trachea and pericardium, and by the spinal column posteriorly. While CT is the primary modality when assessing posterior mediastinal masses, plain chest radiography is often the presenting study. Detection of posterior mediastinal masses on plain radiographs relies on detection of abnormal mediastinal contours. One of these is the azygoesophageal interface, which is formed by the interface between the right lung and the posterior mediastinum. Another important line is the posterior junction line, which is formed by apposition of the left and right lungs posterior to the esophagus but anterior to the vertebral column in the upper thoracic spine. Obliteration of this line may be a clue to a prevertebral mass. The right and left paraspinal lines are formed by pleural reflections over the vertebral column. Abnormal contour of the paraspinal lines is an indicator of a paraspinal mass, commonly neurogenic tumors or lesions originating from the spine.

The differential diagnosis for posterior mediastinal masses includes neurogenic tumors, foregut duplication cysts and neurenteric cysts, hiatal hernias, and esophageal masses. Neurogenic tumors are the most common cause of a posterior mediastinal mass. Aortic aneurysms are the primary vascular etiology of a posterior mediastinal mass. Paraspinal abscesses (usually associated with vertebral diskitis/osteomyelitis) are the predominant infectious cause, and large paraspinal abscesses may be visible on radiographs as a bulging convexity within one of the paraspinal lines. CT is helpful in confirming the presence of a posterior mediastinal mass that may be suspected on a plain radiograph and identifying its organ of origin. Intravenous contrast can help differentiate enhancing masses from cystic lesions such as foregut duplication cysts, which will not enhance and will appear as smoothly marginated masses of fluid density. Additionally, it may help to identify paraspinal abscesses. However, MR (including gadolinium-enhanced sequences) is usually the study of choice for evaluating vertebral diskitis/osteomyelitis, associated paraspinal abscesses, and neurogenic tumors. This is covered further in the neuroradiology chapter. Although CT is not optimal for evaluation of the esophagus (since the esophagus is not usually distended), esophageal wall thickening can sometimes be appreciated despite this, and the presence of a large mass may also be noted. Additionally, CT is helpful for assessing invasion of other mediastinal structures, loss of paraesophageal fat planes, as well as evaluation of distant metastasis. Hiatal hernias will be demonstrated by herniation of the stomach into the posterior mediastinum. This may be seen on plain radiographs of the chest as well, demonstrated by the presence of a gastric air-fluid level in the mediastinum. Achalasia may also

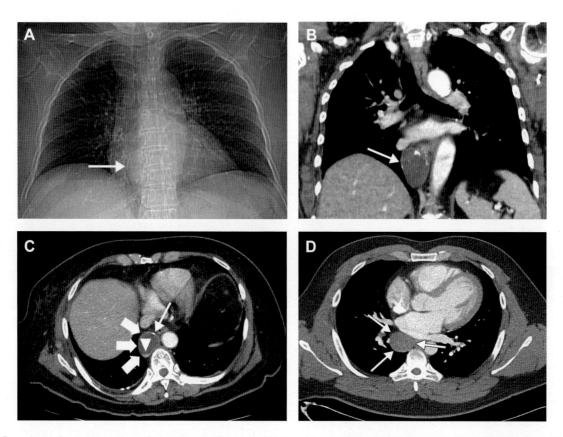

Fig. C21.2 Bronchogenic cyst versus esophageal duplication cyst. (A) Scout image from a CT of the chest demonstrates a smooth bulging of the azygoesophageal recess in the retrocardiac region (white arrow). (B) Coronal chest CT demonstrates a round well-defined fluid attenuation structure in the posterior mediastinum corresponding to the abnormality seen on the scout (white arrow). (C) Axial section demonstrates the posterior mediastinal cystic lesion (thick arrows) with minimal layering debris (arrowhead) and wall calcifications (thin arrow). This could be a bronchogenic cyst or an esophageal duplication cyst as both are similar in appearance and can occur in the posterior mediastinum. (D) Axial section from a chest CT in a different patient demonstrates a smooth well-defined simple appearing fluid attenuation structure in the posterior mediastinum, also consistent with either an esophageal duplication cyst or bronchogenic cyst (white arrows).

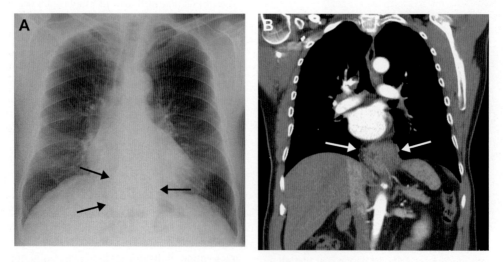

Fig. C21.3 Hiatal hernia. (A) Frontal chest x-ray demonstrates bulging of both paraspinal stripes (black arrows). (B) Coronal reformat from a contrast-enhanced chest CT demonstrates herniation of the stomach into the chest (white arrows), consistent with a hiatal hernia.

present with an air fluid level in the mediastinum, and will be seen at CT as a dilated esophagus with retained food/debris and an air-fluid level in the esophagus as well. An esophagram is the study of choice for evaluating suspected esophageal lesions. Aortic aneurysms will be readily demonstrated by contrast-enhanced CT, typically performed in the arterial phase as a CT angiogram for optimal aortic evaluation and multiplanar evaluation.

Clinical Differential

In an elder male with dysphagia, the differential diagnosis would include a mediastinal mass impinging the esophagus, achalasia, diffuse esophageal spasm, and esophageal cancer. A CNS lesion may also impair the swallowing function.

Imaging Differential

Differential diagnosis for posterior mediastinal masses includes neurogenic tumors, foregut duplication cysts and neurenteric cysts, hiatal hernias, and esophageal masses.

REFERENCES AND SUGGESTED READING

1. Whitten CR, Khan S, Munneke GJ, et al. A diagnostic approach to mediastinal abnormalities. *RadioGraphics*. 2007;27:657-671.
2. Gibbs JM, Chandrasekhar CA, Ferguson EC, et al. Lines and stripes: where did they go? From conventional radiography to CT. *RadioGraphics*. 2007;27:33-48.

CASE 22: THORACIC AORTIC ANEURYSM

PATIENT PRESENTATION

A 70-year-old male with history of smoking, hypercholesterolemia, and hypertension presents with nonspecific chest pain which occasionally radiates to the back.

CLINICAL SUSPICION

Thoracic aortic aneurysm

IMAGING MODALITY OF CHOICE

CT angiogram (Figs. C22.1-C22.4)

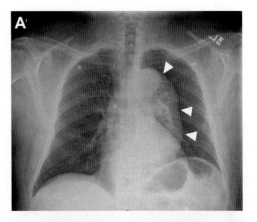

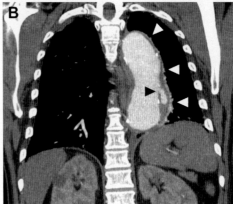

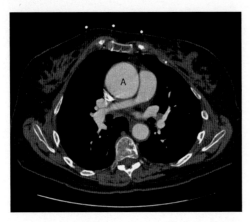

Fig. C22.1 Ascending thoracic aortic aneurysm. Axial CT angiogram of the chest demonstrates an aneurysmally dilated ascending aorta (A).

DISCUSSION

An aneurysm is an abnormal dilation of a blood vessel. The thoracic aorta is normally up to 3 cm in diameter at the mid-ascending aorta up to age 60 and 3.5 cm after age 60. At 4 cm, it is considered aneurysmal. Some authors describe the aorta as "ectatic" between 3 and 4 cm. When the aortic caliber exceeds 5.5 to 6 cm, there is a high risk of rupture, and surgical repair is typically contemplated. Thoracic aortic aneurysms (TAA) can be broadly classified as true aneurysms which contain all 3 layers of the aortic wall, or as false or pseudoaneurysms, which contain less than 3 layers (eg, the blood is contained by only the adventitia). It is not usually possible to differentiate true aneurysms and pseudoaneurysms at imaging, and the terms are often incorrectly used interchangeably. Regardless, most thoracic aneurysms form due to focal weakness in

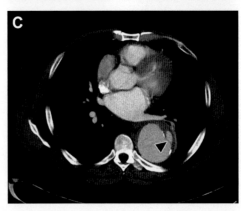

Fig. C22.2 Descending thoracic aortic aneurysm. (A) Frontal chest x-ray demonstrates an abnormally bulging and lobulated contour of the descending aorta (white arrowheads). (B) Coronal reformat from CT angiogram in the same patient demonstrates aneurysmal dilation of the descending aorta (white arrowheads). There is an intramural hematoma in the lateral aortic wall with a focal outpouching of contrast. This is called a penetrating aortic ulcer (black arrowhead). (C) Axial section from CT angiogram also demonstrates the intramural hematoma as a crescentic area of thickening of the aortic wall with luminal displacement of the intimal calcifications. Focal outpouching of contrast (black arrowhead) represents a penetrating aortic ulcer. These may progress to frank dissection and possibly rupture.

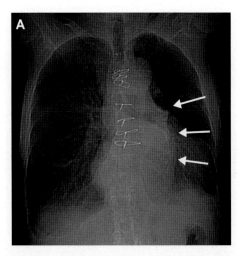
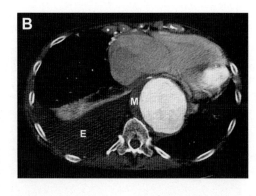

Fig. C22.3 Descending thoracic aortic aneurysm. (A) CT scout image demonstrates a bulging contour of the descending aorta (white arrows). (B) Axial section from CT angiogram demonstrates aneurysmal dilation of the descending aorta with mural thrombus (M). E denotes right pleural effusion.

the aortic wall, which is most often due to either atherosclerosis or cystic medial degeneration. The latter is usually a result of aging and chronic hypertension, although a form of cystic medial necrosis is associated with connective tissue disorders such as Marfan's syndrome. Other etiologies include infection (ie, syphilis, TB, other bacterial infections), congenital weakness, trauma (usually resulting in a pseudoaneurysm), vasculitis, and others. Morphologically, aneurysms can be described as saccular (which appear as a focal outpouching) or fusiform (long segment dilatation). These are purely descriptive terms, and many aneurysms have a more complex morphology that does not neatly fit into either category.

The location of the aneurysm can offer a clue to the etiology. Ascending aortic aneurysms are most commonly due to cystic medial necrosis. Aneurysms of the arch and descending aorta are most commonly atherosclerotic in origin. Posttraumatic aneurysms are typically located near the isthmus (the area on the undersurface of the aortic arch attached to the ligamentum arteriosum), since the aorta is fixed and relatively immobile at this point. Syphilitic aneurysms are more common in the ascending aorta and arch, but may occur anywhere.

At CTA, TAAs are readily identified as focal areas of contrast filled luminal distension or outpouching. The full size and configuration are best evaluated with multiplanar reformatted images, and 3-D reformations are helpful in surgical planning as well. Mural thrombus is readily depicted at CT as areas of irregular typically crescent shaped low attenuation along the wall. Some authors believe that the mural thrombus may act to protect the aneurysm from rupture by decreasing the effective diameter of the lumen. Areas of high attenuation within a mural thrombus, often in

a crescentic shape, are thought to be evidence of impending or high-risk of rupture, possibly due to intravasation of blood into the mural thrombus with resultant instability and loss of the protective function. Surgical consultation should be obtained in this situation. "Draping" of the aorta over the vertebral bodies is also thought to represent an unstable situation at high risk of rupture due to insufficiency of the aortic wall. Ruptured aneurysms are accompanied by the presence of high attenuation blood within the mediastinum, pleural space, or pericardium. Rarely, there may be frank extravasation of intravenous contrast indicative of active hemorrhage, although this situation portends a poor prognosis and these patients do not usually survive long enough to be scanned. Contrast-enhanced or non-contrast-enhanced MRA can also be performed to evaluate the aorta; however, anatomic detail is generally not as good as with CT, and calcifications are not as well demonstrated. Whether CT or MR angiography is performed, the use of ECG-gated technique greatly improves image quality by removing motion artifact due to the beating heart and transmitted aortic pulsations. Transesophageal echocardiography can be performed in certain situations as well, although more invasive and less easily accessible. At plain radiography, abnormal dilation and contour of the aortic shadow is the best clue, although subtler lesions will be missed. Portable chest radiographs may often be the first examination in cases of ruptured aneurysms, and the key finding will be a large mediastinal hematoma. This is discussed further in the section regarding aortic trauma.

Clinical Differential

Many thoracic aortic aneurysms are discovered incidentally during work up of other entities. Those that are symptomatic

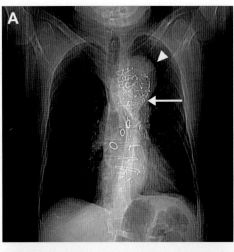

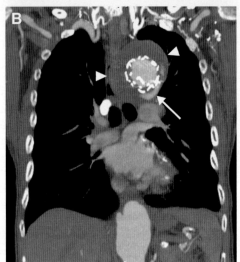

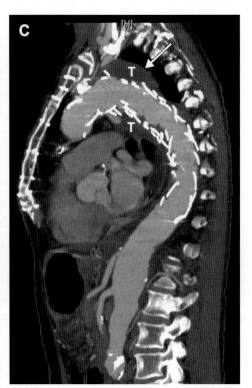

Fig. C22.4 Thoracic aortic aneurysm status post stent-graft repair. (A) Scout image from CT scan demonstrates a bulging aortic knob due to aneurysm involving the aortic arch (arrowhead). The stent-graft is clearly seen (white arrow). (B) Coronal reformat from CT angiogram demonstrates the aneurysm (arrowheads) with a graft and surrounding mural thrombus. Contrast material within the aneurysm sac but outside of the graft (white arrow) indicates endoleak (persistent leakage of blood into the aneurysm sac). There are multiple types of endoleak, and a full discussion is beyond the scope of this text. This was felt to represent a Type II endoleak where the aneurysm sac is fed by collateral vessels, in this case arising from the left subclavian and common carotid arteries (not depicted here). (C) Sagittal reformat also demonstrates the aneurysm and stent-graft with mural thrombus in the aneurysm sac (T). A small amount of extraluminal contrast along the underside of the stent-graft indicates endoleak.

may mimic entities such as myocardial infarction, pulmonary embolism, pneumonia, and even gastroesophageal reflux.

Imaging Differential

When a TAA is encountered at imaging, the main differential consideration is to ascertain whether the aneurysm is due to atherosclerosis or cystic medial degeneration (most common), or something else such as syphilis, mycotic aneurysm, vasculitis, etc. Patients with garden-variety atherosclerotic aneurysms will have evidence of atherosclerotic plaque and calcifications on CT, and will tend to be elderly and have risk factors for atherosclerosis (ie, hypertension, smoking, diabetes, etc). Location can be a clue as well, as discussed above. Inflammatory aneurysms such as those

due to vasculitis or infection may demonstrate nearby fat stranding or thickening of the aortic wall.

REFERENCES AND SUGGESTED READING

1. Schwartz SA, Taljanovic MS, Smyth S, et al. CT findings of rupture, impending rupture, and contained rupture of abdominal aortic aneurysms. *AJR*. 2007;188:W57-W62.

2. Agarwal PP, Chughtai A, Matzinger FRK, et al. Multidetector CT of thoracic aortic aneurysms. *RadioGraphics*. 2009;29:537-552.

3. Atar E, Belenky A, Hadad M, et al. MR angiography for abdominal and thoracic aortic aneurysms: assessment before endovascular repair in patients with impaired renal function. *AJR*. 2006;186:386-393.

CASE 23: ACUTE AORTIC SYNDROME

PATIENT PRESENTATION

A 50-year-old male smoker with uncontrolled hypertension presents with ripping chest pain radiating to the back, of sudden onset.

CLINICAL SUSPICION

Aortic dissection

IMAGING MODALITY OF CHOICE

CT Aortogram. Precontrast and post contrast scans are typically performed, with precontrast scans most helpful in assessing for intramural hematomas (Figs. C23.1-C23.3). ECG gating is optimal to minimize cardiac motion artifact, but availability varies by institution.

DISCUSSION

The aorta is composed of three layers: the innermost intima, the media, and the outermost adventitia. Aortic dissections

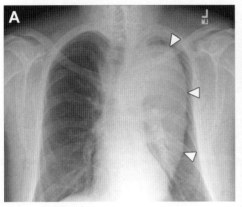
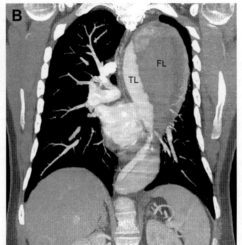
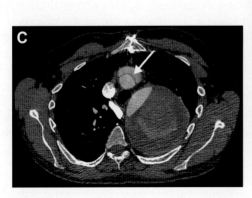
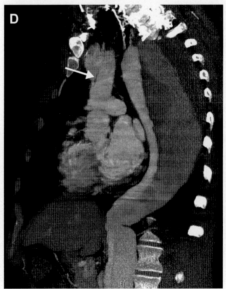

Fig. C23.1 Stanford type A dissection. (A) Frontal chest radiograph demonstrates a grossly enlarged aortic shadow (white arrowheads). (B) Coronal reformation of a CT angiogram demonstrates the aneurysmal aorta, with a dissection as well. The true lumen (TL) and false lumen (FL) are annotated. (C) Axial section from the CT angiogram demonstrates that the dissection flap begins in the ascending aorta, making this a Stanford Type A dissection (white arrow). (D) Sagittal reformation from the same study also demonstrates the dissection beginning in the ascending aorta (white arrow). The dissection flap extends into the abdominal aorta. The patient had Marfan's syndrome.

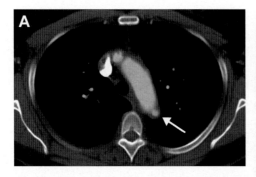

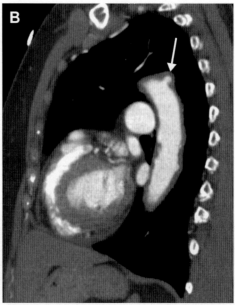

Fig. C23.2 Penetrating aortic ulcer (PAU). (A) Axial contrast-enhanced chest CT demonstrates a small focal outpouching of contrast from the aortic arch (white arrow) consistent with a penetrating aortic ulcer. (B) Sagittal reformation better demonstrates this lesion (white arrow), as well as minimal surrounding intramural hematoma. Also note the diffuse irregularity of the descending aorta due to extensive atherosclerotic plaque. It can sometimes be difficult to differentiate irregularity due to atherosclerosis from a frank PAU. In this case, a PAU was diagnosed as the lesion clearly extends beyond the expected aortic lumen and there is some associated intramural hematoma.

occur when there is a focal tear in the intimal layer (known as an intimal flap or dissection flap), allowing blood to dissect along tissue planes within the media creating a blood filled channel known as a false lumen (as opposed to the true lumen, which is the native lumen). One of several things may then happen to the false lumen: a second intimal tear may be created distally and reenter the true lumen, the false lumen may thrombose (note that the true lumen may thrombose as well), or it may rupture outward (usually at the site of the initial tear). The latter possibility is the most imminently dangerous. Dissections can be broadly classified using the Stanford system, where Type A dissections involve the ascending aorta (and may involve the descending aorta in addition to this) and Type B dissections are limited to the descending aorta only. This is important clinically since dissections of the ascending aorta are typically managed surgically, while dissections of the descending aorta can usually be managed conservatively. Classically, dissection flaps tend to begin along the anterolateral right aspect of the ascending aorta, extend superiorly along the arch, and spiral down to the left posterolateral aspect of the descending aorta. While hypertension is the most common risk factor for aortic dissection in the general population, suspect connective tissue disorders such as Marfan's syndrome in younger patients. On unenhanced CT, the aorta may be entirely normal in appearance, and contrast administration is necessary to assess for and exclude an aortic dissection.

However, if there are atherosclerotic calcifications of the intima involving the dissection flap, these may be seen to be medially displaced, and will appear to be within the lumen of the vessel at noncontrast CT. On contrast-enhanced images, the key finding is direct visualization of the dissection flap. Oblique sagittally reformatted images are extremely helpful in demonstrating involvement of the branch vessels of the aortic arch. It is important to differentiate the true and false lumen of the aorta, with the true lumen being the one that is in continuity with the normal undissected portions of the aorta. Occasionally, curvilinear strands of low attenuation may be seen within the false lumen related to strands of dissected tissue within the media (the "cobweb" sign). The false lumen is also often larger (although this is not always the case) and may be partially or completely thrombosed, in which case the appearance may mimic that of an intramural hematoma (discussed on the next page). The dissection flap may extend into branch vessels, and certain vessels may arise from the false lumen. These findings are important to note for surgical planning. Additional complications which are important to note in the case of Type A dissection include involvement of the coronary arteries or aortic valve and the presence of hemopericardium. On plain radiography, there may be no evidence of dissection, unless the aorta is grossly enlarged and abnormal in contour as a result, and this would merely suggest aneurysm and not necessarily a dissection. Clinical suspicion dictates

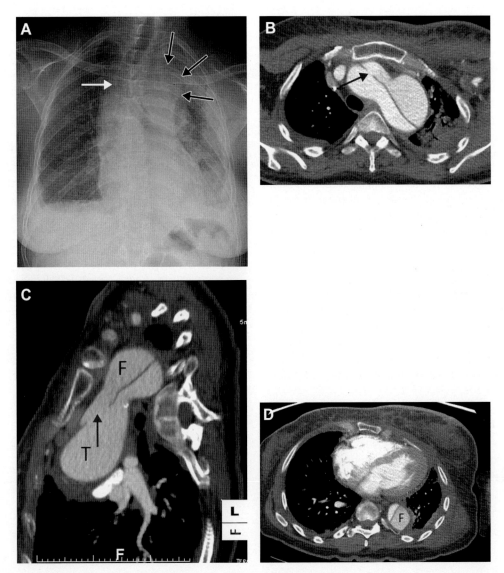

Fig. C23.3 Stanford type A dissection. (A) Frontal chest x-ray demonstrates a grossly enlarged aortic knob (black arrows) with rightward tracheal deviation (white arrow). (B) Axial section from CT angiogram demonstrates a large dissection flap with a focal entry point (black arrow) creating a false lumen where the contrast is slightly less dense (darker) than the true lumen. (C) The dissection flap begins in the ascending aorta, making this a Stanford type A dissection. The entry point is marked (black arrow). T represents the true lumen, and F represents the false lumen. (D) Axial section through the descending aorta. The false lumen is marked F. As in this case, the false lumen is often larger than the true lumen and does not opacify as densely with contrast.

the workup. MR angiography can also be used to assess for aortic dissection, and both contrast-enhanced and noncontrast techniques are possible. Imaging findings are similar to those at CT, although calcifications are not well depicted on MR. Other limitations of MR include higher cost, less availability, and poorer anatomic detail as compared to CT. Also, follow-up imaging after repair is more difficult with MR due to artifacts related to the metallic stents. Traditional catheter based aortography is now used mainly during endovascular repair.

Other acute aortic syndromes include intramural hematoma (IMH), and penetrating atherosclerotic ulcer, which may present with similar clinical symptoms as aortic dissection. Intramural hematoma is caused by spontaneous rupture of vessels within the vasa vasorum of the media with resultant weakening and formation of a hematoma. There is no intimal tear initially, although IMH may progress to frank dissection as well as aneurysm formation. At unenhanced CT, IMH appears as a focal hyperattenuating crescent within the wall of the aorta. After contrast administration, there is no enhancement within the lesion, and it may be difficult to discern the baseline hyperattenuation in relation to the enhancing vessel lumen (which is the primary reason why most CT aortogram protocols include a noncontrast scan through the aorta). Sometimes it may be difficult to differentiate IMH from atherosclerotic plaque or adherent mural thrombus. The high attenuation is key in differentiation, and IMH will also be smooth and crescentic in shape, while atherosclerotic plaque is usually irregular.

Penetrating aortic ulcer (PAU) results from ulceration of an atherosclerotic plaque with dissection of blood through the intima and into the media with creation of a hematoma in the media. This process may be complicated by progression to frank dissection, outward rupture, which may be catastrophic, or by pseudoaneurysm formation. At contrast-enhanced CT, a focal craterlike outpouching may be seen within an atherosclerotic plaque as well as an associated intramural hematoma. It is important to differentiate simple irregular appearing atherosclerotic plaque from a true penetrating aortic ulcer. The presence of an associated mural hematoma is often the key difference. Also, a penetrating aortic ulcer may extend beyond the expected lumen of the aorta.

Clinical Differential

Aortic dissection may mimic entities such as myocardial infarction, pulmonary embolism, pneumonia, and even gastroesophageal reflux.

Imaging Differential

On chest radiographs, aortic dissections are invisible unless there is accompanying dilatation of the aorta. In that case, the differential diagnosis would include a mediastinal mass. The CT appearance of an aortic dissection is essentially pathognomonic.

REFERENCES AND SUGGESTED READING

1. McMahon MA, Squirrell CA. Multidetector CT of aortic dissection: a pictorial review. *RadioGraphics*. 2010;30:445-460.

2. Hayashi H, Matsuoka Y, Sakamoto I, et al. Penetrating atherosclerotic ulcer of the aorta: imaging features and disease concept. *RadioGraphics*. 2000;20:995-1005.

3. Castaner E, Andreu M, Gallardo X, et al. CT in nontraumatic acute thoracic aortic disease: typical and atypical features and complications. *RadioGraphics*. 2003;23:S93-S110.

4. Chao CP, Walker TG, Kalva SP. Natural history and CT appearances of aortic intramural hematoma. *RadioGraphics*. 2009; 29:791-804.

5. Liu Q, Lu JP, Wang F, et al. Three-dimensional contrast-enhanced MR angiography of aortic dissection: a pictorial essay. *RadioGraphics*. 2007;27:1311-1321.

CASE 24: ACUTE TRAUMATIC AORTIC INJURY

PATIENT PRESENTATION

A 35-year-old male status post high speed MVC with multiple broken ribs.

CLINICAL SUSPICION

Traumatic aortic injury

IMAGING MODALITY OF CHOICE

Initial trauma screening is typically performed with plain chest radiograph. CT angiography is the modality of choice to evaluate for traumatic aortic injury (Figs. C24.1-C24.3).

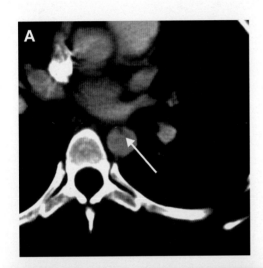

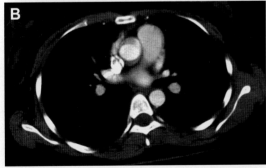

Fig. C24.1 Minimal aortic injury. (A) Axial chest CT from a patient involved in a high speed motor vehicle collision. Note the small intimal flap in the descending aorta (white arrow). There is no stenosis or pseudoaneurysm formation. No mediastinal hematoma was present, and there would be no clue to an injury of this nature on a chest x-ray. This was managed medically. (B) Repeat examination 5 days later demonstrated resolution of the injury.

DISCUSSION

Aortic injuries are typically the result of blunt trauma, especially abrupt deceleration which results in shearing injury. Both head on and side impact motor vehicle collisions are a leading cause. They can be broadly classified as acute traumatic aortic rupture (ATAR), and acute traumatic aortic injury (ATAI). ATAR implies a full thickness tear, which is usually fatal, and these patients rarely make it to the hospital. ATAI implies only partial disruption, which is far more commonly seen, as it is survivable. The thoracic aorta is fixed in place proximally at the ligamentum arteriosum (just distal to the origin of the left subclavian artery) and distally at the diaphragmatic hiatus. The descending aorta is somewhat mobile in between these points. The most common site of injury is in the vicinity of the fixed points, mostly near the ligamentum arteriosum.

The supine chest radiograph is typically the first imaging study obtained in patients suffering major blunt trauma to the chest. While ATAI cannot be directly identified on a chest radiograph, the presence of a mediastinal hematoma can be assessed as indirect evidence of vascular injury. Detection of a mediastinal hematoma on the plain chest radiograph depends on identification of abnormal mediastinal contours. Obscuration of the aortic knob and abnormal convexity in the aortopulmonary window are two important signs. Abnormal thickening of the right paratracheal stripe greater than 5 mm is suspicious. The left paraspinal stripe typically disappears by the level of T4 or T5 superiorly; if it is visible beyond the aortic arch it is suggestive of a mediastinal hematoma. If it continues to extend upward, it may form a left apical pleural cap, suggestive of a massive mediastinal hematoma extending into the left pleural space. Evidence of mass effect such as depression of the left main bronchus, tracheal deviation, and esophageal deviation (typically demonstrated by deviation of an NG tube) should also raise suspicion for mediastinal hematoma in the setting of trauma. It is important to note that the presence of a mediastinal hematoma is rarely due to hemorrhage from the aorta itself, as these patients typically expire in the field. Rather, it is due to hemorrhage from smaller mediastinal vessels including the azygos and hemiazygos systems, spinal and intercostal vessels, and internal mammaries among others. If any of these abnormalities is detected and there is suspicion for mediastinal hematoma, CT angiography should be performed. If there is no evidence of mediastinal hematoma on a good quality radiograph, the probability of a significant aortic injury is significantly reduced. However, CT angiography remains the diagnostic modality of choice for excluding ATAI, and should be performed if suspicion remains for aortic injury.

CT angiography can directly depict ATAI, and has replaced catheter angiography at most institutions for diagnostic purposes. If available, the use of ECG gated techniques greatly improves image quality by removing motion artifact

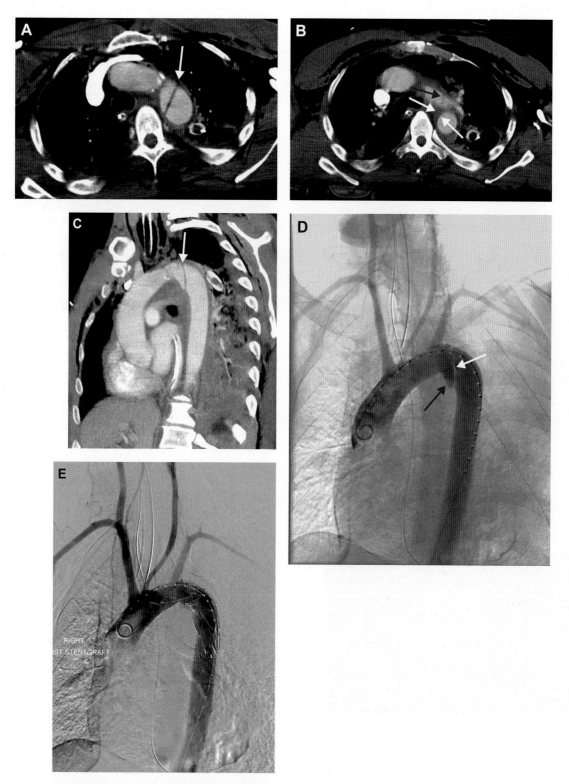

Fig. C24.2 Traumatic aortic dissection and pseudoaneurysm. The patient had suffered a fall of approximately 25 to 40 feet. (A) Initial axial chest CT with contrast demonstrates a dissection flap in the descending aorta (white arrow). A chest tube is present at the left lung apex. (B) Axial section more inferiorly demonstrates a small periaortic hematoma (white arrows). Also, there is an intimal tear in the left pulmonary artery (black arrow). Extensive chest wall emphysema is present in both (A) and (C). Sagittal reformat better demonstrates the dissection flap distal to the origin of the left subclavian artery, in the descending aorta (white arrow). This is the most common site of traumatic aortic injury. Minimal pseudoaneurysm formation is also evident along the undersurface of the aortic arch. (D) Catheter angiogram demonstrates the dissection flap as a linear filling defect (white arrow). The pseudoaneurysm is more evident (black arrow). (E) A stent-graft was placed endovascularly to treat the dissection and pseudoaneurysm, which are no longer visible. The pulmonary artery injury was managed conservatively.

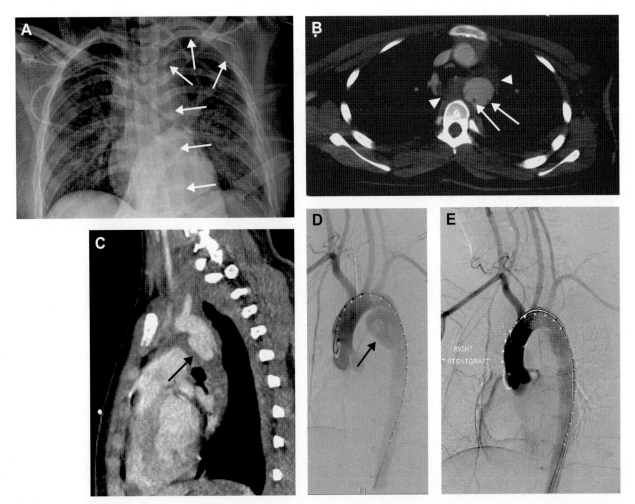

Fig. C24.3 Traumatic pseudoaneurysm of the aorta. (A) Frontal chest x-ray demonstrates medial displacement of the left paraspinal stripe extending superiorly and forming an apical pleural cap (white arrows). The aortic knob is obscured. These findings are suspicious for a mediastinal hematoma in the setting of trauma. (B) Axial chest CT demonstrates multiple intimal tears with aneurysmal dilation of the aorta (white arrows) as well as the mediastinal hematoma (white arrowheads). (C) Sagittal oblique reformat demonstrates the pseudoaneurysm distal to the origin of the left subclavian artery along the undersurface of the aorta, a common site of aortic injury (black arrow). (D) Catheter angiogram redemonstrates the pseudoaneurysm (black arrow). (E) Post stent-graft angiogram no longer demonstrates filling of the aneurysm sac.

due to the beating heart. Direct signs include the presence of an intimal flap, pseudoaneurysm formation, contour abnormality, sudden change in caliber of the vessel, and active contrast extravasation (although this is rare from the aorta, as the patient would typically expire in the field). Mediastinal hematomas are easily demonstrated at CT as well, manifest by soft tissue or higher density infiltrating mediastinal fat planes. If a fat plane is maintained between the hematoma and the aorta, it can be surmised that the hematoma arose due to rupture of smaller mediastinal vessels. However, if there is no clear fat plane between the aorta and the hematoma, it is called a periaortic hematoma and close attention

should be paid for direct signs of aortic injury. In the presence of a periaortic hematoma without direct signs of aortic injury, many authors recommend short-term follow-up CT to assess for evolution of the injury. Intravascular ultrasound (IVUS) and TEE may play a role as well, depending upon the institution. Minimal aortic injuries are those that only affect the intimal layer. With the widespread use of CT angiography, they are being detected with increased frequency. The natural history and management have not been well studied, and currently most authors recommend short-term CT follow-up, at which point most appear to either remain stable or resolve, based on current experience.

Differential Diagnosis

Supine positioning and AP technique may cause apparent widening of the upper mediastinum, making mediastinal hematoma difficult to evaluate. At CT, normal thymic tissue in a young patient may mimic mediastinal hematoma. Additionally, cardiac motion artifact may lead to false positive diagnosis of aortic injury involving the aortic root. Knowledge of these pitfalls will aid in their avoidance. Otherwise, the findings of aortic injury at CT are fairly pathognomonic.

REFERENCES AND SUGGESTED READING

1. Steenburg SD, Ravenel JG, Ikonomidis JS, et al. Acute traumatic aortic injury: imaging evaluation and management. *Radiology.* 2008;248:748-762.

2. Steenburg SD, Ravenel JG. Acute traumatic thoracic aortic injuries: experience with 64-MDCT. *ARJ.* 2008;191:1564-1569.

3. Fishman JE, Nunez D Jr, Kane A, et al. Direct versus indirect signs of traumatic aortic injury revealed by helical CT: performance characteristics and interobserver agreement. *AJR.* 1999;172:1027-1031.

4. Sefczek DM, Sefczek RJ, Deeb ZL. Radiographic signs of acute traumatic rupture of the thoracic aorta. *AJR.* 1983;141:1259-1262.

CASE 25: CORONARY ARTERY DISEASE

PATIENT PRESENTATION

A 55-year-old male presents with atypical chest pain, which is not definitively related to exercise.

CLINICAL SUSPICION

After risk factor analysis, there is an intermediate pretest probability for coronary artery disease (CAD).

IMAGING MODALITY OF CHOICE

Coronary CT angiography (Figs. C25.1-C25.8)

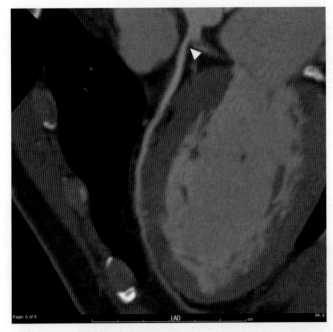

Fig. C25.1 Mild stenosis of the proximal LAD. Sagittal oblique reformatted image from a coronary CT angiogram (CCTA) demonstrates a mild short segment stenosis of the proximal LAD (arrowhead) secondary to noncalcified "soft" plaque.

DISCUSSION

Coronary artery disease is highly prevalent, and its risk factors, etiology, and outcomes have been widely described elsewhere. Here we will focus on nuclear myocardial perfusion imaging (MPI), coronary CT angiography (CCTA), and MRI in the evaluation of CAD. MPI has been a mainstay in the diagnosis of coronary artery disease for a number of years, and relies on the use of radioisotopes (typically thallium-201 or technetium-99m based agents). Images are obtained with a gamma camera both at rest, and after either pharmacologic or exercise induced stress. Stress and rest images are then compared side by side in standardized short axis, horizontal long axis, and vertical long axis orientations. A normal scan demonstrates homogenous myocardial radiotracer uptake on both rest and stress images. Areas that demonstrate decreased uptake on stress images compared to rest images correlate with areas of ischemia, and are described as reversible defects which can benefit from revascularization. Areas that demonstrate decreased or no uptake on both rest and stress images correspond to areas of either infarcted or severely ischemic "hibernating" myocardium. These entities can be differentiated with cardiac PET imaging, with infarcted areas demonstrating no FDG uptake, while hibernating myocardium will demonstrate FDG uptake. Differentiating infarcted from hibernating myocardium is important for treatment planning, as hibernating myocardium may benefit from revascularization, while infarcted myocardium will not. Limitations of MPI include false positives due to attenuation of emitted photons from breast tissue and subdiaphragmatic structures, which may appear as fixed defects. Repeat imaging in the prone position can eliminate these artifacts if the patient can tolerate. Newer attenuation correction techniques and SPECT-CT can also be employed to reduce these artifacts. Also, ECG gated acquisitions can be performed which allow analysis of wall motion. Fixed defects that demonstrate normal wall motion are unlikely to be infarcted, and can then be attributed to attenuation artifact.

Coronary CT angiography has progressed rapidly with the development of CT scanners with increasing numbers of detector rows and faster gantry rotation times. It has become a widely accepted tool in assessing coronary artery anatomy, plaque burden, and evaluation of coronary artery stenosis as well as in the overall assessment of cardiac structure and function. Scanners with 64 or more detector rows are optimal for cardiac imaging due to the increased temporal resolution and resultant image quality. Cardiac CT is performed using a small field of view to increase the spatial resolution, typically on the order of 0.5 mm. By comparison, the resolution of traditional catheter based angiography is on the order of 0.1 mm. Patient preparation involves administration of beta blockers or calcium channel blockers if necessary to bring the heart rate to an acceptable range (optimally <65). Patients with nonsinus rhythms such as atrial fibrillation are not usually considered candidates for CT angiography. Vasodilation is typically achieved just prior to scanning by administration of sublingual nitroglycerine. ECG gating is required, so that coronary artery images may be reconstructed only from time points where there is little to no cardiac motion

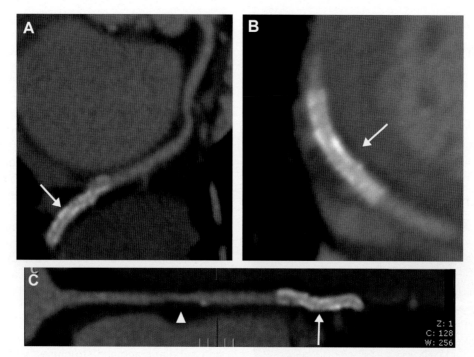

Fig. C25.2 Patent left circumflex artery (Lcx) stent and proximal stenosis. (A, B) Oblique reformatted CCTA images demonstrate a patent stent in the mid portion of the Lcx (white arrow). (C) Curved reformat demonstrates the stent (arrow) as well as a short segment of mild stenosis in the proximal Lcx (arrowhead).

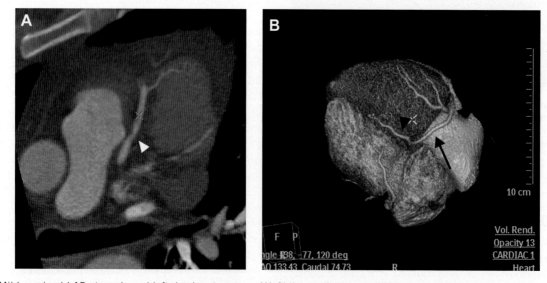

Fig. C25.3 Mild proximal LAD stenosis and left dominant system. (A) Oblique reformatted CCTA image demonstrates a mild proximal LAD stenosis (white arrowhead). (B) Volume rendered image from the same patient demonstrates that the PDA (posterior descending artery, black arrowhead) arises from the left circumflex (black arrow), making this a left dominant system. Dominance is determined by whether the PDA arises from the RCA (most common) versus the left circumflex.

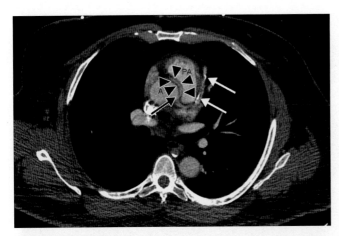

Fig. C25.4 Anomalous origin of the RCA, malignant course. Axial section from a routine chest CT performed for other indications demonstrates anomalous origin of the RCA from the left coronary cusp (black arrow), then passing between the aorta and pulmonary artery (black arrowheads). This is known as the malignant course, and is associated with arrhythmias and sudden cardiac death. There is also a benign course, where the RCA courses posterior to the aortic root rather than anteriorly. Calcified plaque in the LAD is also present (white arrows).

(typically mid to late diastole). Retrospective ECG gating is more common, and involves scanning throughout the cardiac cycle and then retrospectively selecting data from the desired cardiac phase only. Retrospective gating also enables evaluation of cardiac function, as the heart is imaged throughout the cardiac cycle. Prospective ECG gating is a newer development, and reduces radiation dose by scanning only during the desired phase. Regardless of which method is used, an initial noncontrast scan is typically performed for the purpose of calcium scoring. Once the scan is obtained, post processing is performed on a dedicated workstation using various software packages in order to produce curved multiplanar reformatted images and quantify stenotic lesions and calcium burden.

Coronary artery calcification is a marker of underlying atherosclerosis. Quantification and scoring are typically performed based on the Agatston system. Using this system, a calcification is defined as an area of greater than 1 mm^2 (3 consecutive pixels) with an attenuation of greater

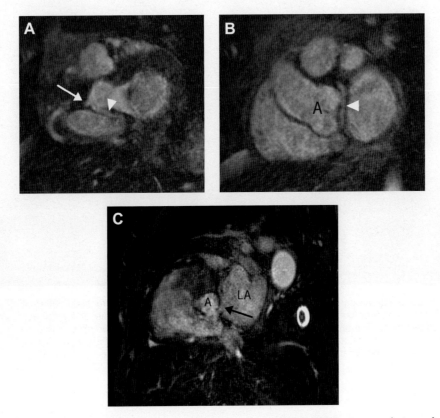

Fig. C25.5 Right-sided origin of the left main coronary artery, retroaortic course. (A) 3-D BTFE sequence (a type of gradient echo or bright blood sequence) demonstrates anomalous origin of the left main coronary artery (white arrowhead) from the right coronary cusp. The RCA origin is denoted by the white arrow. (B) Different section demonstrates aberrant course of the left main coronary artery inferior to the aortic root (white arrowhead). (C) Oblique axial orientation demonstrates retroaortic course (black arrow), between the aorta (A) and left atrium (LA). This variant is typically considered benign, although there are case reports of it being symptomatic.

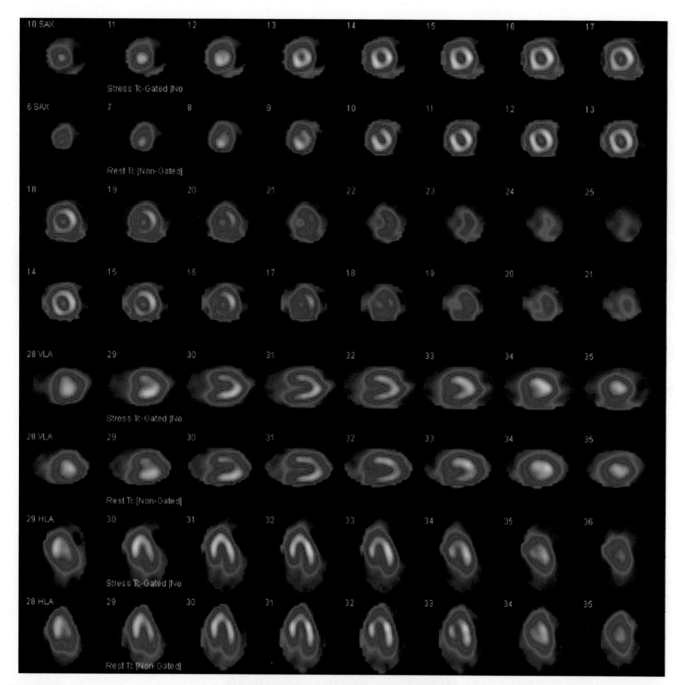

Fig. C25.6 Normal Tc-99m sestamibi myocardial perfusion scan. Stress and rest images are arranged in alternating rows (the top row consists of stress images, the second row consists of resting images, etc). The images are aligned such that each resting image is directly below its corresponding stress image. The top four rows consist of short axis slices, the next two rows consist of vertical long axis slices, and the bottom two rows are the horizontal long axis orientation. These are the standard orientations for viewing MPI images. Note the homogeneous tracer uptake throughout the myocardium, with no mismatches between the stress and rest images.

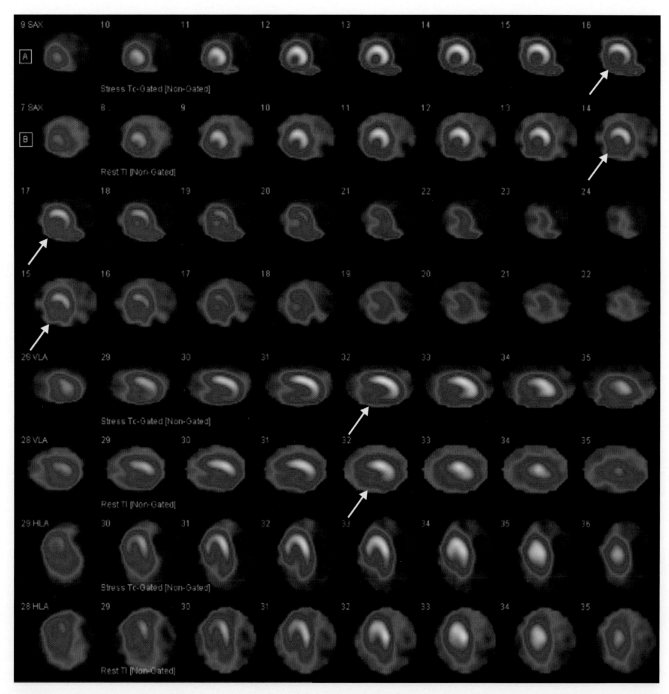

Fig. C25.7 Tc-99m myocardial perfusion scan with fixed inferior wall defect. Both stress and rest images demonstrate an area of decreased tracer uptake in the inferior wall best demonstrated on short axis and vertical long axis views (white arrows). These findings suggest either a fixed infarct or hibernating myocardium. The patient had ECG findings suggestive of an old inferior infarct.

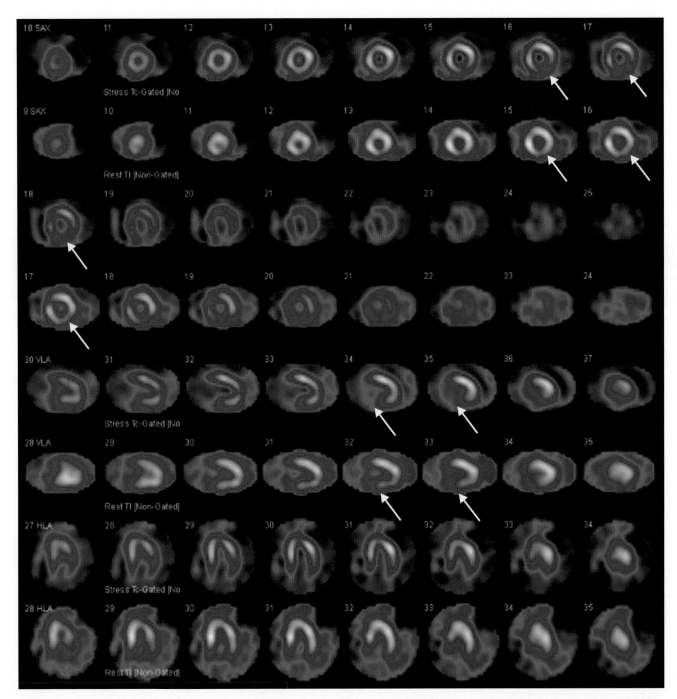

Fig. C25.8 Tc-99m myocardial perfusion scan with reversible inferior wall defect. Stress images demonstrate an inferior wall defect that demonstrates tracer uptake on rest images (white arrows). This is consistent with inferior wall ischemia, in the right coronary artery (RCA) territory. Subsequent cardiac angiography demonstrated a 100% occlusion of the RCA, with collateral supply via septal branches of the left anterior descending artery (LAD).

Table C25.1 Agatston Weighting Factors

Attenuation	Weighting Factor
130-199 HU	1 point
200-299 HU	2 points
300-399 HU	3 points
400+ HU	4 points

than 130 HU. Each calcification is assigned a weighting factor based on the attenuation as in Table C25.1.

The weighting factor is then multiplied by the area of the calcification to arrive at a score for that individual calcification. The scores for each calcification are summed to arrive at a total Agatston score, which are often stratified into 4 groups as in Table C25.2.

The absence of coronary artery calcium argues strongly against coronary artery disease, although a noncalcified or "soft" plaque may still exist. There is also some evidence that the calcium score can be followed to document progression or even regression of disease.

Analysis of the coronary arteries themselves should begin by evaluation of coronary artery anatomy, noting any anatomic variants or congenital anomalies (such as an aberrant origin of the right coronary artery). Coronary artery aneurysms should also be documented if present. Areas of stenosis are then typically reported for each coronary artery segment (based on the American Heart Association scheme) as follows: normal segment, nonobstructive disease (1%-49% stenosis), significant stenosis (50%-74% stenosis), high grade stenosis (75%-99%), and total occlusion. Using 64-detector row systems, a recent meta-analysis estimated 99% sensitivity and 89% specificity for CCTA in detection of CAD on a per-patient basis. On a per-segment basis, the sensitivity was 90%, and specificity was 97%. However, positive predictive value remained low, with a median of 76% across the included studies, indicating a fair amount of false positive studies [5]. Some of this can likely be attributed to the overestimation of the degree of stenosis on CCTA compared to catheter angiography, especially with calcified plaques. This is due to blooming artifact which makes calcifications appear larger than they actually are. One recently introduced technique to reduce this arti-

Table C25.2 Risk Stratification Based on Agatston Score

Agatston Score	Risk Group
<10	Minimal disease
11-100	Mild disease
101-400	Moderate disease
>400	Severe disease

factual effect is the use of iterative reconstruction methods as opposed to the traditional filtered back projection method when reconstructing CT data [7]. Plaque composition (calcified vs noncalcified) is also of significance, and can be reliably determined with CT, an advantage over catheter angiography.

The primary indication for CCTA is to diagnose CAD in patients with a low to intermediate pretest probability, especially in those patients for whom cardiac catheterization would otherwise have been considered. High-risk patients are typically referred straight to catheter angiography by current guidelines. It is also indicated for work up of potential coronary artery anomalies (whether congenital or acquired), congenital heart disease (although echocardiography and cardiac MRI remain the mainstays in this arena), evaluation of cardiac masses, and preoperative assessment of coronary arteries prior to cardiovascular surgery. There is also mounting evidence that CCTA may be helpful to exclude CAD in patients presenting to the emergency department with chest pain who are at low to intermediate risk of acute coronary syndrome, although this requires further study and is not yet widely practiced.

Recently, MRI has emerged as another modality for the evaluation of ischemic heart disease. CMR provides a wide array of sequences for determination and characterization of ischemic insults as a cause for heart disease. Inversion recovery spin echo ("black blood") images suppress signal from blood and produce excellent anatomic detail. Gradient recalled ("bright blood") images, including steady-state free-precession sequences, provide rapid acquisitions that can assess heart motion and function, as well as anatomy. Gadolinium-enhanced perfusion (first pass) images reveal areas of hypoperfusion, which may be seen with ischemia and infarction. Acute and chronically infarcted myocardium will demonstrate delayed hyperenhancement (DHE) after a 10- to 30-minute delay. Conversely, abnormal but viable myocardium that is amenable to revascularization may show abnormal wall motion or immediate hypoperfusion without corresponding DHE. Another way to assess for abnormal, but viable myocardium is to perform rest and stress images pharmacologically in the same way as for MPI. For infarcted myocardium with DHE, the use of fluid sensitive inversion sequences ("edema-weighted images") can help in distinguishing acute infarcts, which should show high signal associated with edema, from chronic ones, which do not. Evaluation of the coronary arteries is also possible with MR, but less commonly used in the setting of ischemic heart disease.

Clinical Differential

The clinical differential for CAD includes many causes of chest pain, including gastroesophageal reflux, pneumonia, pulmonary embolism, and costochondritis.

Imaging Differential

Imaging findings of CAD are characteristic; there is no real differential diagnosis.

REFERENCES AND SUGGESTED READING

1. Jadvar H, Strauss HW, Segall GM. SPECT and PET in the evaluation of coronary artery disease. *RadioGraphics*. 1999;19:915-926.

2. Dvorak RA, Brown RKJ, Corbett JR. Interpretation of SPECT/CT myocardial perfusion images: common artifacts and quality control techniques. *RadioGraphics*. 2011;31:2041-2057.

3. Agatston AS, Janowitz WR, Hildner FJ, et al. Quantification of coronary artery calcium using ultrafast computed tomography. *J Am CollCardiol*. 1990;15:827-832.

4. Chow CK, Sheth T. What is the role of invasive versus non-invasive coronary angiography in the investigation of patients suspected to have coronary artery disease? *Intern Med J*. 2011;41:5-13.

5. Mowatt G, Cook JA, Hillis GS, et al. Sixty-four-slice computed tomography angiography in the diagnosis and assessment of coronary artery disease: systematic review and meta-analysis. *Heart*. 2008;94:1386-1393.

6. Taylor AJ, Cerqueira M, Hodgson JM, et al. ACCF/SCCT/ACR/AHA/ASE/ASNC/NASCI/SCAI/SCMR 2010 appropriate use criteria for cardiac computed tomography. A report of the American College of Cardiology Foundation Appropriate Use Criteria Task Force, the Society of Cardiovascular Computed Tomography, the American College of Radiology, the American Heart Association, the American Society of Echocardiography, the American Society of Nuclear Cardiology, the North American Society for Cardiovascular Imaging, the Society for Cardiovascular Angiography and Interventions, and the Society for Cardiovascular Magnetic Resonance. *J Am Coll Cardiol*. 2010;56:1864-1894.

7. Renker M, Nance JW, Schoepf UJ, et al. Evaluation of heavily calcified vessels with coronary CT angiography: comparison of iterative and filtered back projection image reconstruction. *Radiology*. 2011;260:390-399.

8. Cury RC, Feuchtner G, Mascioli C, et al. Cardiac CT in the emergency department: convincing evidence, but cautious implementation. *J Nucl Cardiol*. 2011;18:331-341.

9. Tamarappoo B, Hachamovitch R. Myocardial perfusion imaging versus CT coronary angiography: when to use which? *J Nucl Med*. 2011;52:1079-1086.

CASE 26: VALVULAR HEART DISEASE

PATIENT PRESENTATION

A 78-year-old male with worsening dyspnea on exertion.

CLINICAL SUSPICION

Aortic stenosis

IMAGING MODALITY OF CHOICE

Echocardiography is the most mainstream modality for evaluation of cardiac valvular disease. However, CT and MR can also effectively image the cardiac valves and are complementary modalities (Figs. C26.1-C26.4).

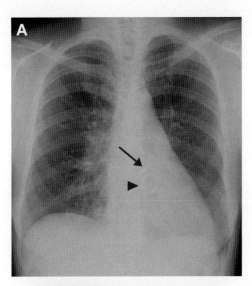

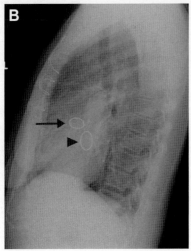

Fig. C26.1 Aortic and mitral valve replacements. (A) Frontal and (B) lateral chest x-rays demonstrate aortic (black arrow) and mitral (black arrowhead) valve replacements. The patient has had a median sternotomy, and the heart is enlarged as well.

DISCUSSION

Echocardiography has long been the traditional imaging modality for imaging the cardiac valves. In the past decade, CT and MRI have become viable alternatives and/or complementary modalities. With the increasing use of CT to assess the coronary arteries, it is not uncommon for it to be the first imaging modality performed, which may yield important information regarding valvular morphology and function. Plain radiographs may offer gross information regarding cardiac chamber enlargement, which can be an indirect sign of valvular disease, although nonspecific.

The interface between the right atrium and the right middle lobe is visible on the frontal chest radiograph. Abnormal bulging of this border can suggest right atrial enlargement, which may be an indicator of tricuspid valve disease among other things. Right atrial enlargement may not be detected on plain radiographs until it is severe. The right ventricle is border forming anteriorly on the lateral view, where right ventricular enlargement may manifest as a bulging anterior cardiac border and filling of the retrosternal clear space. On the frontal view, the cardiac apex may appear to be superiorly displaced, creating a "boot" shaped configuration. Left atrial enlargement can be appreciated on the frontal view of the chest when its right lateral border becomes visible through the right heart border, termed the double density sign. In extreme cases, it may extend beyond the right atrial border and become the border forming structure on the right. Other signs on the frontal view include splaying apart of the carinal angle and superior displacement of the left main bronchus. On the lateral view, the left atrium is border forming postero-superiorly, and there may be posterior bulging of this border. There may also be posterior displacement of the left main bronchus or of the esophagus (which can be seen on a barium esophagram, or inferred by posterior displacement of a nasogastric tube). Left atrial enlargement is often due to mitral valve stenosis or regurgitation. The left ventricle is border forming on the left on a frontal view, and postero-inferiorly on the lateral view. Left ventricular enlargement causes bulging of this border, and rounding of the cardiac apex on frontal view. On the lateral view, the posterior cardiac border will displaced posteriorly, and in advanced cases may overlap the spine. Aortic valve disease can lead to left ventricular hypertrophy and eventual dilatation.

Using retrospectively ECG gated CT angiography of the heart (typically performed for coronary artery evaluation), it is possible to generate cine sequences of the cardiac valves to assess valvular morphology and motion. The primary drawback is the increased radiation dose required for retrospectively gated studies. Thickening or calcification of valvular cusps can be seen, and measurements of the valvular orifice can be obtained. Based on these measurements, the degree of stenosis or regurgitation can be

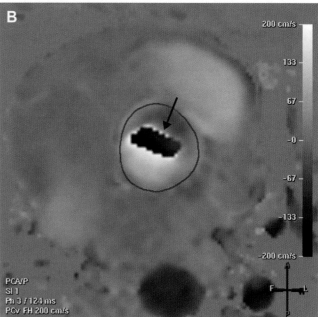

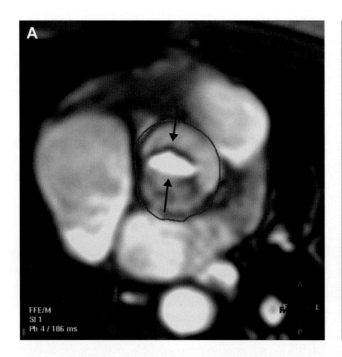

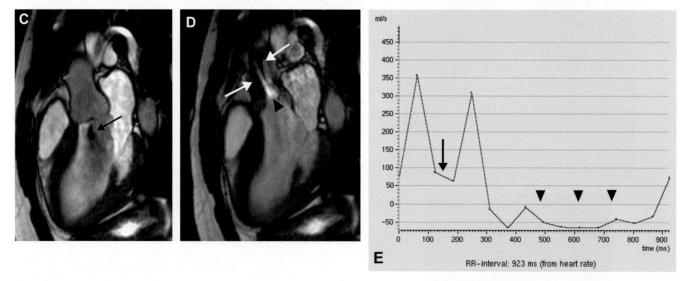

Fig. C26.2 Bicuspid aortic valve with stenosis and regurgitation. (A) Single axial frame from a GRE cine sequence demonstrates a bicuspid aortic valve during systole. The valvular orifice (black arrows) is significantly narrowed. (B) Axial image from phase contrast cine sequence demonstrates high velocity flow across the valvular orifice (bright, high-signal area) with a small area of aliasing (black area annotated with black arrow) where the velocity has gone beyond the preset threshold (in this case 200 cm/s). This is indicative of stenosis. (C) Sagittal oblique GRE cine frame aligned with the left ventricular outflow tract (LVOT) demonstrates a dephasing jet of low signal (black arrow) indicating aortic regurgitation. (D) Different frame from the same sequence now demonstrates a high velocity turbulent jet due to aortic stenosis, with central high-signal laminar flow (black arrowhead) and surrounding turbulent flow at the periphery of the jet manifest by low-signal areas of dephasing (white arrows). (E) Flow quantification curve generated by a software package on the workstation demonstrates artifactually decreased flow during systole due to aliasing (black arrow). Regurgitation is manifest by reversed flow across the valve (black arrowheads). Regurgitant fraction is calculated by the workstation based on the area under the curve.

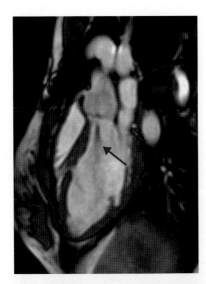

Fig. C26.3 Aortic regurgitation. Sagittal oblique GRE sequence through the LVOT demonstrates an aortic regurgitant jet (black arrow).

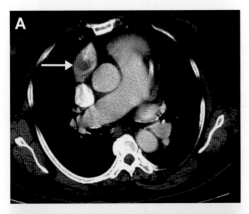

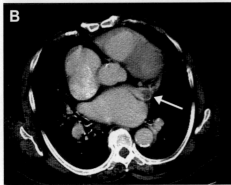

Fig. C26.4 Right and left atrial appendage thrombi. (A) Axial section from a contrast-enhanced CT of the chest. There is a filling defect in the right atrial appendage (white arrow) consistent with thrombus. (B) A similar finding is present in the left atrial appendage as well (white arrow).

inferred. Malcoaptation or fusion of valve leaflets can also be appreciated. Secondary effects including ventricular hypertrophy and chamber dilation can be easily assessed, as well as post stenotic dilation of the aortic root or pulmonary trunk. Large vegetations, valvular tumors, and perivalvular abscesses can also be seen on CT, and it can be useful in evaluation of complications of valvular prostheses including frozen leaflets, vegetations, adherent thrombus, and valvular dehiscence.

During a cardiac MRI exam, cardiac chamber and valvular morphology are usually assessed using a spin echo, "black blood" sequence. Steady-state free precession (SSFP), "bright blood" sequences are used for obtaining cine sequences due to their high temporal resolution so that valvular motion can be observed, and regurgitant jets or areas of turbulence can be qualitatively assessed. Phase contrast imaging provides velocity information that can be used to quantify flow across valvular orifices. Compared to CT, the benefits of MRI are lack of ionizing radiation, no need for intravenous contrast administration, improved temporal resolution of SSFP sequences, and ability to obtain flow velocity information. CT is better for demonstrating valvular calcifications and somewhat better for visualizing valvular anatomy/morphology. Both of these modalities offer benefits over transesophageal echocardiography in terms of better reproducibility, decreased operator dependence, lack of limitations due to acoustic windows, and noninvasiveness as compared to TEE.

DIFFERENTIAL DIAGNOSIS
Clinical Differential
Congestive heart failure, pneumonia, COPD

Imaging Differential
None

REFERENCES AND SUGGESTED READING
1. Vogel-Claussen J, Pannu H, Spevak PJ, et al. Cardiac valve assessment with MR imaging and 64-section multi-detector row CT. *RadioGraphics*. 2006;26:1769-1784.
2. Chen JJ, Manning MA, Frazier AA, et al. CT Angiography of the cardiac valves: normal, diseased, and postoperative appearances. *RadioGraphics*. 2009;29:1393-1412.
3. Ryan R, Abbara S, Colen RR, et al. Cardiac valve disease: spectrum of findings on cardiac 64-MDCT. *AJR*. 2008;190:W294-W303.
4. Morris MF, Maleszewski JJ, Suri RM, et al. CT and MR imaging of the mitral valve: radiologic-pathologic correlation. *RadioGraphics*. 2010;30:1603-1620.

CASE 27: CARDIOMYOPATHY

PATIENT PRESENTATION

A 35-year-old female with palpitations who is found to have episodes of nonsustained ventricular tachycardia on Holter monitoring.

CLINICAL SUSPICION

Arrhythmogenic right ventricular dysplasia/cardiomyopathy (ARVD/ARVC)

IMAGING MODALITY OF CHOICE

Cardiac MRI (Figs. C27.1-C27.9)

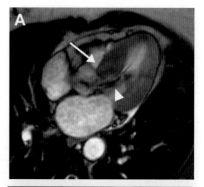

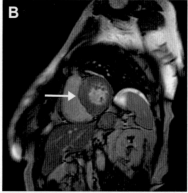

Fig. C27.2 Hypertrophic cardiomyopathy. Axial (A) and short axis (B) gradient echo sequences demonstrate asymmetric thickening of the septum (white arrow) resulting in subvalvular aortic stenosis, with a low-signal turbulent stenotic jet (white arrowhead).

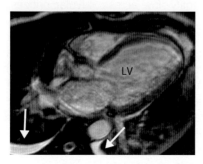

Fig. C27.1 Dilated cardiomyopathy. Horizontal long axis gradient echo sequence demonstrates a dilated left ventricle (LV). This was ischemic in nature as the patient had severe three-vessel coronary artery disease. Also note bilateral pleural effusions (white arrows).

DISCUSSION

Cardiomyopathies are a heterogeneous group of disorders that result in chronic progressive myocardial disease and associated mechanical and/or conductive dysfunction. Cardiac MRI has emerged as an important tool for imaging the myocardium in the evaluation of cardiomyopathies. Cardiomyopathies can be classified morphologically and physiologically as dilated, restrictive, or hypertrophic. ARVC is often discussed as a separate entity, as it does not neatly fit into the above categories. Dilated cardiomyopathy (DCM) can be further classified broadly as ischemic or nonischemic, with the latter being a wastebasket term

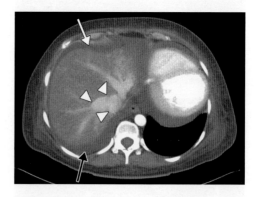

Fig. C27.3 Right heart failure. Axial contrast-enhanced CT through the lung bases/upper abdomen demonstrates opacification of the IVC and hepatic veins (white arrowheads). However, this is an arterial phase study, and contrast has not yet reached the venous system. The IVC and hepatic veins opacified due to contrast refluxing from the right atrium secondary to right heart failure and elevated right heart pressure. Also note the ascites (white arrow) and right pleural effusion (black arrow).

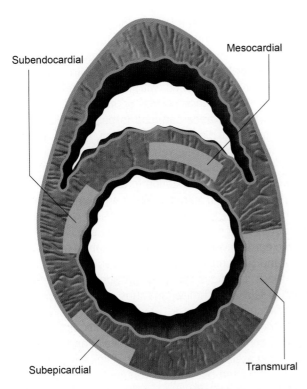

Fig. C27.4 Patterns of myocardial enhancement at cardiac MRI.

encompassing numerous possible etiologies with a similar end result.

Dilated cardiomyopathy is characterized by an enlarged left ventricle, although advanced cases often demonstrate biventricular enlargement. The left ventricular wall may be normal to reduced in thickness. These findings are readily apparent on any form of cross sectional imaging, including CT and MR. Left ventricular ejection fraction is typically decreased, and this can be evident both qualitatively and quantitatively on cine sequences, which are often routinely performed as part of a cardiac MRI protocol. Wall motion can also be evaluated on cine sequences, and global hypokinesis is typical in dilated cardiomyopathy. Differentiating ischemic and nonischemic forms of dilated cardiomyopathy is of central importance in determining treatment. Delayed gadolinium enhanced MRI sequences are helpful in this regard. Areas of delayed hyperenhancement (DHE) represent areas of infarcted myocardium as well as fibrosis and scarring on cardiac MRI. If areas of DHE are confined to one vascular territory and are either subendocardial or transmural in location, they are very likely to be ischemic in nature. If they do not follow typical vascular territories, or are mesocardial (in the mid myocardium) or subepicardial in location, they are not likely to be due to ischemia.

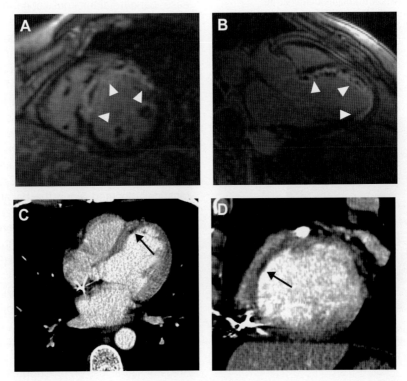

Fig. C27.5 LAD territory infarct. (A) Short axis delayed post contrast MR image demonstrates anteroseptal DHE in a largely transmural distribution, confined to the LAD territory (white arrowheads). (B) Horizontal long axis view. Infarcted territory extends from the base of the ventricle all the way to the apex (white arrowheads). (C, D) Sagittal and axial CT images from the same patient demonstrate a small area of subendocardial fat attenuation (black arrow) within the LV myocardium in the infarcted territory, consistent with a chronic infarction.

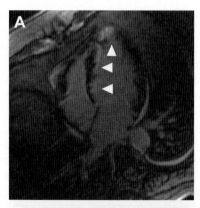

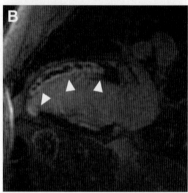

Fig. C27.6 LAD territory infarct. (A, B) Delayed post contrast horizontal and vertical long axis MR images demonstrate anteroseptal DHE in a subendocardial and transmural distribution affecting the LAD territory (white arrowheads), different patient from Fig. C27.5.

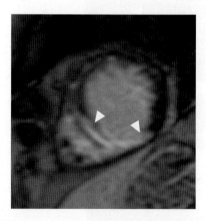

Fig. C27.7 RCA territory infarct. Short axis delayed post contrast MR image demonstrates transmural DHE in the inferoseptal myocardium consistent with infarction in the RCA territory.

A classic location to see DHE in idiopathic dilated cardiomyopathy is in the midwall of the septum.

Hypertrophic cardiomyopathy is characterized by left ventricular wall thickening. The left ventricular volume may be normal to reduced, with the ejection fraction subsequently being either normal or increased. Decreased ventricular compliance can lead to poor ventricular filling and symptoms of diastolic failure. Often, there is asymmetric thickening of the interventricular septum, and this can cause left ventricular outflow tract obstruction that can be dynamic in nature. In addition to the morphologic changes just mentioned, cardiac MRI can demonstrate small patchy areas of DHE, which are thought to represent areas of microinfarction. A classic location to see DHE in hypertrophic cardiomyopathy is where the septum meets the anterior and posterior walls of the left ventricle. It is thought that these fibrotic scars may provide the substrate for eventual fatal arrhythmias, and thus carry some prognostic significance.

Restrictive cardiomyopathy is often difficult to differentiate from constrictive pericarditis clinically, and imaging can be of great assistance in this regard. Clinically, both entities are characterized by reduced ventricular compliance, end diastolic volumes, and poor ventricular filling which may result in diastolic failure, although systolic function is often preserved. As discussed in the section on pericardial disease, pericardial thickness of 4 mm or more is very specific for constrictive pericarditis in this setting. Additionally, the septum maintains its normal convexity in restrictive cardiomyopathy, while it may appear flattened in constrictive pericarditis. Restrictive cardiomyopathy may be idiopathic, or due to a number of diseases affecting the myocardium. Sarcoidosis and amyloidosis are two such infiltrative diseases that will be further discussed here. Sarcoidosis involving the heart leads to thickening of the myocardium. There may be patchy areas of hyperintensity on STIR or fat-suppressed T2-weighted sequences indicating areas of myocardial edema. Areas of DHE, when seen, are characteristically located along the basal portion of the septum and the lateral left ventricular wall. These are often subepicardial or transmural in location. Amyloidosis may also lead to myocardial thickening. Characteristically, there is heterogeneous circumferential DHE of the subendocardial region of the left ventricle.

ARVC (or ARVD) is characterized by fibrofatty replacement of the myocardium of the right ventricular wall. Left ventricular involvement can also be seen, although to a lesser extent. This can be detected by comparing dark blood sequences both with and without fat suppression. Areas of signal loss on fat-suppressed sequences correlate with areas of fatty replacement. These changes characteristically involve the "triangle of dysplasia" made up of the

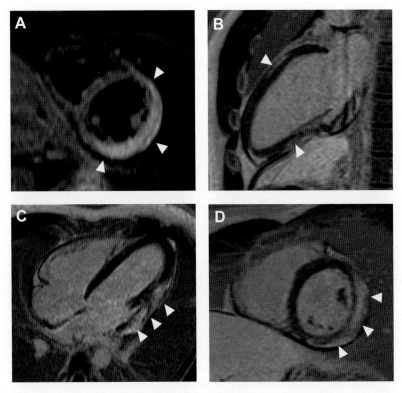

Fig. C27.8 Myocarditis. (A) Short axis STIR sequence demonstrates increased signal in the lateral wall consistent with myocardial edema (white arrowheads). (B) Vertical long axis delayed post contrast sequence demonstrates patchy areas of mesocardial enhancement in the anterior wall and subepicardial enhancement in the inferior wall (white arrowheads). (C) Horizontal long axis view and (D) short axis view demonstrate subepicardial DHE in the lateral wall.

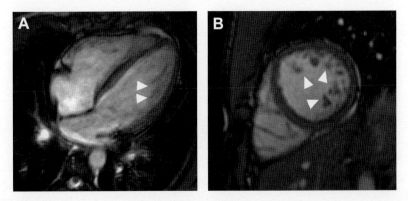

Fig. C27.9 Left ventricular noncompaction. (A) Horizontal long axis and (B) short axis GRE sequences demonstrate abnormally increased trabeculation of the left ventricular myocardium consistent with noncompaction. This is thought to be the result of an arrest in embryologic development, and can result in poor function as well as arrhythmias.

right ventricular outflow tract, inferior wall, and right ventricular apex. Eventually, there is enlargement of the right ventricle, which may be massive. Other less specific findings include regional wall motion abnormalities of the right ventricle and RV dilation or aneurysm formation.

Clinical Differential

Congenital or acquired heart disease, idiopathic right ventricular outflow tract tachycardia, supraventricular tachycardia, bundle branch reentry.

Imaging Differential

Normal fibrofatty infiltration, idiopathic dilated cardiomyopathy and Uhl anomaly (paper-thin right ventricle due to near complete absence of myocardial muscle fibers).

REFERENCES AND SUGGESTED READING

1. Belloni E, Cobelli FD, Esposito A, et al. MRI of cardiomyopathy. *AJR*. 2008;191:1702-1710.
2. Lim RP, Srichai MB, Lee VS. Non-ischemic causes of delayed myocardial hyperenhancement of MRI. *AJR*. 2007;188: 1675-1681.
3. Bluemke DA. MRI of nonischemic cardiomyopathy. *AJR*. 2010; 195:935-940.
4. Murphy DT, Shine SC, Cradock A, et al. Cardiac MRI in arrhythmogenic right ventricular cardiomyopathy. *AJR*. 2010;194: W299-W306.
5. Cummings KW, Bhalla S, Javidan-Nejad C, et al. A pattern-based approach to assessment of delayed enhancement in nonischemic cardiomyopathy at MR imaging. *RadioGraphics*. 2009;29:89-103.
6. Kayser HWM, van der Wall EE, Sivananthan MU, et al. Diagnosis of arrhythmogenic right ventricular dysplasia: a review. *RadioGraphics*. 2002;22:639-648.

CASE 28: PERICARDIAL DISEASE

PATIENT PRESENTATION

A 35-year-old female with lupus presents with chest pain. On examination, a pericardial friction rub is heard. Transthoracic echocardiogram was limited by poor acoustic windows.

CLINICAL SUSPICION

Pericarditis

IMAGING MODALITY OF CHOICE

Transesophageal echocardiography (TEE) and/or cardiac MRI (Figs. C28.1-C28.3)

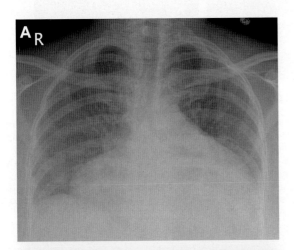

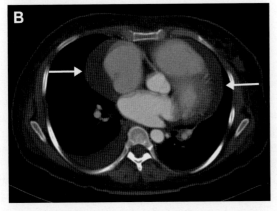

Fig. C28.1 Pericardial effusion. (A) PA view of the chest demonstrates an enlarged cardiac silhouette, with a symmetric water-bottle configuration. (B) Axial contrast-enhanced CT in the same patient demonstrates the pericardial effusion (white arrows).

DISCUSSION

Traditionally, TEE has been the modality of choice for imaging the pericardium; however, it is limited by its invasiveness, operator dependence, and somewhat restricted imaging windows. CT and MRI overcome the operator dependence and limited windows of TEE. ECG gating is required with CT and MRI to produce diagnostic images and eliminate motion artifact when evaluating the pericardium. MR is typically superior to CT when evaluating the pericardium due to its superior soft tissue contrast, although CT is superior in detecting pericardial calcifications. CT and/or MRI should be considered when TEE is nondiagnostic, loculations are suspected, and in imaging pericardial masses. MRI is also performed to evaluate for pericardial thickening in the setting of constrictive pericarditis, especially when surgical pericardiectomy is being contemplated.

A small amount of pericardial fluid is physiologic, as the pericardium normally contains up to 60 mL of serous fluid as demonstrated by early MRI studies. Large pericardial effusions may cause enlargement of the cardiac silhouette on plain chest radiography. Differentiating a pericardial effusion from cardiomegaly on a chest radiograph is not definitively possible, although a globular or bottle-shaped configuration suggest a large pericardial effusion. Pericardial effusions can be directly imaged at CT and MR due to the superior soft tissue contrast and cross sectional nature of these modalities. There are numerous causes of pericardial effusions, and it is helpful to categorize them based on the nature of the fluid. Simple serous fluid is the most common, and may be due to volume overload states, heart failure, and nephrotic syndrome. Purulent fluid may be due to bacterial pericarditis. Hemorrhagic fluid may be due to infection (especially tuberculosis), neoplasm, or trauma. CT attenuation values may be helpful in this characterization, as values close to water attenuation are likely serous fluid, while higher attenuation (>20 HU) values point to hemorrhagic or purulent fluid. On MRI, simple serous fluid will be low signal (dark) on T1-weighted sequences and high signal (bright) on gradient echo (GRE) sequences, while hemorrhagic fluid may be brighter on T1, and lower signal on GRE.

Cardiac tamponade is a complication of pericardial effusions, resulting when the intrapericardial pressure rises high enough to impair ventricular filling and decrease cardiac output. It is related more to the rapidity with which fluid accumulates rather than the total volume of fluid. Gradual accumulation allows the pericardium to distend and maintain a low intrapericardial pressure, whereas rapid accumulation does not allow time for this compensatory mechanism. Although tamponade remains a clinical diagnosis

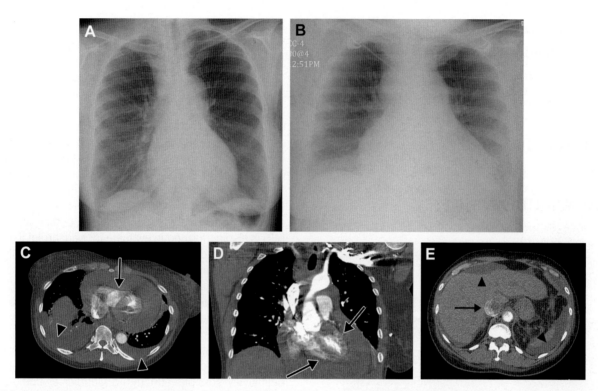

Fig. C28.2 Cardiac tamponade. (A) Baseline PA chest x-ray obtained 6 weeks prior to the patient's presentation for unrelated reasons. (B) AP chest x-ray obtained in the ER when the patient presented with shortness of breath. She was tachycardic and hypotensive upon arrival. The cardiac silhouette is much larger, even accounting for the AP technique. This relatively rapid change in size suggests a pericardial effusion. (C) Axial chest CT demonstrates a large pericardial effusion that compresses upon the right ventricle, suggesting tamponade (black arrow). The pericardial fluid measured 25 HU, suggesting complex or hemorrhagic fluid. There are bilateral pleural effusions as well (black arrowheads) (D) Coronal reformation demonstrates compression of both ventricles (black arrows). (E) Axial CT more inferiorly demonstrates a distended IVC with reflux of high-density contrast, which is seen mixing with unopacified venous blood (black arrow). This is suggestive of increased right heart pressure. The patient also has ascites (black arrowheads). A pericardial window was performed emergently, and vital signs improved. Pericardial biopsy and cytology were positive for metastatic adenocarcinoma, and the patient had a primary adenocarcinoma of the lung.

(Beck's triad of hypotension, muffled or distant heart sounds, and jugular venous distension), there are imaging findings which can suggest tamponade physiology. These include signs of elevated right heart pressures (distended SVC and IVC, reflux of contrast material into the IVC and hepatic veins), and more specifically, flattening of the cardiac chambers (particularly the thinner and more compliant right-sided chambers), and straightening or leftward bowing of the interventricular septum.

Pericarditis may result from many causes. At contrast-enhanced CT and MR, abnormal thickening and enhancement of the pericardium indicate inflammation, and there is often an associated pericardial effusion. At CT, it is sometimes difficult to differentiate a small pericardial effusion from pericardial thickening. Echocardiography or MR can be helpful in this setting. At MR, the normal pericardium

is low in signal on both T1- and T2-weighted sequences due to its fibrous composition. In addition to enhancement, inflammation will result in increased T2 signal of the pericardium. Smooth pericardial thickening suggests a more acute presentation, whereas a more irregular or nodular contour suggests chronicity.

CT and MRI are excellent for imaging of pericardial masses. Pericardial cysts appear as smooth thin-walled structures of homogeneous water attenuation at CT, and homogeneous bright T2 signal with intermediate to low-signal intensity at MRI. They do not demonstrate enhancement on post contrast images. Hematomas may result from trauma or surgery, and demonstrate characteristic evolution on MR sequences. Acute hematomas may demonstrate homogeneously high T1 signal, subacute hematomas will become more heterogeneous in signal, while chronic hematomas

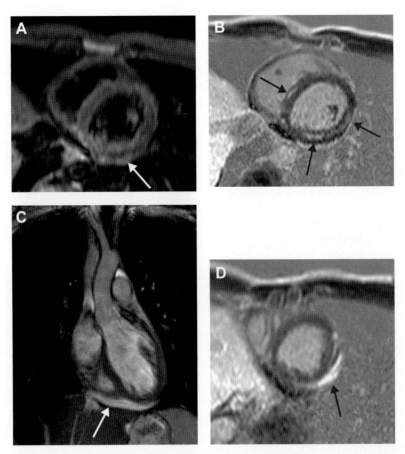

Fig. C28.3 Myocarditis and pericarditis. (A) Short axis STIR sequence demonstrates increased myocardial signal consistent with edema, most prominent in the inferior wall (white arrow), consistent with myocardial edema. (B) Short axis delayed post contrast image demonstrates patchy areas of enhancement (black arrows). These do not conform to any particular vascular territory, and are therefore not consistent with infarction. Rather, this distribution is more typical for entities such as myocarditis or sarcoidosis. (C) Coronal SSFP "bright blood" sequence demonstrates a small pericardial effusion along the inferior border of the heart (white arrow). (D) Delayed post gadolinium sequence demonstrates pericardial enhancement (black arrow). The patient was a 17-year-old male who presented with 2 days of substernal chest pain, and diffuse ST elevations consistent with pericarditis. Cardiac enzymes were elevated, consistent with myocarditis as well.

will be lower in signal and will demonstrate areas of signal loss on GRE sequences due to hemosiderin deposition. Acute hematomas on CT will demonstrate high density due to fresh blood products, and possibly a layering high-density "hematocrit effect." Hematomas will not enhance after contrast administration. Primary pericardial neoplasms are rare, and include benign entities such as lipoma, teratoma, and fibroma, as well as malignant entities such as sarcoma, liposarcoma, and mesothelioma. Teratomas can be identified at CT by the presence of fat density. Lipomas will be of purely fat density at CT, and can be thus identified as well. At MRI, they will be of fairly homogenous high T1 signal. In the absence of these fairly specific findings, histopathologic analysis is often necessary to diagnose pericardial tumors. Metastatic neoplasms may involve the pericardium by direct extension or via lymphatic or hematogenous dissemination.

They appear either as irregular thickening and enhancement of the pericardium, or as discrete pericardial masses that enhance on post contrast images. There is often an associated complex or hemorrhagic effusion.

Constrictive pericarditis results from thickening and loss of compliance of the pericardium that causes impaired ventricular filling. It is often the result of malignancy, tuberculosis, radiation therapy, surgery, hemorrhage, or recurrent infection. The normal pericardium is usually less than 2 mm thick. Thickening to 4 mm or more in the presence of symptoms of constriction is highly suggestive of constrictive pericarditis, and helps to differentiate from restrictive cardiomyopathy, which may have similar clinical symptoms. Thickening may be global or focal in nature. There may be associated pericardial calcifications, adding confidence to the diagnosis. Indeed, the presence of pericardial calcification may suggest the diagnosis in the right clinical setting. As with cardiac tamponade, distension of the IVC, SVC, and hepatic veins suggests constrictive physiology, as does flattening of cardiac chambers.

Clinical Differential

Myocardial infarction, pulmonary embolism, GERD, pneumonia. Pericarditis itself may result for many causes including infection, uremia, connective tissue disease, and drug reaction among others.

Imaging Differential

On imaging, the differential diagnosis for pericarditis includes metastatic disease to the pericardium.

REFERENCES AND SUGGESTED READING

1. Wang ZJ, Reddy GP, Gotway MB, et al. CT and MR imaging of pericardial disease. *RadioGraphics*. 2003;23:S167-S180.
2. Rienmuller R, Groll R, Lipton MJ. CT and MR imaging of pericardial disease. *Radiol Clin N Am*. 2004;42:587-601.
3. Sechtem U, Tscholakoff D, Higgins CB. MRI of the normal pericardium. *AJR*. 1986;147:239-244.
4. Restrepo CS, Lemos DF, Lemos JA, et al. Imaging findings in cardiac tamponade with emphasis on CT. *RadioGraphics*. 2007;27:1595-1610.

CASE 29: CONGENITAL HEART DISEASE

PATIENT PRESENTATION

Newborn with cyanosis on first day of life.

CLINICAL SUSPICION

Congenital heart disease

IMAGING MODALITY OF CHOICE

While echocardiography is the modality of choice, a chest x-ray will often be performed first. Therefore, it is important to recognize clues to congenital heart disease on the chest x-ray even though a definitive diagnosis will probably not be made without advanced imaging including echocardiography and possibly cardiac MRI in complex cases (Figs. C29.1-C29.4).

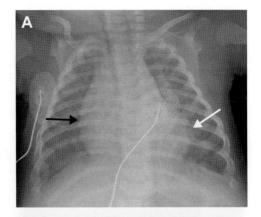

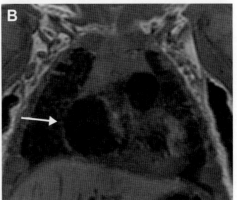

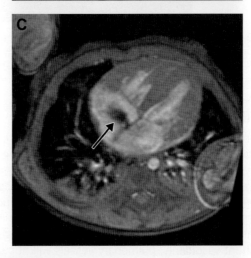

Fig. C29.2 ASD. (A) Frontal chest radiograph demonstrates cardiomegaly. Bulging right heart border suggests right atrial enlargement (black arrow), upturned cardiac apex suggests right ventricular hypertrophy (white arrow). This pattern of enlargement suggests ASD. Pulmonary vascularity is difficult to evaluate in this case due to underlying chronic lung disease. (B) Coronal "black blood" cardiac MRI image confirms right atrial enlargement. (C) Axial "bright blood" sequence demonstrates a dephasing jet in the right atrium (black arrow) indicative of an ASD with left to right shunt.

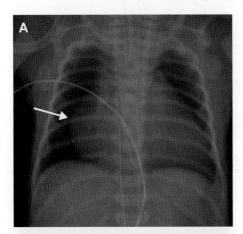

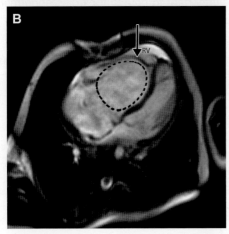

Fig. C29.1 Ebstein's anomaly. (A) Frontal chest radiograph of a neonate demonstrates decreased pulmonary vascularity with cardiomegaly and right atrial enlargement (white arrow). Presence of an endotracheal tube suggests that this may be a cyanotic lesion. (B) Axial "bright blood" cardiac MRI image demonstrates apically displaced septal leaflet of the tricuspid valve (black arrow). Atrialized portion of the RV is outlined with a dashed line. RV annotates the residual tiny RV cavity.

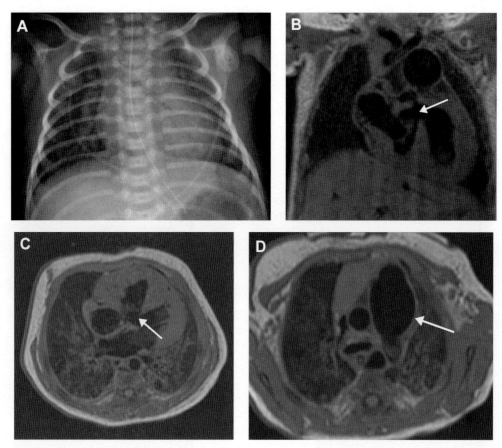

Fig. C29.3 VSD. (A) Frontal chest x-ray demonstrates shunt vascularity and mild cardiomegaly. (B) Coronal and (C) axial "black blood" MRI image demonstrate the VSD (white arrow). (D) Axial "black blood" MRI image demonstrates a massively dilated main pulmonary artery (white arrow) due to left to right shunting and resultant volume overload.

FINDINGS

Congenital heart disease can be broadly categorized as cyanotic ("blue") or acyanotic ("pink") depending upon the oxygenation status of the patient. On the basis of the chest x-ray, it is then helpful to further characterize the pulmonary vascularity into four broad categories: normal, decreased vascularity, increased pulmonary arterial flow ("shunt" vascularity), and pulmonary venous congestion. With shunt vascularity, pulmonary vessels will appear enlarged, but will maintain distinct margins and will extend further into the periphery than normal. In pulmonary venous congestion, vessel margins will be hazy, and there may be other evidence of interstitial or alveolar edema in advanced cases. After knowing clinically whether the child is cyanotic or acyanotic, categorizing the pulmonary vascularity will help to limit the differential diagnosis. Entities listed in Table C29.1 will be discussed here. Bear in mind that this is not a complete list, and a complete discussion of congenital heart disease is beyond the scope of this text.

Also, it is important to note that cardiac abnormalities are often multiple in nature.

Table C29.1 Cyanotic and Acyanotic Congenital Heart Disease

Cyanotic	Acyanotic
Decreased vascularity	Normal vascularity
• Tetralogy of Fallot (TOF)	• Coarctation
• Ebstein's anomaly	• Valvular disease
• Tricuspid atresia	
Increased vascularity	"Shunt" vascularity
• TAPVR (total anomalous pulmonary venous return)	• ASD (atrial septal defect)
	• VSD (ventricular septal defect)
• Truncus arteriosus	• PDA (patent ductus arteriosus)
Variable	Pulmonary venous congestion
• d-TGA (d-transposition of the great arteries)	• CHF (many causes)

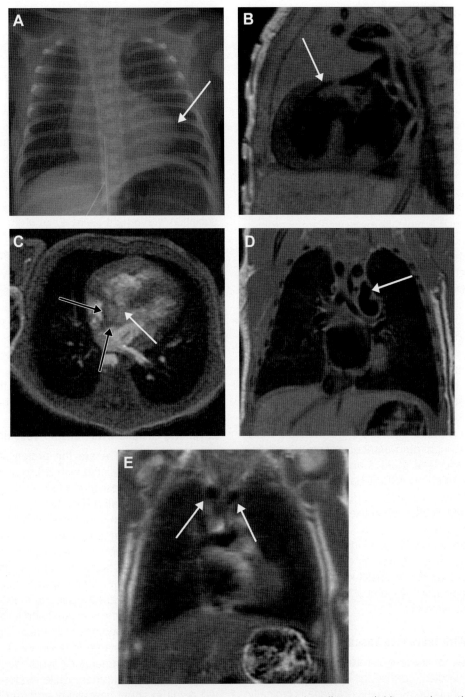

Fig. C29.4 Tetralogy of Fallot. (A) Frontal chest radiograph demonstrates an upturned cardiac apex (white arrow) creating a boot shaped cardiac silhouette. This suggests right ventricular hypertrophy. Pulmonary vascularity is not significantly affected in this case. (B) Sagittal "dark blood" MRI sequence demonstrates pulmonary infundibular stenosis (white arrow). (C) Axial "bright blood" sequence demonstrates a high VSD (white arrow) with an overriding aortic root (black arrows). (D) There is a large PDA feeding the left pulmonary artery (white arrow). (E) There is also a double aortic arch (white arrows). Cardiac anomalies are often multiple.

Cyanotic Lesions With Decreased Pulmonary Vascularity

Pulmonic stenosis is the hallmark of tetralogy of Fallot (TOF) and may occur at the valvular or subvalvular (infundibular) level. The stenosis may be dynamic, with acute episodes of cyanosis known as tet spells. There is an associated high (membranous) VSD with rightward displacement of the aortic root resulting in "overriding" of the VSD. There is right to left shunting across the VSD due to the pulmonic stenosis. Right ventricular hypertrophy results due to the RV outflow stenosis. Chest x-ray findings include a boot-shaped heart due to right ventricular hypertrophy that results in upward displacement of the cardiac apex. Pulmonary vascularity is decreased due to the pulmonic stenosis. The diagnosis is typically made with echocardiography, and MRI may have an adjunctive role as well especially for surgical planning.

Ebstein's anomaly is characterized by maldevelopment of the tricuspid valve with apical displacement of the septal leaflet. This results in atrialization of a portion of the RV and severe tricuspid regurgitation which results in typically massive dilation of the RA. The right ventricular cavity is small and pulmonary vascularity is decreased due to the poor RV function. The diagnosis is typically made with echocardiography, which directly visualizes the displaced septal leaflet, dilated right atrium, and can assess RV size and function to guide therapy.

Tricuspid atresia is due to agenesis of the tricuspid valve with resultant lack of right atrioventricular communication. The RV is hypoplastic, and there is an obligatory right to left shunt, which is often an ASD or patent foramen ovale (PFO). Blood flow to the lungs is via a PDA or VSD typically. Pulmonary vascularity is often decreased, but may be normal or increased if there is a large VSD. Echocardiography may demonstrate an echogenic band in the expected location of the tricuspid valve, as well as right atrial enlargement and a hypoplastic RV. Associated shunts (ie, ASD, PFO, VSD, PDA) can also be demonstrated. Again, MRI may have an adjunctive role.

Cyanotic Lesions With Increased Vascularity

Total anomalous pulmonary venous return (TAPVR) can be classified as supracardiac, cardiac, or infracardiac. In supracardiac TAPVR, pulmonary venous drainage is typically into a left vertical vein that empties into the brachiocephalic (innominate) vein. The left vertical vein in combination with the SVC shadow on the right classically creates a "snowman" appearance of the cardiomediastinal silhouette. Cardiac TAPVR is characterized by drainage of the pulmonary veins into the coronary sinus or right atrium. In infracardiac TAPVR, a common pulmonary vein courses through the diaphragmatic hiatus and typically drains into the IVC, hepatic veins, or portal vein. Infracardiac TAPVR is often associated with obstruction of the pulmonary venous outflow, and resultant pulmonary edema. Echocardiography makes the diagnosis, but MRI may be helpful in evaluating the anatomy in difficult cases.

Persistent truncus arteriosus is due to failed septation of the embryonic truncus into the aorta and pulmonary artery with a resultant overriding high VSD. There is a single truncal valve that is typically malformed and insufficient. Truncus arteriosus is subdivided into multiple types based on the origin of the right and left pulmonary arteries, but this will not be further discussed here. There is "shunt" vascularity due to preferential flow into the low resistance pulmonary vascular system. Additionally, there is a high association with a right-sided aortic arch.

Cyanotic Lesions With Variable Pulmonary Vascularity

In d-TGA, the aorta arises from the RV while the pulmonary artery arises from the LV. This results in two parallel circulations with an obligatory shunt required for survival. The shunt is typically in the form of an ASD, VSD, or PDA. Affected patients are typically cyanotic within 24 hours of birth. Pulmonary vascularity may be decreased due to associated pulmonic stenosis, or may be increased if there is significant left to right shunting. The thymus is often absent, resulting in a narrowed superior mediastinum.

Acyanotic Lesions With "Shunt" Vascularity

ASD, VSD, and PDA are the prototypical lesions in this group. All are associated with left to right shunting as pulmonary vascular resistance falls in the first few weeks to months of life. Small ASDs may go unnoticed while larger shunts will result in shunt vascularity and right atrial and ventricular enlargement due to volume overload. Long-standing large defects can lead to pulmonary hypertension and Eisenmenger's syndrome with eventual shunt reversal. This may result in a pruned appearance of the pulmonary vasculature. VSDs are the second most common congenital cardiac defect after bicuspid aortic valve. As with ASDs, the radiographic findings vary depending on the severity of the shunt, and large long-standing shunts may eventually lead to Eisenmenger's syndrome. Small shunts will be normal in appearance, while moderate to large shunts will result in shunt vascularity and cardiomegaly involving both right- and left-sided chambers. The ductus arteriosus typically closes within the first 24 hours of life. Failed closure may lead to a left to right shunt as pulmonary vascular resistance decreases. Chest x-ray findings include shunt vascularity and cardiomegaly. In all of these cases, echocardiography can make the diagnosis, as well as quantify shunt fraction, which will aid in treatment planning and prognostication. MRI is typically reserved for complicated cases with multiple concomitant anomalies.

Acyanotic Lesions With Pulmonary Venous Congestion

This group includes all entities which result in congestive heart failure, which is a very diverse group. For example, high output heart failure can result from fetal anemia, large high-flow AV malformations, and hyperthyroidism. Anatomic causes of CHF include severe obstructive lesions such as mitral or aortic stenosis and coarctation (although these more commonly have normal vascularity). Left ventricular dysfunction can be due to entities such as hypoplastic left heart syndrome, glycogen storage diseases, and anomalous origin of the left coronary artery.

Acyanotic Lesions With Normal Vascularity

There are many congenital cardiac defects which may produce only subtle radiographic findings. As noted earlier, small ASDs will be radiographically normal. Additionally, many valvular lesions (such as aortic stenosis, bicuspid aortic valve, mitral stenosis, pulmonic stenosis, etc) may go unnoticed. While severe coarctation can result in CHF, milder forms may be essentially normal radiographically or demonstrate only subtle rib notching due to

distended intercostal arteries. Poststenotic dilatation of the descending aorta may be present, resulting in a configuration resembling the number 3.

REFERENCES AND SUGGESTED READING

1. Ferguson EC, Krishnamurthy R, Oldham SAA. Classic imaging signs of congenital cardiovascular abnormalities. *RadioGraphics.* 2007:27;1323-1334.

2. Chen JT, Capp MP, Johnsrude IS, Goodrich JK, Lester RG. Roentgen appearance of pulmonary vascularity in the diagnosis of heart disease. *Am J Roentgenol Radium Ther Nucl Med.* 1971;112(3):559-570.

3. Mirowitz SA, Gutierrez FR, Canter CE, Vannier MW. Tetralogy of Fallot: MR findings. *Radiology.* 1989;171(1):207-212.

4. Deutsch V, Wexler L, Blieden LC, Yahini JH, Neufeld HN. Ebstein's anomaly of tricuspid valve: critical review of roentgenological features and additional angiographic signs. *Am J Roentgenol Radium Ther Nucl Med.* 1975;125(2):395-411.

5. Kellenberger CJ, Yoo SJ, Valsangiacomo Buchel ER. Cardiovascular MR imaging in neonates and infants with congenital heart disease. *RadioGraphics.* 2007;27:5-18.

Chapter 5

Gastrointestinal Imaging

By Patrick Marcin, Eduardo J. Matta, and Khaled M. Elsayes

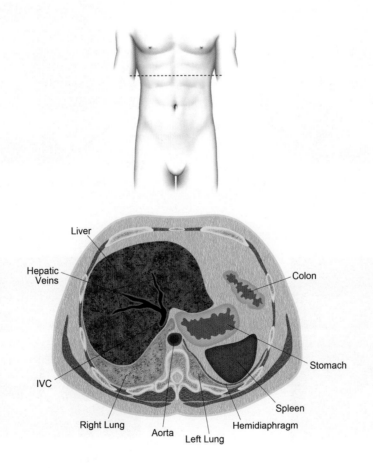

INTRODUCTION

This section serves as an introduction to the basic anatomy of the abdomen.

The human gastrointestinal tract can be divided into upper and lower portions. All structures proximal to the ligament of Treitz can be thought of as the upper GI tract, while structures found distal to it are considered the lower GI tract. We will begin with axial sections depicting the upper abdomen, including the liver and stomach, and work inferiorly toward the pelvis (Figs. 5.1 through 5.9).

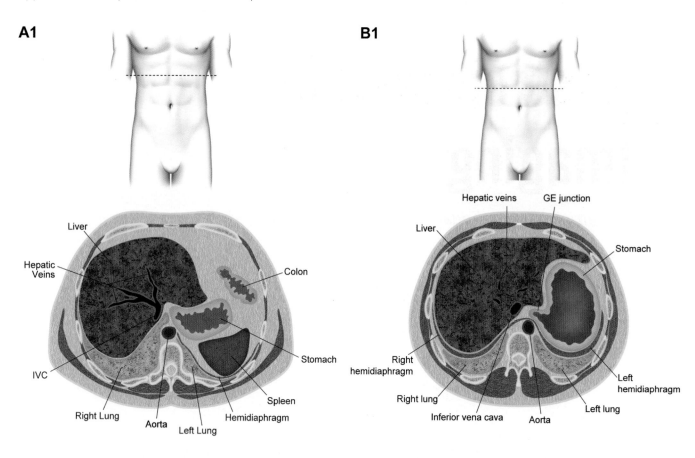

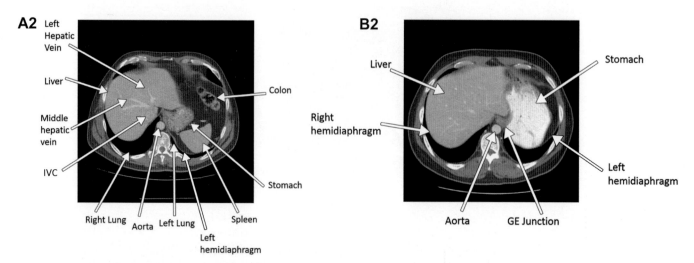

Fig. 5.1 (A) Cross section demonstrating relative anatomy of stomach, liver, aorta, and inferior vena cava. (B) This section offers a clearer view of the hepatic veins, which can be seen within the liver, draining into the inferior vena cava. Axial CT sections correlating with the same level of anatomical cut section.

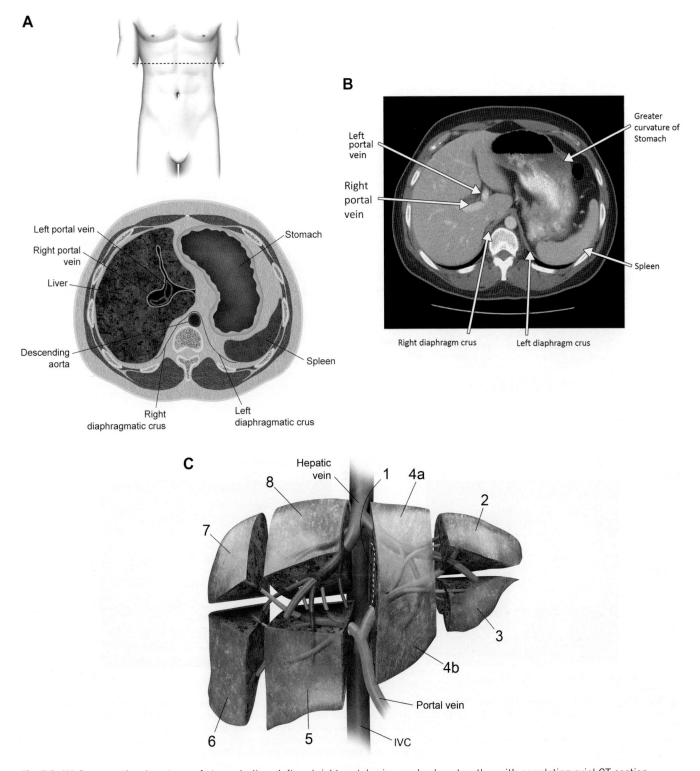

Fig. 5.2 (A) Cross-sectional anatomy of stomach, liver, left and right portal veins, and spleen together with correlating axial CT section (B) correlating with the same level of anatomical cut section. The portal vein is formed by the superior mesenteric vein, inferior mesenteric vein, splenic vein, gastric veins, and cystic veins. The main portal vein splits into the right and left portal vein, then further branches into venules (along with a hepatic arteriole and bile duct, forming a portal triad), and ultimately terminating in the liver sinusoids. (C) Illustration demonstrating the portal vein ascending into the liver, and the hepatic vein joining the IVC. The segments of the liver are demonstrated as well. There are eight segments, each with its own arterial supply, venous drainage, and biliary outflow.

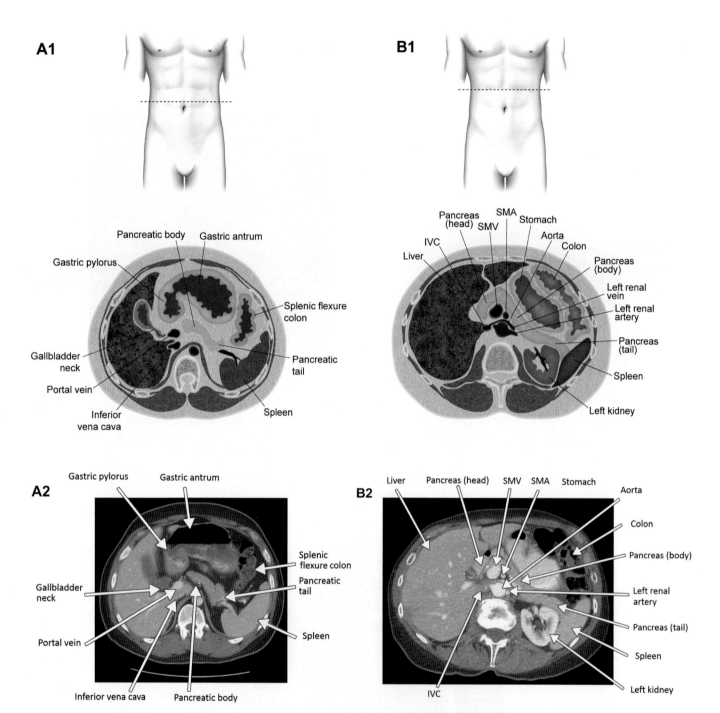

Fig. 5.3 (A) Cross section revealing location of gallbladder in relation to liver, stomach, and pancreatic body and tail. The gallbladder drains into the common hepatic duct via the cystic duct, which later joins the pancreatic duct to form the ampulla of Vater. This empties through the sphincter of Oddi into the duodenum. The portal vein is seen prior to its branching into left and right portal veins. Note the presence of the splenic flexure of the colon as well. (B) Similar cross section revealing anatomy of the pancreatic tail and body. Axial CT section correlating with the same level of anatomical cut section is seen below each pertinent illustration.

A

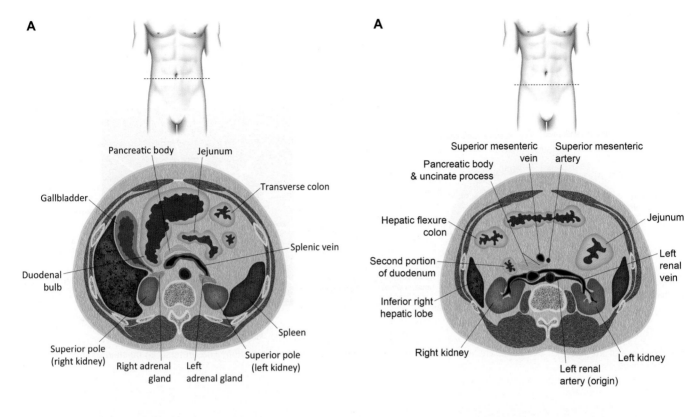

A

Pancreatic body

Jejunum

Gallbladder

Transverse colon

Splenic vein

Duodenal bulb

Superior pole (right kidney)

Right adrenal gland

Left adrenal gland

Superior pole (left kidney)

Spleen

Superior mesenteric vein

Superior mesenteric artery

Pancreatic body & uncinate process

Hepatic flexure colon

Second portion of duodenum

Inferior right hepatic lobe

Right kidney

Jejunum

Left renal vein

Left kidney

Left renal artery (origin)

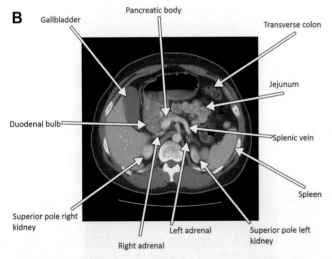

B

Gallbladder

Pancreatic body

Transverse colon

Jejunum

Duodenal bulb

Splenic vein

Superior pole right kidney

Left adrenal

Superior pole left kidney

Right adrenal

Spleen

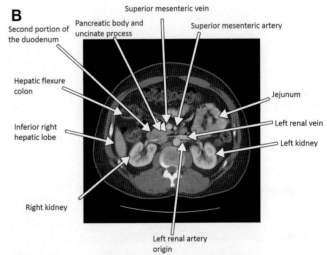

B

Second portion of the duodenum

Pancreatic body and uncinate process

Superior mesenteric vein

Superior mesenteric artery

Hepatic flexure colon

Inferior right hepatic lobe

Jejunum

Left renal vein

Left kidney

Right kidney

Left renal artery origin

Fig. 5.4 The superior poles of the kidneys and the adrenal glands become visible, along with portions of the jejunum, as well as the transverse colon. The splenic vein, which will empty into the portal vein, is seen here also.

Fig. 5.5 More of the kidney is visible, along with the left and right renal arteries and veins. Also the duodenum and the hepatic flexure of the colon become visible.

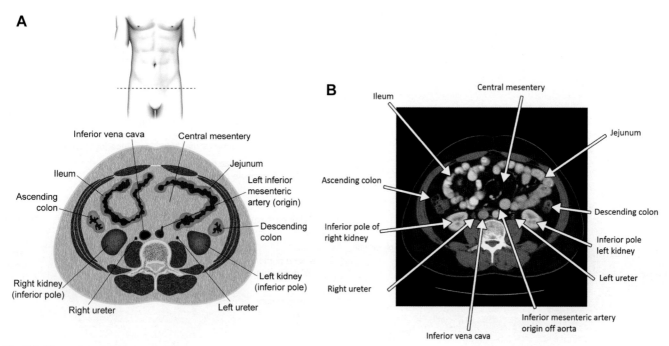

Fig. 5.6 More of the jejunum and ileum are seen along with the ascending and descending colon. The ureters can be seen as they ascend to the kidneys.

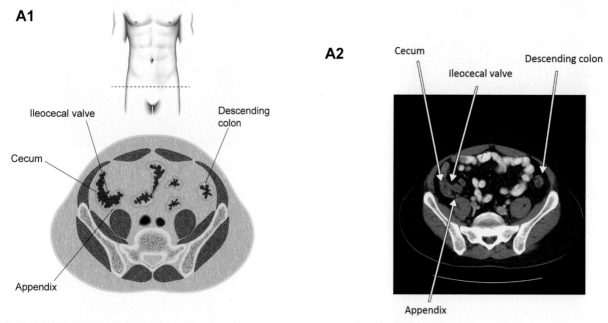

Fig. 5.7 (A) The cecum is visible here along with the ileocecal valve and the appendix.

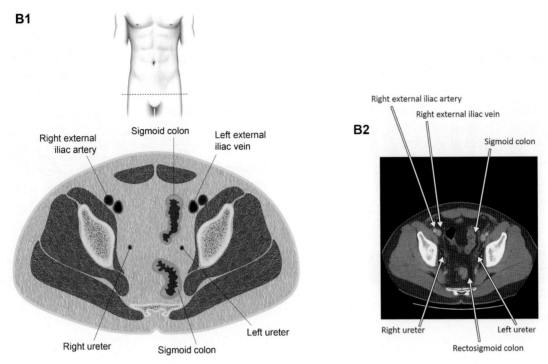

Fig. 5.7 (*continued*) (B) The sigmoid colon is visible as we continue to move more inferiorly in the abdomen. Note the presence of the external iliac artery and vein, as we are below the level of the aorta and inferior vena cava.

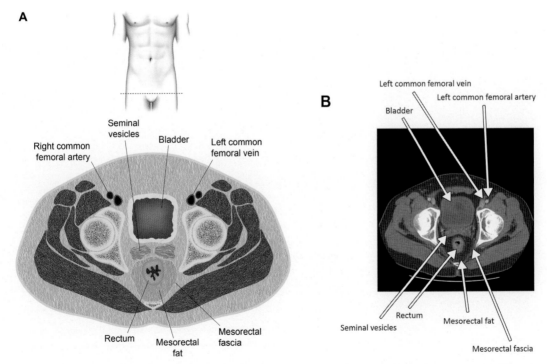

Fig. 5.8 The rectum and its surrounding fat and fascia become visible, adjacent to the seminal vesicles and bladder. The external iliac artery and vein becomes the common femoral artery and common femoral vein, respectively, below the level of the inguinal ligament.

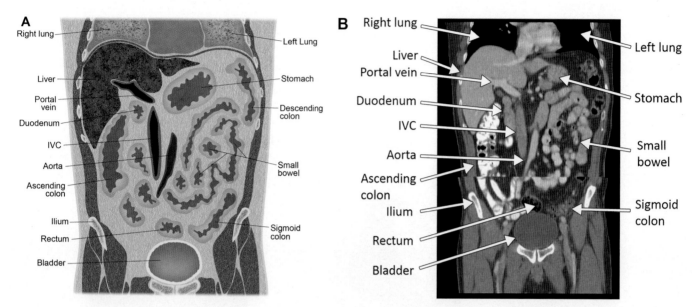

Fig. 5.9 Coronal CT demonstrating the normal anatomy of the GI tract, including the small intestine and ascending colon. The liver, abdominal aorta, and inferior vena cava are demonstrated as well.

CASE 1

PATIENT PRESENTATION

A 72-year-old man presented to an outpatient clinic with halitosis, regurgitation, aspiration, and dysphagia.

CLINICAL SUSPICION

Oropharyngeal dysphagia

IMAGING MODALITY OF CHOICE

Barium swallow examination is the mainstay for the diagnostic workup of dysphagia. The type of study used depends on the clinical presentation. For example, a patient recovering from a recent stroke (or any other disease with neurological sequelae), with a known cause of cough, pneumonia, or suspected aspiration, requires a modified barium swallow, which is performed by a speech pathologist and radiologist. In this, videofluoroscopy is used, usually only in the lateral projection, to evaluate oropharyngeal swallowing, mastication, and the presence and causes of aspiration. It does not evaluate the entire esophagus.

If the cause of oropharyngeal dysphagia is unknown, a more detailed barium study may be performed to assess the functional and structural abnormalities of the pharynx. As in the modified barium swallow, a dynamic examination of the oropharynx with videofluoroscopy allows assessment of the oral and pharyngeal phases of swallowing. However, static images of the pharynx can be obtained to detect structural abnormalities. This portion of the examination uses a double-contrast technique (thick, viscous barium for the mucosal coating and effervescent air crystals for air distention) with spot radiographs in the frontal and lateral projections. The same technique is used to image the entire esophagus and proximal stomach to exclude referred causes of oropharyngeal dysphagia.

STRUCTURAL PHARYNGEAL AND ESOPHAGEAL ABNORMALITIES

Zenker's diverticulum: Zenker's diverticulum is a pulsion diverticulum that occurs in the midline posterior pharynx, above the cricopharyngeus muscle (upper esophageal sphincter). It is believed to occur secondary to a lack of coordination of the cricopharyngeus during swallowing, resulting in increased intraluminal pressure, which creates a diverticulum at a specific anatomic weak point of the posterior pharynx known as Killian's dehiscence. The resulting diverticulum usually extends inferiorly, with a small neck, frequently resulting in trapped food or liquid (Fig. C1.1). This can then compress the ventrally located upper esophagus, resulting in dysphagia. Associated symptoms include aspiration and halitosis due to retained liquids or food.

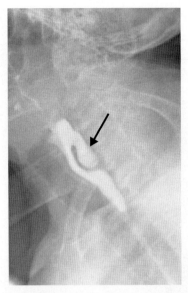

Fig. C1.1 Zenker's diverticulum. Lateral view from barium swallow of the esophagus showing the contrast pooling into the posteriorly positioned Zenker's diverticulum (black arrow). This results in mass effect and effective narrowing of the upper esophagus located anterior to the diverticulum.

Killian-Jamieson diverticulum: Killian-Jamieson diverticulum is a pulsion diverticulum that arises from the anterolateral wall, beginning below the cricopharyngeus muscle and extending along the lateral aspect of the cervical esophagus. This is less common and is usually small and asymptomatic. The location beneath the cricopharyngeus muscle is felt to be a relative protection from aspiration (Fig. C1.2).

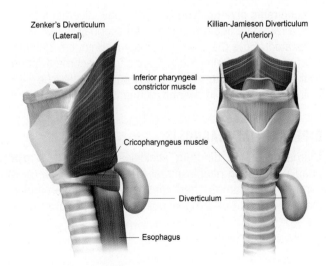

Fig. C1.2 (Left) Zenker's diverticulum arising above the cricopharyngeus (upper esophageal sphincter) from the posterior midline. (Right) A Killian-Jamieson diverticulum arising from the lateral wall and below the cricopharyngeus in contradistinction from the Zenker's diverticulum.

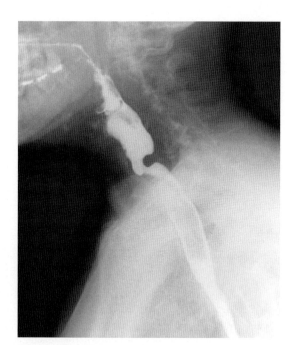

Fig. C1.3 Cricopharyngeus hypertrophy. Lateral radiograph from esophagram shows round smoothly marginated indentation from the posterior wall of the upper esophagus representative of enlargement of the UES.

Cricopharyngeus hypertrophy: Patients with dysphagia may have a history of gastroesophageal reflux. Hypertrophy of the cricopharyngeus or upper esophageal sphincter is believed to represent a protective mechanism from aspiration in the setting of reflux. This should not be confused with a stricture because it has smooth margins (Fig. C1.3).

Epiphrenic diverticulum: An epiphrenic diverticulum is a rare diverticulum of the distal esophagus that is located above the lower esophageal sphincter. Because of the small opening neck, debris can become trapped; if large enough, this debris can compress the true lumen, resulting in dysphagia (Fig. C1.4).

DIFFERENTIAL DIAGNOSIS

Ultimately, many different etiologies can result in dysphagia, including neoplasms of the head and neck (most commonly squamous cell carcinoma) and inflammatory masses (eg, retropharyngeal abscess), trauma, diverticula,

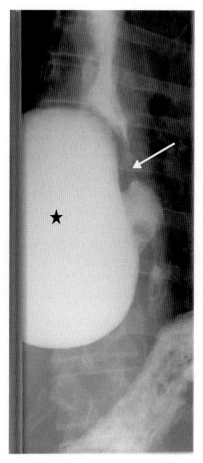

Fig. C1.4 Epiphrenic diverticulum. Upper GI examination shows large epiphrenic diverticulum (*) with mass effect significantly narrowing the lower esophagus (arrow).

esophageal webs, anterior mediastinal masses, cervical spondylosis, or extrinsic structural lesions such as vascular rings. From an imaging standpoint, the differential diagnosis depends on the anatomical location.

REFERENCES AND SUGGESTED READING

1. Rubesin SE, Levine MS. Killian-Jamieson diverticula: radiographic findings in 16 patients. *AJR*. 2001;177:85-89.
2. Brant WE, Helms CH. *Fundamentals of Diagnostic Radiology*. 3rd ed. Philadelphia, PA: Lippincott Williams & Wilkins; 2006.

CASE 2

PATIENT PRESENTATION

A 33-year-old woman presented to a gastroenterology clinic with retrosternal dysphagia, relieved by repetitive swallowing, and several episodes of regurgitation.

CLINICAL SUSPICION

Esophageal dysphagia, achalasia

IMAGING MODALITY OF CHOICE

Barium studies are a vital tool in the initial diagnostic evaluation of dysphagia. When dysphagia is localized to the esophagus rather than the oropharynx and there are no reports of aspiration or coughing immediately after swallowing, video-fluoroscopy of the swallowing reflex in combination with a speech pathologist (modified barium swallow) is usually not necessary. An esophagram study usually entails a double-contrast (thick barium for mucosal detail and effervescent air crystals for distention) examination in the upright position in multiple projections and a single contrast (thin barium) performed in the prone (right anterior oblique) position to evaluate for esophageal distensibility and peristalsis (Fig. C2.1).

Alternative methods for evaluating dysphagia include esophageal manometry, a pH probe, and endoscopy (Fig. C2.2).

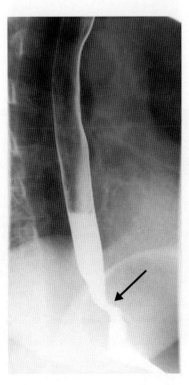

Fig. C2.1 Normal esophagram. Normal double contrast esophagram with air distention and thick barium coating the mucosal surface. Normal GE junction (arrow).

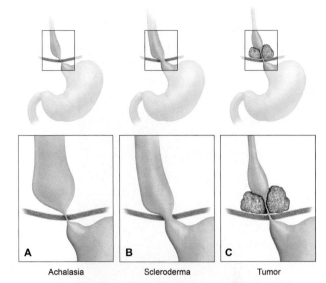

Achalasia   Scleroderma   Tumor

Fig. C2.2 Distal esophagus with achalasia, scleroderma, and tumor. (A) Achalasia results in the most dilated esophagus frequently containing debris related to prior food which has not passed the tight "bird beak" appearance of the LES. (B) Scleroderma results in dilatation of the esophagus, but to a lesser degree than with achalasia. The LES is initially patulous and widened as illustrated, much different than achalasia, but eventually due to reflux esophagitis, can develop a stricture or worse Barrett's esophagitis or adenocarcinoma. (C) Tumors of the GE junction are primarily adenocarcinoma and result in shaggy irregularity of the mucosa with abrupt shouldering and narrowing of the lumen.

NEUROMUSCULAR ESOPHAGEAL ABNORMALITIES

Achalasia: Achalasia is a well-known primary esophageal motility disorder that is characterized by incomplete relaxation of the lower esophageal sphincter (LES) and no primary peristalsis. Men and women are equally affected, with a mean age of 25 to 60 years. Primary achalasia refers to idiopathic loss of inhibitory ganglion cells, resulting in an unopposed excitatory and thus contracted state. Secondary achalasia has a similar appearance but is caused by an underlying disease, such as carcinoma of the gastric cardia or esophagus. Chagas disease is a parasitic infection that can induce secondary achalasia and has many cardiac manifestations.

Long-standing achalasia results in esophageal dilatation. This is often seen on a chest radiograph as a widened mediastinum with an air-fluid level. The classic sign is a dilated esophagus with smooth tapering at the LES, creating the "bird beak" appearance (Fig. C2.3). Other dynamic findings include loss of normal peristalsis.

Scleroderma: Scleroderma is a collagen vascular disease with multiorgan involvement; it is due to immunologic and inflammatory changes. Women are more

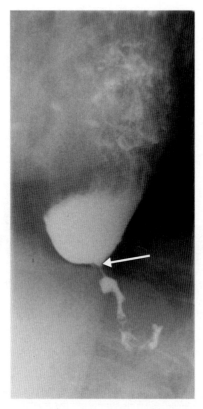

Fig. C2.3 Achalasia. Classic bird beak appearance due to severe narrowing of the LES, with severe dilatation of the proximal esophagus. Notice the mottled appearance (white arrow) due to retained gas, debris, and contrast above the air-fluid level representing contrast mixed with undigested food residing in the dilated esophagus which cannot easily pass through the LES.

commonly affected, at a 3:1 ratio, and the mean age of onset is 30 to 50 years. Scleroderma is usually classified as one of two types:

- Diffuse scleroderma: Diffuse scleroderma is more severe, with interstitial pulmonary fibrosis. It is associated with anti-topoisomerase 1 Ab (anti-Scl 70).
- CREST syndrome (calcinosis of skin, Raynaud phenomenon, esophageal dysmotility, sclerodactyly, and telangiectasia): CREST syndrome is the more benign course. It is associated with anti-centromere Ab.

The radiographic findings include a lack of primary peristalsis of the lower two-thirds of the esophagus, which is controlled by smooth muscle (the proximal one-third is striated muscle). Early in the course of disease, there is a patulous or widened LES, with or without a hiatal hernia (Fig. C2.4). Chronic reflux may lead to reflux esophagitis, which may result in a fusiform peptic stricture at the LES. Proximal to the stricture, the esophagus will be dilated but to a lesser degree than with achalasia. Complications from long-standing reflux esophagitis include Barrett esophagus and adenocarcinoma.

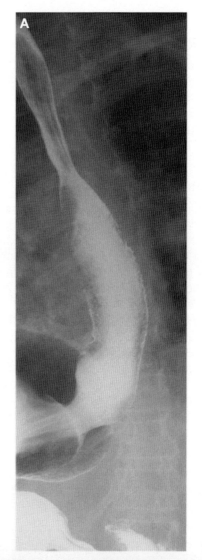

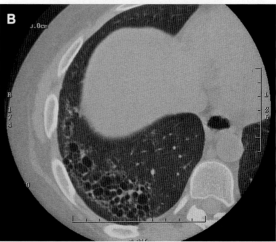

Fig. C2.4 Scleroderma. Esophagram shows the dilated esophagus with a patulous LES which leads to chronic reflux and ultimately strictures. Axial CT in the same patient shows the associated pulmonary fibrosis with honey combing in the lung bases as well as a dilated esophagus.

Diffuse esophageal spasm: Diffuse esophageal spasm is an esophageal motility disorder that can present with chest pain. Similar disorders include nutcracker esophagus and nonspecific esophageal motility disorder. Cardiac disease must be excluded because patients present with anginalike symptoms. Radiographic evaluation plays a lesser role because of the intermittent nature of these diseases. A barium swallow will reveal a classic "corkscrew" esophagus in 30% of the patients. Esophageal manometry remains the gold standard.

Esophageal cancer: Two different subtypes of esophageal cancer exist: squamous cell carcinoma (SCC), involving the proximal two-thirds of the esophagus (Figs. C2.5A,B), and adenocarcinoma, involving the lower one-third (Figs. C2.6A,B). The risk factors for SCC include smoking and alcohol use, and the risk factors for adenocarcinoma are a history of gastroesophageal reflux disease (GERD) and Barrett's esophagus. In the past, SCC was far more common than adenocarcinoma; however, this trend has changed significantly over the past few decades because of a higher incidence of GERD. Barium esophagography

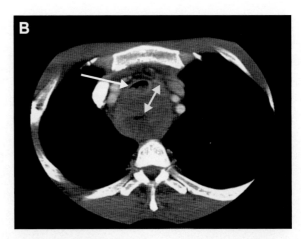

Fig. C2.5 (*continued*) Esophageal SCC. (B) CT shows the diffuse circumferential thickening of the upper esophagus (yellow arrow), invading the trachea (white arrow).

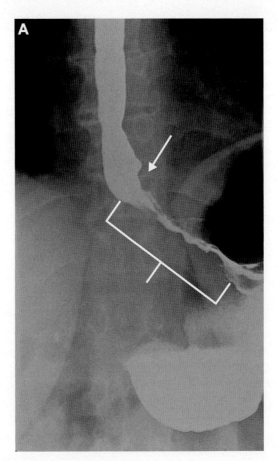

Fig. C2.6 Esophageal adenocarcinoma. (A) Upper GI examination demonstrating an abrupt narrowing of the distal esophagus with shouldering (white arrow) extending to the cardia of the stomach with irregular mucosal nodularity through the strictured segment (bracket).

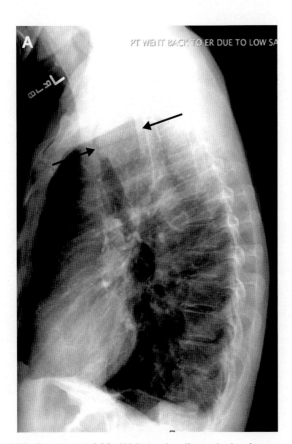

Fig. C2.5 Esophageal SCC. (A) Lateral radiograph showing mass in the middle mediastinum displacing the trachea anteriorly, with extension into the lumen (arrows).

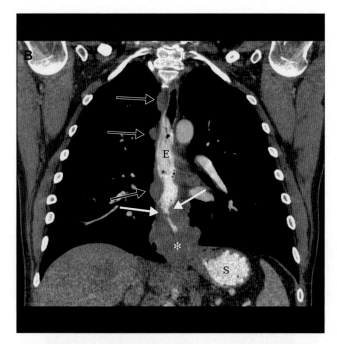

Fig. C2.6 (*continued*) Esophageal adenocarcinoma. (B) Coronal CT with oral and intravenous contrast demonstrates a large circumferential mass (*) centered at the lower esophagus extending to the GE junction. Oral contrast is visualized in the dilated esophagus (E). The mass narrows the esophageal lumen with shouldering proximally (white arrows). Oral contrast does reach the stomach (S). Due to lack of a surrounding serosa of the esophagus, early lymphatic spread occurs frequently; seen as the paraesophageal soft tissue masses representing mediastinal lymphadenopathy (black arrows) within the middle mediastinum.

remains useful for the initial noninvasive evaluation of esophageal complaints; however, endoscopy is the gold standard for diagnosis. A multimodal approach can be used, with endoscopic sonography for T staging and computed tomography (CT) for excluding unresectable disease or diagnosing distant metastasis. PET is more useful for assessing distant metastasis and restaging after neoadjuvant therapy.

DIFFERENTIAL DIAGNOSIS

Many other pathological conditions can result in dysphagia, including strictures, Schatzki rings, esophageal webs, foreign bodies, benign or malignant neoplasms, vascular compression, and mediastinal masses.

REFERENCES AND SUGGESTED READING

1. Levine MS, Rubesin SE. Update on esophageal radiology. *AJR.* 1990;155(5):933-941.

2. Marco G. Achalasia and other esophageal motility disorders. *J Gastrointest Surg.* 2001;15:703-707.

3. Kim TJ. Multimodality assessment of esophageal cancer: preoperative staging and monitoring of response to therapy. *RadioGraphics.* 2009;29:403-421.

CASE 3

PATIENT PRESENTATION

A 42-year-old man with multiple episodes of vomiting and retching presented with severe epigastric and chest pain; he had no cardiac risk factors and normal electrocardiography results.

CLINICAL SUSPICION

Boerhaave's syndrome

IMAGING MODALITY OF CHOICE

A chest radiograph should be the initial imaging study when evaluating patients with chest pain, regardless of whether the source is believed to be cardiac or noncardiac. The presence of air within the mediastinum, known as pneumomediastinum, would indicate a noncardiac process originating from either the esophagus or the lungs. Signs of pneumomediastinum on a chest radiograph are included in Table C3.1.

Many patients with chest pain are not initially suspected of having esophageal perforation and will undergo a standard CT of the chest, which will be more sensitive for pneumomediastinum than a chest radiograph (Fig. C3.1). Fluoroscopic water-soluble contrast esophagography has been the imaging modality of choice for esophageal perforation because extravasation of oral contrast into the mediastinum or pleural space is pathognomonic for perforation. The limitations of fluoroscopic esophagography include difficulty performing the examination in seriously ill patients, the need to transport the patient to a fluoroscopic suite, and potential false-negative results. To improve diagnostic capability for the detection of esophageal perforations, if no gross perforation is identified on initial studies performed with water-soluble agents, many advocate subsequent use of barium to detect subtle leaks that are more likely to be visualized with a high-density contrast agent.

To expedite the diagnosis and minimize the number of examinations that need to be performed, CT esophagram protocols can be performed in several different ways. At our institution, an initial noncontrast examination of the

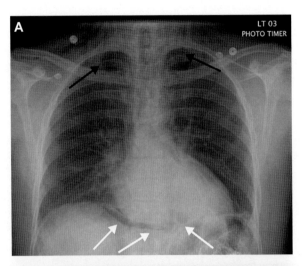

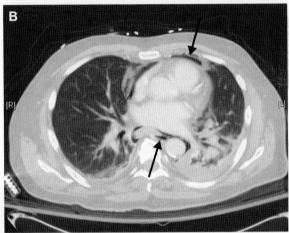

Fig. C3.1 Pneumomediastinum. (A) Frontal chest radiograph demonstrating linear lucencies within the upper mediastinum and neck (black arrows) as well as the "continuous diaphragm" (white arrows) consistent with pneumomediastinum. (B) Same patient as chest radiograph demonstrating how visualizing pneumomediastinum on a CT chest is much easier. Air is tracking around the heart, esophagus, and aorta (back arrows). This was iatrogenic from endoscopic balloon dilatation of an esophageal stricture.

chest is performed as the baseline, followed by a CT of the chest performed immediately after the patient swallows 1 cup of water-soluble contrast. Intravenous contrast can be added to the second scan if needed.

DIFFERENTIAL DIAGNOSIS

Esophageal perforation is an uncommon but potentially life-threatening event. The most common cause is iatrogenic perforation associated with endoscopy and thoracic surgery, which accounts for more than 50% of perforations. Other etiologies include idiopathic, foreign body, and traumatic perforations.

Table C3.1 Signs of Pneumomediastinum

- Linear streaks of lucency in the mediastinum and cervical soft tissues.
- "Continuous Diaphragm"–linear extrapleural air collection outlining the diaphragm.
- "V" sign of Naclerio–sharply marginated area of lucency at the left paraspinal location above the diaphragm.

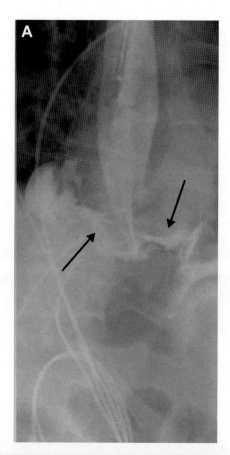

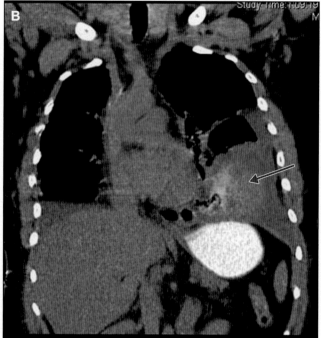

Boerhaave's syndrome refers to the spontaneous rupture of the esophagus secondary to violent episodes of retching or vomiting. This involves a transmural or full thickness tear of the esophageal wall, typically posteriorly near the left diaphragmatic crus. Radiography may reveal pneumomediastinum, a left-sided pneumothorax, or a left pleural effusion (Fig. C3.2).

In contrast to Boerhaave's syndrome, Mallory-Weiss syndrome refers to partial or nontransmural tears of the esophageal wall. This may have a similar clinical presentation because it usually occurs after prolonged and forceful vomiting. However, because this is only a partial or nontransmural tear, it will not be radiographically detectable because no pneumomediastinum or contrast leak should be present.

DIFFERENTIAL DIAGNOSIS

First and foremost, whenever chest pain is the chief complaint, regardless of associated symptoms, cardiac etiologies must first be excluded. Other potential causes of acute noncardiac chest pain include disorders of the esophagus, including gastroesophageal reflux or motility disorders; pulmonary disorders including pneumonia, pneumothorax or pulmonary embolism; and musculoskeletal pain.

Radiologically, a chest radiograph with pneumomediastinum would be suggestive of esophageal perforation in the proper clinical context. More commonly, pneumomediastinum occurs through a sequence of events known as the Macklin effect, which includes: (1) alveolar rupture, (2) air dissection along the interstitium of the bronchovascular sheath, and (3) free air reaching the mediastinum. This occurs not uncommonly with asthmatics, but can also occur from any form of barotrauma including forceful illicit drug inhalation, scuba diving, severe coughing, or in patients who are on assisted respiratory devices.

REFERENCES AND SUGGESTED READING

1. *ACR Appropriateness Criteria: ACR Practice Guideline for the Performance of Esophagrams and Upper Gastrointestinal Examinations in Adults.* Revised 2008.

2. Swanson JO. Usefulness of high-density barium for detection of leaks after esophagogastrectomy, total gastrectomy, and total laryngectomy. *AJR.* 2003;181:415-420.

3. Farhan F. Helical CT esophagography for the evaluation of suspected esophageal perforation or rupture. *AJR.* 2004; 182(5):1177-1179.

Fig. C3.2 Boerhaave's syndrome. (A) Esophagram through NG tube using water-soluble contrast show the distal esophageal perforation with contrast leaking into the mediastinum and pleural spaces bilaterally (back arrows). (B) Coronal CT utilizing oral contrast with perforation distally resulting in extravasation of contrast into the left pleural space (black arrow).

CASE 4

PATIENT PRESENTATION

A 58-year-old man presented with severe left upper quadrant and left chest pain and retching without vomiting; a nasogastric tube could not be inserted.

CLINICAL SUSPICION

Gastric obstruction or volvulus

IMAGING MODALITY OF CHOICE

An initial evaluation may include radiographs of the abdomen or chest. Preferably, a 2-view chest or acute abdominal series should be ordered. The latter includes both supine and upright views of the abdomen to identify gravity-dependent free air and air-fluid levels.

In the past, a diagnosis of gastric volvulus was made with an upper GI series with barium or water-soluble contrast, but the relative availability and timeliness of CT with multiplanar reconstructions may be more suitable in the acute setting. A CT of the chest and abdomen should be performed to image the entire region of interest, preferably with intravenous contrast (a lack of normal enhancement of the gastric mucosa indicates ischemia) and oral contrast. An advantage of an upper GI series is its ability to grade the degree of obstruction.

> **Gastric volvulus:** Gastric volvulus is relatively rare and is an uncommon site of volvulus of the gastrointestinal tract. It is seen in children and adults, but it is far more common in the elderly. The Borchardt triad (acute onset epigastric pain, intractable retching, and an inability to pass a nasogastric tube) is highly suggestive of gastric volvulus. Delays in diagnosis and definitive surgical treatment can lead to serious complications such as gastric ischemia, perforation, internal hemorrhage, splenic rupture, and aspiration pneumonia. The nonoperative mortality rate reaches 80%.

FINDINGS

Gastric volvulus is subdivided into two subtypes, organoaxial and mesenteroaxial (Fig. C4.1). Organoaxial volvulus is far more common, accounting for almost two-thirds of cases; however, mesenteroaxial appears to be more common in children.

- Organoaxial volvulus occurs when the stomach rotates along the long axis (line made from intersecting the gastroesophageal junction with the pylorus) and becomes obstructed. This results in the greater curvature being displaced superiorly and the lesser curvature inferiorly.

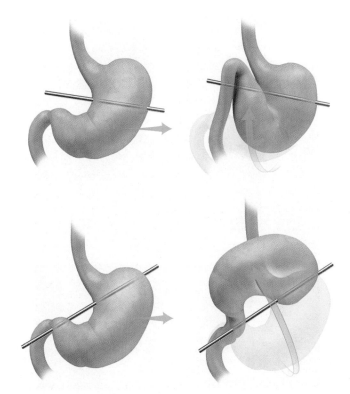

Fig. C4.1 Gastric volvulus may be either mesenteroaxial (top) or organoaxial (bottom).

- Mesenteroaxial volvulus occurs when the stomach rotates along its short axis, with subsequent displacement of the antrum or pylorus above the gastroesophageal junction.

Radiographic Findings

Radiographs may demonstrate a large retrocardiac opacity with two separate air-fluid levels. If completely obstructed, there will be a relative paucity of gas in the small bowel.

An upper gastrointestinal series will reveal the abnormal orientation of the stomach and the degree of intraluminal obstruction or gross perforation. If high-grade obstruction is present, no contrast may enter the stomach. "Beaking," or rapid tapering in the shape of a bird's beak, may be seen at the point of volvulus (twisting).

Multidetector row CT, especially with coronal reformations, will demonstrate the abnormal position of the stomach and the size, location, and extent of commonly associated diaphragmatic defects (Fig. C4.2). More important, CT can illustrate complications such as gastric ischemia, pneumatosis, or perforation.

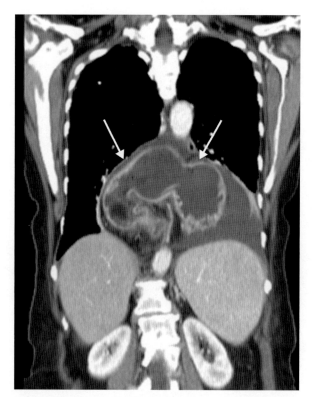

Fig. C4.2 Organoaxial volvulus. Coronal CT image of the chest/upper abdomen shows an organoaxial gastric volvulus, with the greater curvature along the superior border (white arrows).

DIFFERENTIAL DIAGNOSIS

Large sliding hiatal hernias can manifest on a chest radiograph as retrocardiac masses, which can have an air-fluid level. These usually only contain the gastroesophageal junction or cardia and not the entire stomach as in a volvulus (Fig. C4.3). In addition, most will be incidentally detected. Other conditions that can present as retrocardiac masses with an air-fluid level include paraesophageal hernia, epiphrenic diverticulum, large infected bronchogenic or cardiophrenic cyst, mediastinal abscess, and postsurgical changes after a prior esophagectomy with gastric pull-through.

Besides volvulus, several other entities can result in gastric obstruction. The term gastric outlet obstruction can have several etiologies that result in narrowing and obstruction of the gastric antrum or pylorus which inhibit normal empting of the stomach. This process can be the result of tumors or infectious/inflammatory processes such as peptic ulcer disease or Crohn's disease. The imaging appearance across all modalities is a grossly dilated stomach with narrowing at the antral region (Fig. C4.4).

Clinically, just as in the previous case, cardiac causes must be first eliminated. A similar differential of noncardiac chest pain would be included as well as well as epigastric and left upper quadrant pain including, gastritis, peptic ulcer disease, pancreatitis, and/or pyelonephritis or nephrolithiasis of the left kidney.

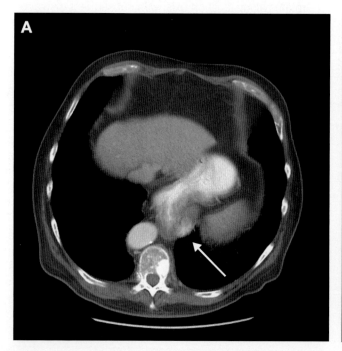
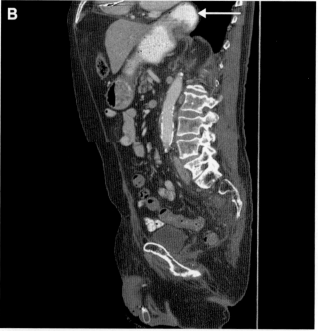

Fig. C4.3 (A) Axial CT demonstrates a large hiatal hernia (white arrow). (B) Sagittal reconstruction of the same CT demonstrates the hernia through widened esophageal hiatus of the diaphragm (white arrow).

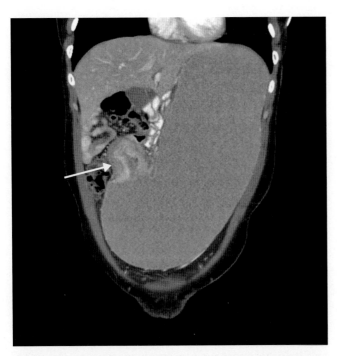

Fig. C4.4 Gastric outlet obstruction. Coronal CT image with intravenous contrast demonstrating a very distended gastric body. No oral contrast was given, with all this fluid representing prior swallowed fluid. Not shown was dependent solid food debris layering posteriorly in the fundus. Focal wall thickening of the antrum (white arrow) is noted which was found to be due a large malignant ulcer from gastric adenocarcinoma.

REFERENCES AND SUGGESTED READING

1. Miller DL, Pasquale MD, Seneca RP. Gastric volvulus in the pediatric population. *Arch Surg.* 1991;126(9):1146-1149.

2. Peterson, CM. Volvulus of the gastrointestinal tract: appearances at multimodality imaging. *RadioGraphics.* 2009;29:1281-1293.

CASE 5

PATIENT PRESENTATION

A 47-year-old man with a 2-week history of dull, gnawing, intermittent epigastric pain that was progressively worsening. The patient was self-medicating his chronic right shoulder pain with ibuprofen as needed.

CLINICAL SUSPICION

Gastritis or gastric or duodenal ulcers

IMAGING MODALITY OF CHOICE

The choice of test to diagnose peptic ulcer disease may depend on the clinical setting. Epigastric pain may be seen in the setting of cardiopulmonary disease; thus, as always, the initial cardiopulmonary workup tests should be performed before the radiologic workup. In the acute setting of severe epigastric pain, an initial radiographic workup may include an acute abdominal series to identify free air from perforation. Free air or pneumoperitoneum has a variable appearance that depends on the position of the patient, with free air rising to the nondependent portion of the peritoneal cavity. For that reason, upright chest radiographs will reveal subdiaphragmatic air as crescentic lucencies (Fig. C5.1); decubitus views will reveal air along the paracolic gutter, which becomes nondependent in this position. Free air on supine films is more difficult to detect because it rises to the anterior abdominal wall and therefore will not be tangential to x-rays. Only when larger volumes of air are present are both the inner and outer bowel walls visible. The inner mucosal wall is always visible, but the outer wall is not because there is no interface between the surrounding peritoneal fat and bowel. The double wall sign, also known as Rigler's sign, is indicative of pneumoperitoneum. Occasionally, the falciform ligament can be visualized when free air outlines both margins of the ligament, resulting in the so-called football sign.

Alternatively, CT of the abdomen and pelvis with intravenous and oral contrast can be performed, especially when the cause of epigastric pain is not readily evident. If there is a possibility of perforation of the gastrointestinal tract, water-soluble contrast (eg, gastroview, omnipaque, or visipaque) should be used in place of barium. Barium is a nonabsorbable substance that can cause chemical peritonitis and remain in the peritoneum indefinitely. The advantages of CT include rapid acquisition time; high sensitivity for pneumoperitoneum; small, contained perforations; and alternative diagnoses. The disadvantages include limited evaluation of the gastric mucosa and frequency of underdistention of the gastric lumen, limiting evaluation of gastric wall thickening.

In the less acute or chronic outpatient setting, an upper gastrointestinal series may be performed as a less invasive test than an endoscopic gastroduodenoscopy. An upper gastrointestinal series consists of a double-contrast evaluation (thick consistency barium and effervescent air crystals) to distend the esophagus, stomach, and proximal small bowel as well as to thinly coat the mucosal surface, followed by single-contrast barium (thin, watery consistency) to identify distention and peristalsis (Fig. C5.2).

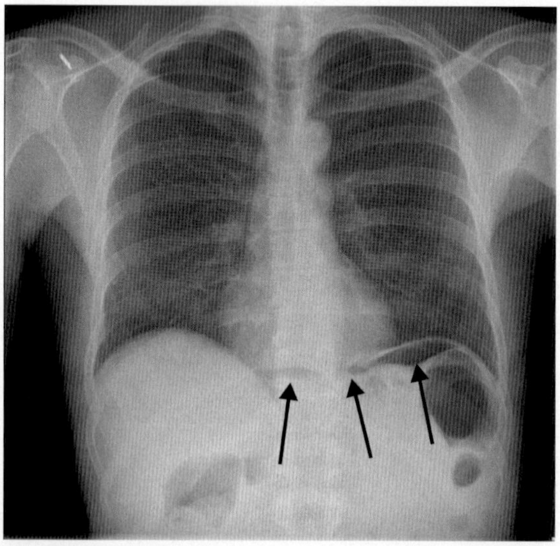

Fig. C5.1 Pneumoperitoneum. Upright chest radiograph demonstrating pneumoperitoneum with subdiaphragmatic free air (arrows) due to perforated duodenal ulcer found at exploratory laparotomy.

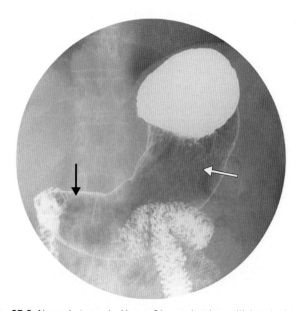

Fig. C5.2 Normal stomach. Upper GI examination utilizing double contrast demonstrating normal contours and mucosa of the stomach. Normal folds are visualized (white arrow). Areae gastricae are normal features of the gastric mucosa producing the fine reticular pattern (black arrow). This image was obtained with the patient in the supine position with the liquid barium layering dependently in the most posterior portion of the stomach, the fundus.

Other tests that test for presence of *Helicobacter pylori*, one of the causes for gastritis, are the nuclear medicine C-14 urea breath test, which is based on the principle that *H pylori* produces urease that breaks down the radioactive urea into C-14 containing CO_2, which can be collected and quantified. Alternative noninvasive tests include the *H pylori* stool antigen test and serum antibodies for *H pylori*; however, antibodies may be positive up to 3 years after eradication.

FINDINGS
Gastritis

Gastritis is inflammation of the stomach; however, it includes numerous disorders with different etiologies, histological types, and clinical presentations. Different forms of gastritis include:

- *H pylori* gastritis (most common)
- Erosive or NSAID-induced gastritis
- Phlegmonous (acute bacterial) gastritis
- Emphysematous gastritis
- Granulomatous gastritis
- Eosinophilic gastritis
- Atrophic gastritis

All forms of gastritis have variable radiological presentations, but in general, they share several common features: thickening of gastric folds, scalloping or nodularity of antral folds, and erosions surrounded by radiolucent halos of edematous, elevated mucosa. CT can reveal a thickened gastric wall (>5 mm) and thickened rugae, with decreased attenuation of submucosa related to edema (Fig. C5.3).

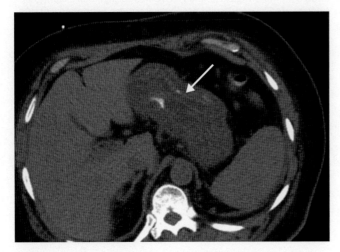

Fig. C5.3 Gastritis. Axial CT image without intravenous contrast, but with oral contrast demonstrates diffusely thickened gastric folds. The oral contrast can faintly be seen between the thickened folds (white arrow).

Ulcers

An ulcer is a focal area of mucosal disruption that penetrates through the muscularis mucosae. Benign gastric ulcers are predominantly caused by *H pylori* infections (approximately two-thirds); the remaining are mostly due to nonsteroidal anti-inflammatory drugs (NSAIDs). On the other hand, 95% of duodenal ulcers are caused by *H pylori* infections. Approximately 20% of gastric ulcers are multiple, whereas multiple postbulbar duodenal ulcers are unusual and raise suspicion for Zollinger-Ellison syndrome.

Gastric ulcers can usually be categorized as benign or malignant, but ultimately, any gastric ulcer identified by imaging would need to be evaluated by endoscopy and most likely a biopsy for definitive diagnosis. Imaging features of both benign and malignant ulcers are included in Table C5.1. Most benign gastric ulcers are located on the lesser curvature or posterior wall (Fig. C5.4). NSAID-induced benign ulcers have a propensity for being located on the greater curvature, making location less reliable for distinguishing benign from malignant. The major complications of ulcers are bleeding, gastric outlet obstruction, and perforation (Fig. C5.5). Bleeding can occur in up to 20% of patients and can present as melena, hematemesis, or hematochezia.

DIFFERENTIAL DIAGNOSIS

Clinically, many disorders can have similar symptoms including functional dyspepsia, GERD, gastroenteritis, esophagitis, cholecystitis, cholangitis, biliary colic, acute coronary syndrome, and pancreatitis.

On imaging, thickened gastric folds can be found with gastritis, lymphoma, Ménétrier disease, and gastric varices (Fig. C5.6).

Table C5.1 Gastric Ulcer Characteristics

Benign
• Smooth, round/ovoid barium collection/ring shadow
• Hampton's line or smooth ulcer collar
• Smooth, straight folds radiating to ulcer's edge
• Projects outside expected luminal contour

Malignant
• Irregular-shaped, abnormally surfaced ulcer
• Mucosal nodularity at ulcer's edge
• Lobulated, enlarged, club-shaped, or pencil point-shaped folds
• Projects into mass (either inside or outside expected luminal contour)

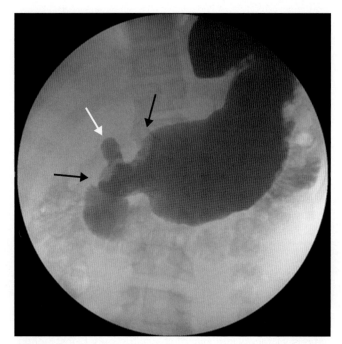

Fig. C5.4 Benign gastric ulcer. Water-soluble contrast upper GI examination showing smooth ovoid ulcer (white arrow) collection as well as Hampton's line with smooth ulcer collar (black arrows) of biopsy-proven benign ulcer.

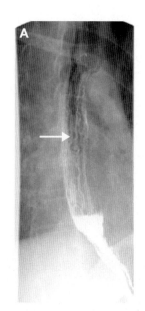

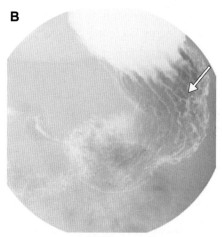

Fig. C5.6 Varices. Double-contrast upper GI examination demonstrates prominent gastric folds as well as serpiginous esophageal folds related to gastric and esophageal varices (white arrows) due to portal hypertension.

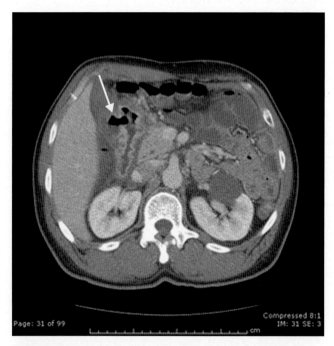

Fig. C5.5 Ruptured duodenal ulcer. Axial CT with intravenous contrast demonstrates a focal disruption of the lateral wall of the second portion of the duodenum with a contained perforation with extraluminal air-fluid level (white arrow). Because the duodenum has portions that are either intraperitoneal or retroperitoneal, depending on the location of the ulcer, perforation could result in pneumoperitoneum or pneumoretroperitoneum.

REFERENCES AND SUGGESTED READING

1. Rubesin SE, Levine MS. Double-contrast upper gastrointestinal radiography: a pattern approach for diseases of the stomach. *Radiology*. 2008;246:33-48.

2. Brant WE, Helms CA. *Fundamentals of Diagnostic Radiology*. 3rd ed. Philadelphia, PA: Lippincott Williams & Wilkins; 2006.

CASE 6

PATIENT PRESENTATION

A 62-year-old woman with a history of right breast cancer treated 2 years earlier with mastectomy and adjuvant chemoradiation therapy presented with progressive nausea, occasional vomiting, a 15-lb unintentional weight loss, and anorexia.

CLINICAL SUSPICION

Gastric cancer

IMAGING MODALITY OF CHOICE

Upper endoscopy has mostly supplanted the routine use of upper gastrointestinal series for initial diagnosis, largely because of the ability to confirm diagnosis with biopsy, but upper gastrointestinal series are still a useful, inexpensive, safe, and noninvasive diagnostic tool.

Multidetector CT has remained the modality of choice for the preoperative staging of gastric cancer and for follow-up. Several newer staging techniques include multiphase dynamic imaging during the arterial and later portal venous phases. The arterial phase is the most useful for determining the arterial supply and the depth of tumor invasion; it is similar to endoscopic ultrasound (EUS). The portal venous phase is the most adequate for detecting distant metastasis. In addition, these techniques use a neutral oral contrast, such as water or a 0.1% barium suspension (VoLumen), for the optimal evaluation of mucosal and mural enhancement, and multiplanar reconstructions and 3-D processing. Gastric distension may be optimal with the use of negative contrast, and gas-producing crystals.

The combination of FDG-PET and CT is useful in the preoperative staging of stomach cancer and in restaging after treatment, but it is still limited in initial locoregional staging.

FINDINGS

Gastric carcinoma is the fourth most common malignancy worldwide and a common cause of cancer mortality. The incidence varies highly across different geographic locations, with much higher rates (5 times higher) seen in Japan, Finland, Chile, and Iceland than in the United States. One reason for a large difference in mortality rate and incidence between developed and undeveloped countries is that gastric cancer is one of a few cancers with can develop due to an infection (H pylori), and therefore without treatment of the underlying infection, more cancers can develop. The mortality rate is dismal because most patients are not diagnosed until the later stages; the 5-year survival rate is 20%.

Adenocarcinoma is the most common malignant gastric neoplasm, comprising more than 90% of cases. Other malignant gastric neoplasms include lymphoma, mucosa-associated lymphoid tissue (MALT) lymphoma, GIST, leiomyosarcoma, carcinoid, small cell carcinoma, and metastasis (lungs, breast, melanoma, colon, prostate, and pancreas). The risk factors for gastric adenocarcinoma include H pylori infection, adenomas, polyposis syndromes, pernicious anemia, atrophic gastritis, and prior partial gastrectomy (Billroth II>I).

Gastric neoplasms have several different radiological presentations. Approximately one-third present as a polypoid mass extending into the gastric lumen, either papillary or broad based (Fig. C6.1). Another one-third present as malignant ulcers, previously characterized in Table C5.1. The remaining tumors present as scirrhous carcinoma or superficial spreading. Scirrhous carcinoma is a cause of "linitis plastica" or "water bottle stomach." These terms describe a narrowed and nondistensible stomach due to diffuse infiltration of the gastric wall with poorly differentiated or undifferentiated neoplastic cells (Fig. C6.2).

Gastric cancer usually spreads by local invasion through the gastric wall into the perigastric fat and adjacent organs, via the lymph nodes, or by seeding the peritoneal cavity. The primary role of CT in imaging of gastric cancer is staging. Newer CT techniques, however, have improved T staging, which is now comparable to EUS. A CT criterion for local staging closely mirrors the American Joint Committee on Cancer's TNM staging system.

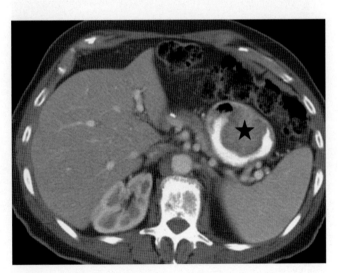

Fig. C6.1 Gastric adenocarcinoma. Axial CT of the abdomen with IV and oral contrast demonstrates a round polypoid mass (*) within the stomach.

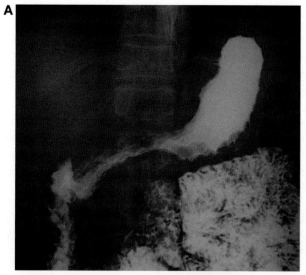

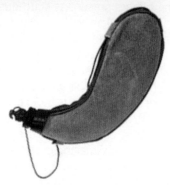

AJCC T Staging

- T1: Tumor invades the lamina propria or submucosa
- T2: Tumor invades the muscularis propria or subserosa
- T3: Tumor penetrates the serosa, with no invasion of adjacent structures
- T4: Adjacent organs involved

CT Staging

- T1: Nontransmural enhancement; inner or middle wall enhancement only
- T2: Transmural enhancement with smooth outer wall
- T3: Transmural enhancement with irregular wall or reticular or linear perigastric opacities
- T4: Extension to adjacent organs

The local lymph nodes that are commonly involved include the perigastric, gastrohepatic, gastrocolic, celiac, and para-aortic nodes. A Virchow node is a metastatic, enlarged left supraclavicular node that receives drainage from lymph vessels in the abdomen. Hematogenous spread is usually to the liver. Intraperitoneal spread or seeding can result in peritoneal carcinomatosis or a Krukenberg ovarian tumor (Fig. C6.3), the original name given for ovarian masses from "drop" gastric metastasis.

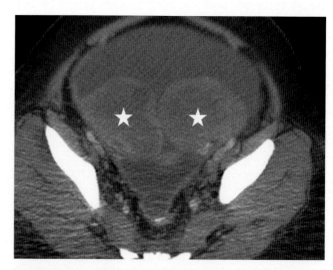

Fig. C6.2 Linitis plastica. (A) Upper GI radiograph demonstrating the nondistensible stomach with a water bottle shape consistent with linitis plastica. (B) Same patient with axial CT showing the thickened nondistensible stomach (white arrow) due to a scirrhous carcinoma.

Fig. C6.3 Krukenberg tumors. Axial CT of the pelvis with large bilateral adnexal masses (*) as well as a large volume of ascites due to metastatic gastric cancer consistent with Krukenberg tumors, gastric cancer metastatic to ovaries.

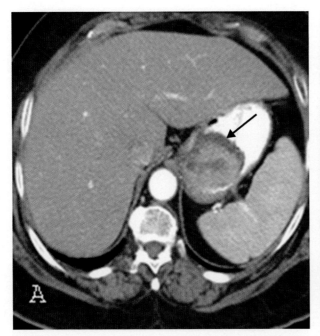 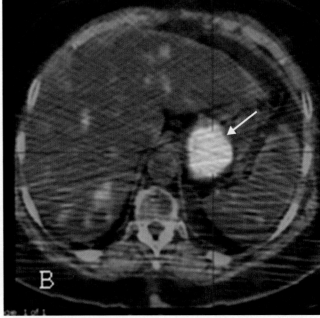

Fig. C6.4 Gastric lymphoma. Axial CT postcontrast (A) and PET/CT axial fusion (B) images shows an endoluminal polypoid mass (arrows) within the cardia that is FDG avid. This appearance is nonspecific from other gastric malignancies.

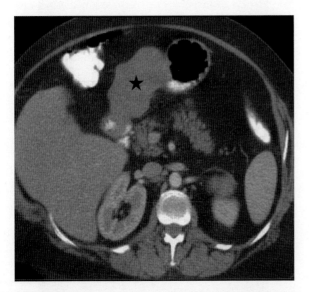

Fig. C6.5 Gastrointestinal stromal tumor. Axial CT with contrast demonstrates an exophytic GIST arising from the antrum (*).

Lymphoma: Lymphoma comprises approximately 2% of gastric malignancies. Most cases are non-Hodgkin's B-cell type. Infection with *H pylori* is a risk factor for MALT gastric lymphoma, which has a better prognosis than the B-cell type because of a more indolent course. Lymphoma has a wide variety of presentations, but marked wall thickening is characteristic of gastric lymphoma; this thickening does not result in luminal narrowing (Fig. C6.4).

Gastrointestinal stromal tumors (GISTs): GISTs are the most common mesenchymal neoplasm from the gastrointestinal tract. GISTs express KIT (CD117), a tyrosine kinase receptor; this distinguishes them from other mesenchymal tumors, such as leiomyomas, leiomyosarcomas, schwannomas, and neurofibromas. These tumors are highly receptive to treatment with KIT tyrosine kinase inhibitors such as imatinib. Common radiologic features include a large predominantly exophytic mass, heterogeneous enhancement, and little lymphadenopathy (Fig. C6.5.).

REFERENCES AND SUGGESTED READING

1. Hargunani R, Maclachlan J. Cross-sectional imaging of gastric neoplasia. *Clin Radiol.* 2009;64:420-429.

2. Van Cutsem E. The diagnosis and management of gastric cancer: expert discussion and recommendations from the 12th ESMO/World Congress on Gastrointestinal Cancer, Barcelona, 2010. *Ann Oncol.* 2011;22(suppl 5):v1-v9.

3. Lim JS. CT and PET in stomach cancer: preoperative staging and monitoring of response to therapy. *RadioGraphics.* 2006;26:143-156.

4. Canon C. *McGraw-Hill Specialty Board Review: Radiology.* New York: McGraw-Hill Companies; 2010.

5. Fishman EK, Urban BA, Hruban RH, et al. CT of the stomach: spectrum of disease. *RadioGraphics.* 1996;16:1035-1054.

CASE 7

PATIENT PRESENTATION

A 32-year-old man presented with nausea, vomiting, generalized abdominal pain, and distention; he had a history of open appendectomy. His abdomen was tympanic to percussion, with high-pitched bowel sounds.

CLINICAL SUSPICION

Small bowel obstruction (SBO)

IMAGING MODALITY OF CHOICE

The choice of imaging modality for a suspected SBO varies among experts and is based on the clinical presentation. Abdominal radiography may be the first modality used because it is relative easy and inexpensive; however, its effectiveness at diagnosing SBO ranges from 30% to 90%. An important early differentiation in SBO is complete or high grade versus low grade, equivocal, or normal. Common radiographic findings include multiple dilated loops more than 2.5 cm in caliber, multiple air-fluid levels, and collapsed distal bowel. Two specific radiographic findings on upright plain films that are predictive of severe SBO are differential air-fluid level heights in the same small bowel loop and a mean air-fluid level width of 2.5 cm or greater (Fig. C7.1).

Standard multidetector CT of the abdomen and pelvis with intravenous contrast and multiplanar reformatting is the American College of Radiology (ACR)'s Appropriateness Criteria Committee's recommended imaging modality. Oral contrast is no longer believed to be necessary in routine cases because of the delay in diagnosis. Intraluminal fluid in the obstructed segment acts as a natural neutral contrast agent, facilitating visualization of the bowel wall. The CT criteria for SBO include dilated SB loops greater than 2.5 cm, with air-fluid levels. A helpful but nonpathognomonic sign is the "small bowel feces" sign, which refers to small gas bubbles intermixed with particulate matter in the dilated loops of small bowel, usually proximal to the transition point. CT can accurately confirm the diagnosis; it can also characterize the severity, identify the cause and the transition point, and most important, identify any complications (Figs. C7.2 and C7.3). Table C7.1 lists the signs of bowel ischemia. Mesenteric ischemia can be due to a variety of causes including strangulating obstruction or volvulus (Fig. C7.4), as well as arterial occlusion due to embolic disease or thrombosis at sites of atherosclerosis, venous occlusion, or hypoperfusion associated with nonvascular disease. Mesenteric ischemia has a high mortality rate.

As a problem-solving tool for partial or low-grade small bowel obstructions, small bowel follow through exams may be performed. This entails administration of oral contrast

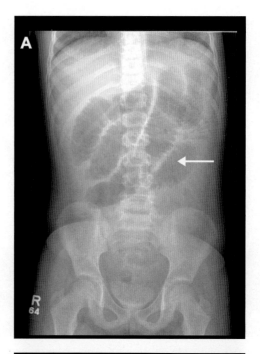

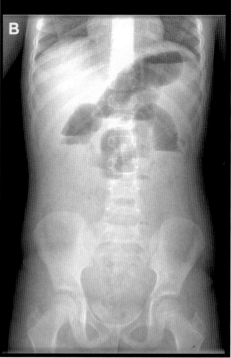

Fig. C7.1 Small-bowel obstruction. (A) AP supine radiograph of the abdomen with SBO with multiple dilated loops. In contrast to large-bowel obstruction (LBO), notice the more central position and mucosal folds extending completely across the loop of bowel, representative of the valvulae conniventes (white arrow). (B) Upright AP radiograph of the abdomen of same patient showing multiple differential air-fluid levels with dilated loops of bowel. Given enough time, with a high grade SBO, the distal bowel including the colon and rectum will be devoid of air as in this case.

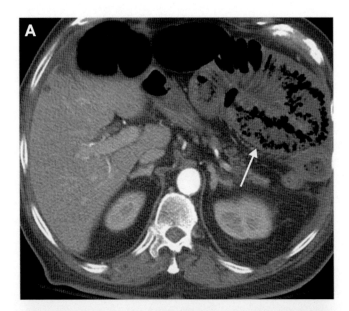

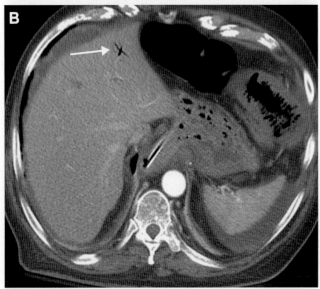

Fig. C7.2 Pneumatosis intestinalis. (A) Axial postcontrast CT images showing pneumatosis intestinalis (white arrow) of the proximal jejunum. Air can be seen along the nondependent wall, but never along the dependent wall as visualized posteriorly in this case. (B) Images slightly superior demonstrate a small amount of linear air collection within the liver representative of portal venous air (white arrow).

with intermittent spot overhead radiographs or direct fluoroscopy to evaluate the contrast transit through the bowel, looking for focal narrowing or strictures. Limitations include overlap of bowel segments and incomplete distention of the small bowel. Other imaging techniques advocated by the ACR Appropriateness Criteria for intermittent or low grade SBO include CT or MR enterography or enteroclysis. Enteroclysis studies are slightly more invasiveness requiring placement of an enteric tube to inject contrast directly

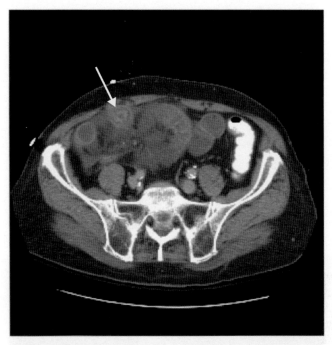

Fig. C7.3 Bowel ischemia. Small bowel ischemia with diffusely thickened bowel wall. Notice target sign of end on bowel (arrow).

into the small bowel which results in greater intraluminal pressure and distention of the bowel to visualize focal narrowing and strictures.

DIFFERENTIAL DIAGNOSIS
Clinical Differential

Adhesions: Adhesions are the most common cause of SBO; most of them are postoperative. Adhesions are usually not identified on imaging but instead are a diagnosis of exclusion.

Hernia: Hernias are also a common cause of SBO. External hernias usually occur in congenital or surgically weakened defects in the abdominal or pelvic wall and are commonly clinically apparent (Fig. C7.5). Internal hernias occur through defects in the mesentery or peritoneum.

Table C7.1 Signs of Strangulation

- Thickening and increased attenuation of bowel wall
- Lack of wall, asymmetric or delayed enhancement
- Halo or "target sign"
- Pneumotosis intestinalis
- Gas in portal vein
- Congestion or hemorrhage of attached mesentery

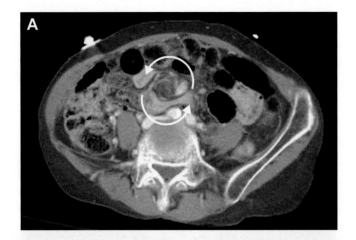

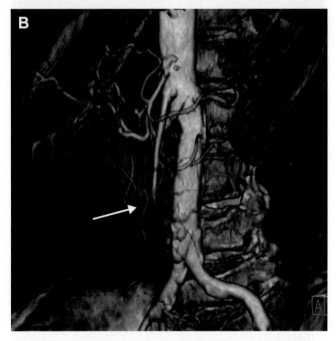

Fig. C7.4 (A) Small bowel volvulus. Axial CT postcontrast showing the "whirl" sign from mesenteric torsion due to the twisting of the mesentery (arrows). This resulted in acute mesenteric ischemia with partial infarction of the small bowel. At surgery an ileal duplication cyst was found as the lead point for the volvulus. (B) Mesenteric ischemia. 3-D reconstruction from the same patient with mesenteric torsion, showing abrupt occlusion of the SMA (white arrow).

Crohn's disease: SBO in Crohn's disease can occur in several ways, including acute inflammatory, cicatricial stenosis from long-standing disease, and secondary to postoperative adhesions, strictures, and incisional hernias.

Mass: Primary neoplasms rarely cause SBO. Metastasis to the small bowel is more common and may occur

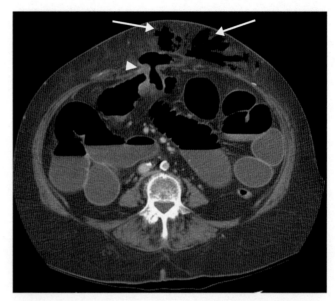

Fig. C7.5 SBO from ventral hernia. Axial CT with small bowel obstruction due to ventral hernia. This ventral hernia has a narrow neck (arrowhead) and could not be reduced manually. The incarcerated segment of bowel perforated resulting in the subcutaneous air throughout the anterior wall (arrows).

hematogenously or by direct spread from peritoneal carcinomatosis.

Intussusception: A condition in which a part of the gastrointestinal tract has invaginated into another section. Intussusception is usually found in children and most commonly is ileum invaginating into the ascending colon (ileocolic). In adults, intussusception may occur and be due to a lead point such as a polyp or other mass. The classic sign of bowel-within-bowel, with or without mesenteric fat and vessels, resulting in the "bulls-eye sign" is pathognomonic. In children, intussusceptions may be imaged initially with ultrasound, which involves no radiation to the child. It can also be imaged and treated with air or contrast enemas. Transient intussusceptions in adults are commonly incidentally identified in the proximal jejunum, but should not be confused with pathologic cases that result in obstruction.

Others: Radiation enteritis, hematomas, vascular causes (mesenteric ischemia or small mesenteric vein thrombosis), foreign body (bezoar), and gallstone ileus.

Closed-loop obstruction: A closed-loop obstruction occurs at 2 points, usually with mesenteric involvement, and is often overlooked because of a lack of dilatation of the upstream proximal bowel loops; it should not be missed because it tends to progress rapidly to ischemia. The involved bowel segment may be completely filled with fluid, with no air-fluid level. A

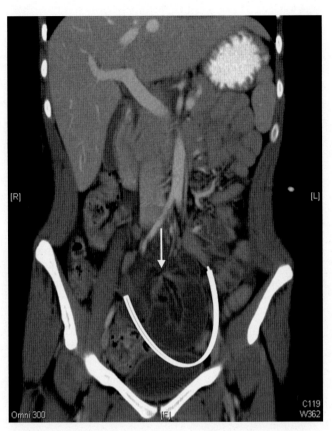

Fig. C7.6 Closed loop small bowel obstruction. Coronal CT with closed loop obstruction due to adhesions. Notice the U-shaped loop of bowel beaking converging to same point (arrow).

characteristic C- or U-shaped bowel configuration is often present, with a "beaking sign" at the point of torsion or obstruction (Fig. C7.6).

Imaging Differential

The differential diagnosis includes multiple air-distended bowel loops: an adynamic or paralytic ileus, aerophagia, or a large bowel obstruction.

REFERENCES AND SUGGESTED READING

1. ACR Appropriateness Criteria. Suspected small-bowel obstruction.
2. Lappas JC. Abdominal radiography findings in small-bowel obstruction: relevance to triage for additional diagnostic imaging. *AJR.* 2001;176:167-174.
3. Boudiaf M. CT evaluation of small bowel obstruction. *RadioGraphics.* 2001;21:613-624.
4. Silva AC. Small bowel obstruction: what to look for. *Radio–Graphics.* 2009;29:423-439.

CASE 8

PATIENT PRESENTATION

A 24-year-old man presented with acute-onset abdominal pain that was localized to the right lower quadrant and was associated with fever and leukocytosis.

CLINICAL SUSPICION

Acute appendicitis

IMAGING MODALITY OF CHOICE

Acute appendicitis is a common cause of acute abdominal pain and requires surgery. Several imaging modalities are available for evaluating right lower quadrant pain; the modality of choice depends on the patient's demographics. In adults, CT is, by far, the best diagnostic test. In children, a few factors favor initial evaluation with sonography, including a small body size, with less body fat, and a high radiosensitivity to ionizing radiation. For similar reasons, in pregnant women, sonography or magnetic resonance imaging (MRI) may initially be used to minimize ionizing radiation exposure (Fig. C8.1).

Abdominal and pelvic CT with intravenous contrast and multiplanar reconstructions is the preferred protocol. The addition of intravenous contrast has been found to increase the sensitivity and specificity, but no significant difference has been found if oral or rectal contrast are used. Contrast is institutional dependent and is favored at our institution. The routine use of CT for appendicitis has been found to decrease the negative appendectomy rate from 43% to 7% among women aged 18 to 45 years.

Findings

The pathogenesis of appendicitis relates to appendiceal lumen obstruction, which results in progressive luminal distention, bacterial overgrowth, and inflammatory cascade activation. If left untreated, the increasing intraluminal pressure and inflammatory changes of the appendiceal wall can lead to perforation and generalized peritonitis. Early CT findings reflect these changes and include a dilated appendix (>6 mm), thickening and enhancement of the appendiceal wall, and surrounding periappendiceal fat stranding (Fig. C8.2). Other helpful signs include an obstructing appendicolith. If rectally or orally administered contrast material opacifies the appendiceal lumen, this in most cases would exclude the diagnosis of appendicitis. Late appendicitis after rupture may no longer demonstrate a dilated appendix, but adjacent inflammatory changes, including a disorganized phlegmonous collection or an

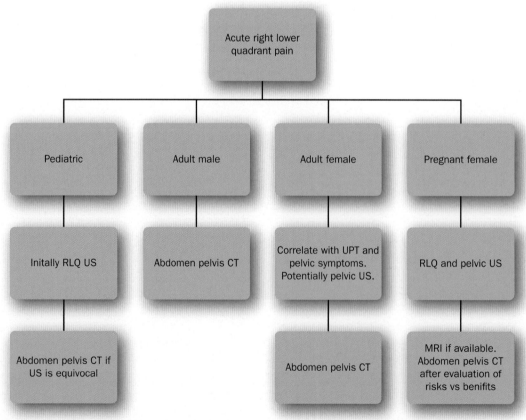

Fig. C8.1 Algorithm for RLQ pain depending on age.

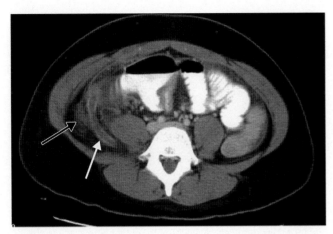

Fig. C8.2 Acute appendicitis. Axial CT of the lower abdomen with intravenous and oral contrast. Acute appendicitis with a dilated appendix with enhancing walls within the right lower quadrant (white arrow). Notice the surrounding inflammation manifested by the stranding or increased density of the periappendiceal fat (black arrow) as opposed to the near uniform black subcutaneous fat.

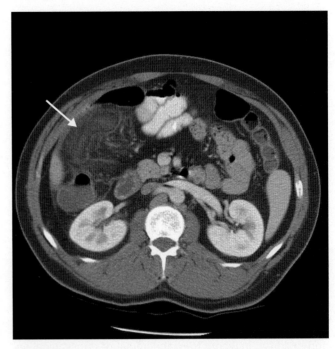

Fig. C8.3 Omental torsion/infarct with extensive stranding in the right abdomen (white arrow) inferior to the right hepatic lobe.

abscess, may be identified. Gross free intraperitoneal air may be present, but is uncommon. In patients with little intra-abdominal fat, the bowel loops are commonly not separated and visualization of the appendix can be difficult; this is particularly true in children. However, nonvisualization of the appendix on an otherwise normal CT scan has a negative predictive value of 98.7%.

DIFFERENTIAL DIAGNOSIS

Numerous disorders present with right lower quadrant pain. The differential considerations are much larger in women because several gynecologic disorders can mimic appendicitis, including pelvic inflammatory disease, tubo-ovarian abscess, ectopic pregnancy, ovarian torsion, ruptured ovarian cyst, and endometriosis. Other differentials include Crohn's disease, diverticular disease, gastroenteritis, renal calculi, and urinary tract infection.

Omental infarct or torsion is another cause of lower abdominal pain; it most commonly occurs on the right side, can mimic appendicitis clinically. Omental torsion occurs when the greater omentum becomes twisted over itself, leading to vascular compromise and infarction. CT may demonstrate swirling fatty tissue around a vessel, indicating torsion or focal fat stranding with hazy soft tissue

infiltration of the involved omental fat (Fig. C8.3). The appendix is not expected to be dilated, but the adjacent stranding may be misinterpreted as periappendiceal fat stranding.

A few neoplasms can mimic appendicitis, including a mucocele of the appendix that is formed by a mucus-producing tumor and can result in a dilated, mucus-filled appendix. This usually lacks surrounding inflammatory changes unless it becomes secondarily infected. Other tumors include carcinoid and adenocarcinoma of the appendix; carcinoid is more common. These can infiltrate the adjacent fat, mimicking inflammatory stranding and regional lymphadenopathy. The mass can eventually obstruct the lumen, resulting in acute appendicitis.

REFERENCES AND SUGGESTED READING

1. Yoo E. Greater and lesser omenta: normal anatomy and pathologic processes. *RadioGraphics*, 2007;27:707-720.

CASE 9

PATIENT PRESENTATION

A 72-year-old woman presented with left lower quadrant pain that was rated 8 on a 10-point pain scale; it had progressively worsened over the past day. The patient was febrile, with slight leukocytosis, guarding, and minimal rebound.

CLINICAL SUSPICION

Diverticulitis

IMAGING MODALITY OF CHOICE

Multidetector CT remains the imaging modality of choice when evaluating older patients with a typical presentation of diverticulitis. It is also indicated when a patient presents with acute, severe left lower quadrant pain, with or without fever or chronic, intermittent low-grade pain. The caveats to this generalization include women of childbearing age and children, in whom transabdominal or transvaginal sonography should be used first to minimize radiation dose and in women exclude any gynecologic abnormalities.

An optimal CT examination uses intravenous, oral, and rectal contrast to improve bowel luminal distension and visualization. Again, if the clinical signs suggest perforation, a water-soluble contrast should be used rather than barium.

Barium contrast enema was the imaging of choice in the past; however, this has been replaced by CT because contrast enemas are more invasive and are insensitive to extramucosal manifestations, including pericolonic inflammation, abscess, and alternative diagnosis. CT is widely available and reproducible; it can be performed rapidly and can help triage patients who can be treated medically versus surgically.

DIFFERENTIAL DIAGNOSIS

Clinical Differential

Diverticulosis: Diverticulosis is common in developed countries because of a diet low in or devoid of fiber; it is uncommon before age 40 years, and the incidence increases with age. A diverticulum is an acquired herniation or outpouching of the mucosa and submucosa through the muscular layers of the bowel wall, usually at the site of penetrating vessels (Fig. C9.1). They are most common in the sigmoid colon, which tends to have more intraluminal pressure. Diverticulosis may be asymptomatic or may present with mild pain, alternating episodes of constipation and diarrhea due to luminal narrowing, or rectal bleeding. Bleeding is believed to be due to a close proximity to penetrating vessels.

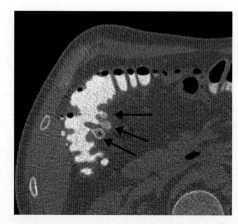

Fig. C9.1 Diverticulosis. Axial CT with rectal contrast filling the hepatic flexure demonstrating many diverticula as small outpouchings (arrows) from the colonic wall.

Diverticulitis: Diverticulitis refers to inflammatory changes in a diverticulum due to obstruction of the neck of the diverticulum by stool, inflammation, or food products, which results in microperforation of the diverticulum and inflammation in the surrounding pericolonic tissues. CT findings of diverticulitis include segmental wall thickening and pericolonic fat stranding (Fig. C9.2). What distinguishes these inflammatory changes from other etiologies of bowel inflammation is the presence of diverticula in the affected

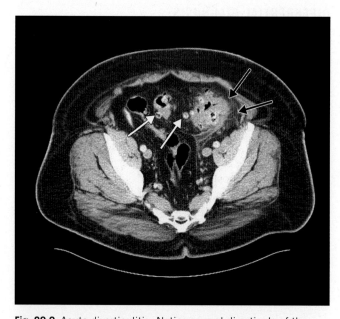

Fig. C9.2 Acute diverticulitis. Notice several diverticula of the sigmoid colon as small round outpouchings (white arrows). These alone would be simply diverticulosis, but notice within the left lower quadrant, the extensive pericolonic fat stranding and wall thickening of that segment of colon (black arrows) consistent with acute diverticulitis.

segment of colon; however, these are sometimes not clearly perceived, and the diagnosis is inferred from other associated findings. Complications of diverticulitis include contained perforations with adjacent pericolonic abscesses, sinus tracts, and colovesical or colovaginal fistula (Fig. C9.3) (air in the bladder or vagina and thickening of the bladder wall adjacent to an affected bowel segment), gross perforation with free air and peritonitis, mesenteric vein thrombosis, and liver abscess. When pericolonic abscesses are found, CT can be used to map placement of a percutaneous drain. Colon carcinoma can occasionally mimic the appearance of diverticulitis. A clear distinction cannot always be made, and a histopathologic correlation may be required. For this reason, following the treatment of diverticulitis and resolution of acute inflammatory changes, patients should have a follow-up colonoscopy to exclude an occult malignancy.

Epiploic appendagitis: The appendices epiploicae are small lobulations of pericolonic fat that occur along the teniae coli of the colon. Epiploic appendagitis refers to an inflammatory condition in which these small fat lobulations become ischemic as a result of torsion or spontaneous venous thrombosis. This results in localized inflammation, with a clinical presentation of severe, focally localized pain in the right or left lower quadrant. The CT findings include pericolonic round or fingerlike fat-containing masses with thin-enhancing or hyperattenuating rims and surrounding mesenteric stranding (Fig. C9.4). These are more common in the sigmoid and distal descending colon. Identification is important to avoid unnecessary surgery because this is a benign, self-limiting process that should be treated conservatively, including use of analgesics.

Others: Several other diseases may present with left lower quadrant pain, including infectious colitis, pseudomembranous colitis, ulcerative colitis, Crohn's disease, ischemic colitis, gynecologic causes (torsion, endometriosis, salpingitis, tubo-ovarian abscess, and

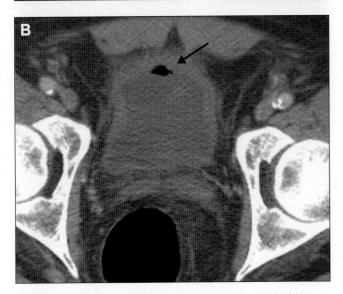

Fig. C9.3 (A) Multiple sigmoid diverticuli (white arrows) with linear tract containing air outside the bowel lumen consistent with a fistula (black arrow) as a complication of diverticulitis. (B) Same patient showing air within the bladder (black arrow) consistent with a colovesical fistula from diverticulitis.

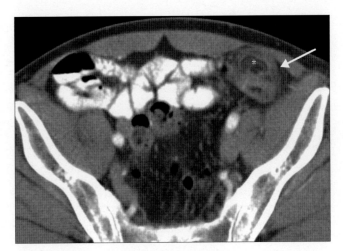

Fig. C9.4 Epiploic appendagitis. Notice the small ovoid mass in the left lower quadrant (*) that is composed of fat, therefore the internal density is low and equal to the subcutaneous fat. Also notice the thin peripheral rim and the surrounding fat stranding (white arrow).

fibroids), renal calculi, sigmoid volvulus, pyelonephritis, spontaneous retroperitoneal hemorrhage, and inguinal hernia.

IMAGING DIFFERENTIAL

Several diseases may present with similar radiographic findings of colonic wall thickening, including colon cancer, all types of colitis (infectious, pseudomembranous, ischemic, and radiation), and inflammatory bowel disease. Each of these diseases may have variations with unique distributions or accompanying signs to suggest a specific diagnosis.

REFERENCES AND SUGGESTED READING

1. Horton KM. CT evaluation of the colon: inflammatory disease. *RadioGraphics*. 2000;20:399-418.
2. ACR Appropriateness Criteria. Left lower quadrant pain.

CASE 10

PATIENT PRESENTATION

An 81-year-old man presented with progressive abdominal pain, distention, and no bowel movements or flatus during the past day.

CLINICAL SUSPICION

Large bowel obstruction (LBO)

IMAGING MODALITY OF CHOICE

In the setting of constipation or obstipation in the elderly, the initial imaging modality should be conventional radiography, which helps distinguish between small bowel and large bowel etiologies. The large bowel can usually be distinguished from dilated small bowel based upon their location and morphology, as it is usually situated predominantly along the periphery of the peritoneal cavity, although the transverse and sigmoid colons can be quite redundant, and morphologically the large bowel has haustra which result in its segmented sacculationlike appearance. Haustra are not circumferential, unlike the small bowel mucosal folds called valvulae conniventes, which are complete circumferential rings. The characteristic findings of a LBO are dilated large bowel loops (>5 cm) and air-fluid levels (Fig. C10.1). In the setting of sigmoid volvulus, radiographs are diagnostic in 75% of cases. If a large bowel obstruction is initially identified, further evaluation could be obtained by CT or water-soluble contrast enema.

CT can differentiate mechanical obstruction from pseudo-obstruction and may identify the underlying etiology, such as an obstructing mass or volvulus. A water-soluble contrast enema may also be considered, as they are not only diagnostic but sometimes therapeutic; however, caution should be exercised because of the risk of perforation in a severely inflamed or ischemic colon.

DIFFERENTIAL DIAGNOSIS

Sigmoid volvulus is the most common colonic volvulus, accounting for 60% to 75% of cases. Predisposing factors include chronic constipation, high-fiber diets that induce sigmoid redundancy, pregnancy, and hospitalization. Radiographically, sigmoid volvulus appears as a large air-filled bowel loop that extends out of the pelvis in an upside-down U-shape, most commonly directed at the right upper quadrant (Fig. C10.2). The "coffee bean" sign refers to the shape the dilated and folded sigmoid colon may assume. The "white stripe" sign refers to the dense line formed by the two apposed walls. CT reveals the dilated loop of colon but may also show the "whirl" sign, in which the mesentery and vessels twist at the site of volvulus (Fig. C10.3). A water-soluble

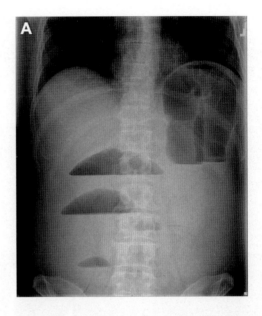

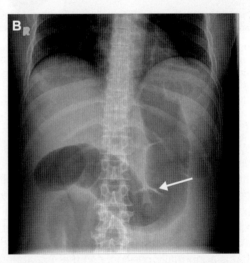

Fig. C10.1 (A) Large bowel obstruction. Upright AP radiograph of the abdomen shows multiple large air-fluid levels within dilated large bowel loops. (B) Supine AP radiograph shows the air within the transverse colon and both flexures, the most nondependent portions of the colon. Haustral markings of the colon can be visualized (white arrow) which are not circumferential, unlike valvulae conniventes of the small bowel.

contrast enema may reveal a beak-shaped narrowing at the site of the volvulus, with no contrast passing beyond.

Cecal volvulus is the next most common site of colonic volvulus, accounting for approximately 30% of cases. Compared with the acquired nature of sigmoid volvulus, most cecal volvulus cases are due to congenital anatomical variants, including incomplete fusion of the right colon to the posterior parietal peritoneum. Radiographically, a cecal volvulus presents as a large dilated bowel loop,

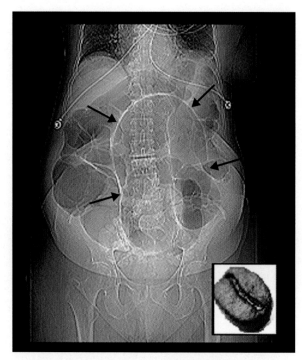

Fig. C10.2 Scout image from abdomen pelvis CT shows large dilated upside down U-shaped loop of bowel (black arrows) emanating from the left lower quadrant consistent with sigmoid volvulus. Notice the similarities with the "coffee bean."

usually in the left upper quadrant or mid-abdomen, with a single large air-fluid level (Fig. C10.4). Dilated gas or small fluid-filled bowel loops may be seen proximally, with collapse of the distal colon and rectum. CT and contrast enema will reveal similar findings as in sigmoid volvulus, including the "whirl" and "beaking" signs, but in the cecum and right colon. A cecal bascule is a distended cecum that is abnormally positioned in the mid-abdomen as a result of upward folding of the cecum, with no twisting.

Ogilvie syndrome, also known as colonic ileus or colonic pseudo-obstruction, refers to a dilated colon with no obstructive lesion. The proximal colon, including the cecum and ascending colon, are distended to a larger degree than the distal colon. Patients present with nonspecific obstructive symptoms, commonly after surgery or severe illnesses. Although no real mechanical obstruction is present, progressive distention can lead to ischemia from diminished venous outflow or even perforation. Therefore, surgery may be indicated for functional obstruction.

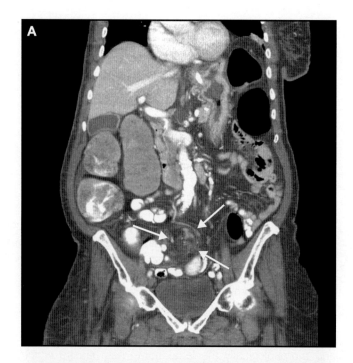

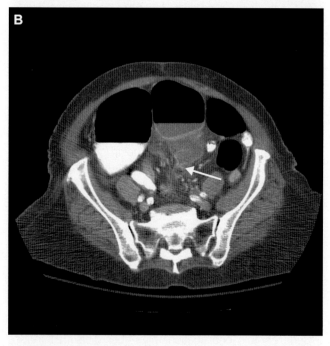

Fig. C10.3 (A) Coronal CT image of same patient shows the round whirling of the mesenteric vessels (white arrows) at the site of volvulus. (B) Axial CT from same patient shows the dilated loops with abrupt tapering at the site of torsion (white arrow) consistent with the beak sign.

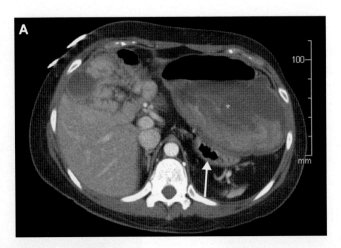

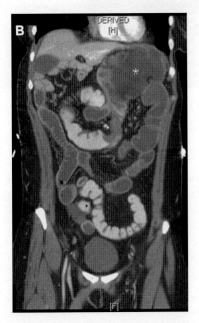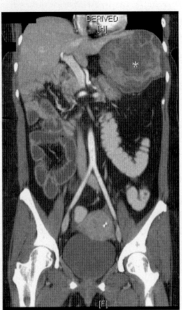

Fig. C10.4 (A) Axial CT with large dilated loop of bowel within the left upper quadrant (*) with air-fluid level representative of cecal volvulus. This should not be confused with the stomach which is collapsed posteriorly (white arrow). (B) Coronal CT depicts the dilated cecum displaced in the left upper quadrant. Mildly dilated small bowel loops are seen proximally (*).

Other differentials for large bowel obstruction include all forms of colitis, diverticulitis, colon carcinoma, and fecal impaction. Other nonmechanical forms of obstruction resulting in ileus include metabolic abnormalities such as hypokalemia.

REFERENCE AND SUGGESTED READING

1. Peterson CM. Volvulus of the gastrointestinal tract: appearances at multimodality imaging. *RadioGraphics*. 2009;29:1281-1293.

CASE 11

PATIENT PRESENTATION

A 25-year-old woman presented to her primary care physician with intermittent lower right quadrant pain, diarrhea, and fever. The patient had an elevated C-reactive protein level.

CLINICAL SUSPICION

Inflammatory bowel disease

IMAGING MODALITY OF CHOICE

CT enterography (CTE) should be used, according to recommendations of the ACR Appropriateness Criteria Committee. CTE is an alternative to the conventional small bowel series for assessing the small bowel. It consists of thin-slice CT with a neutral oral contrast, such as a 0.1% barium suspension (VoLumen), which provides good luminal distension and excellent contrast between the bowel wall and lumen after a bolus injection of intravenous contrast. Multiplanar reformatting is performed in the axial and coronal oblique views (Figs. C11.1 and C11.2).

CTE versus Capsule Endoscopy

Although capsule endoscopy is reported to have high sensitivity for evaluating the small bowel mucosa, CTE provides better visualization of the entire small bowel wall and allows the detection of intramural and extraenteric disease. Additional disadvantages of capsule endoscopy include a higher rate of false-positive findings due to mucosal breaks and erosions, which may occur even in healthy patients,

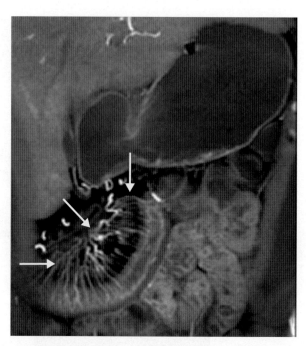

Fig. C11.2 Inflammatory bowel disease. Coronal volume-rendered CT enterographic sections demonstrate prominence of the vasa recta, or "comb sign" (arrows).

and the risk of possible impaction of the capsule proximal to a diseased or strictured bowel segment. CTE is also useful for detecting complications, such as obstruction, strictures abscesses, and fistulae.

MRI Enterography

MRI enterography (MRE) has been gaining popularity for the follow-up of children and young patients. The lack of ionizing radiation is an advantage of MRE over CTE. However, MRE is more time-consuming, expensive, and variable in regard to image quality than CTE. Imaging findings of active inflammatory bowel disease: CT reveals mucosal hyperenhancement and wall thickening (>3 mm). Mural stratification, however, is the most sensitive indicator of active disease. The term *mural stratification* denotes visualization of bowel wall layers in which the edematous wall has a trilaminar appearance: enhanced outer serosal and inner mucosal layers with interposed lower attenuation edematous submucosa.

Prominent vasa recta may be seen in the form of the "comb sign." This sign, along with increased mesenteric fat attenuation, is the most specific CT feature of active disease. Mesenteric fat stranding may be nonspecific but may also be seen with active disease.

Inflammatory bowel disease mainly includes Crohn's (more common) and ulcerative colitis (less common). The main differences between them are shown in Table C11.1.

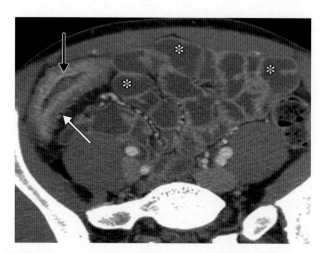

Fig. C11.1 Inflammatory bowel disease. Axial CT enterographic section shows mucosal hyperenhancement (black arrow) and mural stratification (white arrow) of the terminal ileum, an appearance that contrasts nondiseased adjacent ileal segments (*).

Table C11.1 Differentiating Characteristics of Inflammatory Bowel Disease

Crohn's Disease	Ulcerative Colitis
• Predominantly small bowel but may involve the large bowel	• Predominantly large bowel but can extend to the terminal ileum (backwash ileitis)
• Discontinuous (skip lesions)	• Contiguous involvement
• Extraintestinal manifestations: common (eg, fistulas)	• Extraintestinal manifestations: uncommon
• Smaller risk for malignancy	• Greater risk for malignancy

DIFFERENTIAL DIAGNOSIS

Various conditions can cause right lower quadrant pain (eg, acute appendicitis, hernia, ureteric stone, omental torsion, and gynecologic processes such as ectopic pregnancy, hemorrhagic ovarian cyst, endometrioma, and tubo-ovarian abscess). Diarrhea can be caused by diseases such as gastroenteritis, irritable bowel syndrome, and celiac disease.

Radiologically, the above described findings can be characteristic of active Crohn's disease in the proper clinical setting. However, other causes of enteritis can lead to nonspecific findings, including mucosal hyper-enhancement and mural stratification.

REFERENCES AND SUGGESTED READING

1. Elsayes KM, Al-Hawary MM, Jagdish J, et al. CT enterography: principles, trends, and interpretation of findings. *RadioGraphics*. 2010;30:1955-1970.
2. American College of Radiology. ACR Appropriateness Criteria. Reston, VA: American College of Radiology; 2005.
3. Hara AK, Leighton JA, Heigh RI, et al. Crohn disease of the small bowel: preliminary comparison among CT enterography, capsule endoscopy, small-bowel follow-through, and ileoscopy. *Radiology*. 2006;238:128-134.

CASE 12

PATIENT PRESENTATION

A 24-year-old man presented with fever and progressive crampy abdominal pain with watery mucoid diarrhea. He had a history of cellulitis and was being treated with the antibiotic clindamycin.

CLINICAL SUSPICION

Pseudomembranous colitis

IMAGING MODALITY OF CHOICE

Multidetector CT is the preferred imaging modality for initially evaluating diffuse nonlocalizable abdominal pain with fever. Abdominal radiographs have a limited role. Unlike contrast enemas, which only characterize the colonic lumen and mucosal wall, CT can characterize intramural, pericolonic, regional, and distant conditions.

A routine abdominal and pelvic CT with intravenous and oral contrast is the preferred study. If colonic disease is suspected, oral contrast can be administered the night before to adequately opacify the colon; otherwise, in urgent cases, contrast can be administered rectally. Rectally administered contrast also distends the colonic lumen, which results in a more accurate examination because the bowel wall in nondistended segments may appear thickened, simulating disease even when normal. Positive (iodinated) contrast agents and neutral contrast such as water could be used to opacify and distend the colon. The latter has the added advantage of allowing better characterization of wall and mucosal enhancement.

Numerous conditions can lead to colonic inflammation, most of which share common imaging features; however, they may be distinguished on the basis of their location, severity, and clinical history.

Pseudomembranous colitis (PMC) is an acute inflammation of the colon caused by the toxins produced by the bacteria *Clostridium difficile*. Recent exposure to antibiotics is the most common precipitating event. Clindamycin is most commonly associated with PMC; however, ampicillin, tetracycline, erythromycin, and penicillin have also been reported as causes. Antibiotic therapy, after as early as 2 days and rarely up to 6 months, alters the normal bowel microflora, leading to unopposed overgrowth by resistant enteric *C difficile*. In return, *C difficile* produces toxin A (enterotoxin) and toxin B (cytotoxin), which lead to mucosal damage. These toxins form the basis for diagnosis by stool assay; however, the test may require up to 48 hours for confirmation.

PMC commonly causes pancolitis, with markedly thickened colon walls, to a higher degree than other forms of colitis with the exception of Crohn's disease. However, the

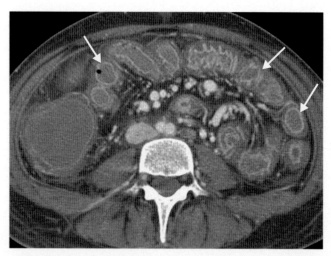

Fig. C12.1 Pseudomembranous colitis. Axial CT of the abdomen showing significantly thickened colonic wall due to PMC. Notice the intense enhancement of the inner mucosa (white arrows).

walls have a more irregular and shaggy appearance than do the uniformly thickened walls typically found in Crohn's disease (Fig. C12.1). Markedly thickened colonic folds resulting in the "accordion" sign, which refers to alternating bands of trapped high-density contrast between low-density thickened and edematous haustra, is more commonly seen in PMC than other forms of colitis. Compared with other forms of colitis, there is relatively little pericolonic fat stranding because of the mucosal pathogenesis of PMC. Severe cases can lead to toxic megacolon and colonic perforation and rupture.

Infectious colitis has fewer specific imaging features and is typically diagnosed clinically. Common bacterial causes include *Shigella*, *Salmonella*, *Yersinia*, *Campylobacter*, *Escherichia coli*, and *Staphylococcus*. CT features usually include wall thickening, mucosal enhancement surrounded by low attenuation from submucosal edema, and pericolonic fat stranding. Different organisms preferentially affect different portions of the colon. For instance, *Salmonella*, *Yersinia*, and *Mycobacterium tuberculosis* typically affect the cecum or right colon and invariably the terminal ileum. *Shigella* and *Schistosomiasis* involve the left colon, whereas *Gonorrhea*, *Chlamydia*, and *Herpes* affect the rectosigmoid region. Immunocompromised patients are susceptible to other organisms such as cytomegalovirus (CMV) which can result in diffuse pancolitis (Fig. C12.2).

Ischemic colitis occurs when blood flow to the colon is compromised. This can be due to hypoperfusion in the setting of shock (septic, hemorrhagic, cardiac, or neurogenic), resulting in shunting of blood away from the splanchnic vessels to perfuse critical organs. A similar pathogenesis can occur with the use of vasopressors to maintain mean arterial pressure at the cost of a reduced splanchnic blood supply. Colonic ischemia can be caused by a thrombus or

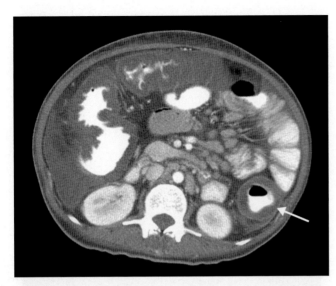

Fig. C12.2 CMV colitis. Axial CT with intravenous, oral and rectal contrast in a young male with AIDS presenting with diarrhea demonstrating diffuse colonic wall thickening (white arrows), ascites, and prominent central mesenteric lymph nodes due to CMV pancolitis.

embolism in the mesenteric arteries or veins. Regardless of the cause, the CT findings include symmetric bowel wall thickening, pneumatosis, or portal venous gas. The "double halo" or "target" sign was initially described in ischemic colitis but is now found with other causes of colitis. This describes concentric layers of differing attenuation, with enhancement of the mucosa and serosa and intervening low attenuation of the submucosa. Whether related to ischemia or other causes, the submucosa appears hypoattenuating because of edema. Thrombus may be directly visualized in the mesenteric arteries or portal vein. With hypoperfusion, watershed segments may be affected; for example, the splenic flexure between the superior mesenteric artery (SMA) and inferior mesenteric artery (IMA) territories or the rectosigmoid between the IMA and hypogastric artery.

DIFFERENTIAL DIAGNOSIS

The clinical presentation of colitis is nonspecific but may include crampy lower abdominal pain and or diarrhea. Depending on the severity, patients may or may not be imaged. If the patients are febrile or have leukocytosis, imaging is recommended by the ACR.

Radiologically, there is much overlap in the appearance, and differentiation based solely upon imaging would be quite difficult, therefore pertinent history is vital in making the correct diagnosis or at least narrowing the differential diagnosis.

REFERENCE AND SUGGESTED READING

1. Horton KM. CT evaluation of the colon: inflammatory disease. *RadioGraphics*. 2000;20:399-418.

CASE 13

PATIENT PRESENTATION

A 63-year-old woman with increasing fatigue was found to have microcytic anemia, with a positive fecal occult blood test.

CLINICAL SUSPICION

Colon cancer

IMAGING MODALITY OF CHOICE

Colon cancer is the most common cancer of the gastrointestinal tract and a common cause of cancer mortality in men and women. The incidence increases with age after age 50 years, with a peak at 65. The natural history of colon cancer is well established, beginning with benign adenomas that undergo malignant transformation over a span of 7 to 10 years. The overall survival rate at 5 years is 50%. When diagnosed early (Dukes stage A), the survival rate is 81% to 85%; however, with late presentation and advanced disease (Duke Stage D), the prognosis is dismal, with only 5% to 14% of patients surviving after 5 years. Early and effective screening is paramount in the treatment of this disease.

Screening entails subjecting healthy or asymptomatic patients to a test with potential physical or psychological harm and financial burden. Colonoscopy remains the gold standard for diagnosing colon cancer because it can detect and simultaneously biopsy lesions, but less invasive tests may be appropriate in certain populations.

The screening population can be divided into three risk categories:

- Average: 50 years old or older with no personal or family history.
- Moderate: First-degree relative with a history of adenoma or carcinoma or a personal history of large adenoma or carcinoma. This increases the risk of colon cancer two- to threefold compared with the general population.
- High: Hereditary syndromes such as hereditary nonpolyposis colorectal cancer, familial adenomatous polyposis, ulcerative colitis, or Crohn's disease.

The current guidelines are for average-risk individuals and are supported by the World Health Organization and the U.S. Preventative Service Task Force; they include an annual or biennial fecal occult blood test, flexible sigmoidoscopy every 5 years, double-contrast barium enema (DCBE) every 5 years, and or colonoscopy every 10 years. A revision by the American Cancer Society and American College of Radiology included CT colonography (CTC) every 5 years for average-risk individuals.

CTC, also known as "virtual colonoscopy," was developed in the early 1990s, and studies have found variable sensitivity and specificity rates for polyp detection, many of which are similar to those of conventional colonoscopy.

Various protocols are available, but patients generally must undergo overnight colon preparation, identical to that of a colonoscopy. During the examination, the colon and rectum are distended by a pressure-regulated CO_2 insufflator through a rectal tube, with subsequent nonintravenous contrast scanning in the prone and supine positions. The images are then evaluated in myriad 2-D and 3-D reformats on vendor-specific and proprietary software (Fig. C13.1).

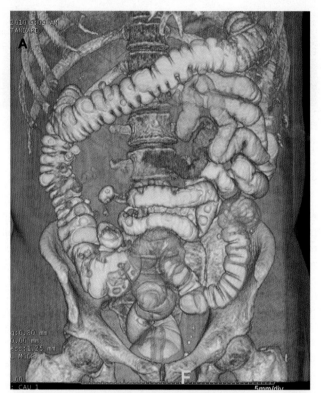

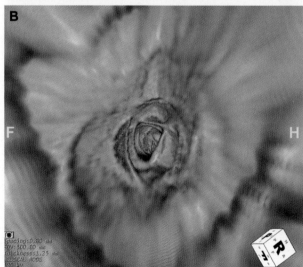

Fig. C13.1 Image on the left is a 3-dimensional reconstruction from the CT colonography, while the image above is also 3-D, but is a virtual view as from inside simulating the colonoscopy.

Conventional CT remains the standard for initial staging of regional and distant disease and follow-up restaging of recurrence. Because local staging of colon cancer is based on the depth of tumor spread through the colon wall rather than on overall size, CT plays a lesser role in staging. Positron emission tomography (PET) also plays in invaluable role in follow-up staging, especially when performed in conjunction with CT (PET/CT).

Findings

Double contrast barium enema (DCBE) was the gold standard in colon cancer screening in the last century but now plays a lesser role because of the widespread availability of colonoscopy and its ability to make a diagnosis of the visualized polyp and or mass. DCBE can still serve as a useful alternative, especially in situations in which colonoscopy or CTC is not available or is suboptimal. For example, it may be useful in patients who have an incomplete colonoscopy or cannot undergo anesthesia. DCBE is a safe procedure, with a perforation rate of 1/25,000 compared with those of other colorectal examinations, including 1/5,000 for flexible sigmoidoscopy and 1/2,000 for diagnostic colonoscopy.

Early cancer findings include sessile (plaquelike) lesions or thick, short polyps. The infamous "apple core" lesion signifies advanced cancer with an annular lesion that results in circumferential narrowing of the bowel, with shelf-like overhanging edges.

CT

The principal pitfall of CTC and routine abdominal CT of the colon is underdistention and presence of retained fecal material. For that reason, a high-quality colon preparation is necessary before CTC to minimize the number of indeterminate or missed findings. Cancer findings include asymmetric mural thickening (distended normal colon <3 mm, 3-6 mm indeterminate, or >6 mm abnormal), an endoluminal polypoid mass (Fig. C13.2), and extracolonic tumor extension. Extracolonic findings can include soft tissue stranding from the serosal surface into pericolic fat or loss of surrounding fat planes. Enlargement of lymph nodes (>1 cm short axis dimension, loss of central fatty hilum, or loss of normal reniform shape architecture) in draining nodal basin is highly suspicious for metastatic disease. Metastatic disease to the liver is the most common, appearing as predominantly hypodense, hypoenhancing masses (Fig. C13.3). As stated earlier, colon cancer is a leading cause of large bowel obstruction in the elderly and a diligent search for the underlying cause is necessary (Fig. C13.4).

DIFFERENTIAL DIAGNOSIS

Screening for colon cancer is necessary because it can frequently be clinically silent therefore delaying the diagnosis.

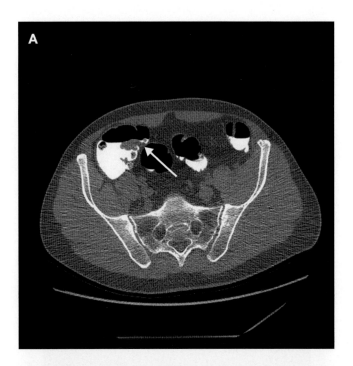
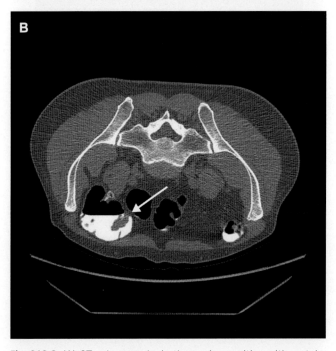

Fig. C13.2 (A) CT colonography in the supine position with rectal contrast and CO_2 distention. Note the 3.5 cm polyp (arrow) arising from the cecum. (B) CT colonography but this time imaged in the prone position. Notice how the rectal contrast layers along the dependent wall, but how the cecal polyp (arrow) attaches to the nondependent wall.

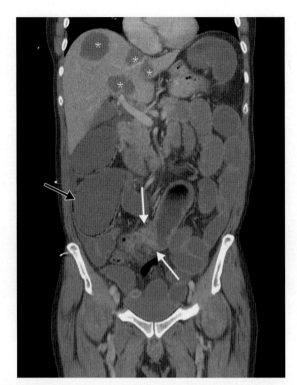

Fig. C13.3 Coronal CT shows a circumferential mass with ill-defined margins obstructing the sigmoid colon (white arrows). Also note the multiple hepatic hypoattenuating masses (*) consistent with metastases as well as thin lucencies within the walls of the cecum (black arrow) consistent with pneumatosis coli from the LBO.

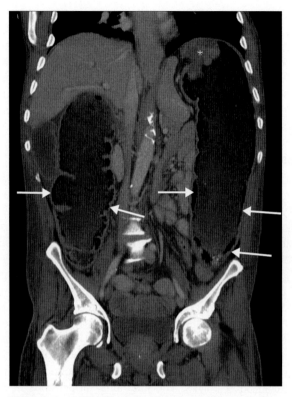

Fig. C13.4 Coronal CT with obstructing polypoid mass in the splenic flexure (*) representing adenocarcinoma. Note the large dilated loops of colon due to severe LBO. The loop of colon on the left is actually redundant transverse colon. The distal left colon is collapsed. This case also demonstrates pneumatosis of the colonic wall.

Rectal bleeding is one particular clinical finding and should always warrant further evaluation. Besides colorectal cancer, causes include diverticulosis or any form of colitis as well as several abnormalities of the anus such as perianal abscesses, fistulae or fissures, or hemorrhoids, necessitating proper clinical evaluation.

Besides colon adenocarcinoma, other colonic "masslike lesions" include GISTs, or lymphoma as well as inflammatory changes secondary to diverticulitis or endometriosis.

REFERENCES AND SUGGESTED READING

1. ACR Appropriateness Criteria. Colorectal cancer screening.
2. Horton KM. Spiral CT of colon cancer: imaging features and role in management. *RadioGraphics*. 2000:20:419-430.

CASE 14

PATIENT PRESENTATION

A 60-year-old man with a history of benign prostatic hyperplasia presented to a urologist for a routine follow-up visit. On digital rectal examination, a palpable rectal mass identified.

CLINICAL SUSPICION

Rectal cancer

IMAGING MODALITY OF CHOICE

Screening and staging of rectal cancer are similar to those of colon cancer; thus, the conditions are commonly referred to as colorectal cancer. Flexible colonoscopy, sigmoidoscopy, or rigid proctoscopy remain the gold standard for diagnosing any rectal cancer.

Incidental cancers may be found on imaging, but diagnostic imaging primarily serves as a staging tool. Once rectal cancer has been a histologically diagnosed, several imaging modalities can be used for staging. MRI of the pelvis can be used for local staging and follow-up after resection for local recurrence. CT of the chest, abdomen, and pelvis is used to evaluate distant metastases.

FINDINGS

Adenocarcinoma accounts for most primary tumors of the rectum (98%), with the remainder being composed of carcinoid, lymphoma, or GIST. With newer surgical techniques, the risk of local recurrence has significantly improved. Depending on the T stage, several different surgical options are available. Surgeries with lower morbidity rates can be used for low-stage tumors without increasing the risk of recurrence or decreasing survival, whereas high-stage tumors require more extensive surgery. The increasing implementation of total mesorectal excision over the past decade has dramatically reduced the risk of recurrence when these tumors are properly preoperatively staged. This technique involves en bloc resection of the entire tumor, along with the rectum and the surrounding mesorectum. The mesorectum is the fat surrounding the rectum that contains blood vessels and lymphatics; it is enveloped by a surrounding fascial border named the mesorectal fascia. The total mesorectal excision technique uses the mesorectal fascia as the boundary of the resection; this is referred to as the circumferential resection margin (CRM).

When using the mesorectal fascia as the CRM, tumors that approach or are in close proximity to the mesorectal fascia (T3+) or extend through the fascia (T4) are known to have a high recurrence rate. Proper preoperative staging with EUS and MRI can help determine the proper surgical technique and can also help identify patients who will benefit from preoperative (neoadjuvant) chemotherapy and radiation therapy (Table C14.1 and Fig. C14.1).

- T1: Tumor grows through the muscularis mucosa and extends to the submucosa.
- T2: Tumor grows through the submucosa and extends into the muscularis propria.
- T3– CRM: Tumor grows through the muscularis propria and extends into the inner mesorectal fat but is some distance from the mesorectal fascia.
- T3+ CRM: Tumor grows through the muscularis propria and extends into the inner mesorectal fat and closely approximates the mesorectal fascia but does not violate it.
- T4: Tumor penetrates the mesorectal fascia and may invade neighboring organs such as the prostate or seminal vesicles.

MRI of the rectum entails multiplanar T2-weighted images in the axial, sagittal, and oblique or orthogonal axial planes. The oblique axial plane is perpendicular to the lumen of the rectum. Other techniques include endorectal coil MRI, in which a wire is placed in the rectum, allowing increased image resolution of the surrounding structures. This allows different layers of the rectal wall to be identified and thus be properly T staged. The muscularis propria manifests

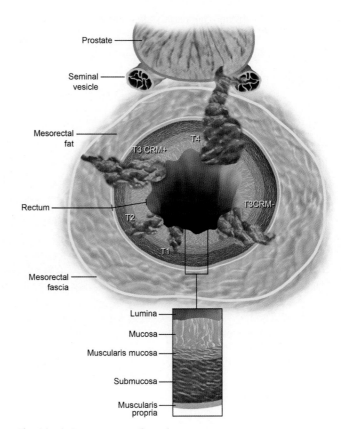

Fig. C14.1 Rectal cancer T-staging.

Table C14.1 TNM Guidelines for the Staging of Rectal Cancer

Descriptor	Definition
Tumor	
TX	Determination of tumor extent is not possible because of incomplete information
Tis	Tumor in situ involves only the mucosa and has not grown beyond the muscularis mucosa
T1	Tumor grows through the muscularis mucosa and into the submucosa
T2	Tumor grows through the submucosa and into the muscularis propria
T3	Tumor grows through the muscularis propria and into the mesorectum
T4a	Tumor penetrates the visceral peritoneum
T4b	Tumor directly invades or is adherent to other organs or structures
Node	
NX	Nodal staging is not possible because of incomplete information
N0	No regional lymph node metastasis
N1a	Tumor in one regional lymph node
N1b	Tumor in 2-3 regional lymph nodes
N1c	Tumor deposits in the subserosa, mesentery, or nonperitonealized pericolic or perirectal tissues without regional nodal metastasis
N2a	Tumor in 4-6 regional lymph nodes
N2b	Tumor in 7 or more regional lymph nodes
Metastases	
M0	No distant metastasis
M1a	Tumor confined to one organ or site (eg, liver, lung, ovary, nonregional node)
M1b	Tumor in more than one organ or site or the peritoneum
Stage	
0	Tis, N0, M0
I	T1-T2, N0, M0
IIa	T3, N0, M0
IIb	T4a, N0, M0
IIc	T4b, N0, M0
IIIa	T1-T2, N1, M0; T1, N2a, M0
IIIb	T3-T4a, N1, M0; T2-T3, N2a, M0; T1-T2, N2b, M0
IIIc	T4a, N2a, M0; T3-T4a, N2b, M0; T4b, N1-N2, M0
IVa	Any T, Any N, M1a
IVb	Any T, Any N, M1b

Adapted with permission from Edge SB. *AJCC Cancer Staging Manual*, 7th ed. New York: Springer; 2010.

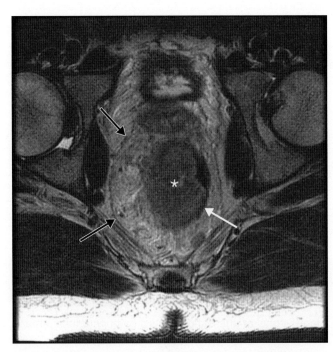

Fig. C14.2 Orthogonal axial high-resolution T2-weighted MR image of the pelvis. Notice the large mass arising from the right lateral wall of the rectum (*). The hypointense left lateral wall (white arrow) can be visualized representing intact muscularis propria, however because of tumor invasion the hypointense line cannot be visualized along the right aspect consistent with a T3 tumor. The mesorectal fascia can be clearly visualized as the hypointense line (black arrows).

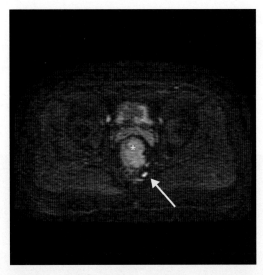

Fig. C14.3 Diffusion weighted image (DWI) shows the mass to be hyperintense because of restricted diffusion (*). Also note how the mesorectal lymph node is hyperintense (white arrow) and more conspicuous than on the T2-weighted sequence. This node abuts the posterior lateral mesorectal fascia and upstages this tumor to a stage T3c or T3+ CRM.

REFERENCES AND SUGGESTED READING

1. Kaur H. MR imaging for preoperative evaluation of primary rectal cancer: practical considerations. *RadioGraphics*. 2012; 32(2):389-409.

2. Iafrate F. Preoperative staging of rectal cancer with MR imaging: correlation with surgical and histopathologic findings. *RadioGraphics*. 2006;26:701-714.

as a thin T2 hypointense layer. The mesorectal fat is T2 hyperintense to allow a sharp contrast between the muscularis propria and the mesorectal fascia, which will also appear as a thin T2 hypointense layer (Figs. C14.2 and C14.3). A large field-of-view T1-weighted sequence can also be obtained to evaluate for pelvic lymphadenopathy.

DIFFERENTIAL DIAGNOSIS

The same differential stated earlier for rectal bleeding pertains to both colon and rectal cancer. MR imaging is usually utilized as a staging examination and not necessarily for screening individuals.

CASE 15

PATIENT PRESENTATION

A 45-year-old woman presented to the emergency department with more than 24 hours of sharp right upper quadrant pain and a subjective fever. The patient had an elevated white blood cell count (Figs. C15.1 and C15.2).

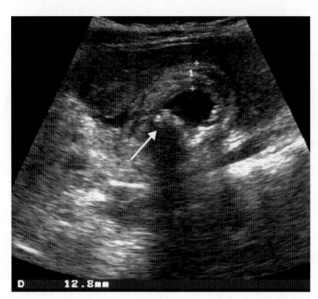

Fig. C15.1 Transverse gray-scale image of the gallbladder shows wall thickening denoted by calipers. Echogenic gallstones with posterior shadowing are seen (arrow). Repositioning the patient during an exam can demonstrate nonmobile stones suggesting impaction within the gallbladder neck/cystic duct.

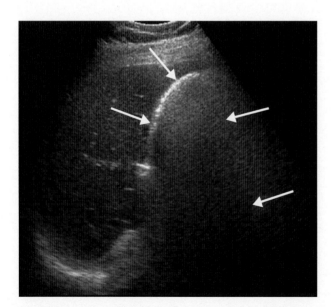

Fig. C15.2 Sagittal sonogram shows a curvilinear echogenic interface in the gallbladder fossa (arrowheads) with reverberation artifact (arrows). Findings are suggestive of gas in the gallbladder wall in the setting of emphysematous cholecystitis.

CLINICAL SUSPICION

Acute cholecystitis

IMAGING MODALITY OF CHOICE

Sonography. Advantages: Readily available, low cost, reasonably sensitive without radiation exposure.

FINDINGS

Sonographic findings of acute cholecystitis:

- Gallstones (calculous cholecystitis)
- Gallbladder wall thickening (>3 mm)
- Gallbladder distension
- Pericholecystic fluid
- A stone impacted in the gallbladder neck
- Focal tenderness (sonographic Murphy's sign)

Alone, none of these findings is pathognomonic, but a combination of several of these findings is highly suggestive (gallbladder stone and Murphy's sign, 92% positive predictive value).

Several subtypes and complications of acute cholecystitis have been described; some of these have a prognosis that is significantly poorer than that of the typical form, such as gangrenous and emphysematous cholecystitis.

Emphysematous cholecystitis: Emphysematous cholecystitis is caused by gas-forming bacteria usually in older patients with diabetes. There is a fivefold increased risk of gangrene or perforation. Air in the gallbladder wall, as evidenced by echogenic foci with reverberation artifacts on ultrasound, is pathognomonic (Fig. C15.2).

Gangrenous cholecystitis: Gangrenous cholecystitis is gallbladder wall ischemia that leads to necrosis. Murphy's sign is often negative because of denervation. The gallbladder wall appears asymmetrically thickened, and intraluminal sloughed membranes may be seen.

Perforation: Perforation is a serious complication with an increased mortality rate, generally due to peritonitis. A focal wall defect may be seen on sonography.

If the sonographic examination is equivocal, cholescintigraphy should be performed by intravenous injection of technetium-labeled hepatic iminodiacetic acid (HIDA), which is taken up by the hepatocytes and excreted into the bile. After 30 to 60 minutes, the scan will show (excretion of isotope) the flow of bile through the biliary tree, including the common bile duct, cystic duct, and gallbladder. A diagnosis of acute cholecystitis is made when no isotope accumulation is visible in the gallbladder, indicating obstruction of the cystic duct, with normal excretion noted into the duodenum.

HIDA scans can be false positive when the gallbladder does not fill in the absence of cholecystitis. These situations include severe liver disease, total parenteral nutrition, hyperbilirubinemia, and alcohol or opiate abuse.

DIFFERENTIAL DIAGNOSIS

Acalculous cholecystitis: Acalculous cholecystitis involves gallbladder wall thickening and distension in the absence of stones. It is often seen in pediatric and severely ill patients. Cholescintigraphy is a useful tool.

Mimics: Disease mimics include acute pancreatitis, perforated duodenal ulcer, hepatitis, diverticulitis, pyelonephritis, and gallbladder wall edema due to systemic conditions, such as heart failure or hypoalbuminemia.

REFERENCES AND SUGGESTED READING

1. Smith EA, Dillman JR, Elsayes KM, et al. Cross-sectional imaging of acute and chronic gallbladder inflammatory disease. *AJR.* 2009;192:188-196.
2. O'Connor OJ, Maher MM. Imaging of cholecystitis. *AJR.* 2011;196(4):W367-W374.

CASE 16

PATIENT PRESENTATION

A 42-year-old woman presented to the emergency department with symptoms of severe biliary colic. The pain was localized to the epigastric and right upper quadrant. The white blood cell count was normal, but the bilirubin and transaminase levels were slightly elevated.

CLINICAL SUSPICION

Obstructive biliary disease

IMAGING MODALITY OF CHOICE

Sonography should be the initial diagnostic imaging technique for all patients who present with abdominal pain localized to the right upper quadrant and an obstructive liver function test (LFT) pattern. Sonography can be performed quickly and is easily reproduced, less expensive, and safer because it lacks ionizing radiation (Fig. C16.1). It is also excellent for ruling out acute cholecystitis. Supplemental imaging modalities are available for diagnosis or confirmation. Noninvasive diagnostic examinations include magnetic resonance cholangiopancreatography (MRCP), multidetector CT (MDCT), and nuclear HIDA scan, and minimally invasive examinations include endoscopic retrograde cholangiopancreatography.

FINDINGS

The most common cause of acute right upper quadrant pain and biliary dilatation with partial or complete biliary obstruction is choledocholithiasis. This can be categorized as primary when a stone forms in the biliary tract and secondary when a stone forms in the gallbladder and passes into the biliary tract. The most common location of an obstructing stone is the distal common bile duct, near the ampulla of Vater. The degree of obstruction and thus the degree of intrahepatic or extrahepatic biliary dilatation depend on the size and location of the stone. Most large stones are highly echogenic on sonography, resulting in posterior acoustic shadowing. Unfortunately, the overlying bowel commonly obscures stones in the distal common bile duct. Smaller stones may be isoechoic, with no shadowing; therefore, the only sonographic finding may be biliary dilatation. The normal common bile duct can measure up to 6 or 7 mm up to age 60 years and an additional 1 mm for each decade afterward. Because of the anatomy of the portal triad, bile ducts run parallel to the portal vein. Peripheral bile ducts should not be more than 2 mm in diameter or 40% of the adjacent portal vein (Fig. C16.2). A color Doppler signal is probably the easiest method of distinguishing dilated bile ducts (no signal) from intrahepatic vessels with flow.

CT is often used to evaluate right upper quadrant pain; however, CT has inherent limitations for detecting intraductal stones. MRCP takes advantage of MRI sequences that are heavily T2 weighted so that only free fluid such as bile will result in high signal intensity (Fig. C16.3A). Intraductal stones will not produce any signal and will therefore appear as a dark filling defect. MRCP has high sensitivity and specificity (97%-99% and 95%-99%, respectively) for

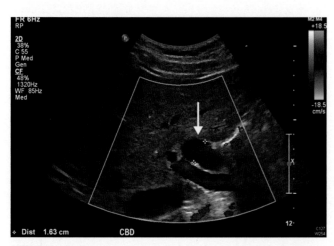

Fig. C16.1 Dilated common bile duct. Color Doppler ultrasound image in the sagittal or long axis of the liver centered over the porta hepatis. The portal vein is visualized (red vessel) with an adjacent parallel tubular structure (arrow) representing the extremely dilated CBD measured at 1.6 cm (normally <0.6 cm).

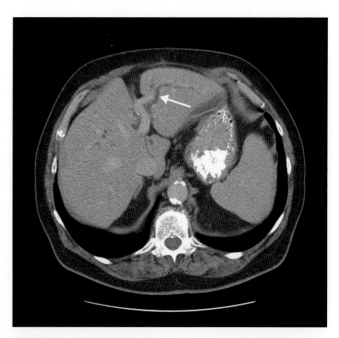

Fig. C16.2 Intrahepatic biliary dilatation. Axial CT postcontrast showing dilated intrahepatic biliary ducts (arrow), which can be seen running parallel to the intrahepatic portal veins as part of the portal triads. Intrahepatic bile ducts should not normally be visible by CT.

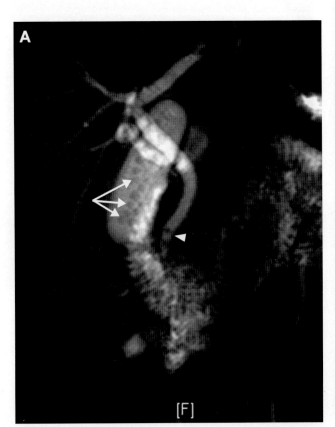

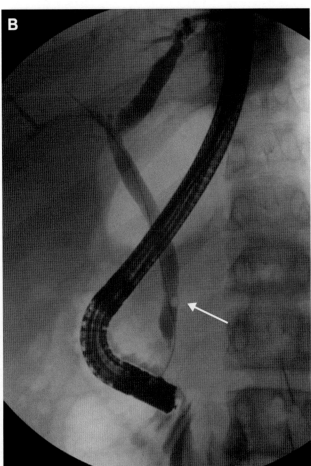

Fig. C16.3 Choledocholithiasis. (A) MRCP thick slab image showing two small filling defects within the distal CBD representing stones (arrowhead). Numerous gallstones are also seen (arrows). There is proximal extrahepatic and intrahepatic biliary dilatation due to obstruction. (B) ERCP radiograph of the same patient shows the same filling defect representative of the obstructing stone (arrow). A sphincterotomy and balloon sweep then cleared the stone.

bile duct abnormalities and is similar to ERCP, but less invasive. However, ERCP allows therapeutic intervention with sphincterotomy and stone removal (Fig. C16.3B).

Cholecystitis will usually not cause biliary obstruction; however, occasionally, an impacted stone in the distal cystic duct that causes cholecystitis may also result in obstruction of the common bile duct. This is referred to as Mirizzi syndrome and occurs frequently in patients with a low insertion of the cystic duct, which runs in a common sheath with the common bile duct (Fig. C16.4). The obstruction can be due to overall mass effect from the stone or due to surrounding inflammation. MRCP is accurate for diagnosis and presurgical identification is crucial for avoiding common bile duct ligation or injury.

Once a stone has been excluded, the other likely cause of a biliary obstruction is strictures. The differential diagnosis for biliary strictures includes benign inflammatory disorders (post pancreatitis, post chemoradiation therapy, AIDS cholangiopathy, and biliary parasites) and neoplasms

(cholangiocarcinoma, pancreatic or gallbladder carcinoma, and metastasis).

Cholangiocarcinoma (adenocarcinoma of the bile ducts) is an uncommon tumor that usually occurs in individuals with an underlying benign biliary disorder. Risk factors include primary sclerosing cholangitis, ulcerative colitis, primary biliary cirrhosis, congenital biliary anatomical anomalies, and biliary infections. It is traditionally classified as extrahepatic or intrahepatic, with intrahepatic being further subdivided into peripheral and central. Central and hilar intrahepatic cholangiocarcinomas are specifically referred to as Klatskin tumors. These tumors have an infiltrative growth pattern that results in a desmoplastic reaction, and they lack a surrounding capsule. Because of this, on CT, these will demonstrate slight enhancement on the arterial and portal venous phases. The central area will not enhance during these phases; however, on delayed sequence, there is prolonged central enhancement when associated fibrosis is present. Traditionally, these tumors have

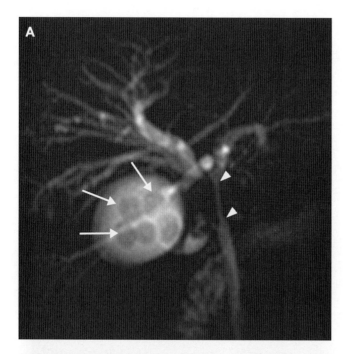

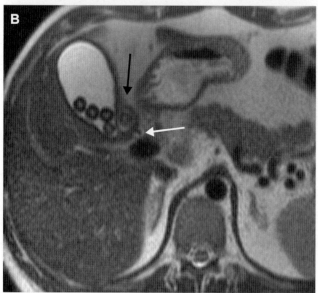

Fig. C16.4 Mirizzi syndrome. (A) MRCP image showing multiple stones in the distended gallbladder (white arrows). The distal common hepatic duct is severely narrowed (arrowheads) to an impacted stone in the cystic duct. The cystic duct stone is not visualized because only fluid based structures are seen on MRCP images. (B) Corresponding axial T2-weighted image demonstrates the relationship of the stone within the cystic duct (black arrow) abutting the common hepatic duct (white arrow).

been evaluated with ERCP or percutaneous transhepatic cholangiography (Fig. C16.5); however, MRCP, along with multiplanar and multiecho sequence liver protocol MRIs, allow excellent identification, characterization, and staging of these tumors.

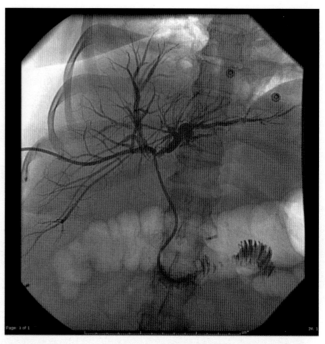

Fig. C16.5 Klatskin tumor. AP radiograph from a percutaneous transhepatic cholangiogram (PTC). An internal-external drainage catheter bridges the obstructing cholangiocarcinoma within the central hilum. Notice the diffuse dilatation of both the left and right biliary branches.

DIFFERENTIAL DIAGNOSIS

When presented with a jaundiced patient, the first step is to determine if the abnormal LFTs are suggestive of an obstructive versus a nonobstructive etiology. The more common nonobstructive pattern will be due to underlying cirrhosis and poor hepatic function. The other causes of nonobstructive jaundice include a whole host of hemolytic related disorders that are beyond the scope of this radiology text. Clinically, the obstructive pattern patients can be further subdivided based upon the presentation of jaundice with associated pain versus painless jaundice. Painless jaundice is usually associated with an underlying mass that has slowly resulted in obstruction rather than an acute obstructing process that results in pain.

REFERENCES AND SUGGESTED READING

1. Han JK. Cholangiocarcinoma: pictorial essay of CT and cholangiographic findings. *RadioGraphics*. 2002;22:173-187.
2. Tkacz, JN. MR imaging in gastrointestinal emergencies. *RadioGraphics*. 2009;29:1767-1780.
3. ACR Appropriateness Criteria. Jaundice.

CASE 17

PATIENT PRESENTATION

A 35-year-old woman presented with intermittent episodes of nausea, diaphoresis, and tremors. She was found to be hypoglycemic during episodes.

CLINICAL SUSPICION

Pancreatic endocrine tumor, insulinoma

IMAGING MODALITY OF CHOICE

The diagnosis of an insulinoma or any other pancreatic endocrine tumor is primarily a clinical diagnosis based on clinical presentation and biochemical testing, but radiographic evaluation is integral to confirmation, treatment planning, and follow-up. The image modality of choice is multiphase CT, using a dedicated multiphasic technique. This technique involves imaging the abdomen during several phases after contrast administration; thus, it should only be used in patients with high clinical suspicion of a neuroendocrine tumor because of the higher radiation dose. Scans are done during the arterial phase (20 seconds), the pancreatic parenchymal phase (40 seconds), and the portal venous phase (70 seconds). Multiplanar reconstructions in the sagittal and coronal planes are essential. A neutral oral contrast such as water or a 0.1% barium suspension VoLumen) is used to distend the stomach and the duodenum to visualize any masses in the bowel wall. Using positive water-soluble contrast or barium will obscure bowel wall masses. A similarly thorough assessment can be made with multiphasic MRI, which has the added benefit of multiple other sequences that further characterize these lesions but is more expensive.

Several other imaging modalities can be used but are usually supplemental. They include endoscopic sonography, a nuclear medicine somatostatin receptor isotope octreoscan, and an interventional radiology venous sampling procedure.

FINDINGS

Pancreatic endocrine tumors neuroendocrine neoplasms that are hormonally functioning or nonfunctioning and can be associated with syndromic or nonsyndromic forms. They can be either well differentiated or poorly differentiated. They were formerly named islet cell tumors but have recently been found to arise from ductal pluripotent stem cells and not from the islets of Langerhans. These tumors include (in order of decreasing frequency) insulinoma, gastrinoma, glucagonoma, vipoma, and somatostatinoma. Each has its own unique clinical presentation based on the manifestation of excess hormone production. For this reason, it is believed that functioning tumors are usually found earlier in their course and are thus smaller in size. Conversely, nonfunctioning tumors may continue to grow, unnoticed, until sufficiently large enough to cause mass effect or metastatic disease. The syndromic forms are associated with multiple endocrine neoplasia type 1, von Hippel-Lindau, and neurofibromatosis type 1.

These tumors share common imaging appearances and can usually only be differentiated from one another clinically. They present as hypervascular masses, best seen during the arterial phase (Fig. C17.1A). They are commonly overlooked during the pancreatic or portal venous phases because the surrounding pancreatic parenchyma demonstrates a similar degree of contrast enhancement (Fig. C17.1B). Thin-section reformats are critical for detection because these masses can be very small despite excessive hormone production. Imaging during different phases of contrast enhancement is not only important for visualizing the mass but also for defining its relationship with critical surrounding structures, such as the splenic and mesenteric vasculature. Their intimacy with these structures may preclude or change surgical options. Larger masses may demonstrate variable degrees of necrosis, hemorrhage, or calcification. They have similar enhancement patterns on MRI and are usually T2 hyperintense.

DIFFERENTIAL DIAGNOSIS

Each of these tumors has a distinct clinical presentation. Insulinomas, for instance, may present with Whipple's classic triad of low blood glucose; hypoglycemia symptoms, including dizziness, blurry vision, confusion, tachycardia, and diaphoresis; and symptom relief with glucose administration. These tumors are usually quite small at the time of diagnosis (<2 cm); tumors larger than 3 cm are more likely to be metastatic, most commonly to the peripancreatic lymph nodes and the liver (Fig. C17.2). These are occasionally multiple and are frequently associated with multiple endocrine neoplasia type 1.

Gastrinomas were described by Zollinger and Ellison as a triad of gastric acid hypersecretion, unusual location or number of peptic ulcers, and a small tumor. Later, gastrin was found to be the causative hormone. These are the second most common pancreatic endocrine tumors (PETs). They are found in extrapancreatic locations, within the gastrinoma triangle, most commonly related to the duodenum.

DIFFERENTIAL DIAGNOSIS

Many other hyperenhancing masses or pseudomasses can be found in the pancreas, including hypervascular metastases from primary tumors such as renal cell carcinoma, thyroid cancer, choriocarcinoma, and melanoma. Other lesions include vascular abnormalities, such as splenic

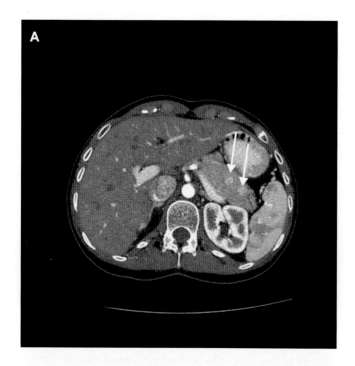

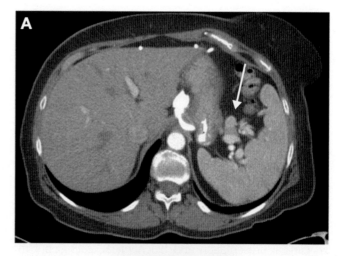

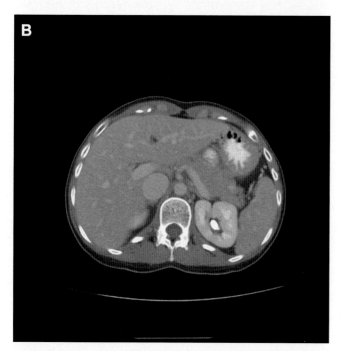

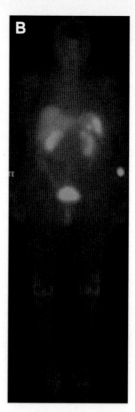

Fig. C17.1 Insulinoma. (A) Axial CT arterial phase from pancreatic protocol showing two small hypervascular enhancing masses in the tail of the pancreas (white arrows). These represented insulinomas, based upon biochemical and ultimately histologic evaluation. The imaging appearance alone is nonspecific amongst neuroendocrine tumors. (B) Axial CT delayed phase of the same patient at the same level. Notice how much more difficult it is to identify the masses because they have become isodense with the surrounding pancreatic parenchyma.

Fig. C17.2 Insulinoma. (A) Axial CT arterial phase with a small hypervascular mass in the pancreatic tail (white arrow). Notice that its degree of enhancement almost reaches the same density as the splenic vein located slightly posteriorly. The high-density ringlike object around the GE junction is a partially visualized lap band for bariatric surgery. (B) Indium-111-pentetreotide scintigraphy (Octreoscan). Whole-body planar images in the anterior projection shows a small focus of abnormal increased uptake in the left upper quadrant corresponding to the hypervascular mass on CT. This scan can result in false negatives when the tumors do not express somatostatin receptors. The normal biodistribution of the radiotracer is within the spleen, liver, kidneys, and bladder. The focal uptake in the left wrist is the site of injection.

artery pseudoaneurysms and intrapancreatic splenules. Vascular lesions should be easily distinguishable on arterial and portal phase imaging and thin-section multiplanar reformats. A splenule shares similar enhancement to the adjacent spleen and can be distinguished with a damaged Tc-99m RBC scan, which will demonstrate focal uptake by normal splenic parenchyma.

REFERENCES AND SUGGESTED READING

1. Horton KM. Multi-detector row CT of pancreatic islet cell tumors. *RadioGraphics*. 2006;26:453-464.
2. Lewis RB. Pancreatic endocrine tumors: radiologic-clinicopathologic correlation. *RadioGraphics*. 2010;30:1445-1464.

CASE 18

PATIENT PRESENTATION

A 33-year-old woman with right flank pain was found to have a nonobstructing ureteropelvic junction stone on noncontrast renal stone CT and an incidental low-density mass in the body of the pancreas.

CLINICAL SUSPICION

Cystic pancreatic mass

IMAGING MODALITY OF CHOICE

Several different cystic lesions can be found in the pancreas that may have significant overlap in imaging appearance, resulting in a diagnostic dilemma. Some of these are benign, but some have malignant potential. Thus, proper identification is crucial for proper management. More and more of these lesions are being incidentally found because of an increasing frequency in the use of cross-sectional imaging. A routine abdomen pelvis CT may identify one of these lesions but may not be optimized for proper characterization because of inadequate timing of contrast bolus and thick slices, resulting in volume averaging and loss of spatial resolution. Thus, a pancreatic protocol CT with multiphase contrast, as well as acquisition with thinner slice thickness, will improve characterization of these lesions. MRCP is superior to MDCT for identifying and characterizing these lesions and can be performed in addition to multiphase contrast-enhanced MRI. MRCP is useful for characterizing the relationship between these lesions and the pancreatic duct and lacks ionizing radiation but is a more limited resource because of availability, cost, and longer imaging times. Invasive procedures such as ERCPs and EUS can also be used. Modern EUS can provide high-resolution images and the ability to aspirate or biopsy these often indeterminate lesions, ultimately leading to a histopathologic diagnosis.

FINDINGS

Pancreatic pseudocysts are one of the common cystic lesions of the pancreas. Therefore, the first step in narrowing down the differential diagnosis is determining whether the lesion is a pseudocyst. Other cystic lesions include serous cystadenoma, intraductal papillary mucinous neoplasm (IPMN), and mucinous cystic neoplasms. Other neoplasms, including solid and papillary epithelial neoplasms (SPEN) and rarely, pancreatic adenocarcinoma, can present as partially cystic lesions, as can neuroendocrine tumors or metastases. Finally, true pancreatic cysts are associated with several syndromes, including von Hippel-Lindau, autosomal dominant polycystic kidney disease, and cystic fibrosis.

A pancreatic pseudocyst is defined as an amylase-rich fluid collection that typically arises in or adjacent to the pancreas with a thick fibrous wall with no epithelial lining.

Unusually, pseudocysts can be found at extrapancreatic locations remote from the pancreas such as in the thorax or pelvis. The CT appearance of these entities includes a round, oval, or irregular fluid collection with a uniformly thin or thick wall that enhances on contrast-enhanced scans (Figs. C18.1A-D). They are usually diagnosed when there is a clinical history of pancreatitis or when prior examination demonstrates a temporal evolution of acute pancreatitis, with organizing fluid collections over time. They may also be found where the pancreas demonstrates the stigmata of chronic pancreatitis, including atrophy, ductal dilatation,

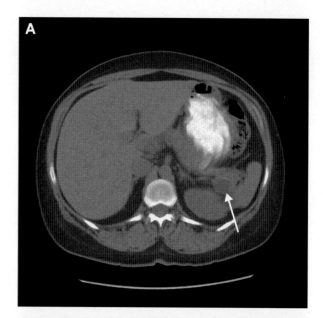

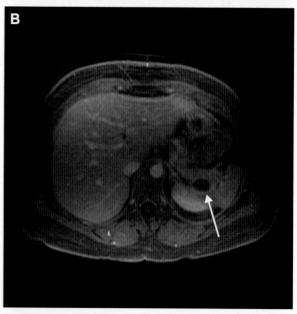

Fig. C18.1 Pseudocyst. (A) Axial noncontrast CT shows a nonspecific hypodense cystic lesion in the tail of the pancreas (white arrow) with a thin rim. Patient reported no history of pancreatitis. (B) Follow-up MRI of the abdomen postcontrast T1 weighted demonstrating a nonenhancing T1 hypointense lesion (white arrow).

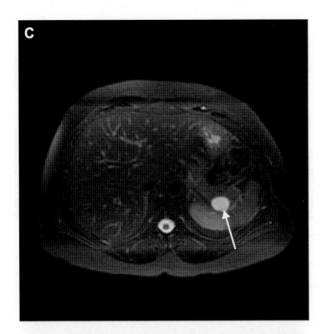

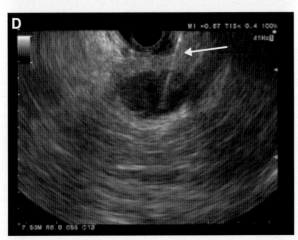

Fig. C18.1 (*continued*) Pseudocyst. (C) Fat-saturated T2-weighted shows a simple appearing, centrally nonenhancing T2-hyperintense cyst (white arrow) in the tail of the pancreas with a thin peripherally enhancing rim. These findings remained nonspecific due to the absence of a history of pancreatitis. (D) EUS also showed a simple appearing anechoic round fluid collection in the tail of the pancreas. FNA yielded high concentration of amylase with no mucin consistent with a psuedocyst. The linear echogenic structure (arrow) represents the needle extending from the endoscope into the cyst.

and calcifications; however, if there is no history to corroborate these findings, it may be difficult to distinguish a pseudocyst from other cystic lesions especially mucinous tumors. Diagnosis can be more difficult without a history of pancreatitis; these cases may require aspiration/biopsy.

A pancreatic serous cystadenoma, also known as a microcystic cystadenoma, is usually asymptomatic and presents as an incidental finding in older women. Occasionally, these are large enough to cause pain or obstructive symptoms, thus requiring surgery, but they are rarely

malignant. They are lobulated cystic masses, composed of multiple small cysts, resulting in a honeycomb appearance (Figs. C18.2A-C). Depending on the size of the cysts, they can appear solid or cystic on sonography or CT. A central stellate scar-containing calcification is a rather specific and distinguishing finding, but is seen infrequently. A macrocystic or oligocystic variant is rare but may be difficult to distinguish from a mucinous cystic neoplasm.

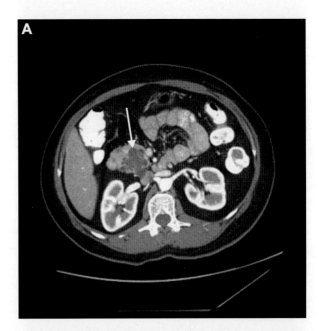

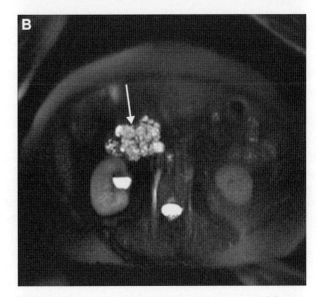

Fig. C18.2 Serous cystadenoma. (A) Axial postcontrast CT shows a complex cystic lesion in the head of the pancreas (white arrow). Notice the lobulated contour due to composition of multiple smaller cysts, with intervening septations. (B) Axial T2-weighted fat-saturated image with the same complex cystic lesion in the pancreatic head (white arrow). The honeycomblike appearance due to the internal septations is more easily appreciated.

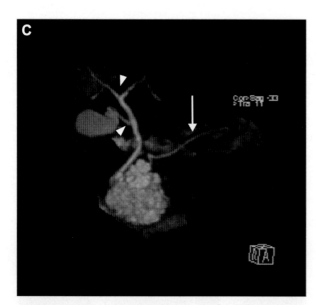

Fig. C18.2 (*continued*) Serous cystadenoma. (C) MRCP image demonstrates how this mass is composed of numerous smaller individual cysts. It also clearly demonstrates the normal caliber of the main pancreatic duct (arrow) as well as CBD, cystic duct, and common hepatic ducts (arrowheads).

Mucinous cystic neoplasms are the most common cystic neoplasm; they can be benign or malignant (eg, a cystadenoma or cystadenocarcinoma, respectively). Imaging can at times differentiate between the two; as both have malignant potential they are grouped together and are considered malignant, requiring resection. These lesions are oval or rounded in configuration, have larger cysts, and can be multilocular or unilocular. They can have enhancing septae, small mural nodularity, and peripheral calcifications that distinguish cystadenomas from cystadenocarcinomas. Calcifications in mucinous tumors are usually located in the tumor periphery in contrast to the distinct central stellate calcifications of serous cystadenoma (Fig. C18.3).

An intraductal papillary mucinous neoplasm results from papillary proliferation of the ductal epithelium, producing mucin. They are divided into main duct, side branch, or combined subtypes, and all have malignant potential. Intraductal papillary mucinous neoplasms result in cystic dilatation of the involved pancreatic ducts that contain mucin. They are more common in elderly men, with vague abdominal symptoms and occasional hyperamylasemia. The gold standard for diagnosis has been ERCP, which demonstrates bulging of the ampulla of Vater into the duodenum, mucin pouring out of the ampulla, and communication of these cystic lesions with the pancreatic ducts. However, thin-section multiplanar CT and MRCP can demonstrate communication with the main pancreatic duct, offering a noninvasive alternative (Fig. C18.4).

Finally, solid and papillary epithelial neoplasms of the pancreas are a low-grade tumor with minimal malignant potential that usually presents in young women. These masses are composed of solid and cystic components

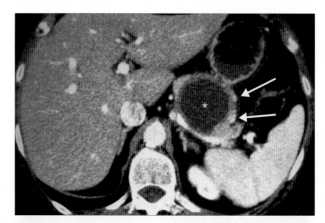

Fig. C18.3 Mucinous cystic neoplasm. Axial CT postcontrast image shows a unilocular cyst in the tail of the pancreas (*) consistent with a mucinous cystadenoma that was proven at surgery. This has a thick surrounding rim with faint calcifications visualized along the peripheral margin (white arrows).

and are commonly associated with central necrosis with hemorrhage and fluid-fluid levels (Fig. C18.5). They are usually large at the time of diagnosis, causing nonspecific symptoms such as nausea, vomiting, or abdominal fullness resulting in their resection.

All lesions require clinical correlation for proper diagnosis. Management not only varies by histologic type but also by symptoms, size, and location; therefore, a multidisciplinary approach and close follow-up are usually required.

DIFFERENTIAL DIAGNOSIS

As stated earlier, the main clinical distinction that has to be made is whether there is a history of pancreatitis, which would suggest the cystic lesion is a pseudocyst. In the absence of that clinical history, these are quite difficult to distinguish because they do not always demonstrate the characteristic features listed above and there is an overlap in the imaging appearances (Fig. C18.6).

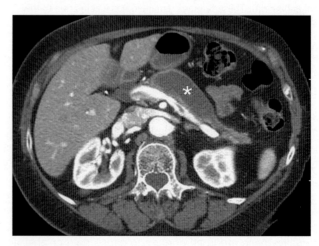

Fig. C18.4 IPMN. Axial CT postcontrast image demonstrates diffuse dilatation of the main pancreatic duct (*). This extends to the ampulla.

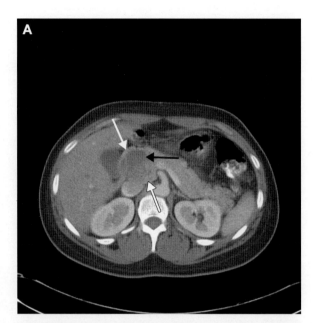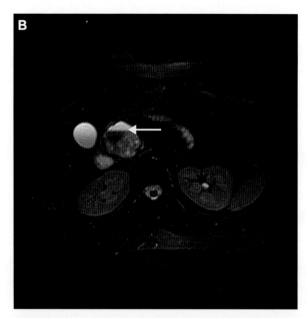

Fig. C18.5 SPEN. (A) Axial CT postcontrast image from a 19-year-old female showing a complex mass in the head of the pancreas (white arrows). The ventral aspect appears cystic while the dorsal aspect appears solid and enhancing. A layering hematocrit line can be seen with hyperdense RBC's layering dependently below the less dense plasma (black arrow). (B) Axial T2-weighted fat saturated respiratory trigged image demonstrating the same SPEN within the pancreatic head. The layering hematocrit line (white arrow) within the ventral cystic component is more easily detected on the MRI.

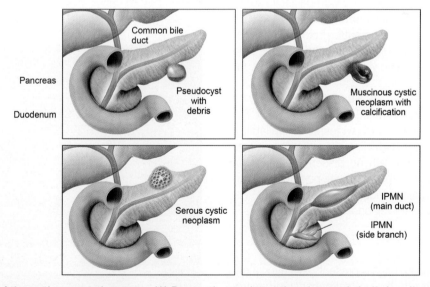

Fig. C18.6 Illustrations of the cystic pancreatic masses. (A) Pancreatic pseudocyst that characteristically is unilocular. (B) Mucinous cystic neoplasm that is characteristically either unilocular or multilocular (<5 cysts) with thick walls and peripheral curvilinear calcifications. (C) Serous cystadenoma with honeycomb appearance due to numerous tiny microcysts with a central stellate fibrotic region containing calcification. (D) IPMN including the main duct type with diffuse dilatation of the pancreatic main duct as well a side branch type with a focal cystic mass with continuity to the main duct.

REFERENCES AND SUGGESTED READING

1. Kim YH. Imaging diagnosis of cystic pancreatic lesions: pseudo-cyst versus nonpseudocyst. *RadioGraphics.* 2005;25:671-685.

2. Sahani SV. Cystic pancreatic lesions: a simple imaging-based classification system for guiding management. *RadioGraphics* 2005;25:1471-1484.

CASE 19

PATIENT PRESENTATION

A 62-year-old man presented with painless jaundice; initial abdominal sonography demonstrated dilatation of the distal common bile duct and the pancreatic duct ("double duct sign").

CLINICAL SUSPICION

Pancreatic cancer

IMAGING MODALITY OF CHOICE

Multiphase MDCT is the imaging modality of choice for diagnosing and staging pancreatic adenocarcinoma. Pancreatic adenocarcinoma is the fourth leading cause of cancer-related death in the United States. The overall 5-year survival rate is dismal, at less than 5%. The only curative treatment is complete resection with negative margins. Whipple surgery or pancreaticoduodenectomy, the surgical treatment for tumors of the head and uncinate process of the pancreas, has significant morbidity; therefore, it is crucial to preoperatively identify proper surgical candidates. Surgery of incompletely resectable tumors provides no survival advantage compared with palliative surgical procedures; it only increases morbidity.

MDCT with a multiphase pancreatic protocol has a reported sensitivity of 80% to 91% for detecting unresectable disease and positive predictive values of 76% to 100% for identifying unresectable tumors.

Dynamic contrast MRI is an alternative especially to those who cannot receive iodinated contrast, but MDCT is more commonly used because of its widespread availability. Occasionally, when there is high clinical suspicion, such as pancreatic ductal dilatation with no discernible mass on MDCT, further workup with endoscopic sonography is warranted because of its ability to identify smaller lesions, especially in the periampullary region.

FINDINGS

Pancreatic adenocarcinoma usually presents as a hypoattenuating focal mass relative to the normal-enhancing pancreatic parenchyma. For this reason, pancreatic protocol MDCT attempts to image during the pancreatic parenchymal or late arterial phase to achieve maximal parenchymal enhancement and increase the relative contrast conspicuity between the mass and background parenchyma (Figs. C19.1 and C19.2). When these masses are relatively isodense, additional radiographic findings may include a focal change in normal parenchymal lobulations or texture; an abrupt change in the caliber of the pancreatic duct or bile duct, or abrupt termination of a dilated pancreatic duct, particularly when associated with a density or texture change; and modification

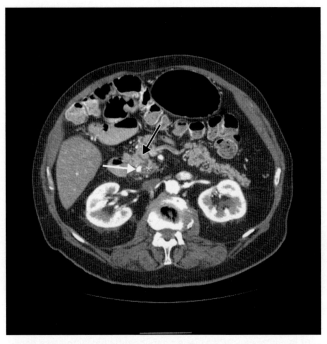

Fig. C19.1 Pancreatic adenocarcinoma. Axial CT in the late arterial phase through the head of the pancreas shows an ill-defined hypodensity (*) in the pancreatic head representing primary pancreatic adenocarcinoma. Notice the dilated pancreatic duct (black arrow) and the biliary stent (white arrow) inserted because of obstruction of the CBD from this infiltrating mass.

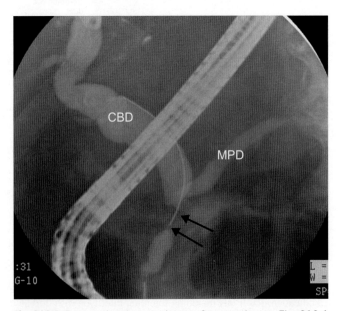

Fig. C19.2 Pancreatic adenocarcinoma. Same patient as Fig. C19.1 with ERCP image showing the double duct sign with abrupt short segment narrowing (between two black arrows) involving the confluence of the distal common bile duct and pancreatic duct.

of the contours of the pancreas. The main objective of preoperative MDCT is staging to identify potential surgical candidates. In terms of TMN staging, T1 through T3 tumors are considered potentially resectable. This includes tumors that have extended into the peripancreatic soft tissues, without invasion into the stomach, colon, celiac axis, or SMA. Invasion into any of these structures constitutes T4 disease and is usually regarded as unresectable. Extension into the duodenum is not a criterion for unresectability, as this is removed en bloc with the pancreas during Whipple surgery. Because of the intimate anatomical relationship of the pancreas to many visceral vessels, including the small mesenteric vein–portal confluence, SMA, and celiac axis, and because resectability frequently hinges on their noninvolvement, these must be closely evaluated (Fig. C19.3). Sometimes the only clue to vascular involvement is a small faint soft tissue cuff around the vessels as opposed to the more striking appearance of complete encasement or occlusion. Depending on the degree of vascular involvement, different institutions determine which tumors are resectable. Table C19.1 lists the criteria used at our institution.

Obviously, metastatic disease precludes surgery as an option; however, presence of local peripancreatic lymphadenopathy is not considered a sign of unresectability. MDCT has not been found to be accurate in staging lymph node involvement, and in potentially resectable cases, questionable lymph node involvement is best assessed by EUS and biopsy.

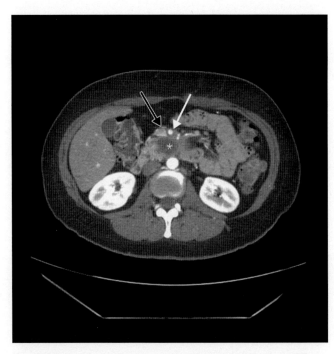

Fig. C19.3 Unresectable pancreatic adenocarcinoma. Axial CT image of pancreatic adenocarcinoma. The hypodense mass is primarily within the pancreatic uncinate process (*), but notice the ventral extension and complete encasement of the SMA (white arrow) consistent with infiltrative unresectable tumor. The SMV is abutted but not encased (black arrow).

DIFFERENTIAL DIAGNOSIS

Numerous other pancreatic lesions, both neoplastic and nonneoplastic, may mimic adenocarcinomas. One of the more common problematic lesions is focal pancreatitis.

Chronic pancreatitis has a variable presentation, including atrophy or enlargement of the organ and ductal dilatation. With focal enlargement and parenchymal changes due to chronic inflammation, this may be identical to the features

Table C19.1 Criteria for Resectability of Pancreatic Cancer at the M.D. Anderson Cancer Center

Affected Vessel	Characterization		
	Resectable	Borderline Resectable	Locally Advanced
SMA	No extension, normal fat plane between tumor and artery	Tumor abutment affecting less than or equal to 180° of the circumference of the artery, periarterial stranding and tumor points of contact forming a convexity against the vessel improve chances of resection	Encased (>180° of the circumference of the artery)
Celiac axis or hepatic artery	No extension	Short-segment encasement or abutment of the common hepatic artery (typically at the gastroduodenal origin), surgeon should be prepared for vascular resection or interposition grafting	Encased and no technical option for reconstruction (usually due to extension to the junction of the celiac axis, splenic vein, and left gastric artery or to the origin of the celiac axis)
SMV-PV	Patent	Short-segment occlusion with suitable vessel condition superiorly and inferiorly, segmental venous occlusion alone without SMA involvement is rare and should be apparent at CT	Occluded and no technical option for reconstruction

of adenocarcinoma. Compounding the problem, the inflammatory changes of pancreatitis may result in adjacent lymphadenopathy and perivascular changes, mimicking neoplasm.

Primary pancreatic lymphoma is quite rare, representing less than 1% of primary extranodal lymphomas. It may present as a large mass that is hypoattenuating relative to the normal pancreatic parenchyma. A distinguishing feature from adenocarcinoma is displacement of the ducts and vessels rather than invasion.

Patients presenting clinically with painless jaundice need an extensive work up to find the underlying etiology. If the patient has an obstructive pattern then some obstructing cancer should be first on the clinical differential list. This could include any masses along the course of the biliary system resulting in obstruction including pancreatic neoplasms, cholangiocarcinoma, other primary liver masses such as HCC, stomach or duodenal malignancies, and distant metastases.

REFERENCES AND SUGGESTED READING

1. Darren DD. Comprehensive preoperative assessment of pancreatic adenocarcinoma with 64-section volumetric CT. *RadioGraphics*. 2007;27:1653-1666.

2. Bronstein YL. Detection of small pancreatic tumors with multiphasic helical CT. *AJR*. 2004;182:619-623.

3. Tamm EP. Staging of pancreatic cancer with multidetector CT in the setting of preoperative chemoradiation therapy. *Abdom Imaging*. 2006;31:568-574.

4. To'o KJ, Raman SS, Yu NC, et al. Pancreatic and peripancreatic diseases mimicking primary pancreatic neoplasia. *RadioGraphics*. 2005;25:949-965.

CASE 20

PATIENT PRESENTATION

A 45-year-old man presented with new-onset acute epigastric abdominal pain that was constant and burning in nature.

CLINICAL SUSPICION

Pancreatitis

IMAGING MODALITY OF CHOICE

The clinical course of acute pancreatitis varies widely. Thus, it has been categorized as mild or severe. The initial diagnosis is usually made easily with the typical presentation of severe unrelenting epigastric abdominal pain and elevation of serum amylase and lipase levels (<3 times normal). As severe pancreatitis can lead to bad outcomes, several clinical scoring systems, such as the Ranson's score, APACHE II score, and SIRS score have been developed to predict the morbidity and mortality. Table C20.1 lists the criteria used by Ranson for grading the severity of acute pancreatitis.

Advanced imaging may not be necessary in patients with a low clinical score, the caveat being the use of sonography to evaluate the biliary system to exclude gallstone pancreatitis. However, evaluation of the actual pancreatic parenchyma is limited with sonography because it is often obscured by overlying bowel gas.

MDCT with intravenous contrast is superior in its ability to evaluate for pancreatitis, determine the extent of disease, identify complications, and plan treatment, such as interventional procedures. Balthazar created a CT severity

Table C20.1 Ranson Criteria

On Admission:	At 48 Hours after Admission:
• Age >55	• Hematocrit decrease of more than 10%
• WBC count >16,000 (16 x 10^9 / L)	• BUN level increase of more than 5 mL/dL (1.8 mmol/L)
• Serum glucose level > 11.1 mmol/L	• Calcium <2 mmol/L
• SLDH/ALT >350 IU/L	• PaO$_2$ <60 mmHg
• AST level >250 IU/L	• Base deficit >4 mmol/L
	• Fluid sequestration >6 L

At admission 5 objective measurements are made, then at 48 hours after presentation 6 additional objective measurements are obtained. The morbidity and mortality rate increases with the number of risk factors. <3 positive signs has a mortality rate of zero, while ≥6 positive signs is associated with a mortality rate >50%.

Table C20.2 CT Severity Index for Acute Pancreatitis

CT Grade	Description	Points
A	Normal pancreas	0
B	Enlarged pancreas	1
C	Pancreatic inflammation or peripancreatic fat stranding	2
D	Single peripancreatic fluid collection	3
E	≥2 peripancreatic fluid collections ± retroperitoneal gas	4

Necrosis	Points
<33%	2
33%-50%	4
>50%	6

Total Points	Morbidity	Mortality
0-3	8%	3%
4-6	35%	6%
7-10	92%	17%

Data from Balthazar EJ. Acute pancreatitis: value of CT in establishing prognosis. *Radiology.* 1990 Feb;174(2):331-336.

index based on imaging findings to predict not only severity but also clinical outcome (Table C20.2). MRI with MRCP can also be sued to evaluate both the pancreatic parenchyma and biliary and pancreatic duct.

FINDINGS

Acute pancreatitis is acute inflammatory process of the pancreas caused by intracellular activation of proteolytic enzymes, which autodigest the pancreatic parenchyma. The most common causes include alcohol, gallstones, metabolic disorders, trauma, drugs, and infection. The imaging findings of mild acute edematous pancreatitis include localized or diffuse enlargement of the pancreas and uniform enhancement of the parenchyma. There may be a variable degree of adjacent peripancreatic and retroperitoneal fat stranding and peripancreatic fluid collections.

Pancreatitis can lead to pancreatic necrosis, which is characterized by heterogeneous or diminished enhancement of the pancreatic parenchyma (Fig. C20.1). Several vascular complications can occur, including development of pseudoaneurysms and thrombosis of the splenic, superior mesenteric, or portal vein (Fig. C20.2). Acute peripancreatic fluid collections commonly resolve spontaneously, making drainage unnecessary; in fact, because these are usually sterile, percutaneous drainage can actually be detrimental if it results in infection. Those that do not spontaneously resolve will become organized over time, eventually

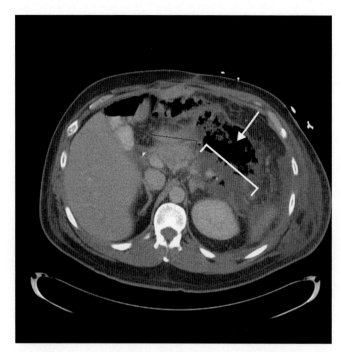

Fig. C20.1 Necrotizing pancreatitis. Axial CT postcontrast of hemorrhagic pancreatitis. Notice how the parenchyma of the pancreatic head is enhancing (black bracket) while the pancreatic tail is not (white bracket). This bout of pancreatitis was secondary to perforated gastric ulcer with free air located ventral to the pancreas (arrow).

developing a fibrous capsule that enhances after contrast. When they occur at least 4 weeks after acute pancreatitis, these rim-enhancing collections are referred to as pancreatic pseudocysts. These can also spontaneously regress and are usually sterile; therefore, asymptomatic pseudocysts do not require drainage. However, if they become symptomatic, causing pain from mass effect or infection, drainage may be indicated. Unfortunately, imaging cannot readily differentiate between sterile and infected pseudocysts unless gas bubbles have developed inside the collection, indicating infection due to a gas-forming organism.

Chronic pancreatitis, usually in the setting of chronic alcohol abuse in Western countries, refers to chronic inflammatory disease of the pancreas, with irreversible damage to the morphological characteristics and function of the pancreas. Diagnostic features include gland atrophy, main pancreatic duct dilatation and beading, and intraductal calcifications. Pseudocysts and vascular complications may also be present.

Autoimmune pancreatitis, which is also known as lymphoplasmacytic sclerosing pancreatitis, is an uncommon variant of pancreatitis that has a different clinical course and imaging features. It usually occurs without the classic attacks of acute pancreatitis, has elevated immune markers (IgG4), and responds dramatically to steroid therapy. Patients may present with jaundice, abdominal pain, or weight loss, mimicking the presentation of pancreatic carcinoma. They commonly have a coexisting autoimmune disorder, such as sclerosing cholangitis, primary biliary cirrhosis, inflammatory bowel disease, retroperitoneal fibrosis, sclerosing mesenteritis, or Sjogren syndrome. Imaging findings include diffuse enlargement, with loss of lobular contour resulting in a "sausage" shape, a diffusely narrowed main pancreatic duct, and a peripheral "rind" or hypoattenuation with delayed enhancement (Fig. C20.3).

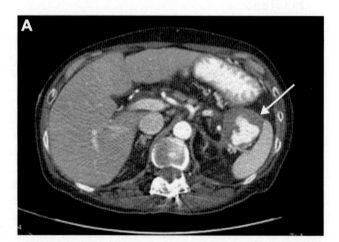
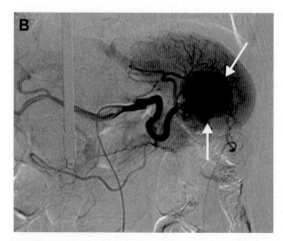

Fig. C20.2 Splenic artery pseudoaneurysm. (A) Axial postcontrast CT demonstrates a round mass within the splenic hilum. The central aspect enhances to an equal degree as the contrast within the aorta consistent with a vascular etiology. Scrolling through images shows it arising from the distal splenic artery in the patient with several bouts of prior pancreatitis. The nonenhancing soft tissue component along the ventral and medial walls of the pseudoaneurysm (white arrow) represents thrombus. (B) Digital subtraction angiogram with selection of the splenic artery demonstrates the large pseudoaneurysm as the densely opacifying round mass (arrows) with the normal splenic parenchyma enhancing posteriorly. This was subsequently treated with endovascular coiling.

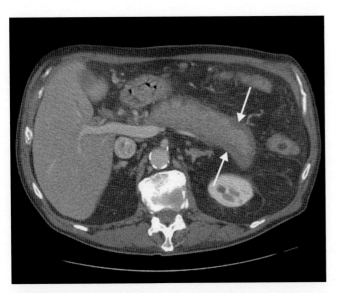

Fig. C20.3 Autoimmune pancreatitis. Axial postcontrast CT showing diffuse enlargement of the pancreas with loss of lobular contour resulting in a "sausage" shape and a peripheral "rind" or hypoattenuation (white arrows).

DIFFERENTIAL DIAGNOSIS

The clinical differential for adult patients presenting with localized epigastric pain besides pancreatitis, includes peptic ulcer disease, GERD, gastritis, cardiac related (MI, angina, pericarditis) or vascular abdominal aortic aneurysm or dissection. Elevated levels of serum amylase and lipase will confirm the suspected diagnosis.

REFERENCES AND SUGGESTED READING

1. Balthazar EJ. Acute pancreatitis: value of CT in establishing prognosis. *Radiology.* 1990;174(2):331-336.
2. ACR Appropriateness Criteria. Acute pancreatitis.

CASE 21

PATIENT PRESENTATION

A 32-year-old Hispanic man presented for routine follow-up to his family practice physician for type II diabetes and obesity and was found to have slightly elevated LFTs.

CLINICAL SUSPICION

Liver dysfunction

IMAGING MODALITY OF CHOICE

There is a wide range of clinical entities that can present with abnormalities of LFTs. Many of these can be deduced clinically, but imaging plays an important role in evaluating any structural changes of the hepatobiliary system. Sonography is the imaging modality of choice in any initial workup of suspected hepatobiliary disease because of its safety with lack of ionizing radiation, low cost, and versatility. A focused right upper quadrant sonography can evaluate the size, texture, and morphological characteristics of the liver and the patency and caliber of the main portal vein, gallbladder, intrahepatic and extrahepatic biliary system, and right kidney. A routine abdominal sonogram will also include evaluation of the spleen, pancreas, left kidney, and bladder. A more in-depth evaluation of the liver can be performed with a Doppler sonography, which evaluates the hepatic vasculature in more detail, including the direction and waveforms of the main, left, and right portal veins; the hepatic artery; and the left, right, and middle hepatic veins.

After initial sonography, many other modalities are available, including CT, MRI, and nuclear medicine HIDA to evaluate the liver and its functional status. Routine multidetector CT of the abdomen with intravenous contrast usually involves imaging the abdomen during the portal venous phase of contrast enhancement. This is performed to optimize the parenchymal enhancement of the liver because of its dual blood supply, with majority of the blood coming from the portal vein (80%) and the remainder from the hepatic artery. Important information may be derived from a noncontrast examination of the abdomen, but the routine use of "without and with" examinations should be avoided to minimize the overall radiation dose. Multiphase liver protocol CTs are primarily reserved for instances when a liver mass is known or suspected and needs further characterization. MRI allows for an even more detailed evaluation of the liver without ionizing radiation but with higher costs and longer imaging times.

DIFFERENTIAL DIAGNOSIS

Hepatic steatosis or fatty infiltration of the liver is now the most common cause of elevated LFTs, primarily because of the obesity epidemic. There are several variant forms: When associated with inflammation, it is termed steatohepatitis. When occurring with alcohol use, it is known as alcohol-related fatty liver. When no history of alcohol is present, the term used is nonalcoholic fatty liver disease (NAFLD), or nonalcoholic steatohepatitis (NASH) if inflammation is also present. Besides alcohol and obesity, other risk factors include diabetes, hyperlipidemia, total parenteral nutrition, and drugs (ie, tetracycline, amiodarone, corticosteroids, antiretrovirals, salicylates, and tamoxifen). Previously thought to be a benign condition, steatohepatitis may rarely progress to liver fibrosis and cirrhosis and ultimately hepatocellular carcinoma (HCC). Benign steatosis may be diffuse (more common) or focal, and steatohepatitis is usually diffuse. Unfortunately, noninvasive imaging can only detect the presence of fat, not inflammation; therefore, a liver biopsy is ultimately required for a definitive diagnosis.

Imaging Features of Hepatic Steatosis

Sonographic evaluation of the liver parenchymal echogenicity can be subjective, and it varies depending on the settings or gain used during acquisition. To aid in this dilemma, the echogenicity of the liver can be compared with that of the adjacent right kidney parenchyma. The normal liver should be equally or slightly more echogenic than the renal cortex or spleen. Fatty liver is suspected if the liver's echogenicity is higher (brighter) than that of the renal cortex or spleen. Another finding that should be used in conjunction with increased liver echogenicity is increased attenuation of the sonographic wave, resulting in poor delineation of intrahepatic vessels, posterior liver margin, and diaphragm.

On noncontrast CT, the liver attenuation will be decreased. An absolute attenuation of 40 Hounsfield units (HU) or less suggests the diagnosis. Usually, the liver is 10 HU, higher than the spleen. If the liver attenuation is less than that of the spleen, fatty liver may be present (Fig. C21.1). Attenuation measurements are less reliable

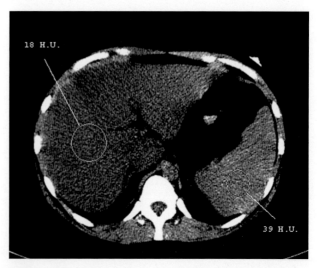

Fig. C21.1 Hepatic steatosis. Noncontrast axial CT showing diffuse hepatic steatosis of the liver. Note that the spleen is denser visually. Regions of interests (ROIs) which measure the density in Hounsfield units, show that the liver measures 18 HU and the spleen 39 HU.

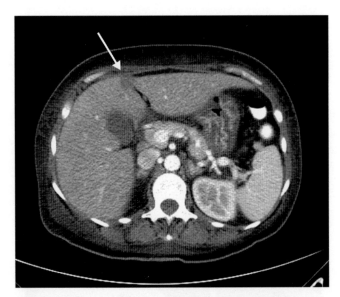

Fig. C21.2 Focal hepatic steatosis. Axial postcontrast CT image showing focal low density located near the falciform ligament (white arrow), which is due focal hepatic steatosis. This is thought to be secondary to altered perfusion.

for contrast-enhanced CT because the appearance of the liver and spleen depends on timing and technique. When a fatty liver evaluation is performed after contrast enhancement, the equilibrium phase is preferred if available because it decreases attenuation differences due to vascular phenomena.

The focal form of steatosis is commonly found at characteristic locations, including adjacent to the falciform ligament, porta hepatis, and gallbladder fossa (Fig. C21.2). This is believed to be due to variations in venous drainage. Other imaging features suggestive of focal fat rather than true hepatic lesions include vessels running through the lesion with no mass effect or displacement, a geographic pattern rather than a round or oval shape, poorly delineated margins, and an enhancement pattern similar to that of the adjacent parenchyma (Fig. C21.3). However, focal fat deposition can be difficult to distinguish from more aggressive lesions, and may require use of chemical shift MRI to make the diagnosis (Fig. C21.4).

The most sensitive imaging modality for assessing hepatic steatosis remains MRI, which uses specific sequences that take advantage of the differing relaxation times of fat and water during in-phase and out-of-phase timing. The out-of-phase sequence cancels out the signal of microscopic fat so that when viewed side by side, the out-of-phase sequence of an area that contains microscopic fat or lipids will have a lower signal than will the in-phase sequence (Fig. C21.5). The out-of-phase sequence can be easily identified by the signature India ink artifact, which is a black rim of no signal surrounding the abdominal organs and results from cancellation of fat-water signal at interface of the organs with the peritoneal fat.

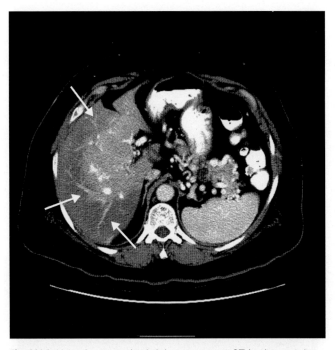

Fig. C21.3 Hepatic steatosis. Axial postcontrast CT in the portal venous phase demonstrates that the peripheral right hepatic lobe is lower in attenuation than the more central portion. The noncontrast exam demonstrated similar findings. Notice how normal branching vessels (white arrow) are seen crossing through the regions of steatosis.

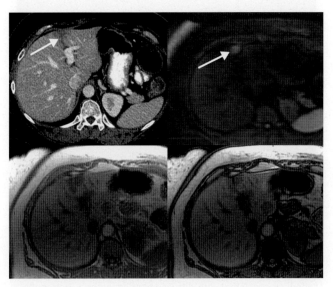

Fig. C21.4 Breast metastasis mimicking focal steatosis. Top left: Axial postcontrast CT demonstrates ill-defined hypoenhancing lesion (arrow) near the falciform ligament, a common site of focal steatosis, but new from prior baseline exam. Bottom images: Axial T1 in (left) and-out-of phase (right) imaging shows focal T1 hypointensity that does not drop in signal on the out-of-phase sequence. Top right: Diffusion weighted image (DWI) shows a focal area of restricted diffusion, which is nonspecific but in this case consistent with a metastasis from known breast primary.

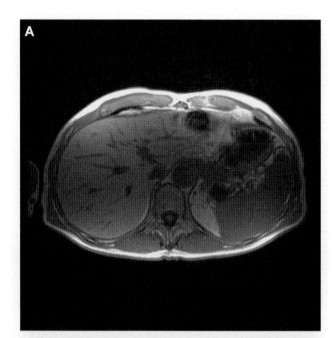

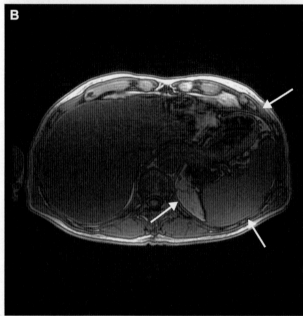

Fig. C21.5 Diffuse hepatic steatosis. (A) Axial T1-weighted in-phase image of the abdomen demonstrates normal high signal intensity of the liver relative to the musculature. (B) Axial T1-weighted out-of-phase image which is simultaneously attained with the in-phase images demonstrates significant drop in signal of the liver consistent with diffuse hepatic steatosis. Notice the India ink artifact (thin black line) surrounding the organs.

Imaging Features of Hepatic Iron Overload

Hepatic iron overload, due to conditions such as hemochromatosis or multiple blood transfusions, has imaging features that differ from those of fatty infiltration. On CT, the liver parenchyma will be hyperdense—usually more than 75 HU on noncontrast examination. MRI not only is more

sensitive at detecting hepatic iron overload but can actually quantify the amount of iron deposition; in the past, the only alternative was an invasive liver biopsy. Iron causes a magnetic susceptibility artifact, which results in decreased signal intensity on MRI sequences. This can be seen with a dramatically low signal intensity of the liver on T2-weighted images. On T1-weighted in- and out-of-phase imaging, the signal will drop out during the in-phase sequence rather than the out-of-phase, the reverse of what is seen in diffuse hepatic steatosis (Fig. C21.6). (This is generally true with 1.5 tesla MRI scanners, but differing imaging parameters on 3 tesla scanners may alter this principle.)

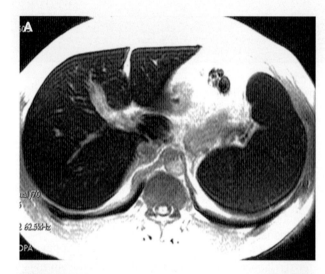

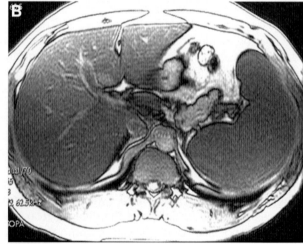

Fig. C21.6 Hemosiderosis due to multiple transfusions. (A) Axial T1 in phase image shows extremely low signal of both the liver and the spleen. Compare this to the case of diffuse hepatic steatosis (Fig. C21.5) earlier. (B) Axial T1 out-of-phase images shows the significant increase in signal of the liver relative to the in-phase consistent with iron deposition. Notice how the change in signal is the opposite to that seen in the case of diffuse hepatic steatosis. The spleen will not be involved with hemochromatosis, which is a distinguishing feature from secondary forms of hemosiderosis.

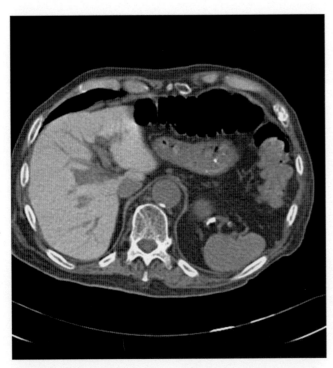

Fig. C21.7 Hyperdense liver due to Amiodarone. Axial CT without contrast with hyperdense liver secondary to amiodarone therapy. As a reference, look at the spleen and the paraspinal musculature. Also notice how the hepatic venous structures stand out.

Patients receiving amiodarone (an anti-arrhythmic drug) can develop a hyperdense liver on CT; however, this is secondary to the iodine content of the medication rather than iron (Fig. C21.7). In addition, iron overload will eventually lead to cirrhosis, whereas a hyperdense liver due to amiodarone therapy does not necessarily indicate toxicity.

DIFFERENTIAL DIAGNOSIS

There are numerous causes of elevated liver function tests, but in general, when approached with this problem a short differential list will cover a majority of the causes. The first step should be to identify any medications the patient might be taking that can cause elevation of LFTs. Second, a social history about alcohol use should be obtained. Serological testing for viral hepatitis could then be obtained and finally imaging studies could be obtained to diagnose hepatic steatosis or hemochromatosis.

REFERENCES AND SUGGESTED READING

1. Queiroz-Andrade M. MR imaging findings of iron overload. *RadioGraphics*. 2009;29:1575-1589.
2. Hamer OW. Fatty liver: imaging patterns and pitfalls. *RadioGraphics*. 2006;26:1637-1653.

CASE 22

PATIENT PRESENTATION

A 42-year-old man presented to his primary care physician with increasing abdominal girth and jaundice. The patient had a history of drug and alcohol abuse.

CLINICAL SUSPICION

Cirrhosis

IMAGING MODALITY OF CHOICE

Cirrhosis is the result of usually chronic but also acute insults to the liver. In the Western world, alcohol abuse remains the most common cause of cirrhosis, followed by viral hepatitis. Several other etiologies include congenital metabolic disorders such as glycogen storage diseases, hematologic disorders such as hemochromatosis, and medication side effects such as acetaminophen toxicity or Reye's syndrome with salicylates. There is an increasing awareness of the long-term consequences of fatty infiltration of the liver. Once considered benign, the steatohepatitis variant of fatty liver is now known to sometimes progress to cirrhosis.

Unfortunately, once cirrhosis has been diagnosed, there is no treatment to reverse the damage. Treatment mainly consists of eliminating further exposure to the offending agents (eg, through alcohol abstinence or antivirals for hepatitis B or C). Other medications are used to mitigate metabolic derangements and minimize symptoms such as ascites or encephalopathy. Ultimately, the only definitive treatment is liver transplantation.

A variety of imaging modalities are available to aid in the diagnosis and follow the course of disease. Sonography is highly effective for evaluating direct and indirect signs of cirrhosis; it is also cost effective and safe. Liver protocol multiphase CT and MRI have become instrumental in screening for HCC in patients on transplantation lists.

FINDINGS

The direct sonographic findings of cirrhosis include coarsened echotexture of the hepatic parenchyma and an irregular nodular contour. Later in the disease course, the right hepatic lobe frequently becomes atrophic, with hypertrophy of the caudate lobe. However, early in the course, the liver may be enlarged, making the size less specific. The secondary signs are usually related to the development of portal hypertension, including enlargement of the main portal vein (>1.5 cm), reversal of flow in the portal vein (normally hepatopetal, but when reversed, hepatofugal), splenomegaly (maximum length >12 cm), portosystemic collaterals, and ascites. Other nonspecific findings include gallbladder wall and bowel wall thickening, which

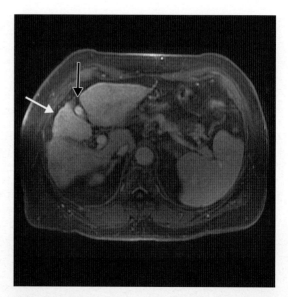

Fig. C22.1 Cirrhosis. Axial MR postcontrast T1-weighted image during the portal venous phase demonstrates a nodular contour along the periphery of the right lobe (white arrow) as well as recanalization of the umbilical vein (black arrow) representative of a portosystemic collateral due to portal hypertension.

are thought to result from passive congestion in the absence of intrinsic causes of edema.

With the exception of vascular flow direction, these findings are more evident on CT and MRI of the abdomen. For example, large gastric or esophageal varices are easily seen on CT and MRI but may be difficult to visualize on sonography because of overlying ribs and air in the stomach and lungs (Fig. C22.1). Multiphasic CT or MRI are predominantly used to characterize liver lesions but are also useful for characterizing variant hepatic anatomy and venous structure and collateral patency.

Another etiology of liver dysfunction that can be diagnosed on imaging is passive hepatic congestion due to heart failure. This occurs when the venous pressures in the right heart are elevated; these high pressures are transmitted back to the liver sinusoids, preventing normal blood flow. On imaging, this is commonly detected when an intravenous contrast bolus injected through the upper extremity refluxes into the inferior vena cava and hepatic veins instead of entering the right ventricle. The hepatic veins may be distended as well.

Portal vein thrombosis can result from a variety of conditions but is most commonly caused by cirrhosis, in which diminished flow results in stagnation (Fig. C22.2). Unfortunately, this can further exacerbate portal hypertension. In some cases, such as in patients with no liver disease but a prothrombotic genetic condition, it can result in portal hypertension. The clinical outcome is quite variable, ranging from being incidentally detected to being life threatening

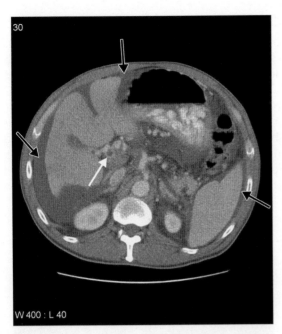

Fig. C22.2 Portal vein thrombosis. Axial postcontrast CT demonstrating portal vein thrombosis (white arrow) as filling defect in the opacified portal vein. Notice the ascites (black arrows).

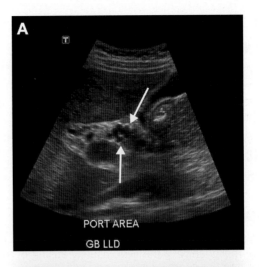

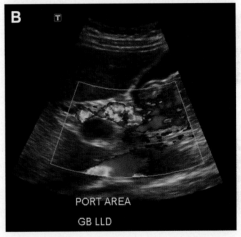

Fig. C22.3 Cavernous transformation of the portal vein. (A) Grayscale ultrasound of the liver evaluating the porta hepatis. Notice instead of a single large anechoic portal vein, there appears to be multiple cystic lesions (white arrows), representing the serpiginous tangle of collateral vessels. (B) Color Doppler image shows flow within these vessels with a turbulent appearance due to the tortuous course of the vessels.

as a result of acute bowel ischemia from a large thrombus extending into the superior mesenteric vein. After portal vein thrombosis, the portal vein may recanalize to reestablish portal blood flow to the liver, or more frequently in patients with cirrhosis, the portal vein will undergo cavernous transformation. Cavernous transformation refers to the development of several small collateral vessels in the porta hepatis that provide an alternate path for the blood around the main portal vein obstruction. This cavernous transformation can be visualized on color sonography or contrast-enhanced CT or MRI (Fig. C22.3).

DIFFERENTIAL DIAGNOSIS

Several diseases can mimic the appearance of cirrhosis, most infamously pseudocirrhosis, which refers to a nodular appearing liver that develops after chemotherapy treatment of widespread hepatic metastases, usually from such primaries as breast, lung, or colorectal cancer.

REFERENCES AND SUGGESTED READING

1. Gupta AA. CT and MRI of cirrhosis and its Mimics. *AJR*. 2004;183:1595-1601.
2. Tchelepi H. Sonography of diffuse liver disease. *J Ultrasound Med*. 2002;21(9):1023-1032.

CASE 23

PATIENT PRESENTATION

A 42-year-old man with a history of chronic hepatitis B underwent biannual screening sonography, which demonstrated a new hypoechoic 3 cm nodule; the alpha-fetoprotein was 50 ng/mL.

CLINICAL SUSPICION

Hepatocellular carcinoma (HCC)

IMAGING MODALITY OF CHOICE

HCC also known as a hepatoma, is the most common primary malignancy of the liver, usually arising in a background of chronic liver disease that is most commonly caused by alcoholism or chronic hepatitis B or C. Because of the obesity epidemic, HCC is increasingly arising in a background of steatohepatitis. Early-stage HCC is often clinically silent and is commonly advanced at presentation. Complete surgical resection or liver transplantation offers the best chance at survival, but these options are frequently not available because of advanced disease at the time of diagnosis. Consensus guidelines were created by several large international groups to standardize the surveillance, diagnosis, and management of HCC. The screening recommendations for high-risk patients include 6-month sonography, with serum AFP levels. Because of the large population of at-risk individuals, the recommendation is for ultrasound screening. This is partly based on overall cost-effectiveness and worldwide availability. Multiphase MDCT or MRI offers significantly higher sensitivity and specificity at detecting HCC, but because of the higher cost, radiation, and limited availability, they are used as confirmatory tests. Institutions may follow different guidelines, depending on their patient populations and availability of resources. A liver protocol MDCT consists of a noncontrast examination to detect calcifications and determine the background parenchymal density, followed by dynamic imaging performed in the arterial, portal venous, and equilibrium phases of contrast enhancement. Many advances have been made in the field of MRI of the liver, including newer sequences and contrast agents that allow detailed characterization of lesions. On MRI, HCC is typically T1 hypointense or isointense, with a relatively high T2 signal. Using techniques such as parallel imaging and volumetric acquisitions, MRI can now provide similar or better dynamic contrast enhancement characterization than CT, in addition to standard multisequence evaluation. The consensus guidelines do not advocate MDCT or MRI over one another in terms of diagnosing HCC; however, not accounting for cost, availability, or imaging time, MRI appears to offer improved characterization of liver lesions.

FINDINGS

Before considering the differential diagnosis of a liver mass, one should be familiar with the patient's demographics, including sex, age, race, and baseline disease status of the liver. The "classic" imaging appearance of a small HCC is a hypervascular mass that homogeneously hyperenhances during the arterial phase and demonstrates subsequent washout of contrast during the portal venous and equilibrium phases, making the mass relatively hypodense to the surrounding parenchyma (Fig. C23.1). Occasionally, they

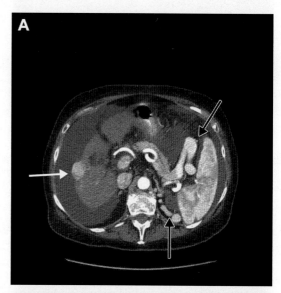

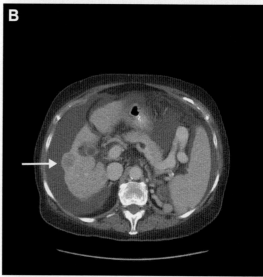

Fig. C23.1 Hepatocellular carcinoma. (A) Axial CT during arterial phase (notice high density of contrast in the aorta and hepatic artery as well as heterogeneous enhancement of the spleen). Large hypervascular nodule (white arrow) representative of HCC. The liver is cirrhotic (atrophic right lobe with accompanying signs of ascites, enlarged splenic vein, and large splenorenal collaterals (black arrows). (B) Axial CT during the delayed equilibrium phase. The HCC mass (white arrow) has washed out, now being hypoattenuating relative to the liver parenchyma.

are isodense on the portal venous and equilibrium phase, and therefore go unnoticed on a routine abdominal CT without an arterial phase. The pattern of arterial enhancement and rapid subsequent washout carries over to all imaging modalities, including dynamic MRI and conventional angiography. Larger HCC (>5 cm) may have a heterogeneous appearance on both CT and MRI; other characteristic findings include a mosaic pattern, tumor capsule, vascular invasion, necrosis, and fatty metamorphosis.

There are several subtypes of HCC, with variable appearances; however, only fibrolamellar HCC is covered here because it has an appearance that could mimic that of focal nodular hyperplasia (FNH). Unlike other HCCs, the fibrolamellar variant occurs in young individuals (second or third decade) without underlying liver disease. These lobulated, fairly well defined, solitary masses demonstrate heterogeneous arterial enhancement with progressive homogeneity during later phases, surrounding a central stellate or amorphous scar. On MRI, the masses are T1 isointense, with a variable T2 signal. Distinguishing features of the central scar include calcifications, and hypointensity on T1 and T2 sequences (Fig. C23.2).

Focal nodular hyperplasia (FNH) is the second most common benign tumor of the liver, after hemangioma. It most commonly occurs in women of reproductive age and is usually asymptomatic. It demonstrates homogeneous enhancement during the arterial phase, with subsequent isodensity to normal liver parenchyma in later phases. If present, the central scar will demonstrate delayed enhancement and will be T2 hyperintense, differing from fibrolamellar HCC. Because FNH is composed of hyperplastic hepatocytes and small bile ducts, imaging with hepatobiliary-specific MRI contrast agents will allow differentiation from other lesions on delayed (1-3 hours with gadobenate dimeglumine and 20 minutes with gadoxetate disodium) scans. These tumors will remain isointense or hyperintense to the background liver, which also excretes the contrast agent (Fig. C23.3). This can help differentiate

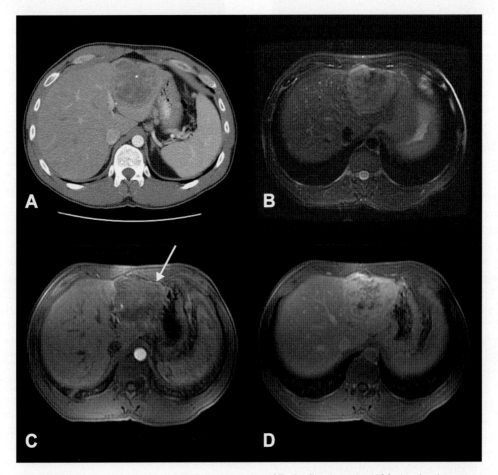

Fig. C23.2 Fibrolamellar hepatocellular carcinoma. (A) Axial postcontrast CT of a fibrolamellar HCC showing heterogenous peripheral enhancement with a punctate central calcification. (B) Axial T2-weighted fat-saturated (FS) MR image with peripheral hyperintensity and a hypointense central scar. (C) Arterial phase of dynamic 3-D LAVA MR series with enhancement of the faint surrounding capsule (arrow). (D) Portal venous phase of dynamic 3-D LAVA series with heterogeneous enhancement but persistent hypoenhancement of the central region. Note, the absence of signs of cirrhosis with a smooth contour of the background liver.

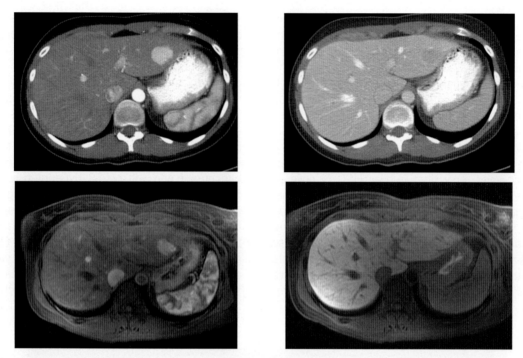

Fig. C23.3 Focal nodular hyperplasia. Multiphase CT with arterial (top left) and portal venous (top right) phases demonstrate an early homogeneously arterial enhancing mass in the left hepatic lobe. This becomes isodense to slightly hypodense on the later portal venous phase. These features are nonspecific, so a multiphase MRI using Eovist contrast, a hepatobiliary imaging agent was performed. The dynamic arterial phase (bottom left) reproduces the arterial enhancing mass in a similar fashion as the CT. The 20-minute postcontrast delayed sequence (bottom right) demonstrates that this mass has normal functioning hepatic parenchyma and takes up the contrast to the same degree as the surrounding parenchyma becoming "isointense": these findings are consistent with a diagnosis of focal nodular hyperplasia. HCC would be hypointense on the delayed sequence.

FNH from other lesions, including adenomas, which will be hypointense on the delayed sequences because of a lack of functioning hepatocytes.

Hepatic adenomas are most common in women taking oral contraceptives. Complications include hemorrhage with hepatic rupture and rarely, malignant transformation to HCC. Adenomas have a variable appearance on CT or MRI, depending on the presence or degree of hemorrhage and fat. They are usually hyperenhancing during the arterial phase, but to a lesser degree than FNH, and can become isodense during the equilibrium phase. They have no bile ducts; therefore, they are hypointense on delayed imaging with hepatobiliary agents.

Hemangiomas are the most common benign primary tumors of the liver. These are well-circumscribed masses with blood-filled channels that are lined by endothelium and supported by a fibrous stroma. Small hemangiomas will demonstrate early flash filling and are isointense to the blood pool (reference aorta) during all imaging phases. Medium-sized hemangiomas demonstrate early discontinuous, peripheral nodular enhancement, which becomes uniformly enhancing to the blood pool in later phases (Fig. C23.4). A characteristic feature of hemangiomas is their intense T2 signal intensity, which is commonly referred to as being "light bulb bright."

Giant cavernous hemangiomas (>5 cm) demonstrate the same early discontinuous, peripheral nodular enhancement, but may also have a nonenhancing central scar. The central scar is T2 hyperintense.

Lastly, while the majority of metastases to the liver result in hypodense masses relative to the normal enhancement of the liver parenchyma, hyperenhancing masses can be found with metastatic disease from a few typical primary malignancies such as renal cell carcinoma (RCC), thyroid cancer, neuroendocrine tumors (Fig. C23.5) (carcinoid, pancreatic NET, pheochromocytoma), choriocarcinoma, and melanoma. These metastases are hypervascular during the arterial phase of imaging.

DIFFERENTIAL DIAGNOSIS

Many of these masses will be asymptomatic and are therefore often incidentally detected. Some masses such as adenomas may present due to right upper quadrant pain secondary to internal hemorrhage and or rupture, especially in young females on oral contraceptives. Giant cavernous hemangiomas can present clinically with a bleeding disorder secondary to a consumptive thrombocytopenia known as Kasabach-Merritt syndrome.

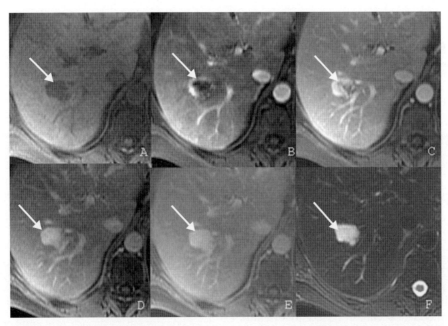

Fig. C23.4 Hepatic hemangioma. Dynamic postcontrast T1-weighted image of the liver demonstrating a hemangioma (white arrows) including precontrast (A), early arterial (B), late arterial (C), portal venous (D), and equilibrium (E) phases showing initially T1 hypointense mass with early discontinuous peripheral nodular enhancement that progressively fills in until uniformly enhancing on the later phase. Axial T2-FS image (F) shows the intense T2 signal intensity described as "light bulb bright."

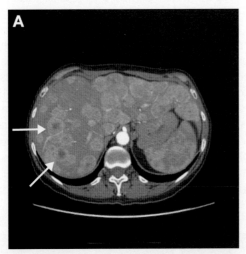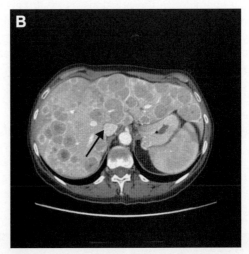

Fig. C23.5 Metastatic carcinoid. (A) Axial CT postcontrast during the arterial phase (note the high density of contrast within the aorta and celiac trunk) with numerous arterial enhancing masses throughout the liver, some with central necrosis (white arrows). (B) Axial CT postcontrast during the portal venous phase with relative increase in enhancement of the hepatic parenchyma and homogeneous enhancement of the spleen. The density of the contrast in the aorta is less and the density of contrast in the IVC has increased (black arrow). The innumerable masses show washout and are now hypodense compared to the parenchyma except for persistent enhancing capsule.

REFERENCES AND SUGGESTED READING

1. Silva AC. MR Imaging of hyper-vascular liver masses: a review of current techniques. *RadioGraphics*. 2009;29:385-402.

2. Chung YE. Hepatocellular carcinoma variants: radiologic-pathologic correlation. *AJR*. 2009;193:W7-W13.

3. Clark HP. Staging and current treatment of hepato-cellular carcinoma. *RadioGraphics* 2005;25:S3-S23.

4. Baron RL. From the RSNA refresher course: screening the cirrhotic liver for hepatocellular carcinoma with CT and MR imaging: opportunities and pitfalls. *RadioGraphics* 2001;21:S117-S132.

5. Tan CH. APASL and AASLD consensus guidelines on imaging diagnosis of hepatocellular carcinoma: a review. *Int J Hepatol*. 2011;2011. Article ID 519783, 11 pages.

CASE 24

PATIENT PRESENTATION

A 56-year-old woman with renal colic pain was evaluated with noncontrast CT. A small ureteropelvic junction stone was found, along with numerous cysts throughout the liver.

CLINICAL SUSPICION

Cystic hepatic lesions

IMAGING MODALITY OF CHOICE

Cystic lesions of the liver are common and have several causes, loosely grouped as congenital, infectious, neoplastic, and other. The lesions can be singular or multifocal and simple or complex. Because many of these lesions overlap in their imaging appearance, the clinical history is useful to narrow down the differential diagnosis.

Various imaging modalities can be used to evaluate cystic hepatic lesions, including sonography, MDCT, and MRI with MRCP. Many lesions have classic appearances on CT and MRI, providing a definitive diagnosis. MRI with fluid-sensitive T2-weighted sequences, including MRCP, can accurately characterize these lesions as cystic, even when extremely small, and define their relationship with the biliary system. However, CT's advantages include the highest sensitivity at detecting calcifications, which is often a distinguishing feature.

FINDINGS

Simple hepatic cysts are one of the most common incidental findings; they are sharply circumscribed, water-attenuating (−10 to 10 HU), T1 hypointense, T2 hyperintense lesions with no postcontrast enhancement. On sonography, they are anechoic fluid collections with increased posterior through transmission. No complex features such as mural modularity or wall thickening or septations are present. Simple hepatic cysts are quite common and may be singular or more often multiple and usually asymptomatic (Fig. C24.1). They can be of variable sizes. Occasionally, these can hemorrhage internally, becoming hyperdense on CT, and of variable signal intensity on MRI. Layering of serous fluid and blood products of varying age may occur, resulting in a hematocrit level. Autosomal polycystic liver disease, alone or coexisting with autosomal dominant polycystic kidney disease, will present as innumerable morphologically simple cysts or complex cysts.

Bile duct hamartomas, also known as von Meyenburg complex, are residual remnants of small interlobular embryonic bile ducts that fail to regress. They are usually asymptomatic and are incidentally found as numerous morphologically simple cystic lesions; their only distinguishing feature is that they tend to be uniformly smaller than 1.5 cm (Fig. C24.2).

Choledochal cysts are rare entities caused by embryonic ductal plate abnormalities; their appearance depends on their involvement with the intrahepatic or extrahepatic biliary system. Todani created a classification system based on which portion of the biliary tree was involved (Fig. C24.3). Most of these cysts are diagnosed during infancy, with a classic triad of abdominal pain, jaundice, and an abdominal mass; however, some may go undetected until adulthood, with variable presentations. The most common form (Todani type I) results from fusiform dilatation of the extrahepatic bile duct (Fig. C24.4). Caroli disease (Todani type V) involves the large intrahepatic ducts, which retain their communication with the biliary tree. This results in large saccular and fusiform dilatation of the intrahepatic bile ducts, which unlike the previously described multicystic diseases, communicate with the biliary tree; they are best appreciated on MRCP. Another distinguishing

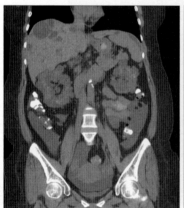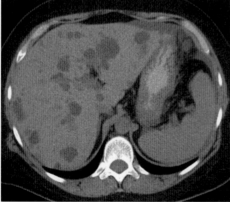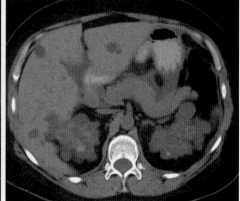

Fig. C24.1 Multiple hepatic cysts in the setting of ADPKD. Axial noncontrast CT shows multiple simple hepatic cysts that are well circumscribed with a low internal density equal to fluid. Also present are innumerable cysts within bilateral kidneys in this patient with autosomal dominant polycystic kidney disease (ADPKD).

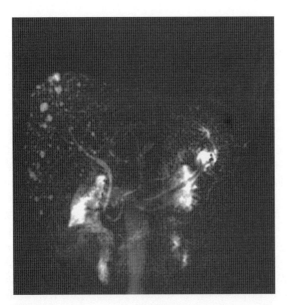

Fig. C24.2 Biliary duct hamartomas. MRCP image demonstrating numerous small T2 hyperintense cystic lesions; majority are less than 1.5 cm in size. They also do not communicate with the biliary tree.

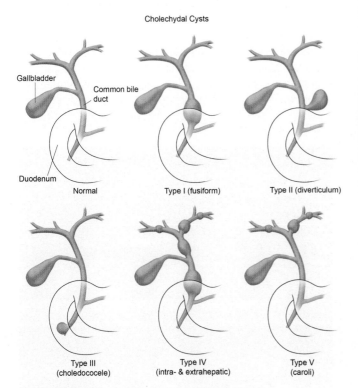

Fig. C24.3 Todani classification of choledochal cysts.
Type I: Most common variety (80%-90%) involving saccular or fusiform dilatation of a portion or entire CBD with normal intrahepatic ducts.
Type II: Isolated diverticulum protruding from the CBD.
Type III or choledochocele: Arise from dilatation of duodenal portion of CBD.
Type IV: Characterized by multiple dilatations of the intrahepatic and extrahepatic biliary tree.
Type V or Caroli's disease: Cystic dilatation of intra hepatic biliary ducts.

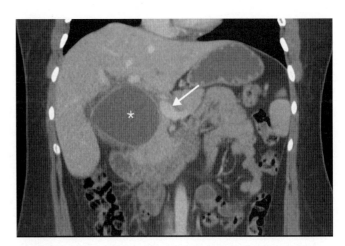

Fig. C24.4 Type 1 choledochal cyst. Coronal CT image demonstrating a large cystic lesion (*) in the porta hepatis adjacent to the portal vein (white arrow) representing fusiform dilatation of the CBD.

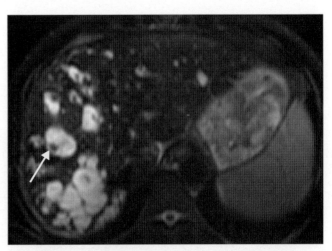

Fig. C24.5 Caroli's disease (Type V). Axial T2 weighted FS image showing Caroli's disease with numerous intrahepatic T2 hyperintense cystic lesions. Notice the "central dot" sign (white arrow) representing the encased portal vein branches.

feature related to their embryogenesis is their relationship to the portal veins. Insufficient resorption of the embryonic duct causes it to dilate and encase the adjacent portal vein. This results in the characteristic "central dot" sign seen on contrast-enhanced CT and MR examinations, representing a cystic lesion surrounding a central portal vein (Fig. C24.5). These can be of variable size, measuring up to 5 cm, and can contain calculi or sludge. Complications from biliary stagnation include recurrent bouts of cholangitis, liver abscesses, or obstructing stones, resulting in jaundice. Caroli syndrome occurs when these findings are coexistent with congenital hepatic fibrosis, which can lead to cirrhosis, portal hypertension, and an increased risk of cholangiocarcinoma.

Mucinous cystic neoplasms, formerly known as biliary cystadenomas or cystadenocarcinomas, are considered premalignant or malignant neoplasms. They usually present in middle-aged white women, accompanied by abdominal pain, nausea, vomiting, or obstructive jaundice. They are described as complex, multilobulated cystic lesions with internal septations, mural nodularity, and a thick outer capsule, all of which may demonstrate contrast enhancement (Fig. C24.6). The density or signal intensity in the cystic portions depends on the proteinaceous content. They are grouped together because imaging cannot reliably distinguish between benign cystadenomas and malignant cystadenocarcinomas; the treatment of all these lesions is surgical resection.

Metastases to the liver are rarely cystic in nature, usually arising from primary tumors such as mucin-producing ovarian or colonic adenocarcinomas or rapidly growing tumors with central necrosis, such as sarcomas or melanoma. Treated metastases from other primary tumors can also undergo degeneration of necrosis and can result in cystic lesions. This is especially true for treated metastases from GISTs. These can occur singularly but are more commonly multiple complex cystic lesions with variable degrees of enhancement.

Infectious causes include pyogenic, amebic, and fungal abscesses. The clinical history and presentation are extremely important in differentiating these entities, which all require different treatment. These usually manifest as low-density lesions, albeit not as low as simple fluid (10-40 HU), with a thick enhancing rim. A characteristic CT finding is the "cluster of grapes" sign, which represents a conglomeration of multiple small pyogenic abscesses in a large multiloculated cavity (Fig. C24.7). Intracavitary gas is also a reliable sign of a pyogenic abscess. A hydatid cyst is caused by the larval tapeworm *Echinococcus granulosus*. Hydatid cysts may be difficult to distinguish on imaging alone, but a clinical history of right upper quadrant pain, eosinophilia, positive serological findings, and travel to endemic areas simplifies the diagnosis. These may manifest as unilocular or multilocular cysts, occasionally with crescentic mural calcifications, small daughter cysts, and little peripheral enhancement.

Hematomas or bilomas may be found; however, these will often have a precedent history of trauma, surgery, or interventional procedure. A large spontaneous hematoma should raise the concern for an underlying mass, such as

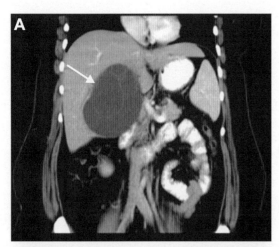

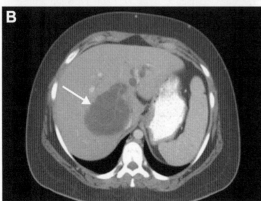

Fig. C24.6 Biliary cystadenoma of the liver. (A) Coronal and (B) axial CT image of a biliary cystadenoma (white arrows). Notice the complexity with internal septations. While this looks very similar in location to the earlier example of the type 1 choledochal cyst, this can be identified as an intraparenchymal lesion, using the "claw" sign. This is the thin tapering rim of parenchyma visualized at the inferior margin of the mass.

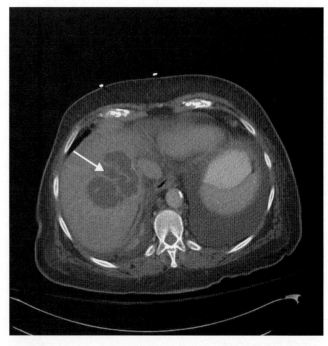

Fig. C24.7 Hepatic abscess. Axial CT postcontrast showing a pyogenic abscess. Notice the thick enhancing, irregular septations (white arrows). Also bilateral reactive pleural effusions.

hepatocellular carcinoma or adenoma. Acute hematomas will be hyperdense but will gradually decrease in attenuation over time. Likewise, their MRI signal intensity will depend on the age of the blood products.

DIFFERENTIAL DIAGNOSIS

As you can see, several entities can present with cystic liver lesions. Some of these may be asymptomatic with no clinical consequence (biliary hamartomas and simple hepatic cysts). Recognizing these as benign lesions when incidentally detected is probably the most important thing to remember. When the lesions become more complex, a much wider differential exists and the clinical context will likely be the distinguishing feature. These could all present with vague right upper quadrant pain, thus imaging will be performed to exclude other acute causes of right upper quadrant pain including hepatitis, cholangitis, biliary colic, pancreatitis, pneumonia, or subdiaphragmatic abscess.

REFERENCES AND SUGGESTED READING

1. Vachha B. Cystic lesions of the liver. *AJR*. 2011;196:W355-W366.
2. **Mortele KJ**. Cystic focal liver lesions in the adult: differential CT and MR imaging features. *RadioGraphics*. 2001;21: 895-910.
3. Brancatelli G. Fibropolycystic liver disease: CT and MR imaging findings. *RadioGraphics*. 2005;25:659-670.

CASE 25

PATIENT PRESENTATION

A 45-year-old man with HIV presented with fever, chills, and left upper quadrant pain.

CLINICAL SUSPICION

Splenic abscess

IMAGING MODALITY OF CHOICE

Sonography could be considered a first-line method for evaluating the spleen for focal or diffuse abnormalities. Occasionally, visualization of the spleen is limited on sonography because of body habitus, bowel gas, and the costophrenic sulcus.

As numerous other etiologies can result in left upper quadrant pain. MDCT may be warranted. New MRI techniques also have increased MRI's role in detecting and characterizing splenic diseases. MRI is an excellent tool for diagnosing and evaluating focal lesions and pathologic conditions of the spleen. Finally, because of the unique physiologic function of the spleen, two different nuclear medicine scans can be used to evaluate it. These include Tc-99m-labeled sulfur colloid, which will be rapidly phagocytized by the reticuloendothelial cells in the liver, spleen, and bone marrow, and imaging with Tc-99m-labeled, heat-damaged red blood cells, which are taken up selectively by functioning splenic tissue.

FINDINGS

The spleen has the same relationship to the circulatory system that the lymph nodes have to the lymphatic system. A wide range of diseases can affect the spleen. Pathologic conditions of the spleen can be classified into the following categories: congenital diseases (accessory spleen, polysplenia, and asplenia); trauma; inflammation and infection (abscess, candidiasis, histoplasmosis, and sarcoidosis); vascular disorders (infarction, diseases affecting the splenic vasculature, and arteriovenous malformation); hematologic disorders (sickle-cell disease and extramedullary hematopoiesis); benign tumors (cysts, hemangioma); malignant tumors (sarcoma, lymphoma, and metastases); and other disease processes that affect the spleen diffusely (portal hypertension, Gaucher disease, and sickle-cell disease).

Many of these diseases share common imaging appearances; therefore, the clinical history is vital to the diagnosis. Accessory splenules are commonly found incidentally and should not be confused with lymphadenopathy. Similarly, splenosis will demonstrate nodules in various locations within the thorax, abdomen, or pelvis with the same enhancement pattern as that of the spleen. Splenosis results from deposition of splenic parenchyma throughout the intraperitoneal cavity or the thoracic cavity after traumatic diaphragm disruption. These entities can also be confirmed with radiolabeled sulfur colloid or heat-damaged red blood cell scans.

One of the more challenging radiologic findings is to determine the etiology of single or multiple low-attenuating lesions within the spleen. The frequency of splenic abscesses has increased due to the higher number of individuals are immunosuppressed. Large bacterial abscesses may demonstrate a rim of enhancement around a necrotic, low-attenuating center. The presence of gas in an intrasplenic lesion is diagnostic for an abscess; however, this finding is infrequently present. Multiple small low-density lesions may be found with fungal microabscesses (Fig. C25.1), especially in individuals with a compromised immune systems. The common organisms include *Candida*, *Aspergillus*, and *Cryptococcus*. Histoplasmosis can affect individuals with an intact immune system but has a higher propensity for those that are immunocompromised. Old granulomas may demonstrate calcification on CT or a characteristic blooming artifact on gradient echo sequences with Gamna-Gandy bodies. Sarcoidosis of the spleen can present with multiple splenic lesions mimicking abscesses. Metastases to the spleen are relatively uncommon; this is somewhat nonintuitive because the spleen is highly vascular and filters the blood. When metastases are present, they are often in the setting of widespread multiorgan metastatic disease.

Splenic infarctions present as low-attenuating or nonenhancing foci but are more easily discernible from these conditions because of their specific morphological characteristics: peripheral location and wedged shape (Fig. C25.2). A search should then be performed for a source, either systemic such as left ventricular thrombus or local such as splenic artery pseudoaneurysm.

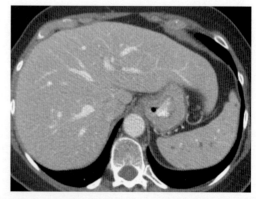

Fig. C25.1 Microabscesses. Axial CT postcontrast with multiple microabscesses. The finding of multiple low attenuating splenic lesions was nonspecific and only after correlation with history of AIDS and *Cryptococcus* infection was the diagnosis of microabscesses due to *Cryptococcus* made.

The most common primary benign neoplasm of the spleen is a hemangioma. These are characterized on MRI as low-attenuating lesions that are T1 hypointense and T2 hyperintense, with variable enhancement. Unfortunately, they are less likely to demonstrate characteristic early, discontinuous nodular centripetal enhancement, followed by uniform enhancement on delayed phases, unlike their hepatic counterparts (Fig. C25.3). A malignant angiosarcoma of the spleen may have a similar appearance to that of a hemangioma, with variable enhancement. Aggressive features such as local invasion, splenic rupture, or distant metastases may be the only clues to this exceedingly rare but ominous tumor (Fig. C25.4).

Finally, diffuse enlargement of the spleen, defined as more than 12 cm in maximum dimension or 215 cc in volume, can be caused by a wide spectrum of diseases. The most common cause of splenomegaly in the United States is portal hypertension from cirrhosis (Fig. C25.5). Other causes of splenomegaly include splenic vein occlusion, or thrombosis, infiltrative diseases (Gaucher disease),

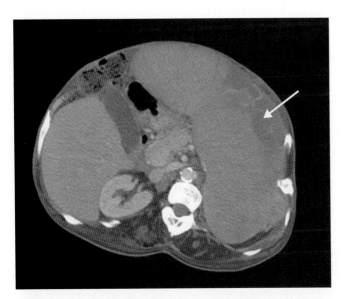

Fig. C25.2 Splenic infarct. Axial CT with splenomegaly due to myelofibrosis with large peripheral hypodensity representative of infarcts (white arrow).

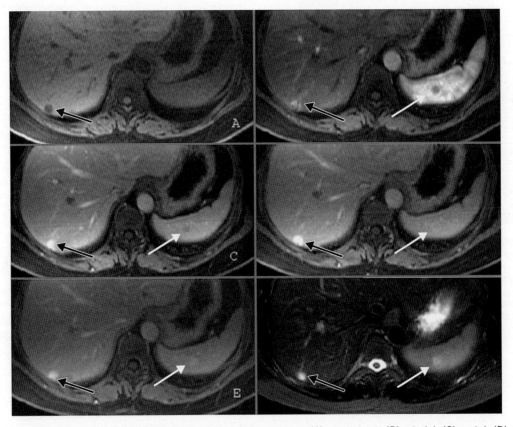

Fig. C25.3 Splenic hemangioma. MRI of abdomen with dynamic LAVA sequence: (A) precontrast, (B) arterial, (C) portal, (D) equilibrium, (E) delayed, and T2-weighted fat-saturated (F). The black arrow points to a hepatic hemangioma with the classic signal characteristics and enhancement pattern of a cavernous hemangioma being T1 hypointense (A), T2 hyperintense with early discontinuous peripheral centripetal enhancement (B), with progressive fill on later phases (C-E). The white arrow points to a splenic hemangioma. This is equal in T1 signal to the hepatic lesion, but because the spleen itself is lower in T1 signal, it is isointense (A) and not visualized. It is also T2 hyperintense, but because the spleen itself has higher intrinsic T2 signal there is less contrast and it does not stand out as well as the hepatic counterpart (E). Enhancement-wise, it appears hypointense on the arterial phase due to early intense normal splenic parenchymal enhancement (B), and progressively fills in becoming isointense (C-D) and later hyperintense, similar to the hepatic hemangioma, but to a slightly lesser degree.

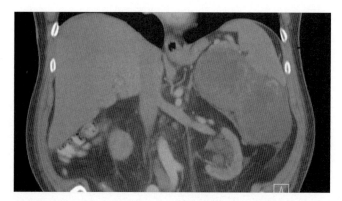

Fig. C25.4 Splenic angiosarcoma. Coronal CT postcontrast with large heterogenously enhancing splenic mass with perisplenic extension.

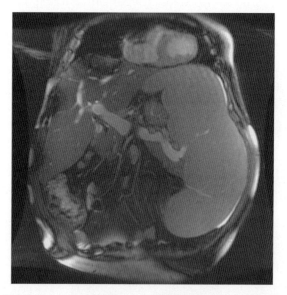

Fig. C25.5 Splenomegaly. Coronal FIESTA MR image with a massively enlarged spleen along with an enlarged liver (to a lesser degree) and dilated portal and splenic vein due to portal hypertension. With cross-sectional imaging, the axial images may not represent the largest splenic dimension, making coronal or sagittal sequences invaluable. The coronal image also allows greater correlation with physical exam findings.

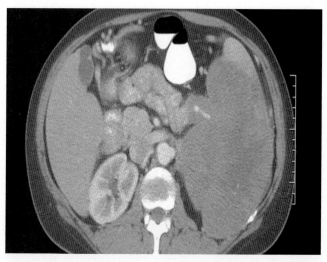

Fig. C25.6 Primary B-cell lymphoma. Axial CT postcontrast showing a large heterogeneously enhancing mass centered within the spleen. Note imaging overlap with angiosarcoma.

hematologic disorders (eg, polycythemia vera, idiopathic thrombocytopenic purpura, or myelofibrosis), inflammatory disease (eg, infectious mononucleosis or Felty syndrome), or tumors such as leukemia or lymphoma (Fig. C25.6).

DIFFERENTIAL DIAGNOSIS

Other entities that may result in left upper quadrant pain besides the previously mentioned splenic abnormalities include gastritis, gastric ulcer, pancreatitis, referred pain from cardiac causes, pneumonia, or pleuritis. A thorough physical examination with special attention for an enlarged palpable spleen is essential during the initial evaluation, however just as with the limitations of imaging studies, different patient characteristics such as body habitus may limit the physical examination findings.

REFERENCES AND SUGGESTED READING

1. Elsayes KM. MR imaging of the spleen: spectrum of abnormalities. *RadioGraphics*. 2005;25:967-982.
2. Rabushka LS. Imaging of the spleen: CT with supplemental MR examination. *RadioGraphics*. 1994;14:307-332.

CASE 26

PATIENT PRESENTATION

A 46-year-old woman presented with recurrent episodes of vague abdominal pain, diarrhea, wheezing, flushing, and diaphoresis.

CLINICAL SUSPICION

Carcinoid syndrome (small bowel and mesenteric masses)

IMAGING MODALITY OF CHOICE

MDCT is the imaging modality of choice for evaluating suspected small bowel or mesenteric masses. MDCT enterography provides more detail in evaluating small-bowel lesions due to even distention of the bowel lumen to evaluate for focal wall thickening or mural modularity, as well as for changes in lumen caliber. Small bowel follow-through studies following an upper gastrointestinal series can be used as a supplemental examination to characterize the mucosal relief pattern of the small bowel. Because most of the small bowel cannot be visualized by conventional endoscopy, imaging plays a crucial role in noninvasively characterizing small bowel lesions. The other alternatives for evaluation of the small bowel are balloon enteroscopy and capsule endoscopy.

FINDINGS

There are several common benign and malignant masses of the small bowel and mesentery which have some overlap in imaging features, but like pancreatic cystic masses, these masses may exhibit a few specific characteristics enabling accurate diagnosis, especially when clinical history is available.

Benign lesions of the small bowel, similar to those of the remainder of the gastrointestinal tract, include adenomas, which are most common in the ampullary region of the duodenum. These are usually solitary but can be multiple with syndromes such as the polyposis syndromes. Lipomas, can act as a lead point for intussusception, and are easily identified by their fat attenuation or signal intensity.

Primary malignant tumors of the small bowel, in order of decreasing frequency, include carcinoid, adenocarcinoma, lymphoma, and gastrointestinal stromal tumors (GISTs). Metastases make up the largest group of small-bowel tumors, usually arising hematogenously from primary tumors such as melanoma, lung, breast, or renal and through direct or peritoneal spread from ovarian or other GI primaries.

Carcinoid tumors arise from neural crest cells and are part of the spectrum of neuroendocrine tumors. Carcinoids of the duodenum are frequently grouped with pancreatic endocrine tumors, which secrete excess gastrin. Carcinoids of the jejunum or ileum are usually aggressive

and when functionally active, produce excessive serotonin. Classic carcinoid syndrome, including repeated bouts of flushing, sweating, wheezing, diarrhea, and right heart failure, occurs in only 10% of patients. This usually only occurs in patients with metastases to the liver (see Fig. C23.5 in case 23). When the carcinoid originates from a primary small bowel mass, the excess serotonin is metabolized by the liver. When the serotonin arises from liver metastases, the excess serotonin can reach the systemic circulation and produce the symptoms of carcinoid syndrome. The imaging appearance can be variable, including a mural or polypoid lesion, focal wall or fold thickening, and/or an abnormal "hairpin" turn of the bowel. None of these in themselves are specific; however, metastatic spread to mesenteric lymph nodes has several distinguishing characteristics. These involved mesenteric nodes produce a desmoplastic reaction that results in a spiculated mass producing a fairly characteristic appearance (Fig. C26.1). This fibrosis also results in retraction of the surrounding mesentery producing a sunburst pattern of the adjacent mesenteric vasculature. Finally, calcifications are seen in up to 70% of these spiculated mesenteric masses. For confirmation or staging, carcinoid tumors can also be imaged with a nuclear medicine octreoscan with indium-111 pentetreotide, which is a somatostatin receptor analogue. This has a high sensitivity, but false negatives

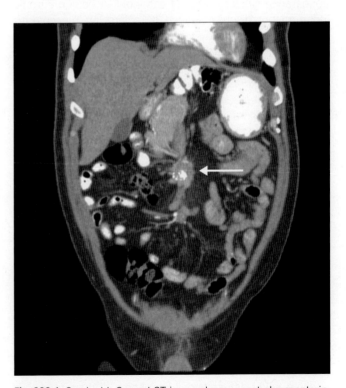

Fig. C26.1 Carcinoid. Coronal CT image shows a central mesenteric mass (arrow) with spiculated margin and central calcifications representative of carcinoid tumor. This represents metastases to the mesentery from a small, undetected tumor most often located in the small-bowel wall.

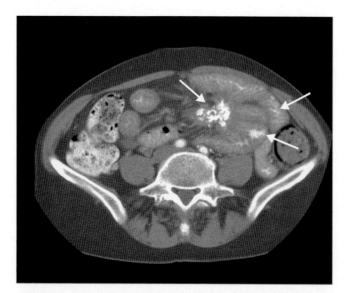

Fig. C26.2 Sclerosing mesenteritis. Axial CT with a mesenteric mass with spiculated margins and coarse dystrophic calcifications (arrows).

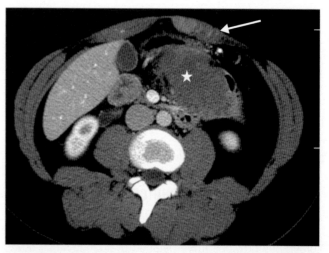

Fig. C26.3 Desmoid. Axial CT with somewhat heterogeneously enhancing soft tissue mass in the central mesentery (*). No calcifications are present. Also notice the irregular enhancement of the left rectus abdominis muscle (white arrow) due to local invasion by the desmoid tumor. No colon is visualized because the patient has had a total colectomy due to Familial adenomatous polyposis (FAP). This constellation of findings represent desmoid tumor in a patient with Gardner's syndrome.

can occur if the tumor does not express the somatostatin 2 or 5 receptor. More recently 68Ga-DOTATOC PET/CT has been used with more impressive results.

A few benign entities of the mesentery can have an appearance similar to that of carcinoid. A benign chronic inflammatory disorder known as sclerosing mesenteritis encompasses a spectrum of benign disorders (Fig. C26.2). Early on, it may present as mesenteric panniculitis, which is characterized by focal mesenteric stranding known as "misty mesentery" and is often sharply marginated region of fatty proliferation with a pseudocapsule. In the more advanced stages, including mesenteric lipodystrophy and retractile mesenteritis, a spiculated mesenteric mass with calcifications from fat necrosis may be present, which can tether or kink the adjacent bowel.

An abdominal desmoid, also known as mesenteric fibromatosis, is a benign fibrous proliferative process usually of unknown etiology but occasionally arises in the setting of prior abdominal surgery. This is associated with familial adenomatous polyposis (FAP) and Gardener's syndrome. This may present as a mass within the abdominal wall, or as an intraperitoneal mass with well-circumscribed borders with a homogeneous or whorled appearance (Fig. C26.3). It has no malignant potential but can be locally aggressive, and it often recurs after resection.

Lymphoma of the small bowel has a varietal appearance and age at presentation, depending on the subtype. It is almost exclusively non-Hodgkin, with the most common subtype being diffuse B-cell lymphoma. It may appear as solitary or multiple lesions, which can be hypoattenuating or isoattenuating, with homogeneous enhancement. With respect to the bowel wall, there can be focal mural

nodularities, a polypoid lesion, or a focal or diffusely infiltrating lesion. The diffusely infiltrating lesions result in significant bowel wall thickening, but in contradistinction to other causes of bowel wall thickening, they cause bowel lumen dilatation rather than narrowing (Fig. C26.4). This "aneurysmal" dilatation of the small-bowel lumen can be appreciated in small bowel studies as displacement or

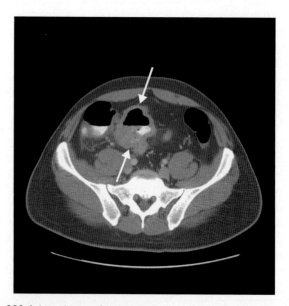

Fig. C26.4 Lymphoma of the small bowel. Axial CT with wall thickening but also focal aneurysmal dilatation (white arrows) of the terminal ileum, which is equal in diameter to the adjacent cecum.

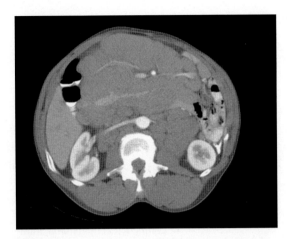

Fig. C26.5 Lymphoma. Axial CT with extensive lymphomatous involvement of both retroperitoneal and mesenteric nodes resulting in a large conglomerate mass. This illustrates the characteristic "pancaking" or "sandwich" sign in which the vessels are encased, but not narrowed.

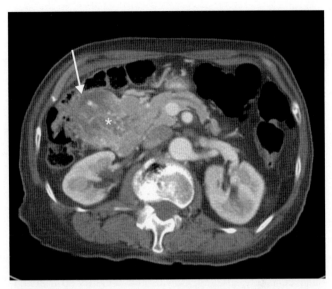

Fig. C26.6 GIST of the duodenum. Axial CT with large exophytic hypervascular mass (large internal vessels) arising from the second portion of the duodenum representative of a GIST. Due to its exophytic nature, this was not visualized during EGD, but actually detected at colonoscopy because of direct invasion of the hepatic flexure (white arrow).

separation of adjacent opacified loops. Lymphoma more commonly presents as diffuse enlargement of the mesenteric and or retroperitoneal lymph nodes leading to a large conglomerate nodal mass. These confluent masses will encase but not narrow the mesenteric vasculature and other major aortic branches (Fig. C26.5). The retroperitoneal nodes also tend to lift the aorta anteriorly off the spine.

The small bowel is the second most common site of involvement, after the stomach. In general, these are similar to the previously described gastric GISTs; their characteristic feature is a large hypervascular, exophytic mass (Fig. C26.6).

DIFFERENTIAL DIAGNOSIS

Small bowel and central mesenteric masses can have a variable clinical presentation. They could present as an obstructing mass leading to small-bowel obstruction (SBO) or could act as a lead point resulting in intussusception. Other clinical features such as the B-symptoms of lymphoma or carcinoid syndrome may help to narrow the differential diagnosis of these masses.

REFERENCES AND SUGGESTED READING

1. Buckley JA. CT evaluation of small bowel neoplasms: spectrum of disease. *RadioGraphics.* 1998;18:379-392.

2. Levy AD. Benign fibrous tumors and tumorlike lesions of the mesentery: radiologic-pathologic correlation. *RadioGraphics.* 2006;26:245-264.

CASE 27

PATIENT PRESENTATION

A 35-year-old man presented after an unrestrained high-speed motor vehicle collision. The patient had an obvious deformity of the right femur, with a GCS score of 13, heart rate of 105 bpm, and blood pressure of 135/90 mmHg.

CLINICAL SUSPICION

Blunt abdominal injury, polytrauma

IMAGING MODALITY OF CHOICE

Trauma is the leading cause of death in individuals aged 1 to 44 years. Blunt trauma accounts for 70% of cases, with the single most common cause being motor vehicle collisions. Triaging polytrauma patients so that major life-threatening injuries can be promptly recognized and treated is of the utmost importance. The imaging modality should be based on the hemodynamic stability of the patient. With unstable patients, radiographs of the chest, abdomen, or pelvis may be obtained quickly. The Focused Assessment with Sonography for Trauma (FAST) is a rapid, bedside sonographic examination performed to identify intraperitoneal hemorrhage or pericardial tamponade. This is primarily used as a tool in unstable patients; when positive, it requires intervention. However, in hemodynamically stable patients or those who have responded favorably to volume replacement, MDCT is considered the imaging modality of choice for evaluating blunt trauma. Sonography is much less sensitive at detecting solid organ and bowel injuries and has a false-negative rate of at least 15%. The high sensitivity of MDCT in detecting injuries that require hospitalization means that a negative CT scan may be sufficient to release the patient in selected cases. Many advocate whole body imaging or "pans-canning" when the mechanism of injury is severe because even in the absence of obvious injuries in stable patients, one study stated an overall change in treatment in 19% of patients after pan-scanning.

FINDINGS

Nonoperative treatment of blunt abdominal trauma is more common because this MDCT can accurately characterize solid organ injuries and exclude major vasculature or bowel injuries that require immediate intervention. In order of decreasing frequency, injuries to the solid organs involve the spleen, liver, kidneys, adrenal glands, and pancreas. Many radiologists include the American Association for the Surgery of Trauma solid organ injury scoring system into their reports as trauma surgeons use this is a guide to patient management. Table C27.1 lists the grading scale utilized for liver injuries. However, this grading system does not

Table C27.1 AAST Liver Injury Scale

Grade*	Type of Injury	Description of Injury
I	Hematoma	Subcapsular, <10% surface area
	Laceration	Capsular tear, <1 cm parenchymal depth
II	Hematoma	Subcapsular, 10%-50% surface area
		intraparenchymal <10 cm in diameter
	Laceration	1-3 parenchymal depth, <10 cm in length
III	Hematoma	Subcapsular, >50% surface area or expanding; ruptured subcapsular or parenchymal hematoma; intra-parenchymal hematoma >10 cm or expanding
	Laceration	>3 cm parenchymal depth
IV	Laceration	Parenchymal disruption involving 25%-75% hepatic lobe or
		1-3 Couinaud's segments within a single lobe
V	Laceration	Parenchymal disruption involving >75% of hepatic lobe or >3 Couinaud's segments within a single lobe
	Vascular	Juxtahepatic venous injuries; ie, retrohepatic vena cava/central major hepatic veins
VI	Vascular	Hepatic avulsion

*Advance one grade for multiple injuries up to grade III.

include vascular injuries such as pseudoaneurysms and active bleeding, which usually require an interventional procedure or surgery. Therefore, this grading system alone is a poor predictor of the need for surgery. For instance, someone with a grade 1 or 2 injury but with active extravasation will likely fail observation alone.

One of the most critical findings that needs to be relayed promptly to treating physicians is the presence of active extravasation. The classic appearance of active extravasation is best visualized on multiphase MDCT, with an early arterial or portal venous phase followed by a delayed scan. With a dual-phase examination, a focal area of hyperattenuation is present that is similar in density to that of the adjacent vessels on early-phase images; it then fades into an enlarged, enhanced hematoma on delayed images. In contrast, a pseudoaneurysm is contained and will appear as a round or ovoid hyperattenuating focus of density that is similar in density to vascular structures in the early phase and fades to the same degree as does the vasculature in the delayed phase, while remaining the same size. Even if the early contrast accumulation is not identified, active extravasation can be diagnosed when a hematoma demonstrates enhancement on the delayed phase. Therefore, when injuries are identified on the early arterial or portal venous phase, a scan should be performed in the delayed phase, albeit with a slightly lower radiation dose. Dense foreign bodies or bone fragments will be hyperdense but will not change on delayed images. Other signs of vasculature injuries include vessel irregularity, caliber change, intimal flap (which signifies dissection), and lack of vessel enhancement (caused by occlusion, dissection, or spasm). Occasionally, the only clue to the source of bleeding is the "sentinel clot" sign, which appears as a focal hyperdense portion of a hematoma because blood at that site has had longer to form into a clot, which becomes denser with time in the acute phase.

Parenchymal injuries to solid organs, mainly in the form of lacerations, appear morphologically similar. These linear hypodensities extend through the normally enhancing parenchyma, with irregular margins (Fig. C27.1). Lacerations are usually graded by depth or extent of involvement and by whether they cross certain anatomical landmarks, such as the intrahepatic inferior vena cava and hepatic veins in the case of the liver, the splenic hilum in the spleen, and the main pancreatic duct in the pancreas. If the main pancreatic duct is disrupted or transected, surgery is necessary to prevent spillage of the pancreatic enzymes throughout the abdomen. Subcapsular hematomas have also been described for encapsulated organs, including the liver, spleen, and kidneys. These appear as peripheral hematomas, confined to the shape of the organ.

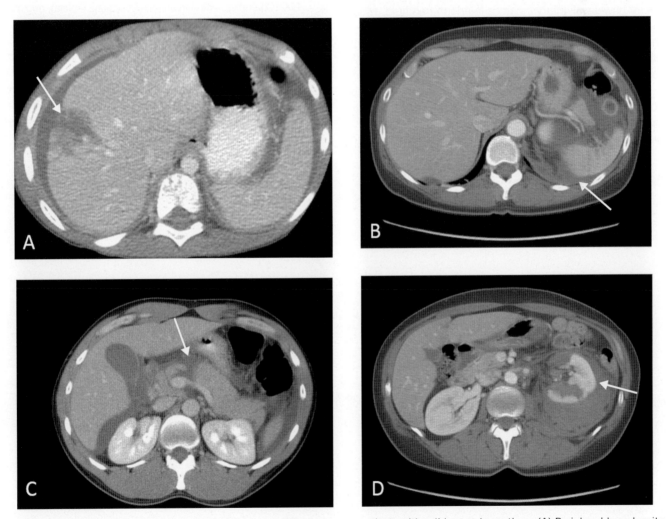

Fig. C27.1 Lacerations. Axial postcontrast CT images of 4 different trauma patients with solid organ lacerations. (A) Peripheral hypodensity with angular margins within segment VIII of the liver consistent with a grade III laceration. The hypodensity along the right liver margin is a subcapsular hematoma as well (arrow). (B) Splenic laceration with linear hypodensity crossing the spleen and surrounding perisplenic hematoma (arrow). (C) Linear hypoenhancement involving full thickness of the body of the pancreas. Subsequent MRCP-confirmed disruption of the pancreatic duct representing high-grade laceration (arrow). (D) Two lacerations through the left kidney with large perinephric hematoma displacing the kidney anteriorly (arrow).

Surgery is necessary in patients with full-thickness bowel wall perforation or active mesenteric extravasation; however, visualization of frank bowel wall discontinuity is rare. Likewise, visualization of extravasation of oral contrast is also rare, because due to the urgent clinical setting of trauma, most protocols do not include the use of oral contrast. Unfortunately, pneumoperitoneum may not be specific for GI tract injury as barotrauma with the Macklin effect (process following trauma producing alveolar rupture, air dissecting along bronchovascular sheaths [interstitial emphysema] extending into the mediastinum as pneumomediastinum) can result in subdiaphragmatic air. Focal bowel wall thickening greater than 3 to 4 mm is another helpful sign indicating bowel injury. Mesenteric stranding or infiltration may represent mesenteric contusion or hematoma and when associated with adjacent bowel wall thickening is highly suggestive of a significant bowel injury. Another sign suggestive of bowel wall injury includes interloop free fluid, which usually appears as a polygonal collection within the folds of the mesentery. A combination of these signs together with clinical assessment will ultimately decide whether a laparotomy is necessary to correct or evaluate for a bowel injury.

In severe traumatic settings when patients with hypovolemic shock are imaged, several imaging features may be present that have been described as the "hypoperfusion complex." This was initially described in children, because children in early shock may appear hemodynamically stable as they are well compensated, but when further stressed, their cardiopulmonary reserve may drop drastically. Hypotension is typically a late finding among children in shock and therefore should not be the only assessment to judge hemodynamic status. The findings of "hypoperfusion complex" include vascular findings of decreased caliber of the abdominal aorta, slitlike appearance of the inferior vena cava; bowel changes including diffuse dilatation of the bowel containing fluid and intense enhancement of the mucosa; solid organ changes including intense prolonged enhancement of the kidneys and pancreas; and moderate to large intraperitoneal fluid collections.

REFERENCES AND SUGGESTED READING

1. Moore EE, Cogbill TH, Jurkovich GJ, Shackford SR, Malangoni MA, Champion HR. Organ injury scaling: spleen and liver (1994 revision). *J Trauma.* 1995:38:323-324.

2. Brody JM. CT of blunt trauma bowel and mesenteric injury: typical findings and pitfalls in diagnosis. *RadioGraphics.* 2000;20:1525-1536.

3. Dreizin D. Blunt polytrauma: evaluation with 64-section whole body CT angiography. *RadioGraphics.* 2012;32:609-631.

4. Taylor GA. Hypovolemic shock in children: abdominal CT manifestations. *Radiology.* 1987;164:479-481.

Chapter 6

Genitourinary System

By Usama Salem, Eduardo J. Matta, Ayda Youssef, and Khaled M. Elsayes

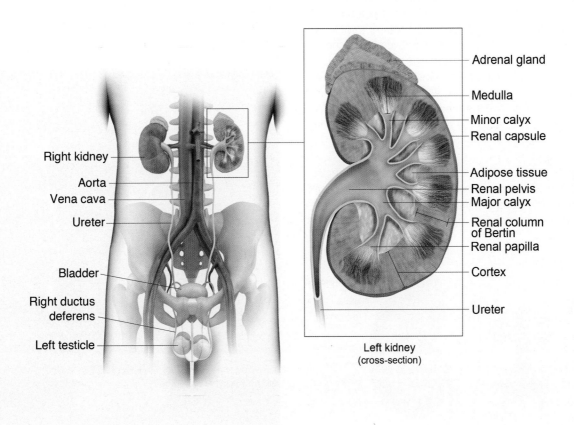

Left kidney
(cross-section)

BASIC ANATOMY OF THE URINARY SYSTEM

THE KIDNEY

The kidneys are located in the retroperitoneum on either side of the spine. The left kidney is slightly higher than the right one and it typically extends from the level of T12 to the level of L3 vertebral body. The adrenal gland is located on top of each kidney. Both the kidney and adrenal gland are surrounded from the inside to the outside by the perinephric fat, the renal fascia (Gerota fascia), and the paranephric fat.

The kidney is a bean-shaped structure harboring the hilum on the medial side. Through the hilum, the renal artery enters the kidney posterior to the renal vein and anterior to the renal pelvis.

The internal structure of the kidney, the renal parenchyma, is composed of a superficial cortex and a deep medulla. The medullary pyramids are triangular with the base directed outward toward the cortex and the apex directed inward toward the renal pelvis. The renal columns of Bertin are an invagination of the renal cortex between the medullary pyramids. The tip of the pyramid extends to the collecting system and is called the renal papilla. The renal papilla is surrounded by the minor calyx, which collects the urine coming from the papilla of the renal pyramids. Two or three minor calyces unite to form the major calyx. Major calyces in turn unite forming the renal pelvis, which gives forth the ureter (Fig. 6.1).

The ureter is a muscular tube, 25 to 30 cm in length. It descends in the retroperitoneum downward and medially in front of the psoas muscle, opposite the tips of the lumbar transverse processes up to the pelvic brim, where it crosses over the end of the common iliac artery or the beginning of the external iliac artery. The ureter then runs along the lateral pelvic wall until it reaches the level of the ischial spine, where it courses anterior and medially to enter the urinary bladder at its posterior inferior surface at the vesicoureteral junction. The ureter has three areas of relative narrowing in its course. These are common sites for stone impaction: at the pelviureteric junction, where it crosses the pelvic brim and at the ureterovesical junction.

THE URINARY BLADDER

The urinary bladder lies in the pelvis with the peritoneum covering only its superior surface. On its posterior surface, the ureters pass through the bladder wall for 2 cm in an oblique course before they open into the urinary bladder cavity by slitlike apertures. The two ureteric orifices are joined with the interureteric ridge. The openings of the ureters together with the opening of the urethra define the boundaries of the bladder trigone (Fig. 6.2).

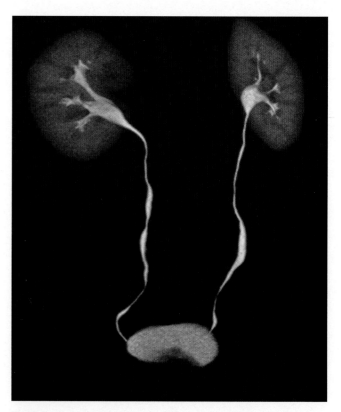

Fig. 6.2 CT urography (CTU) in 3D volume rendering in the excretory phase reveals a normal renal pelvis, ureters, and urinary bladder.

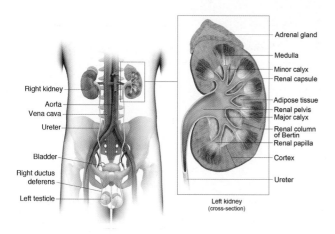

Fig. 6.1 Normal anatomy of the genitourinary system.

CASE 1: RENAL STONE

PATIENT PRESENTATION

A 40-year-old woman presents to the emergency department with a sudden onset of colicky left flank pain radiating to the upper thigh and hematuria that started 12 hours previously.

CLINICAL SUSPICION

Ureteral stone

IMAGING MODALITY OF CHOICE

Noncontrast computed tomography (CT) is the most accurate technique, according to American College of Radiology appropriateness criteria. Advantages of CT:

- High sensitivity (95%-98%) and specificity (96%-100%)
- Short examination time
- No need for contrast
- No patient preparation and not operator-dependent like sonography
- Ability to obtain coronal reformatted images
- Can detect extraurinary causes of flank pain such as appendicitis, diverticulitis, and gynecological problems

   Disadvantages of CT: Radiation exposure. A low-dose protocol has been developed for young patients, pregnant patients in the second and third trimester, and patients who require repeated imaging.

FINDINGS

Imaging Findings in Ureteral Stone.   Direct detection of the stone as a rounded or oval CT-dense structure in the urinary tract (Fig. C1.1) (except stones complicated by indinavir, a protease inhibitor used in HIV-positive patients, which is CT radiolucent). CT can accurately determine the stones' size, location (Fig. C1.2), and number, which are the most important factors affecting clinical decision.

   If obstructive, the following findings can be seen (Fig. C1.3):

- Dilation of the proximal ureter and renal pelvis (hydro-ureter and hydronephrosis).
- Unilateral renal enlargement.
- Stranding of the perinephric and periureteral fat.
- In chronic obstruction, some patients may develop hydronephrosis, with thinning of the renal parenchyma in chronic cases.
- If seen on contrast-enhanced CT, the affected kidney can have decreased or delayed concentration and excretion of contrast material.

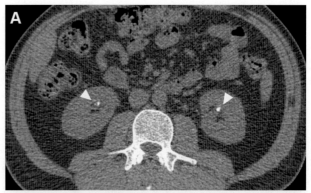
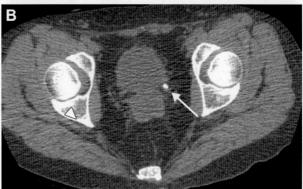

Fig. C1.1 Axial noncontrast CT of the urinary tract (A, B) reveals small bilateral hyperdense stones in the renal pelves (arrow-heads). Another stone is seen lodged in the left vesicoureteric junction (arrow).

Future Perspectives: Implication of Dual-Energy CT

Dual-energy CT is an evolving technique that can be used to detect the chemical composition of the stone, which may affect the choice of therapy, by providing information about how the stone behaves in different energies. For example, to differentiate calcium-containing stone from uric acid-containing stone, the postprocessing algorithm can provide color-coded images in which the voxels containing calcium are coded in blue and those containing urate are coded in red. Dual-energy CT can also be used to detect urinary stones in the contrast-filled collecting system through its ability to generate virtual unenhanced images from the original contrast-filled images.

DIFFERENTIAL DIAGNOSIS

Clinical Differential

Ureteral stones should be differentiated from other causes of flank pain in women, including appendicitis, diverticulitis, ruptured ectopic pregnancy, torsion of ovarian cyst, and enterocolitis.

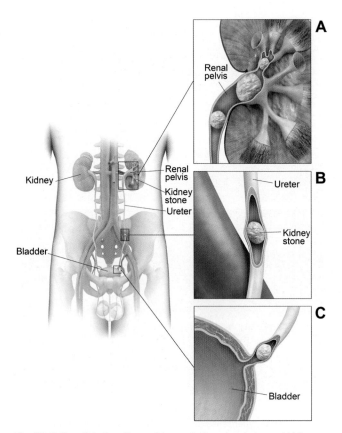

Fig. C1.2 Possible locations of impacted ureteral stone: (A) in the renal calyx, (B) in the middle portion of the ureter where it crosses the iliac vessels, (C) at the vesicoureteric junction.

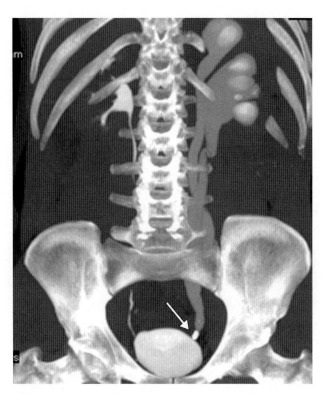

Fig. C1.3 CTU with 3D reformatting shows left ureteric stone (arrow) with proximal hydronephrosis in an incomplete duplicate left kidney. The decrease in the density of the urine within the dilated pelvis and ureter is due to either decreased or delayed contrast excretion secondary to obstruction.

Imaging Differential

- Phlebolith, which is a calcification within a vein. Differentiated by:
  1. Anatomical location outside the urinary tract.
  2. Absence of secondary signs of obstruction.
  3. Tissue rim sign: This sign is specific for stone. It refers to the presence of a halo of soft tissue surrounding the stone representing the mural edema of the ureter (Fig. C1.4).
  4. Comet tail sign: Can be seen with phlebolith. It refers to the presence of eccentric soft tissue extending from the phlebolith representing the collapsed vein.
  5. Central lucency present in phlebolith and absent in stones.
- From noncalcular causes of hydroureter and hydronephrosis such as urinary tract malignancies and external compression.

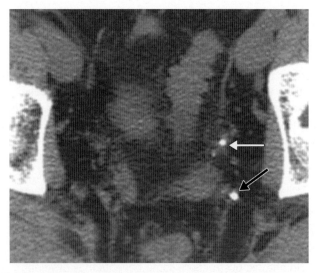

Fig. C1.4 Tissue rim sign: A rind of soft tissue surrounding a stone in the left pelvic ureter (white arrow). Note the presence of a phlebolith simulating a stone below (black arrow).

REFERENCES AND SUGGESTED READING

1. Eisner BH, McQuaid JW, Hyams E, Matlaga BR. Nephrolithiasis: what surgeons need to know. *AJR*. 2011;196(6):1274-1278.

2. Kambadakone AR, Eisner BH, Catalano OA, Sahani DV. New and evolving concepts in the imaging and management of urolithiasis: urologists' perspective. *RadioGraphics*. 2010;30(3):603-623.

3. Yilmaz S, Sindel T, Arslan G, et al. Renal colic: comparison of spiral CT, US and IVU in the detection of ureteral calculi. *Eur Radiol*. 1998;8(2):212-217.

4. Grosjean R, Sauer B, Guerra RM, et al. Characterization of human renal stones with MDCT: advantage of dual energy and limitations due to respiratory motion. *AJR*. 2008;190(3): 720-728.

CASE 2: ACUTE PYELONEPHRITIS

PATIENT PRESENTATION

A 35-year-old woman presents at the emergency department with increased burning micturition, right flank pain, costovertebral angle tenderness, a high-grade fever (102°F), and rigors.

CLINICAL SUSPICION

Acute pyelonephritis

IMAGING MODALITY OF CHOICE

CT of the abdomen and pelvis, with and without contrast.

FINDINGS

Usually, patients with acute pyelonephritis are diagnosed on a clinical basis, without imaging. However, imaging is indicated if there is no response to treatment within the first 72 hours; the patient is at high risk of developing serious complications, such as with diabetic and immunocompromised patients; when the patient has congenital or anatomic genitourinary anomalies; or to assess the severity of complications.

Women are affected more often than men. The source of infection is usually from the lower urinary tract, with *E coli* being the most common causative organism.

Imaging Findings

The goal is to confirm the diagnosis and detect complications.

The CT protocol includes unenhanced followed by contrast-enhanced images taken 50 to 90 seconds after contrast injection to image the kidney in the nephrographic phase. A delayed phase may also be needed when obstruction of the urinary tract is suspected.

Unenhanced images may reveal mild renal enlargement, stranding of the perirenal fat planes, and thickened Gerota's fascia. Mild cases may have no abnormal findings, however.

When focal, acute pyelonephritis typically includes wedge-shaped areas of low attenuation or hypoenhancement that extend from the renal papilla to the cortical surface. The diffuse form may demonstrate a striated nephrogram (Fig. C2.1).

Abscesses can complicate acute pyelonephritis, especially in diabetic patients. An abscess is clinically suspected when the appropriate treatment does not resolve symptoms. CT usually demonstrates parenchymal or extraparenchymal rounded or oval cystic lesions with marginal enhancement. The inflammatory process can spread to adjacent structures, such as the psoas muscle.

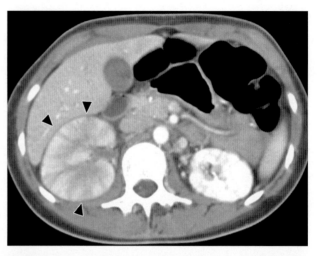

Fig. C2.1 Postcontrast axial CT of the abdomen in a patient with acute pyelonephritis reveals a swollen right kidney with a characteristic striated nephrogram (arrowheads).

UNUSUAL AND LIFE-THREATENING SUBTYPES OF ACUTE PYELONEPHRITIS

Emphysematous pyelonephritis: This severe necrotizing form of pyelonephritis occurs in diabetics, immunocompromised patients, and patients with urinary tract obstruction. The most common organism is *Escherichia coli;* less common organisms include *Klebsiella, Pseudomonas,* and *Candida.* The characteristic finding is the presence of gas foci in renal parenchyma or surrounding the kidney

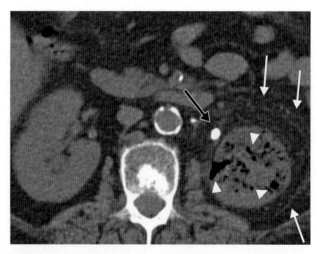

Fig. C2.2 Noncontrast axial CT of the abdomen in a patient with emphysematous pyelonephritis reveals multiple foci of gas density in the left kidney (arrowheads) and stranding of the perinephric fat (white arrows). Note the presence of a left ureteric stone (black arrow), which may be a predisposing factor for this severe type of renal infection.

(Fig. C2.2). Emphysematous pyelonephritis is a medical emergency, and prompt treatment with IV antibiotic is needed as early as possible and relief of urinary obstruction. In severe cases, nephrectomy is performed. If not properly treated, rapid progression with fulminant sepsis can occur.

Emphysematous pyelitis: In this less aggressive type of emphysematous pyelonephritis, gas is not involving the renal parenchyma and is localized within calyceal system and the ureter.

Fungal pyelonephritis: Fungal pyelonephritis is less common than is bacterial. *Candida albicans* is the most common pathogen. CT may reveal fungus balls in the collecting system and multiple hypodense lesions in the renal parenchyma, which represent microabscesses.

DIFFERENTIAL DIAGNOSIS
Clinical Differential
Pyelonephritis should be differentiated from other causes of flank pain in women, including appendicitis, diverticulitis, ruptured ectopic pregnancy, torsion of ovarian cyst, enterocolitis, and ureteric stone.

Imaging Differential
Pyelonephritis should be differentiated from other causes of focal hypodense parenchymal lesions, including renal infarcts and renal masses, such as renal lymphoma and renal cell carcinoma (RCC).

REFERENCES AND SUGGESTED READING

1. Craig WD, Wagner BJ, Travis MD. Pyelonephritis: radiologic-pathologic review. *RadioGraphics*. 2008;28(1):255-277.
2. Rucker CM, Menias CO, Bhalla S. Mimics of renal colic: alternative diagnoses at unenhanced helical CT. *RadioGraphics*. 2004;24(suppl 1):S11-28.
3. Stunell H, Buckley O, Feeney J, Geoghegan T, Browne RF, Torreggiani WC. Imaging of acute pyelonephritis in the adult. *Eur Radiol*. 2007;17(7):1820-1828.

CASE 3: XANTHOGRANULOMATOUS PYELONEPHRITIS

PATIENT PRESENTATION

A 40-year-old diabetic woman with a history of recurrent urinary tract infection presents with right flank pain, hematuria, a low-grade fever, and malaise.

CLINICAL SUSPICION

Pyelonephritis

IMAGING MODALITY OF CHOICE

CT of the abdomen and pelvis with IV contrast

FINDINGS

The classic imaging findings of xanthogranulomatous pyelonephritis are renal enlargement, staghorn stone, and partial or complete renal function compromise. There is destruction and replacement of the renal parenchyma, with multiple low-attenuating areas that represent xanthomatous tissue and dilated calyces filled with debris (Fig. C3.1).

Xanthogranulomatous pyelonephritis is an uncommon atypical form of chronic infection due to an abnormal immune reaction to bacterial infection. *E coli* and *Proteus mirabilis* are the most common pathogens. Risk factors include chronic urinary tract obstruction and diabetes mellitus.

Patients are usually middle-aged women with a fever, malaise, weight loss, and flank pain. An examination may reveal a renal mass, and urinalysis reveals hematuria and pyuria.

The inflammatory process can be localized to the kidney (stage 1), extend to the perirenal space (stage 2), or spread to the pararenal spaces (stage 3). The disease process can be focal; however, most cases have diffuse involvement of the whole kidney.

Nephrectomy is the definitive treatment. A partial nephrectomy is indicated for the focal form, whereas total nephrectomy is indicated for the diffuse form.

DIFFERENTIAL DIAGNOSIS

Clinical Differential

The clinical differential diagnosis includes renal inflammatory lesions such as pyelonephritis and renal abscess.

Imaging Differential

The disease can simulate a renal neoplasm, especially when focal. These neoplasms include renal cell carcinoma, transitional cell carcinoma, renal lymphoma, and metastases. Diffuse form can be simulated by obstructive hydronephrosis caused by large calculus.

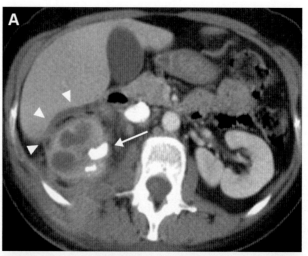

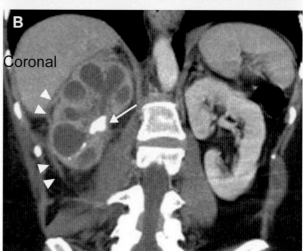

Fig. C3.1 Axial (A) and coronal (B) postcontrast CT scan of the abdomen in a patient with xanthogranulomatous pyelonephritis reveals enlargement of the right kidney with a large staghorn stone (arrow) in the renal pelvis causing hydronephrosis with multiple low-attenuation areas. There is thickening of the Gerota's fascia (arrowheads), which is seen in all types of inflammatory conditions of the kidney.

REFERENCES AND SUGGESTED READING

1. Craig WD, Wagner BJ, Travis MD. Pyelonephritis: radiologic-pathologic review. *RadioGraphics.* 2008;28(1):255-277.

2. Hayes W, Hartman D, Sesterbenn I. From the archives of the AFIP: xanthogranulomatous pyelonephritis. *RadioGraphics.* 1991;11(3):485-498.

3. Kawashima A, Sandler CM, Goldman SM, Raval BK, Fishman EK. CT of renal inflammatory disease. *RadioGraphics.* 1997; 17(4):851-866.

4. Pickhardt PJ, Lonergan GJ, Davis CJ Jr, Kashitani N, Wagner BJ. From the archives of the AFIP. *RadioGraphics.* 2000;20(1):215-243.

5. Rodriguez-de-Velasquez A, Yoder IC, Velasquez PA, Papanicolaou N. Imaging the effects of diabetes on the genitourinary system. *RadioGraphics.* 1995;15(5):1051-1068.

CASE 4: RENAL ABSCESS

PATIENT PRESENTATION

A 44-year-old woman with a history of diabetes presents to the emergency room with a 1-week history of high fever, chills, left flank pain, and dysuria. The patient has a history of recurrent urinary tract infections.

CLINICAL SUSPICION

Renal infection/inflammatory condition

IMAGING MODALITY OF CHOICE

CT of the abdomen and pelvis, with and without contrast

FINDINGS

Intravenous drug abusers and patients with diabetes mellitus, AIDS, and urinary tract anomalies and obstruction are at increased risk for developing renal abscesses. The infection can reach the kidney, most commonly through an ascending infection from a lower urinary tract infection; however, hematogenous spread can also occur, as in patients who are intravenous drug abusers.

On unenhanced CT, the kidney is usually enlarged, showing a single or, less commonly, multiple ovoid, well-defined parenchymal or extraparenchymal (perinephric) hypoattenuating lesions with thick walls. Occasionally, gas density can be seen in the lesion. Gerota's fascia is thickened, with stranding of the perinephric fat (Fig. C4.1). The perinephric abscess is usually confined by the Gerota's fascia although it can extend to adjacent structure (Fig. C4.2). Intravenous contrast is important to differentiate the abscess from a tumor. A renal abscess has rim enhancement of the abscess wall, with no internal enhancement, whereas renal cell carcinoma (RCC) has enhancement of the whole mass, which may acquire a heterogeneous pattern because of areas of hemorrhage and necrosis. However, the most important key of differentiation remains the clinical history and urinalysis, as RCC can be cystic and demonstrate enhancement of its outer thickened wall, which may simulate the appearance of abscess.

DIFFERENTIAL DIAGNOSIS

Clinical Differential

- Acute pyelonephritis: Renal abscesses usually develop as a complication of acute pyelonephritis. Imaging is needed to diagnose the abscess after treatment failure.
- Other causes of intra-abdominal abscess, such as pancreatic and pericolic abscesses.

Imaging Differential

- Cystic RCC, which usually presents as a solitary hypervascular or complex cystic mass with thickened.

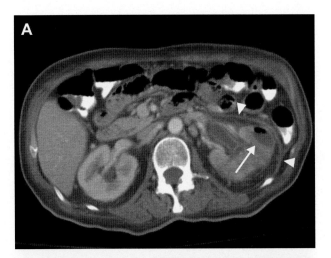

Fig. C4.1 Postcontrast CT scans of the abdomen in (A) axial and (B) coronal planes in a patient with a renal abscess reveal a thick-walled, hypoattenuating lesion in the anterior aspect of the left kidney (arrow) that contains gas. There was notable thickening of the Gerota's fascia (arrowheads).

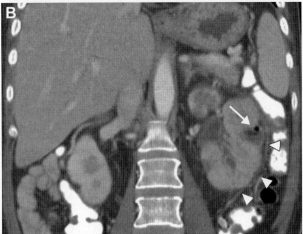

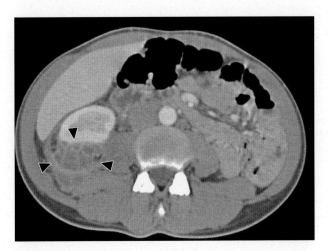

Fig. C4.2 Postcontrast axial CT scan of the abdomen in a patient with a perinephric abscess reveals a thick-walled, complex lesion directly related to the posterior surface of the right kidney (arrowheads), with stranding of the surrounding fat planes.

septations or solid components with no inflammatory symptoms.

- Complicated renal cyst, such as a hemorrhagic or infected cyst, presents with no perinephric inflammatory reaction and is hyperattenuating on unenhanced CT.

- Renal lymphoma, which more commonly presents with multiple lesions and occasionally as diffuse infiltration. Involvement of the perinephric region may be seen.

- Metastases, for which a history of primary tumor is essential. The lesions are usually multiple and show contrast enhancement.

REFERENCES AND SUGGESTED READING

1. Israel GM, Bosniak MA. Pitfalls in renal mass evaluation and how to avoid them. *RadioGraphics*. 2008;28(5):1325-1338.

2. Federle MP, Anne VS, Chen JJ-S. Renal abscess. In: Federle MP, ed. *Diagnostic Imaging: Abdomen*. Utah: Amirsys; 2004:III-3-32-35.

3. Kawashima A, Sandler CM, Goldman SM, Raval BK, Fishman EK. CT of renal inflammatory disease. *RadioGraphics*. 1997; 17(4):851-866.

4. Miller FH, Parikh S, Gore RM, Nemcek AA Jr, Fitzgerald SW, Vogelzang RL. Renal manifestations of AIDS. *RadioGraphics*. 1993;13(3):587-596.

CASE 5: NEPHROCALCINOSIS

PATIENT PRESENTATION

A 34-year-old man with back pain underwent plain radiography of the lumbar spine, which revealed an osteoporotic spine and calcification in the renal pyramids. A laboratory investigation reveals increased PTH and serum calcium.

CLINICAL SUSPICION

Hyperparathyroidism with nephrocalcinosis

IMAGING MODALITY OF CHOICE

Unenhanced CT scan of the abdomen and pelvis is the modality of choice. It has a higher sensitivity than plain radiography.

FINDINGS

Nephrocalcinosis is a condition in which there is a large amount of calcium deposition in the renal parenchyma. It can be classified, according to the site of calcium deposition, as medullary or cortical (Fig. C5.1). Medullary nephrocalcinosis is the most common form and can be seen in patients with hyperparathyroidism, type 1 renal tubular acidosis, medullary sponge kidney, and sarcoidosis. Cortical nephrocalcinosis usually develops secondary to chronic glomerulonephritis, renal cortical necrosis, Alport syndrome, and chronic rejection of transplanted kidneys. Rarely, nephrocalcinosis involves both the renal medulla and cortex.

CT reveals calcification in the renal parenchyma. The location and pattern of calcification differs in each type. In cortical nephrocalcinosis, the calcification is seen in the periphery of the renal parenchyma, either as a peripheral

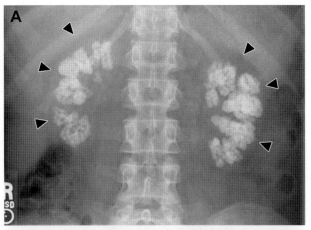

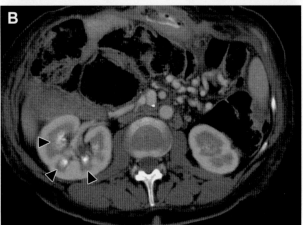

Fig. C5.2 (A) Plain x-ray of medullary nephrocalcinosis reveals a bilateral coarse, confluent, radiopaque calcification, which is seen projecting over the renal shadows (arrowheads). (B) Axial CT scan of the abdomen of another patient reveals calcification in the medullary pyramids of the right kidney (arrowheads).

rim or tram-track appearance. In medullary nephrocalcinosis, the calcification is seen only involving the renal pyramids, with unaffected areas in between representing the column of the renal cortex (Fig. C5.2).

DIFFERENTIAL DIAGNOSIS

Papillary necrosis: The clinical scenario and imaging play important roles in differentiating it from medullary nephrocalcinosis. Papillary necrosis can be caused by analgesic nephropathy, diabetes mellitus, alcoholism, and sickle-cell anemia. There is damage of the renal papilla, with resultant necrosis, cavitation, and calcium deposition. Calcium deposition can occur in a nonsloughed necrotic papilla, in a completely detached papilla which remain in the calyx or at the periphery of a necrotic sloughed papilla. Unenhanced CT reveals a triangular or ring-shaped calcification in the sloughed papilla (Fig. C5.3).

Renal tuberculosis: In patients with pulmonary tuberculosis, the organism can reach the kidneys hematogenously.

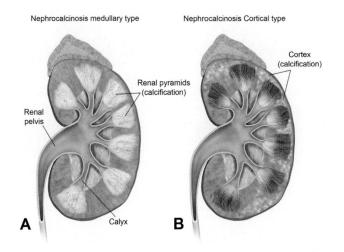

Fig. C5.1 Types of nephrocalcinosis. (A) The medullary type (on the left side) has calcification in the renal pyramids, and (B) the cortical type (on the right side) has calcification in the renal cortex.

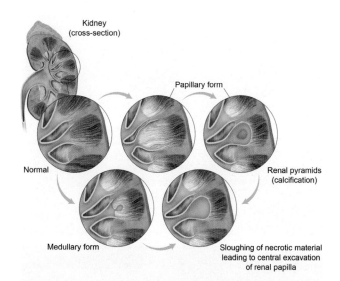

Fig. C5.3 Types of calyceal deformities in papillary necrosis. In the papillary form, the necrosis starts at the fornices and the necrotic papilla may remain in the calyx giving a signet ring appearance. In the medullary form, the necrosis starts in the center of the papilla and sloughing of the dead tissue leads to a blunted calyx. Note the presence of calcification in necrotic papilla, which is common in patient with analgesic nephropathy.

The disease is unilateral, with focal amorphous or granular calcification. The kidney is atrophic, with stricture of the pelvicalyceal system.

Renal infection with *Pneumocystis jiroveci*: This condition occurs only in AIDS patients with low CD4 counts. It can reach the kidneys through hematogenous or lymphatic routes. The calcification is usually punctate and involves the cortex and medulla.

REFERENCES AND SUGGESTED READING

1. Dyer RB, Chen M, Zagoria RJ. Abnormal calcifications in the urinary tract. *RadioGraphics.* 1998;18(6):1405-1424.

2. Dyer RB, Chen MY, Zagoria RJ. Classic signs in uroradiology. *RadioGraphics.* 2004;24(suppl 1):S247-S280.

3. Desser TS. Nephrocalcinosis. In: Federle MP, ed. *Diagnostic Imaging: Abdomen.* Utah: Amirsys; 2004:III-3-52.

4. Harisinghani MG, McLoud TC, Shepard JAO, Ko JP, Shroff MM, Mueller PR. Tuberculosis from head to toe. *RadioGraphics.* 2000;20(2):449-470.

5. Schepens D, Verswijvel G, Kuypers D, Vanrenterghem Y. Renal cortical nephrocalcinosis. *Nephrol Dial Transplant.* 2000; 15(7):1080-1082.

6. Jung DC, Kim SH, Jung SI, Hwang SI. Renal papillary necrosis: review and comparison of findings at multi-detector row CT and intravenous urography. *RadioGraphics.* 2006;26(6): 1827-1836.

CASE 6: ACQUIRED CYSTIC DISEASE OF UREMIA

PATIENT PRESENTATION

A 48-year-old man presents with a long history of chronic renal failure; he is on dialysis. An abdominal sonographic evaluation for flank pain reveals multiple bilateral renal cysts.

CLINICAL SUSPICION

Acquired renal cystic disease

IMAGING MODALITY OF CHOICE

Abdominal sonography can be used as a screening examination to establish the diagnosis; however, contrast-enhanced CT is required to detect complications, especially renal cell carcinoma (RCC), which develops in about 7% of these patients.

Acquired renal cystic disease refers to the development of three or more renal cysts in each kidney in patients with end-stage renal disease. The condition is more common in men and patients undergoing dialysis, irrespective of the method. Its incidence increases with dialysis duration.

Sonography reveals multiple bilateral renal cysts (at least 3 on each side) that appear as anechoic structures with posterior acoustic enhancement. Imaging features of end-stage renal disease are also seen, including bilaterally small kidneys, increased parenchymal echogenicity, and loss of corticomedullary differentiation.

A CT scan reveals atrophic kidneys with multiple parenchymal cysts. Sometimes hemorrhage inside a cyst or calcification in a cyst wall can be seen. CT can detect RCC, which requires intravenous contrast administration and appears as a focal, solid hypervascular lesion (Fig. C6.1).

DIFFERENTIAL DIAGNOSIS

Clinical Differential

The patient is usually asymptomatic and diagnosis is often made in the workup of other complaints

Imaging Differential

Adult Polycystic Kidney Disease.   It is characterized by autosomal dominant inheritance and massive enlargement of both kidneys, with bilateral, innumerable noncommunicating cysts. The cysts usually begin to appear by age 30 and increase in size over time. They diffusely involve the whole kidney, changing its normal renal contour (Figs. C6.2 and C6.3). Complicated cysts, such as hemorrhagic or infected cysts, can be identified on CT by increased attenuation or the presence of gas, respectively. Cysts can also involve the liver, spleen, pancreas, and ovaries. There is no association between adult polycystic kidney disease and RCC. Adult polycystic kidney disease can however lead to end-stage renal disease.

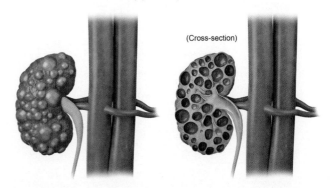

Fig. C6.2 Exterior and the interior appearance of the polycystic kidney.

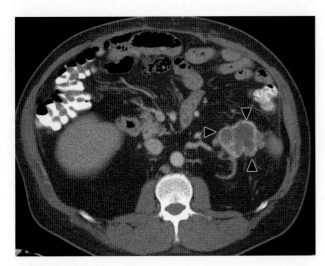

Fig. C6.1 Postcontrast axial CT scan of the abdomen in a patient with end-stage renal disease reveals a hypervascular soft tissue lesion arising from the left kidney (arrowheads) representing RCC on top of ESRD.

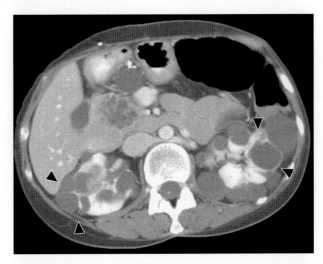

Fig. C6.3 A postcontrast axial CT scan of the abdomen of a patient with polycystic kidney disease reveals multiple bilateral variable-sized cysts that have caused contour irregularities (arrowheads).

Von Hippel Lindau Disease.   It is an autosomal dominant disorder that affects multiple systems. The condition is due to a mutation of the VHL tumor suppressor gene located on chromosome 3. Patients with this mutation can develop hemangioblastomas in the retina, cerebellum, and spine and pancreatic cysts, pancreatic cystic neoplasms, pheochromocytoma, and epididymal cystadenomas. The kidneys are of normal size and function, with multiple bilateral, variable-sized cysts. Complex cysts or cysts with mural nodules can be seen and can suggest malignancy. RCC can develop at a younger age and, along with neurological complications, is a cause of death in these patients.

Tuberous Sclerosis.   It is an autosomal dominant disorder characterized by bilateral renal cysts, multiple renal angiomyolipomas (see case 10), and CNS lesions, including cerebral periventricular calcifications, cortical tubers, and subependymal nodules. Patients may present with seizures due to CNS lesions.

Multiple Simple Renal Cysts.   See case 7.

REFERENCES AND SUGGESTED READING

1. Torres VE, Harris PC, Pirson Y. Autosomal dominant polycystic kidney disease. *Lancet.* 2007;369(9569):1287-1301.

2. Leung RS, Biswas SV, Duncan M, Rankin S. Imaging features of von Hippel–Lindau disease. *RadioGraphics.* 2008;28(1):65-79.

3. Katabathina VS, Kota G, Dasyam AK, Shanbhogue AKP, Prasad SR. Adult renal cystic disease: a genetic, biological, and developmental primer. *RadioGraphics.* 2010;30(6):1509-1523.

CASE 7: RENAL CYSTS

PATIENT PRESENTATION

A 38-year-old man presents with vague left-side abdominal pain; abdominal sonogram was normal, apart from large left renal cysts.

CLINICAL SUSPICION

Simple renal cyst

IMAGING MODALITY OF CHOICE

CT of the abdomen, with and without intravenous contrast, is the modality of choice for assessing indeterminate renal lesions. Sonography can be used to distinguish a simple benign cyst that needs no further workup from a complicated cyst that requires further evaluation by CT. However, multiple factors can affect proper sonographic evaluation, such as the patient's body habitus, small lesions, and cyst wall calcification.

On sonography, simple cysts appear as well-defined, thin-walled anechoic lesions with posterior acoustic enhancement and no internal echoes, septations, or solid nodules. On CT, simple cysts appear as fluid density lesions with no wall enhancement after intravenous contrast.

Dr. Morton Bosniak created the Bosniak classification system on the basis of CT imaging findings to categorize cystic renal lesions into 5 categories (Fig. C7.1). This classification helps in clinical management by classifying these lesions as surgical or nonsurgical.

Category I: Simple uncomplicated cyst, which contains water density fluid and has a thin wall, with no septations, calcifications, solid components, or cyst wall enhancement after intravenous contrast (Fig. C7.2). Cysts in this group are benign and no follow-up is needed.

Category II: Minimally complicated cyst, including homogenous high-attenuation cysts and cysts with few thin septae, a fine rim of calcifications, or a short segment of thickened calcifications. Cysts in this group are benign and no follow-up is needed.

Category IIF: Lesions in this category require follow-up and include cysts with increased numbers of septae, minimal mural or septal thickening, or thick calcium in the wall. Follow-up is done by CT or MRI after 6 months, then every year. If the lesion remains stable for 5 years, it is considered benign.

Category III: More complicated cyst that contains a thickened, enhancing wall or internal septations. Lesions in this group are indeterminate and require surgical excision (partial nephrectomy).

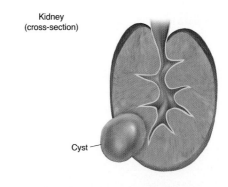

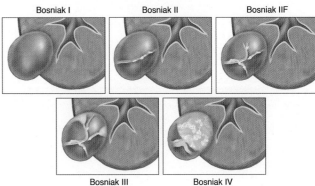

Fig. C7.1 Bosniak classification of renal cyst.

Category IV: Clearly malignant cystic lesion. In addition to the criteria in group III, the cyst contains solid and soft tissue components. Lesions in this group are managed by nephrectomy.

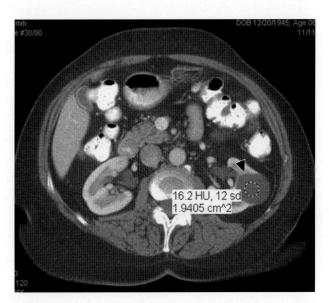

Fig. C7.2 Postcontrast axial CT scan of the abdomen in a patient with a simple cortical cyst (Category I) reveals an oval-shaped hypoattenuating lesion in the left kidney (arrowhead). The lesion measures 16 HU (below 20 HU), denoting fluid content.

DIFFERENTIAL DIAGNOSIS
Clinical Differential
Symptomatic renal cysts must be differentiated from other causes of abdominal pain, such as cholecystitis.

Imaging Differential
- Cystic RCC
- Renal abscess
- Cystic metastases

REFERENCES AND SUGGESTED READING

1. Bosniak MA. The Bosniak renal cyst classification: 25 years later. *Radiology*. 2012;262(3):781-785.
2. Hartman DS, Choyke PL, Hartman MS. From the RSNA refresher courses a practical approach to the cystic renal mass. *RadioGraphics*. 2004;24(suppl 1):S101-S115.
3. Israel GM, Hindman N, Bosniak MA. Evaluation of cystic renal masses: comparison of CT and MR imaging by using the Bosniak classification system. *Radiology*. 2004;231(2):365-371.

CASE 8: RENAL TRANSPLANT DYSFUNCTION

PATIENT PRESENTATION

A 51-year-old man underwent a live donor renal transplant and presents with hypertension 2 weeks later. Laboratory studies revealed a high creatinine level.

CLINICAL SUSPICION

Complicated dysfunctioning transplant due to rejection or vascular compromise

IMAGING MODALITY OF CHOICE

Color and power Doppler sonography

FINDINGS

Renal artery stenosis is the most common vascular complication after renal transplantation. The underlying mechanism includes atherosclerosis of the donor or recipient arteries and iatrogenic causes, such as faulty suture technique, surgical injury to the vessel, or vascular kink. The site of stenosis can be in the recipient iliac artery, at the anastomotic site, or in the donor renal artery (Fig. C8.1).

The condition can be suspected clinically if there is severe hypertension that is refractory to treatment or unexplained impaired renal function after renal transplantation.

Sonography is used to visualize blood flow, measure its speed, and characterize its waveform. Normally, the peak systolic velocity is less than 150 cm/s at the main renal artery. Spectral analysis of the normal Doppler waveform demonstrates rapid systolic upstroke peak and low-resistance continuous forward flow throughout the cardiac cycle.

In case of renal artery stenosis, the site of stenosis will demonstrate increased peak systolic velocity of the flowing blood with a focal area of color aliasing, which can be simply defined as color mixture and spill outside the vessel lumen at the narrowed area (Fig. C8.2A). The velocity gradient between the stenotic and prestenotic segments is increased. Poststenotic turbulent flow is also present. Intrarenal waveforms will also be abnormal, demonstrating presence of a small amplitude waveform with a prolonged systolic rise (slow upstroke), known as parvus tardus waveform (Fig. C8.2B).

The renal artery can also be evaluated using MR angiography (Fig. C8.3). The artery can be visualized without contrast administration, but artifacts from surgical clips may affect image quality.

DIFFERENTIAL DIAGNOSIS

Clinical Differential

Other causes of graft failure include:

• Rejection
• Urinary obstruction

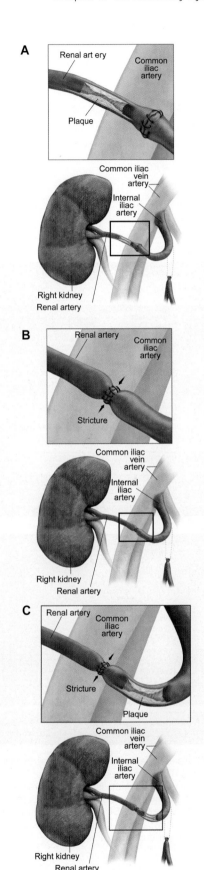

Fig. C8.1 Possible sites of posttransplant renal artery stenosis: (A) The donor renal artery, (B) the anastomotic site, (C) the recipient iliac artery.

- Acute tubular necrosis
- Large hematoma

Imaging Differential

Other vascular complications of renal transplantation include:

- Intrarenal arteriovenous fistula
- Renal artery thrombosis
- Renal graft torsion
- Renal vein thrombosis
- Renal infarction

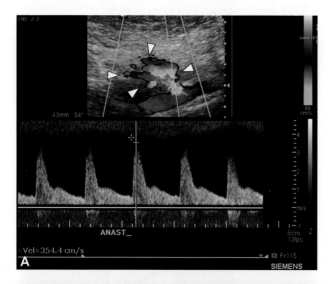

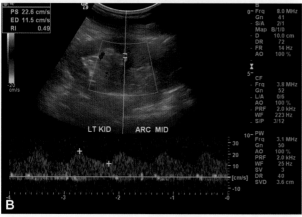

Fig. C8.2 A 24-year-old male presented with hypertension following renal transplant. (A) Spectral Doppler sonogram of transplant renal artery at site of anastomosis demonstrates focal area of color aliasing (arrowheads) with significantly increased systolic upstroke; elevated PSV (peak systolic velocity of 354 cm/s). (B) Longitudinal sonogram of renal transplant shows parvus tardus waveforms in segmental artery with mildly decreased color flow in kidney.

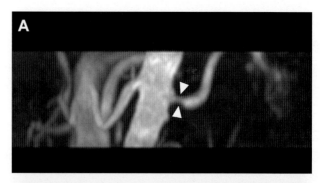

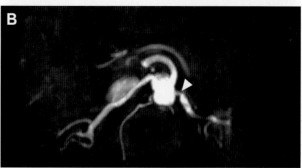

Fig. C8.3 MR angiography of the renal arteries in (A) coronal and (B) axial planes reveals stenosis of the left renal artery (arrowhead).

REFERENCES AND SUGGESTED READING

1. Kobayashi K, Censullo ML, Rossman LL, Kyriakides PN, Kahan BD, Cohen AM. Interventional radiologic management of renal transplant dysfunction: indications, limitations, and technical considerations. *RadioGraphics*. 2007;27(4):1109-1130.

2. Akbar SA, Jafri SZH, Amendola MA, Madrazo BL, Salem R, Bis KG. Complications of renal transplantation. *RadioGraphics*. 2005;25(5):1335-1356.

3. Brown ED, Chen MYM, Wolfman NT, Ott DJ, Watson NE Jr. Complications of renal transplantation: evaluation with US and radionuclide imaging. *RadioGraphics*. 2000;20(3):607-622.

4. Sebastià C, Quiroga S, Boyé R, Cantarell C, Fernandez-Planas M, Alvarez A. Helical CT in renal transplantation: normal findings and early and late complications. *RadioGraphics*. 2001;21(5):1103-1117.

5. Hohenwalter MD, Skowlund CJ, Erickson SJ, et al. Renal transplant evaluation with MR angiography and MR imaging. *RadioGraphics*. 2001;21(6):1505-1517.

CASE 9: RENAL CELL CARCINOMA

PATIENT PRESENTATION

A 55-year-old man presents with fatigue, painless hematuria, and unexplained weight loss.

CLINICAL SUSPICION

Renal cell carcinoma (RCC)

IMAGING MODALITY OF CHOICE

Multiphasic CT scan of the abdomen and pelvis is the modality of choice. Imaging is important for accurate staging, which affects treatment options and surgical planning (Table C9.1). The scanning protocol consists of unenhanced CT, followed by intravenous contrast administration and image acquisition in the corticomedullary and nephrographic phases. The corticomedullary phase is performed after 60 seconds of contrast injection and is important for visualizing the renal vein and detecting distant organ metastases, whereas the nephrographic phase is performed after 80 seconds of contrast injection and is the most sensitive for tumor detection. The excretory phase is optional and performed after 2 to 5 minutes.

Unenhanced CT may reveal a circumscribed, usually solid mass arising from the renal cortex. Depending on the size of the mass, it may cause distortion of the normal renal contour. The attenuation of the lesion may be heterogeneous because of the presence of intratumoral hemorrhage, necrosis, and, less commonly, calcification. After intravenous contrast, the tumor usually enhances, albeit less than the renal parenchyma (Fig. C9.1A,C). Enhancement more than 15 to 20 HU after intravenous injection of contrast is considered significant and highly raises the suspicion of RCC. The papillary type of RCC is hypovascular and can be mistaken for a cyst.

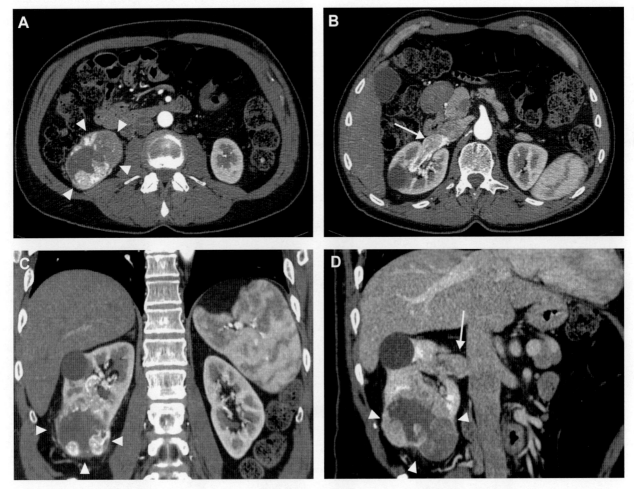

Fig. C9.1 Postcontrast CT scan of the abdomen in axial (A,B) and coronal (C,D) planes of a patient with RCC demonstrated as a hypervascular lesion of the lower pole of the right kidney (arrowheads) with extension of the tumor into the renal vein (arrow).

Table C9.1 The American Joint Committee on Cancer (AJCC) Staging of Renal Cell Cancer

Stage	Description
T0	No evidence of primary tumor
T1a	Tumor is limited to the kidney and is <4 cm in greatest diameter
T1b	Tumor is limited to the kidney and is 4-7 cm in greatest diameter
T2a	Tumor is limited to the kidney and is 7-10 cm in greatest diameter
T2b	Tumor is limited to the kidney and is >10 cm in greatest diameter
T3a	Tumor invades: renal vein or its segmental branches. Perirenal and/or renal sinus fat (no extension beyond Gerota's fascia or to the ipsilateral adrenal gland).
T3b	Tumor invade the IVC below the level of the diaphragm
T3c	Tumor invade the IVC above the level of the diaphragm
T4	Invasion beyond Gerota's fascia or to the ipsilateral adrenal gland
N0	No nodal involvement
N1	Regional lymph node involvement
M0	No distant metastases
M1	Distant metastases

Adapted with permission from Edge SB. *AJCC Cancer Staging Manual*, 7th ed. New York: Springer; 2010.

CT is important in disease staging. It can detect multifocal lesions, perinephric tumor extension, renal sinus fat invasion, and extension to the adjacent organs, including the ipsilateral adrenal gland (Fig. C9.2). Although uncommon, it is important to evaluate the contralateral kidney to exclude bilateral RCC.

Furthermore, the tumor can grow directly into the renal vein, reaching the IVC; it may even extend to the right side of the heart (Fig. C9.3). This is best visualized in the corticomedullary phase of enhancement, which demonstrates a filling defect in the enhanced vein in direct continuity with the primary tumor (Fig. C9.1B,D).

Lymphatic spread occurs to the regional lymph nodes. Hematogenous spread can lead to the development of hypervascular metastasis, most commonly involving the lungs, liver, bones, and brain. Rare locations include the pancreas and thyroid gland.

Clinical Differential

RCC should be differentiated from other causes of gross hematuria, such as those originating from the collecting system, ureter, or a urinary bladder carcinoma.

Imaging Differential

RCC should be differentiated from other renal masses, including:

- Angiomyolipoma (AML): AML are predominantly fatty lesions (see case 10).

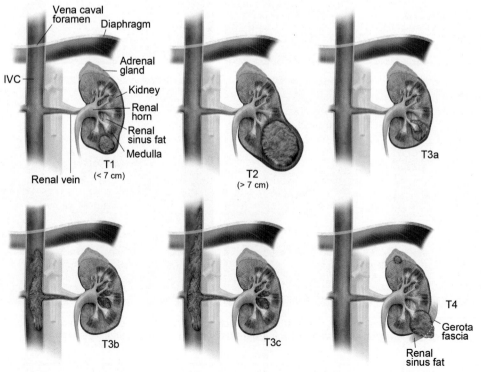

Fig. C9.2 The staging of RCC.

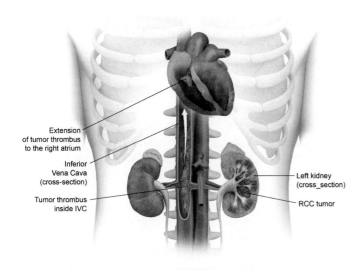

Fig. C9.3 RCC invading the renal vein with formation of tumor thrombus reaching the right atrium.

- Oncocytoma: Oncocytoma is a benign epithelial tumor arising from the collecting ducts. this lesion is usually homogenous and solid, yet pathological diagnosis is usually needed.

- Lymphoma: Lesions are usually multiple and bilateral.
- Hemorrhagic renal cyst: This can be differentiated from tumor by lack of significant enhancement on postcontrast series.

REFERENCES AND SUGGESTED READING

1. Sheth S, Scatarige JC, Horton KM, Corl FM, Fishman EK. Current concepts in the diagnosis and management of renal cell carcinoma: role of multidetector CT and three-dimensional CT. *RadioGraphics.* 2001;21(suppl 1):S237-S254.

2. Prando A, Prando D, Prando P. Renal cell carcinoma: unusual imaging manifestations. *RadioGraphics.* 2006;26(1):233-244.

3. Prasad SR, Humphrey PA, Catena JR, et al. Common and uncommon histologic subtypes of renal cell carcinoma: imaging spectrum with pathologic correlation. *RadioGraphics.* 2006; 26(6):1795-1806.

CASE 10: RENAL ANGIOMYOLIPOMA

PATIENT PRESENTATION

A 43-year-old woman presents with vague abdominal pain. Sonography reveals an incidental hyperechoic mass lesion within the left kidney.

CLINICAL SUSPICION

Renal angiomyolipoma

IMAGING MODALITY OF CHOICE

CT of the abdomen, with and without contrast

FINDINGS

Angiomyolipoma (AML) is the most common benign tumor of the kidney. These tumors are composed of macroscopic fat, blood vessels, and smooth muscles in different proportions (Fig. C10.1). It ranges in size from a few millimeters to several centimeters or even larger. Angiomyolipoma can be single or multiple. Multiple angiomyolipomas can be seen in patients with tuberous sclerosis (Fig. C10.2).

On CT, AML appears as a well-defined cortical lesion. The presence of intralesional fat density (low-density areas of –30 to –100 HU) is an important clue for diagnosis. However, when the lesion is small, it may be difficult to differentiate from small cyst or other lesions.

On MRI, AML will demonstrate bright signal on non-fat-suppressed T1-weighted images in both in and opposed phase and will lose signal only in fat-suppressed sequences because the fat in AML is macroscopic (Fig. C10.3).

Angiomyolipomas may be fat-poor, especially in the setting of tuberous sclerosis, as up to one-third do not demonstrate macroscopic fat on CT. Calcification is rare.

AML can be complicated with rupture and hemorrhage (Fig. C10.4). This can be seen in large tumors (diameter greater than 4 cm). Patient will present with acute abdominal pain and CT will demonstrate perinephric hematoma. Control of hemorrhage can be done by embolization of the bleeding vessel followed by partial or complete nephrectomy.

Spontaneous renal bleeding secondary to an AML usually occurs in tumors larger than 4 cm.

Clinical Differential

AML is usually asymptomatic. However, in cases of spontaneous rupture it will present with acute abdomen, and workup should be performed to differentiate it from other causes of acute abdomen.

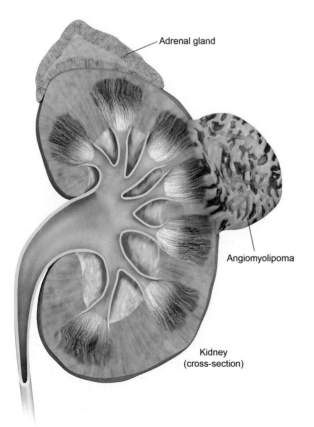
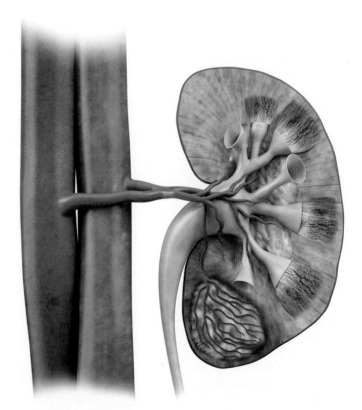

Fig. C10.1 Cross section in renal angiomyolipoma composed of fat, blood vessels, and smooth muscles.

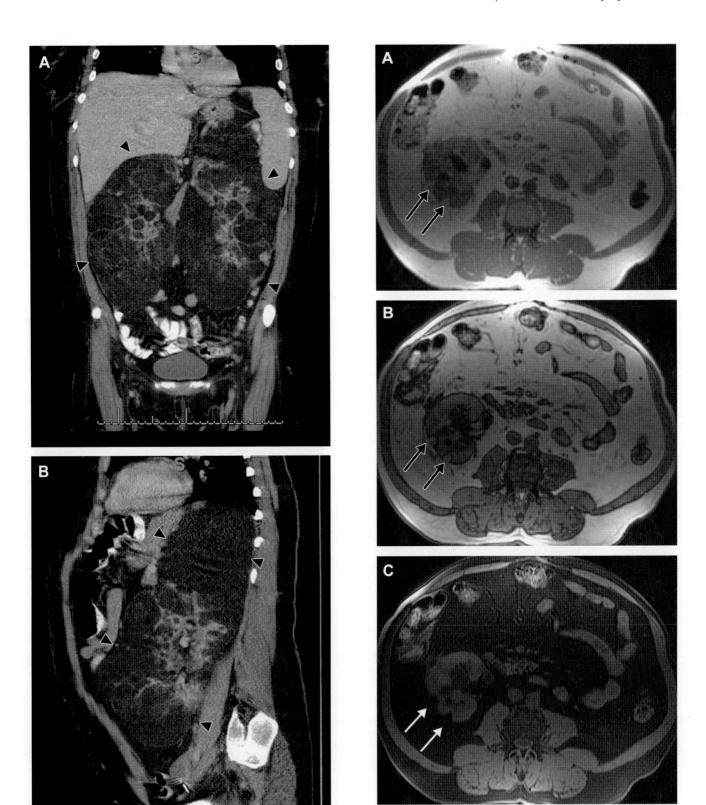

Fig. C10.2 Postcontrast CT scan of the abdomen in coronal (A) and sagittal (B) reconstruction reveals huge bilateral angiomyolipomas in a patient with tuberous sclerosis (arrowheads).

Fig. C10.3 Axial T1WI in-phase (A), out-of-phase (B) and fat suppression of the abdomen in a patient with angiomyolipomas reveals two well-defined left renal fat-containing mass lesions with a bright signal on T1WI in-phase and out-phase (black arrow, A and B). Note the loss of signal of the lesion in the fat suppressed (white arrow, C) but not in the out of phase image denoting the presence of macroscopic fat within.

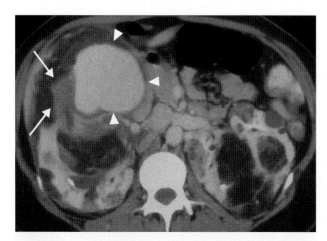

Fig. C10.4 Postcontrast axial CT of the abdomen in a patient with bilateral angiomyolipoma reveals multiple variable-sized fatty renal mass lesions; the largest, in the right kidney, has a hyperdense area of acute (arrowheads) and subacute blood (arrow).

Imaging Differential

There is essentially no differential diagnosis for typical AML (as the dominant presence of macroscopic fat is virtually pathognomonic for angiomyolipoma). In atypical AML, especially fat-poor, other lesions to consider include RCC, retroperitoneal sarcoma invading the kidney, oncocytoma, Wilms' tumor, metastases, and lymphoma.

- Retroperitoneal liposarcoma invading the kidney: The center of the lesion is outside the kidney and the kidney appears compressed by the lesion.
- RCC: The absence of fat and presence of calcification within the lesion make AML less likely and raise suspicion of RCC.
- Oncocytoma: It is a benign renal tumor and may contain fat. The lesion is usually solid, and demonstrate homogenous enhancement.
- Wilms' tumors: It may contain fat. However, this tumor occurs in the pediatric age group.

REFERENCES AND SUGGESTED READING

1. Prando A. Radiological classification of renal angiomyolipomas based on 127 tumors. *Int Braz J Urol.* 2003;29(3):208-216.
2. Silverman SG, Mortele KJ, Tuncali K, Jinzaki M, Cibas ES. Hyperattenuating renal masses: etiologies, pathogenesis, and imaging evaluation. *RadioGraphics.* 2007;27(4):1131-1143.
3. Helenon O, Merran S, Paraf F, et al. Unusual fat-containing tumors of the kidney: a diagnostic dilemma. *RadioGraphics.* 1997;17(1):129-144.

CASE 11: SEPSIS-INDUCED ADRENAL HEMORRHAGE

PATIENT PRESENTATION

A 10-year-old boy with a recent history of meningitis presents with fatigue, anorexia, nausea, and vomiting.

CLINICAL SUSPICION

Adrenal hemorrhage caused by sepsis, especially meningococcemia (also known as Waterhouse-Friderichsen syndrome)

IMAGING MODALITY OF CHOICE

CT scan examination of the abdomen (without and with intravenous contrast)

FINDINGS

Sonography: The pattern of echogenicity of an adrenal hematoma depends on its age.

- An early-stage hematoma appears solid, with diffuse or inhomogeneous echogenicity. As liquefaction occurs, the mass demonstrates mixed echogenicity with a central hypoechoic region and eventually becomes completely anechoic and cystlike.

- Calcification may be seen in the walls of the hematoma as early as 1 to 2 weeks after onset and gradually becomes more compact as the blood is absorbed.

Color Doppler and power Doppler imaging allow confirmation of the avascular nature of the mass.

CT

Adrenal hematomas characteristically appear round or oval, often with surrounding stranding of the periadrenal fat.

The attenuation value of adrenal hematoma depends on its age:

- Acute to subacute hematomas contain areas of high attenuation that usually range from 50 to 90 HU (Fig. C11.1).

- Adrenal hematomas decrease in size and attenuation over time, and most resolve completely.

- Organized chronic adrenal hematomas appear as masses with hypoattenuating centers, with or without calcifications (also known as adrenal pseudocysts).

- Adrenal hematomas may calcify after 1 year.

DIFFERENTIAL DIAGNOSIS

Clinical Differential

Causes of adrenal hemorrhage:

- Trauma is a common cause of unilateral adrenal hemorrhage.

- Bilateral adrenal hemorrhage is frequently attributed to adrenal vein spasm or thrombosis.

Predisposing risk factors include:

- Disseminated intravascular coagulation

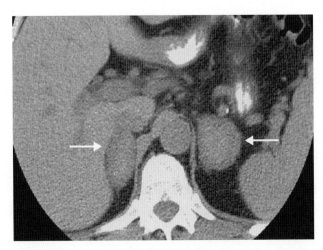

Fig. C11.1 Noncontrast axial CT study of the abdomen in a patient with bilateral adrenal hematomas reveals bilateral well-defined hyperdense soft tissue masses occupying the region of the adrenal gland (arrows).

- Primary antiphospholipid syndrome
- Heparin-induced thrombocytopenia
- Steroid usage
- Anticoagulation
- Underlying adrenal tumor

Imaging Differential

Adrenal hematoma can be differentiated from other adrenal masses by lack of enhancement. They also contain blood with expected attenuation or signal intensity of blood. All the lesions listed below shows contrast enhancement (see case 12).

- Adenoma: the most common adrenal lesion; can be diagnosed by multiphasic CT
- Adrenal metastasis
- Pheochromocytoma
- Asymmetric adrenal cortical hyperplasia
- Adrenal granulomatous disease
- Adrenal myelolipoma
- Adrenal cortical carcinoma
- Neuroblastoma, ganglioneuroblastoma, ganglioneuroma
- Adrenal abscess
- Adrenal hemangioma
- Adrenal lymphoma

REFERENCES AND SUGGESTED READING

1. Elsayes KM, Mukundan G, Narra VR, et al. Adrenal masses: MR imaging features with pathologic correlation. *RadioGraphics*. 2004;24(suppl 1):S73-S86.

2. Mayo-Smith WW, Boland GW, Noto RB, Lee MJ. State-of-the-art adrenal imaging. *RadioGraphics*. 2001;21(4):995-1012.

CASE 12: ADRENAL MASS

PATIENT PRESENTATION

A 34-year-old woman presents with vague abdominal pain. Sonographic findings are normal except for an incidental right adrenal lesion.

CLINICAL SUSPICION

Adrenal mass (adrenal incidentaloma)

IMAGING MODALITY OF CHOICE

Multiphasic precontrast and postcontrast CT or MRI of the adrenal glands

FINDINGS

CT

Adrenal adenomas can be either lipid rich (70% of cases) or lipid poor (30% of cases). In case of lipid rich adenoma, the low attenuation value of the lesion (<10 HU) measured on the noncontrast CT scan of the abdomen is sufficient for the diagnosis (Fig. C12.1). However, lipid-poor adenomas have a higher attenuation on the noncontrast CT and a dedicated CT study of the abdomen is required to assess the adrenal mass and to differentiate it from malignant lesions. This study should include a noncontrast scan, an early venous postcontrast scan 60 seconds after contrast injection, and a delayed scan after 15 minutes. The density of the adrenal lesion is measured in every scan, and the absolute and relative enhancement washout are calculated (Fig. C12.2). Values above 40% for the relative washout and 60% for the absolute washout are 98% sensitive and 92% specific for diagnosing adrenal adenomas, while lower values are indeterminate and further follow-up or biopsy may be required (Fig. C12.3).

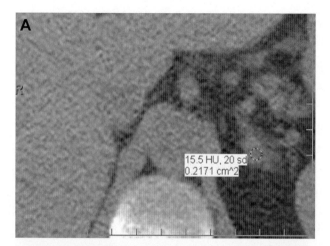

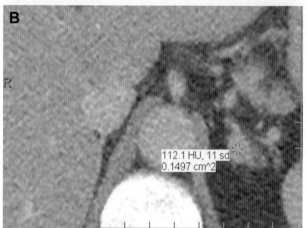

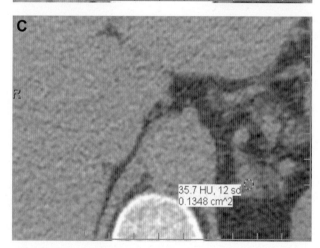

Fig. C12.2 Multiphasic axial precontrast (A) and postcontrast CT study, venous phase (B), and delayed phase (C) in a patient with left lipid-poor adrenal adenoma showing well-defined left adrenal lesion with calculated relative washout of 68% and absolute washout 79%.

$$\text{Absolute washout} = \frac{\text{(venous attenuation} - \text{delayed attenuation)}}{\text{(venous attenuation} - \text{precontrast attenuation)}} \times 100$$

$$\text{Relative washout} = \frac{\text{(venous attenuation} - \text{delayed attenuation)}}{\text{(venous attenation)}} \times 100$$

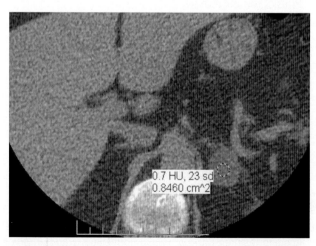

Fig. C12.1 Noncontrast axial CT scan in a patient with left lipid-rich adrenal adenoma. The lesion is well defined with low attenuation (<10 HU) diagnostic for lipid-rich adrenal adenoma.

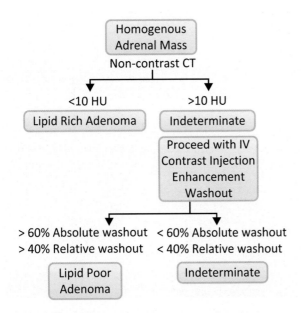

Fig. C12.3 Characterization of homogenous adrenal mass.

MRI

MRI can be used to diagnose adrenal adenoma based on the fact that adrenal adenomas contain intracellular fat. This is especially useful if the adrenal mass is heterogeneous, which limits the diagnostic accuracy of the CT. Intracellular fat can be detected using MRI through chemical shift imaging (in-phase and out-phase sequences). Loss of signal intensity of the adrenal mass on out-of-phase compared to in-phase pulse sequences is diagnostic of the presence of intracellular lipid. Through calculating signal intensity index, more than 16.5% signal loss is highly specific for diagnosis of adrenal adenoma.

$$\text{Signal intensity index} = \frac{(\text{SI of in phase} - \text{SI of out of phase})}{(\text{SI of in phase}) \times 100}$$

REFERENCES AND SUGGESTED READING

1. Zeiger MA, Thompson GB, Duh Q-Y, et al. American Association of Clinical Endocrinologists and American Association of Endocrine Surgeons medical guidelines for the management of adrenal incidentalomas. *Endocr Pract.* 2009;15:1-20.

2. Elsayes KM, Mukundan G, Narra VR, et al. Adrenal masses: MR imaging features with pathologic correlation. *RadioGraphics.* 2004;24(suppl 1):S73-S86.

3. Mayo-Smith WW, Boland GW, Noto RB, Lee MJ. State-of-the-art adrenal imaging. *RadioGraphics.* 2001;21(4):995-1012.

CASE 13: ADRENAL MYELOLIPOMA

PATIENT PRESENTATION

A 50-year-old woman presents with vague abdominal pain.

CLINICAL SUSPICION

Adrenal myelolipomas are usually asymptomatic and discovered incidentally on workups for other complaints.

IMAGING MODALITY OF CHOICE

Cross-sectional imaging by CT or MRI is the modality of choice; ultrasound can also be helpful in diagnosis. This uncommon tumor is composed of a fatty component and a hematopoietic component. Imaging appearances depend on the proportion of each component—the more the fatty component the more homogenous is the lesion.

FINDINGS

US

Sonographic findings: Soft tissue mass at the adrenal region demonstrates heterogeneous mixed hyperechoic and hypoechoic components, with the former primarily resulting from fatty portions.

CT

The CT appearance is usually characteristic. Myelolipomas typically appear as relatively well-circumscribed adrenal masses with macroscopic fat-containing components (Fig. C13.1). Variable amounts of macroscopic fat are seen, ranging from only a few small regions in an otherwise mostly soft tissue density mass (10%) to masses made up of roughly equal components of fat and soft tissue (50%) or almost completely composed of fatty tissue (40%). Small punctate calcifications are seen in 25% to 30% of cases. If hemorrhage is present, regions of higher attenuation may be seen. This is more common in large lesions (>10 cm). Myelolipoma is a benign lesion with no recognized malignant potential, but large lesions carry the risk of rupture and retroperitoneal hemorrhage.

MRI

Because myelolipoma contains macroscopic fat, the lesion will a hyperintense signal on non-fat-suppressed T1 weighted with loss of signal intensity on fat suppression but not on out-of-phase.

DIFFERENTIAL DIAGNOSIS

Fat-containing lesions of the retroperitoneum include:

- Lipomas: Lipomas rarely occur in the retroperitoneum, do not enhance with contrast, and may have thin septations.

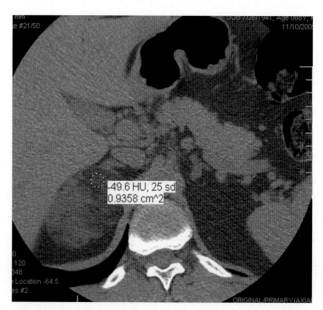

Fig. C13.1 Noncontrast axial CT study in a patient with a right adrenal myelolipoma reveals an ill-defined adrenal lesion that contains areas of macroscopic fat.

- Pelvic lipomatosis: Pelvic lipomatosis is the overgrowth of histologically normal fat in the extra-abdominal compartments of the pelvis along the perirectal and perivesicular spaces.
- Lipoblastomas: Lipoblastomas occur in infants and young children.
- Liposarcomas: Liposarcomas typically occur in patients 50 to 70 years old. They may have thick septations, variable enhancement, and areas of necrosis.
- Hibernomas: Hibernomas are a rare benign soft tissue tumor composed of brown fat.
- Teratomas: Teratomas are neoplasms that originate in pluripotent cells; they contain calcifications, fat, fluid, and soft tissue components.
- Renal angiomyolipomas: Renal angiomyolipomas are composed of varying admixtures of blood vessels, smooth muscle cells, and adipose tissue; any one or two of these elements may predominate.

REFERENCES AND SUGGESTED READING

1. Lee JK. *Computed Body Tomography with MRI Correlation.* Lippincott Williams & Wilkins. 2006. ISBN:0781745268.
2. Craig WD, Fanburg-Smith JC, Henry LR, Guerrero R, Barton JH. Fat-containing lesions of the retroperitoneum: radiologic-pathologic correlation. *RadioGraphics.* 2009;29(1):261-290.
3. Mayo-Smith WW, Boland GW, Noto RB, Lee MJ. State-of-the-art adrenal imaging. *RadioGraphics.* 2001;21:995-1012.

CASE 14: ADRENAL CARCINOMA

PATIENT PRESENTATION

A 45-year-old man presents with a palpable mass in the right flank.

CLINICAL SUSPICION

Renal or adrenal mass

IMAGING MODALITY OF CHOICE

Precontrast and postcontrast CT study of the abdomen

FINDINGS

- Adrenal carcinomas tend to be large (> 6 cm), irregularly shaped, ill-defined heterogeneous masses with central areas of necrosis and hemorrhage, resulting in variable enhancement (Fig. C14.1). Calcification is seen in up to 30% of cases.

- Direct extension into the renal vein, inferior vena cava, and liver are relatively common, with some series finding renal vein involvement in up to 40% of patients.

- Metastasis to regional lymph nodes, the liver, and the lungs can occur.

- Usually unilateral; is bilateral in 10% of cases.

MRI

MRI is used if CT is inconclusive and helps in determining hepatic invasion and more accurately detecting extension into the renal vein and IVC.

Renal and adrenal masses usually appear as relatively hypointense on T1-weighted images and hyperintense on T2-weighted images compared with the liver, with heterogeneous enhancement (often with tumor necrosis) on postcontrast studies.

DIFFERENTIAL DIAGNOSIS

Clinical Differential

Adrenal cortical carcinoma typically present with a palpable flank mass.

A flank mass can arise from various organs on the right side, such as:
- Liver
- Right Kidney
- Right adrenal gland
- Bowel

On the left side, such as:
- Spleen
- Left Kidney
- Left adrenal gland
- Bowel

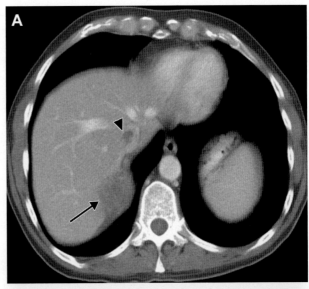

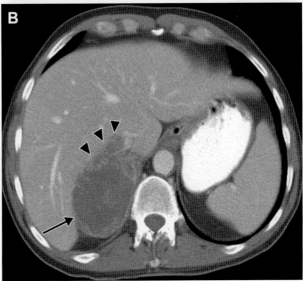

Fig. C14.1 Postcontrast axial CT of the abdomen (A, B) of a patient with adrenocortical carcinoma reveals an ill-defined heterogeneous soft tissue mass lesion occupying the right adrenal region (arrow) and extending into the hepatic segment of the inferior vena cava (arrowheads).

On either side, adrenal cortical carcinoma can be mimicked by large retroperitoneal masses such as retroperitoneal sarcoma, teratoma, or lymphoma.

The clinical history of the patient, physical examination, and imaging help to detect the origin of the mass.

Imaging Differential

Adrenal cortical carcinoma is the most likely diagnosis for large lobulated adrenal mass in adults. If infiltrative, the organ of origin may not be determined and other retroperitoneal masses can be included in the differential diagnosis, such as retroperitoneal sarcomas, lymphoma and seminoma.

On imaging, it is likely that the mass could be localized to the surprarenal region displacing the kidney inferiorly. Thus, the imaging differential diagnosis can be that of large adrenal mass. Although, adrenal cortical carcinoma in the most likely diagnosis for large adrenal mass, other masses can rarely present as large adrenal mass such as:

- Pseudocyst (well circumscribed, non-invasive)
- Metastasis
- Lymphoma
- Pheochromocytoma
- Ganglioneuroma
- Hemorrhage

In children, adrenal cortical carcinoma is not common, neuroblastoma and ganglioneuroblastoma are the likely diagnoses for large adrenal mass.

REFERENCES AND SUGGESTED READING

1. Rosenthal TC, Kraybill W. Soft tissue sarcomas: integrating primary care recognition with tertiary care center treatment. *Am Fam Physician*. 1999;60(2):567-572.
2. Sanyal R, Remer EM. Radiology of the retroperitoneum: case-based review. *AJR*. 2009;192(6)(suppl):S112-117 (Quiz S118-121).

CASE 15: PHEOCHROMOCYTOMA

PATIENT PRESENTATION

A 40-year-old man presents with uncontrolled paroxysmal hypertension and an elevated VMA level.

CLINICAL SUSPICION

Pheochromocytoma

IMAGING MODALITY OF CHOICE

Due to high incidence of incidental adrenal lesions, imaging is done after the diagnosis is made on clinical and laboratory background. The role of imaging is the localization and staging of the tumor before surgery is planned. MIBG is performed for detection and then MRI for characterization.

An MIBG scan is a scintigraphic study that uses metaiodobenzylguanidine (MIBG) labeled with iodine-123 or iodine-131. MIBG was introduced by Sisson, et al in 1981 as a radiopharmaceutical for the diagnosis of pheochromocytoma. It is a marker for norepinephrine storage and shares the same mechanism of adrenergic tissue uptake as norepinephrine. It provides specific noninvasive evidence of pheochromocytomas; detects recurrent tumors at previous surgery sites; detects small lesions at extra-adrenal sites, especially in multicentric and syndromic cases; and helps in the evaluation of metastatic pheochromocytomas.

MRI

MRI is a sensitive modality for identifying pheochromocytomas and is particularly useful in cases of extra-adrenal location. The overall sensitivity is reported to be 93.3% to 100% [4].

FINDINGS
MR

The scan for extra-adrenal tumors ranges from the diaphragm to the symphysis pubis. MRI characteristics of pheochromocytoma:

T1-weighted image: Slightly hypointense to the remainder of the adrenal gland. If necrotic or hemorrhagic, the signal will be more heterogeneous. It maintains its signal intensity on out-of-phase gradient echo chemical shift images (with no drop of signal, as seen with adrenal adenoma).

T2-weighted image: Hyperintense. This is a helpful feature, but not specific. Some other tumors, such as adenomas and carcinomas, exhibit a moderate signal on T2WI.

T1-weighted image after contrast: Heterogeneous enhancement is prolonged, persisting for as long as 50 minutes.

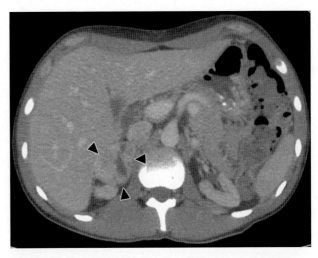

Fig. C15.1 Postcontrast axial CT of the abdomen in a patient with uncontrolled hypertension and elevated plasma and urine catecholamine reveals a well-defined, heterogeneously enhancing right adrenal mass lesion representing the pheochromocytoma (arrowheads).

CT

Pheochromocytoma usually appears as a solid mass with intense enhancement. Heterogeneous attenuation due to tumor hemorrhage and necrosis (Fig. C15.1). Some tumors may show calcification. Rarely, pheochromocytoma has been characterized as cystic mass.

DIFFERENTIAL DIAGNOSIS
Clinical Differential

Essential hypertension is the most common cause of hypertension worldwide. However, hypertension in a young patient or hypertension refractory to multiple drug treatment points toward secondary hypertension. The most common causes of secondary hypertension are renal such as renal artery stenosis or glomerulonephritis. Other less common causes are Cushing's syndrome, Conn's syndrome, hypothyroidism, and pheochromocytoma. Pheochromocytoma causes episodes of hypertension, headache, palpitation, and sweating due to release of epinephrine and norepinephrine from the tumor into the bloodstream.

Imaging Differential

MIBG-positive lesions include neuroblastoma, carcinoid tumor, pheochromocytoma, medullary thyroid carcinoma, ganglioneuroma, and ganglioneuroblastoma. On MRI, solid adrenal tumors in may be adrenal adenoma (characterized by decreased signal intensity in out-of-phase gradient images), adrenal carcinoma (see case 14), or adrenal metastasis.

Differentiating large tumors, especially malignant ones, from RCC can be difficult.

REFERENCES AND SUGGESTED READING

1. Sisson JC, Frager MS, Valk TW, et al. Scintigraphic localization of pheochromocytoma. *N Engl J Med*. 1981;305(1):12-17.

2. Blake MA, Cronin CG, Boland GW. Adrenal imaging. *AJR*. 2010;194(6):1450-1460.

3. Elsayes KM, Mukundan G, Narra VR, et al. Adrenal masses: MR imaging features with pathologic correlation. *RadioGraphics*. 2004;24(suppl 1):S73-S86.

4. Blake MA, Kalra MK, Maher MM, et al. Pheochromocytoma: an imaging chameleon. *RadioGraphics*. 2004;24(suppl 1): S87-S99.

5. Lumachi F, Tregnaghi A, Zucchetta P, et al. Sensitivity and positive predictive value of CT, MRI and 123I-MIBG scintigraphy in localizing pheochromocytomas: a prospective study. *Nucl Med Commun*. 2006;27(7):583-587.

CASE 16: BLADDER DIVERTICULUM

PATIENT PRESENTATION

A 20-year-old male presents with recurrent urinary tract infections.

CLINICAL SUSPICION

Urinary tract structural abnormality leading to stasis and repeated infection (such as bladder diverticulum)

IMAGING MODALITY OF CHOICE

Ultrasound or CT of the abdomen and pelvis, without and with intravenous contrast

FINDINGS

CT, with and without intravenous contrast, has been described as the "examination of choice" for evaluating complicated urinary tract infections and detecting underlying structural problems or complications.

Unenhanced CT is used to determine the presence or absence of calculi throughout the urinary tract, which are sometimes associated with recurrent UTIs.

Reduced-radiation protocols for CT are being used and developed that result in similar renal stone detection while reducing patient radiation exposure.

Ultrasound, a noninvasive, inexpensive diagnostic tool that carries no risk of ionizing radiation, can detect a urinary bladder diverticulum as an anechoic outpouching, define its location, and diagnose any associated complications such as stones or debris (Fig. C16.1). In addition, the postvoiding residual urine can easily and accurately be determined by ultrasound.

Bladder diverticula are acquired abnormalities in most instances, usually forming as a result of bladder outlet obstruction or a neurogenic bladder. Only rarely are they congenital. Acquired bladder diverticula are false diverticula because they represent herniations of bladder mucosa through the submucosa (Fig. C16.2). They may occasionally be difficult to detect on anteroposterior radiographs obtained during excretory urography or cystography because most bladder diverticula extend posteriorly, such that the normal bladder is superimposed over them.

Several complications of bladder diverticula are possible. Urine can accumulate in acquired diverticula during voiding, resulting in the desire to urinate again immediately after initial voiding is complete. Bladder diverticula can also serve as a cause of urinary stasis, resulting in an increased likelihood of urinary tract infections. Bladder calculi may also form (Fig. C16.1). Finally, bladder neoplasms may develop; when this happens, the neoplasms may be

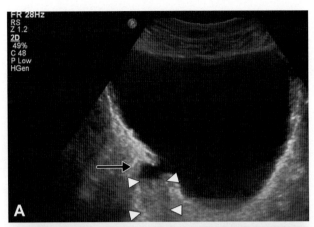

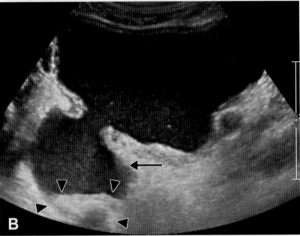

Fig. C16.1 Transverse transabdominal sonography of two patients with complicated bladder diverticulum. (A) Sedimentation of infected urine (arrowheads) and thickening of the diverticular wall (arrow). (B) Another patient with diverticulum (arrow) and a stone is seen in the dependent portion of the diverticulum (arrowheads).

aggressive because they are not contained by submucosal, muscular, or serosal layers.

DIFFERENTIAL DIAGNOSIS

Urinary bladder diverticula arise from a number of causes.

Primary (Congenital or Idiopathic)

- Hutch diverticulum (in paraureteral region)

Secondary

- Bladder outlet obstruction
- Bladder neck stenosis
- Neurogenic bladder
- Posterior urethral valve
- Prostatic enlargement (hypertrophy, carcinoma)

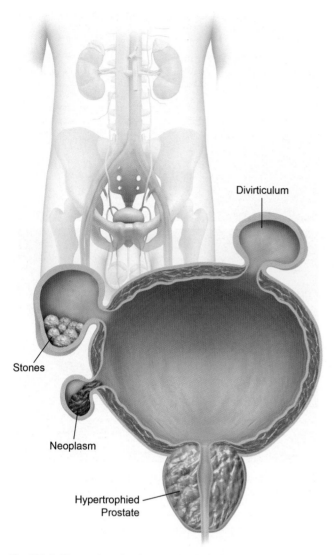

Stones

Neoplasm

Hypertrophied
Prostate

Divirticulum

Fig. C16.2 Illustration showing acquired bladder diverticula.

- Ureterocele (large)
- Urethral stricture
- Congenital syndromes
- Diamond-Blackfan syndrome
- Ehlers-Danlos syndrome
- Menkes syndrome (kinky hair syndrome)
- Prune-belly syndrome (Eagle-Barrett syndrome)
- Williams syndrome (idiopathic hypercalcemia)

REFERENCES AND SUGGESTED READING

1. Vaddi S, Pogula V, Devraj R, Sreedhar A. Congenital bladder diverticulum-a rare adult presentation. *JSCR*. 2011;4:8.

2. Berrocal T, López-Pereira P, Arjonilla A, Gutiérrez J. Anomalies of the distal ureter, bladder, and urethra in children: embryologic, radiologic, and pathologic features. *RadioGraphics*. 2002;22(5):1139-1164.

CASE 17: BLADDER CANCER

PATIENT PRESENTATION

A 45-year-old man presents with painless hematuria. The patient has a history of long-term use of cyclophosphamide for treatment of lymphoma.

CLINICAL SUSPICION

Bladder cancer

IMAGING MODALITY OF CHOICE

CT of the abdomen and pelvis, with and without contrast (CT urography)

FINDINGS

Bladder carcinoma has variable appearances, including focal regions of mural thickening of the bladder wall, masses protruding into the bladder lumen (Fig. C17.1), or, in advanced cases, masses extending into adjacent tissues.

Mural wall thickening on imaging has many causes and depends on the degree of bladder distension, but asymmetric mural thickening should be viewed with suspicion.

Transitional cell carcinoma (TCC) tumors have soft tissue attenuation and may be encrusted with small calcifications.

MRI is superior to CT in detecting and staging (Table C17.1) early tumors and can distinguish between T1 (invasion of the subepithelial connective tissue), T2 (invasion of the muscle layer), and T3a (microscopic extravesical

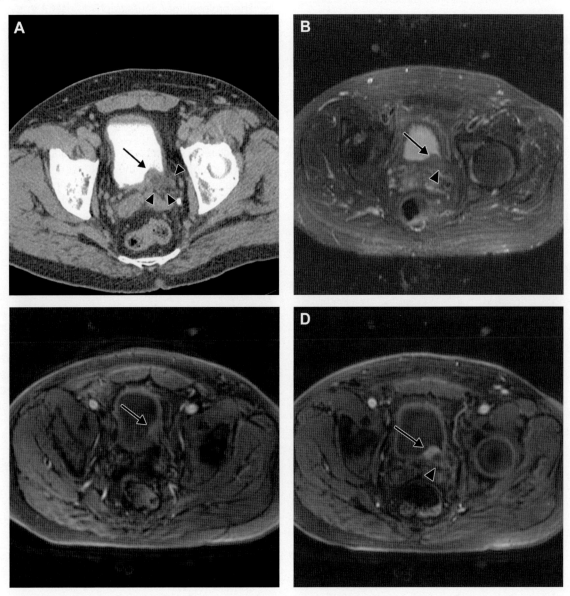

Fig. C17.1 (A) Axial CT, (B) axial T2WI, (C) axial T1WI, and (D) axial T1WI postcontrast MRI of a patient with transitional cell carcinoma of the left vesico-ureteric junction; the images reveal an ill-defined, irregularly shaped soft tissue mass at the left vesico-ureteric junction (arrow), with invasion of the wall and extension into the perivesical fat planes (arrowheads).

Table C17.1 The American Joint Committee on Cancer (AJCC)
T Staging of Bladder Cancer

T Stage	Description
Tis	Tumor is limited to the epithelium and is flat
Ta	Tumor is limited to the epithelium and protrude into lumen
T1	Tumor extend to the subepithelial connective tissue
T2a	Tumor invades the inner half of the muscle layer
T2b	Tumor invades the outer half of the muscle layer
T3a	Microscopic invasion of the perivesical tissues
T3b	Macroscopic invasion of the perivesical tissues
T4a	Invasion of the adjacent organs such as prostate
T4b	Invasion of the pelvic wall

Adapted with permission from Edge SB. *AJCC Cancer Staging Manual*,
7th ed. New York: Springer; 2010.

spread). MRI and CT are used to distinguish T3b (macroscopic extravesical spread with extravesical mass, stranding, nodules in perivesical fat) and T4 tumors (involvement of the adjacent organs) (Fig. C17.2).

Nodal metastases are common, seen in 30% of T2 tumors and 60% of T3 and T4 tumors.

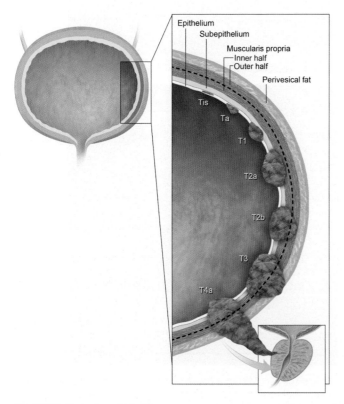

Fig. C17.2 T staging of bladder cancer.

CT or Conventional Urography

The main role of urography is to assess the urinary tract for urothelial lesions and rule out metachronous or synchronous lesions of the renal pelvis or ureter.

Approximately 30% of TCC patients present with multifocal disease in the bladder, including widespread areas of squamous metaplasia and carcinoma in situ.

CT urography is now the first-line study for the evaluation of the collecting systems, ureters, and bladder. CT also helps in the detection of back-pressure changes in the kidneys and in metastatic workup. When tumors are large and of the papillary type, contrast filling the interstices between papillary projections can lead to a dappled appearance referred to as the stipple sign.

The protocol for CT urography is useful in evaluation of the upper and lower urinary tract for any pathology. It consists of 4 phases. After the unenhanced phase, noniodinated contrast is injected and scans are taken for the corticomedullary phase, nephrographic phase, and pyelographic or excretory phase after 25 to 50 seconds, 50 to 90 seconds, and 4 to 5 minutes, respectively. The unenhanced phase is important to determine stones, calcification, renal cysts, or masses. The corticomedullary phase is important for detection of renal tumors and their enhancement as well as for the demonstration of the anatomy of the renal arteries. The nephrographic phase is best for renal tumor detection and vascular invasion. The excretory phase is important for detection of lesions in the collecting system, ureters, and urinary bladder.

Clinical Differential

Patients presenting with hematuria need a thorough workup including physical examination, laboratory testing, and imaging studies. This is because hematuria can be caused by a wide range of pathologies including renal and nonrenal causes. The most common renal causes are stones, infection, trauma, and tumors. Nonrenal causes include bleeding diathesis such as hemophilia and intravascular hemolysis such as paroxysmal nocturnal hemoglobinuria.

Imaging Differential

Other causes of focal bladder masses or diffuse mural thickening that may mimic malignancy include:

• Various types of cystitis (cystitis cystica, cystitis glandularis, and eosinophilic cystitis) that require pathologic diagnosis.

• Bladder infection with tuberculosis and schistosomiasis, which produces nonspecific bladder wall thickening and ulceration.

• Chemotherapy cystitis and radiation cystitis, which should be clinically evident.

- Inflammatory pseudotumor, a rare disorder that produces ulcerated, bleeding polypoid bladder masses.
- Bladder endometriosis, which involves submucosal masses with hemorrhagic foci and reactive fibrosis.
- Bladder malacoplakia, an inflammatory condition that has nonspecific imaging features and characteristic Michaelis-Gutmann bodies on pathologic evaluation.
- Extrinsic inflammatory diseases such as Crohn's disease and diverticulitis, which may be associated with fistulas to the bladder and focal bladder wall abnormalities.

- Extrinsic masses arising from the prostate or distal ureter, which may cause filling defects, that can be confused with intrinsic bladder masses.

REFERENCES AND SUGGESTED READING

1. Vikram R, Sandler CM, Ng CS. Imaging and staging of transitional cell carcinoma: part 1, lower urinary tract. *AJR.* 2009;192(6):1481-1487.

2. Dyer RB, Chen MY, Zagoria RJ. Classic signs in uroradiology. *RadioGraphics.* 2004;24 (suppl 1):S247-280.

3. Tekes A, Kamel IR, Imam K, Chan TY, Schoenberg MP, Bluemke DA. MR imaging features of transitional cell carcinoma of the urinary bladder. *AJR.* 2003;180(3):771-777.

CASE 18: BLADDER RUPTURE

PATIENT PRESENTATION

A 30-year-old patient presents with blunt pelvic trauma and hematuria.

CLINICAL SUSPICION

Bladder rupture

IMAGING MODALITY OF CHOICE

CT pelvis with bladder contrast (CT cystography) is sensitive and accurate, provided that adequate bladder distention (with at least 350-400 mL of contrast material administered in retrograde fashion) is achieved before the study is performed.

A conventional cystogram may be performed in the acute setting.

Important note: Bladder catheterization is performed only after a trauma surgeon determines urethral continuity on the basis of clinical or retrograde urethrographic findings.

FINDINGS

There are 5 types of injury:

- Type I: Bladder contusion
  - Most common form
  - Results from incomplete tear of bladder mucosa
  - Presents with hematuria
  - Cystography is normal
- Type II: Intraperitoneal rupture (Fig. C18.1)
  - Results from trauma to the lower abdomen when the bladder is distended.
  - Because the bladder dome is the weakest part, it ruptures more easily.
  - CT demonstrates intraperitoneal contrast material around bowel loops, between mesenteric folds, and in the paracolic gutters (Fig. C18.2).
- Type III: Interstitial injury (rare)
  - Caused by a tear of the serosal surface
  - Intramural hemorrhage and submucosal extravasation of contrast material without transmural extension
- Type IV: Extraperitoneal (Fig. C18.1)
  - Almost always associated with pelvic fractures
  - Usually close to the base of bladder anterolaterally

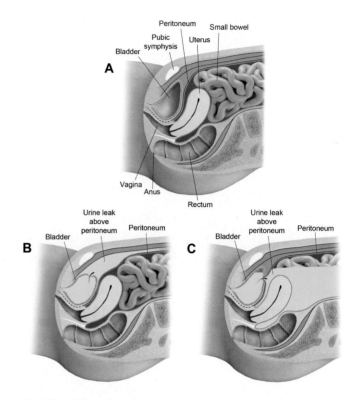

Fig. C18.1 (A) Normal bladder, (B) extraperitoneal bladder rupture, and (C) intraperitoneal bladder rupture.

  - Subdivided into simple, with extravasation limited to the prevesical space (Fig. C18.3A), complex, with extravasation extending to the thigh, scrotum, or perineum (Fig. C18.3B)
- Type V: Combined extraperitoneal and intraperitoneal rupture
  - Usually demonstrates extravasation patterns that are typical of both types of injury

DIFFERENTIAL DIAGNOSIS

Rupture should be differentiated from other bladder injuries (see Findings). Identification of intraperitoneal rupture is important as it carries higher complication and it needs surgical intervention.

Management of patient with blunt abdominal trauma is summarized in Fig. C18.4.

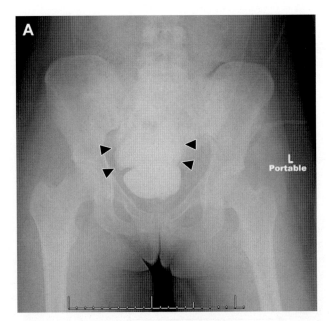

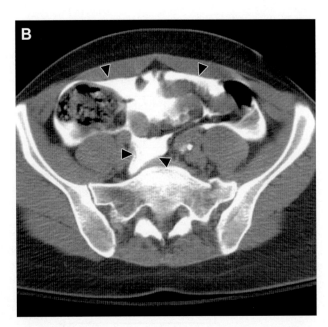

Fig. C18.2 (A) Conventional and (B) CT cystography of a patient with intraperitoneal bladder rupture reveals extension of the contrast upward around the bowel loops within the peritoneal cavity (arrowheads).

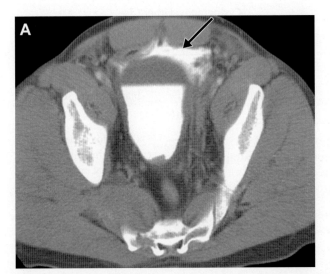

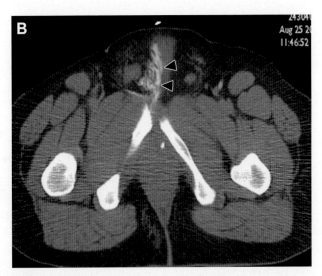

Fig. C18.3 (A,B) CT cystography of a patient with extraperitoneal bladder rupture reveals extension of the contrast within the pelvic cavity, prevesical space (arrow) and downward into the scrotum (arrowheads).

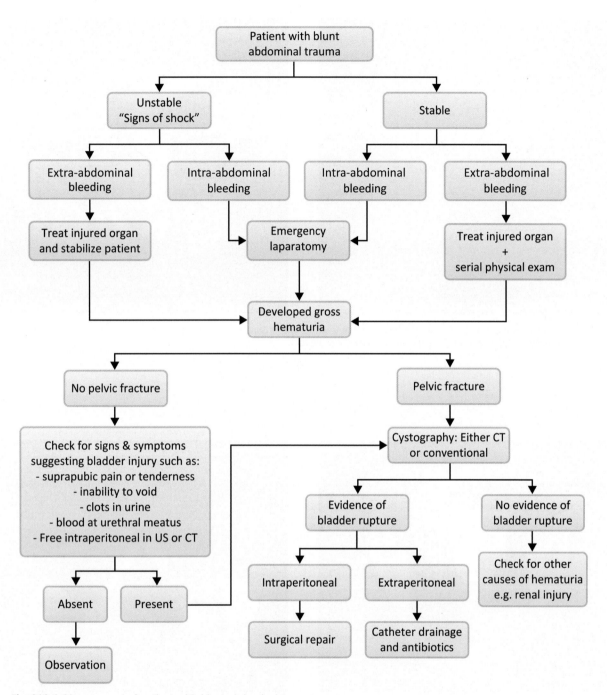

Fig. C18.4 Management of patient with blunt abdominal trauma

REFERENCES AND SUGGESTED READING

1. Vaccaro JP, Brody JM. CT cystography in the evaluation of major bladder trauma. *RadioGraphics*. 2000;20(5):1373-1381.

2. Chan DP, Abujudeh HH, Cushing GL Jr, Novelline RA. CT cystography with multiplanar reformation for suspected bladder rupture: experience in 234 cases. *AJR*. 2006;187(5): 1296-1302.

3. Morey AF, Iverson AJ, Swan A, et al. Bladder rupture after blunt trauma: guidelines for diagnostic imaging. *J Trauma*. 2001;51(4):683-686.

4. Isenhour JL, Marx J. Advances in abdominal trauma. *Emerg Med Clin North Am*. 2007;25(3):713-733, ix.

CASE 19: BENIGN PROSTATIC HYPERTROPHY

PATIENT PRESENTATION

A 65-year-old man presents with urinary hesitancy, frequency, and incomplete emptying of the bladder.

CLINICAL SUSPICION

Benign prostatic hypertrophy

IMAGING MODALITY OF CHOICE

Sonography of the pelvis and kidneys

FINDINGS

Transrectal sonography has become the standard first-line investigation method after a digital rectal examination.

Sonography usually reveals an increase in the prostate volume, with a calculated volume exceeding 30 cc using the formula to approximate the volume of an ellipsoid,

$$\left(\frac{A \times B \times C}{2}\right).$$

The enlargement is mainly noted at the central gland, which is hypoechoic or of mixed echogenicity. Calcification can be seen in the hypertrophied gland and the pseudocapsule (representing the compressed peripheral zone).

The postmicturition residual volume is typically increased as well.

The urinary bladder has uniform mural thickening, secondary to chronic bladder outlet obstruction.

Sonography of both kidneys is indicated in patients who present with concomitant hematuria, a history of urolithiasis, an elevated creatinine level, or a history of upper urinary tract infection to evaluate the effect of prostatic enlargement and secondary hydroureteronephrosis.

Clinical Differential

Symptoms that are often attributed to benign prostatic hyperplasia (BPH) can be caused by:

- Cystitis
- Prostatitis
- Prostatodynia
- Prostatic abscess
- Overactive bladder
- Bladder carcinoma
- Foreign bodies in the bladder (stones or retained stents)
- Urethral stricture due to trauma or a sexually transmitted disease
- Prostate cancer
- Neurogenic bladder
- Pelvic floor dysfunction

Excluding these entities on the basis of findings from a thorough history and appropriately directed diagnostic studies is essential.

Imaging Differential

Prostate Carcinoma. Prostate carcinoma typically involves the peripheral zone (70%); is hypoechoic on endorectal sonography, with increased color Doppler flow; and has a low signal mass on T2 MRI, among other characteristics.

REFERENCES AND SUGGESTED READING

1. Mueller-Lisse UG, Thoma M, Faber S, et al. Coagulative interstitial laser-induced thermotherapy of benign prostatic hyperplasia: online imaging with a T2-weighted fast spin-echo MR sequence—experience in six patients. *Radiology*. 1999;210(2):373-379.

2. Grossfeld GD, Coakley FV. Benign prostatic hyperplasia: clinical overview and value of diagnostic imaging. *Radiol Clin North Am*. 2000;38(1):31-47.

3. Geboers AD, Giesen RJ, Huynen AL, Aarnink RG, Wijkstra H, Debruyne FM. Imaging in BPH patients. *Arch Esp Urol*. 1994;47(9):857-864; discussion 864-855.

CASE 20: PROSTATE CANCER

PATIENT PRESENTATION

A 60-year-old man presents with hematuria, increased urinary frequency, and a hard prostatic mass by rectal examination.

CLINICAL SUSPICION

Prostate cancer

IMAGING MODALITY OF CHOICE

Transrectal ultrasound (TRUS) and MRI with endorectal coil

Advantages of TRUS

- Available
- Cheap
- May detect the actual tumor
- Helps guide biopsies and brachytherapy seed placement

Advantages of MRI

- Used when TRUS is inconclusive
- Used in accurate cancer staging, especially the extra-capsular extension
- Used to differentiate recurrent tumor from posttherapeutic changes

FINDINGS

The prostate is triangular. It is composed of a base directed superiorly toward the urinary bladder, apex directed inferiorly toward the urogenital diaphragm, and mid gland in between. Histologically, the prostate is divided into 4 zones: the peripheral zone, the central zone, the transitional zone, and the anterior fibromuscular stroma (Fig. C20.1).

The peripheral zone forms the posterior and posterolateral parts of the gland, and its volume increase toward the apex of the gland. It contains 70% to 80% of the glandular tissue, and it is the origin of 70% of prostate cancer. On T2WI, the peripheral zone exhibits bright signal.

The central zone lies within the superior portion of the gland just posterior to the proximal prostatic urethra. It contains 20% of the glandular tissue. The transitional zone is located anterior and on both sides of the proximal prostatic urethra. It contains 5% of the glandular tissue. On imaging, the central and transitional zones are indistinguishable, so they are called the central gland. They exhibit lower T2 signal in relation to the peripheral zone.

The anterior fibromuscular stroma is located anterior to the transitional zone. It does not contain any glandular tissue, and therefore it does not give rise to any malignancy. It exhibits low signal intensity on T2WI.

The prostate capsule is readily visible as a low signal in T2WI along the posterior and posterolateral aspect of the gland as it stands against the bright T2 signal of the peripheral zone. The integrity of the capsule is an important factor in determination of extraprostatic extension of prostate carcinoma. The neurovascular bundles are seen along the posterolateral aspect of the capsule in 5 and 7 o'clock location.

Sonography: Prostate cancer is usually seen as a hypoechoic lesion (60%-70%) in the peripheral zone of the gland (Fig. C20.2), but can be hyperechoic or isoechoic (30%-40% of lesions).

Color Doppler: Cancer foci are usually hypervascular.

MRI: In MRI prostate cancer usually appears as a region of low signal in a normally high signal peripheral zone on T2WI (Fig. C20.3). This is not always easily identified.

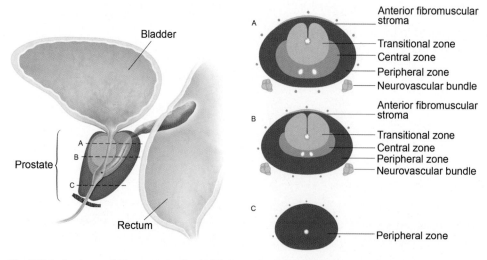

Fig. C20.1 Anatomy of the prostate gland. (A) Cross section through the base. (B) Cross section through mid-zone. (C) Cross section through apex.

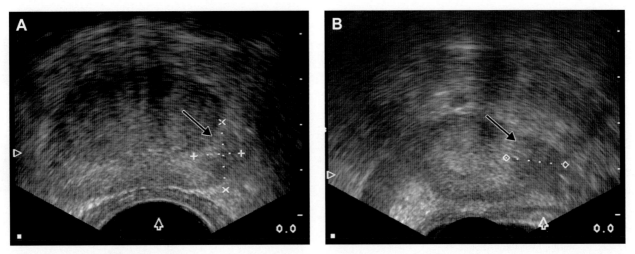

Fig. C20.2 Transrectal sonography of transverse (A) and longitudinal (B) planes in a prostate cancer patient reveal a well-defined focal lesion at the peripheral zone (arrow).

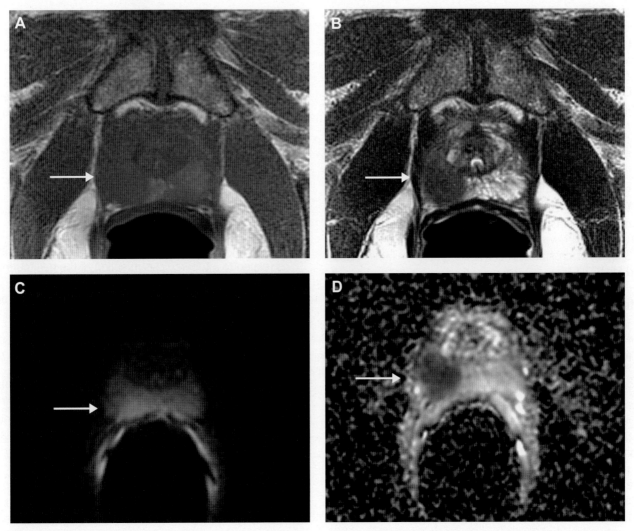

Fig. C20.3 MRI with endorectal coil of a patient with prostate cancer. (A) Axial T1WI. (B) Axial T2WI. (C) DWI. (D) ADC map reveals a well-defined focal lesion exhibiting an isointense signal on T1WI and hypointense on T2WI, with restricted diffusion (arrow).

Table C20.1 T Staging of Prostate Cancer

T Stage	Description
T1	Tumor is within the prostate but not detectable by palpation or imaging.
T2	Tumor is within the prostate and can be detectable by palpation or imaging.
T2a	Tumor is involving not more than one half of one lobe.
T2b	Tumor is involving more than one half of one lobe.
T2c	Tumor is involving both lobes.
T3	Tumor extends beyond the prostatic capsule.
T3a	Extra capsular extension.
T3b	Seminal vesicle invasion.
T4	Tumor invades other adjacent structures sucha as the rectum, bladder neck levator muscle or pelvic wall.

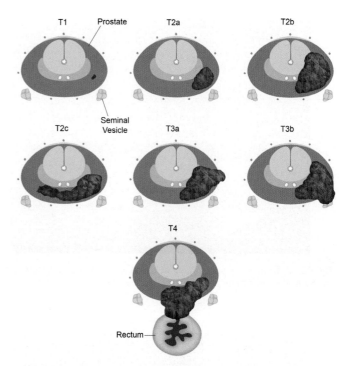

Fig. C20.4 T-staging of prostate cancer.

Furthermore, cancer in the central gland is more difficult to perceive using T2 techniques alone. Diffusion restriction, MR spectroscopy, and dynamic contrast enhancement have all been instrumental in increasing the accuracy of prostate MRI.

Extracapsular extension is associated with a poor prognosis. Assess for:

- Asymmetry or extension into neurovascular bundles
- Obliteration of the rectoprostatic angle
- Involvement of the urethra
- Extension into the seminal vesicles (normal seminal vesicles have a high signal on T2)

Lymphadenopathy is best appreciated on postcontrast, fat-suppressed, T1-weighted images.

Staging of prostate cancer is illustrated in Table C20.1 and Fig. C20.4.

Future Perspectives

Sonographic contrast agents are presumed to play a role in identifying prostate cancer. By demonstrating tumor vascularity, they play a role in establishing prognosis in patients with biopsy-detected prostate cancer. On the other hand, they increase the time and cost of sonography-guided prostate biopsy procedures. These agents remain experimental and have not been adopted into standard uroradiologic practice.

Sonoelastography is a noninvasive new imaging technique that can be useful for differentiating tumor from normal tissue by measuring tissue stiffness using the sonographic waves. The value of elastography in the diagnosis of prostate cancer is under investigation; however, its role is still unclear.

MR spectroscopy is an area of research that holds promise for the detection of disease. It is a noninvasive imaging technique that is able to analyze the metabolic changes in the tissue of interest. The normal prostate produces a large of amount of citrate from the peripheral zone, which tumors do not.

Clinical Differential

Palpable abnormalities that simulate prostate cancer include prostatitis and BPH.

Imaging Differential

- Granulomatous prostatitis. Granulomatous prostatitis is related to a tuberculosis infection of the genitourinary tract or is a reaction after local BCG instillation for a superficial bladder tumor. It involves the peripheral or transitional zones, has a nodular hypoechoic appearance, and has no vascularity.
- Chronic prostatitis. Chronic prostatitis uncommonly simulates a palpable tumor. The appearance is a palpable hypoechoic peripheral zone nodule after an episode of acute prostatitis.
- Palpable calcifications. Palpable calcifications without hypoechoic nodules correspond to corpora amylacea (transitional zone calcifications) or postinflammatory changes (peripheral zone calcifications).
- BPH nodules. BPH nodules that develop in the peripheral zone are present in approximately 20% of cases at pathological examination of radical prostatectomy specimens and are visible in approximately 6% of cases on TRUS.

Whatever the cause, a biopsy is mandatory to exclude malignancy. If the result is benign, a repeat biopsy can be avoided if the TRUS features are typical of BPH.

REFERENCES AND SUGGESTED READING

1. Carroll PR, Coakley FV, Kurhanewicz J. Magnetic resonance imaging and spectroscopy of prostate cancer. *Rev Urol*. 2006;(8)(suppl 1):S4-S10.

2. Turkbey B, Pinto PA, Choyke PL. Imaging techniques for prostate cancer: implications for focal therapy. *Nat Rev Urol*. 2009;6(4):191-203.

3. Naik KS, Carey BM. The transrectal ultrasound and MRI appearances of granulomatous prostatitis and its differentiation from carcinoma. *Clin Radiol*. 1999;54(3):173-175.

4. Casciani E, Polettini E, Bertini L, Pansadoro V, Gualdi GF. Granulomatous prostatitis: a pitfall in endorectal MR imaging and 3D MR spectroscopic imaging. *Eur J Radiol Extra*. 2005;54(3):111-114.

CASE 21: PROSTATITIS OR PROSTATE ABSCESS (PA)

PATIENT PRESENTATION

A 35-year-old immunocompromised man presents with acute onset of fever, chills, malaise, perineal pain, dysuria, urinary frequency, and urinary urgency.

CLINICAL SUSPICION

Prostatitis or PA

IMAGING MODALITY OF CHOICE

TRUS

FINDINGS

Imaging reveals one or more variable hypoechoic areas containing thick liquid, mainly located in the transition and central zones of the prostate; these are permeated by hyperechogenic areas and anatomic distortion. The lesion may have internal septa or solid portions. The outer margin of the hypoechoic area may be well defined and thick.

Color Doppler reveals diffusely increased blood flow peripheral to the hypoechoic area and in the remaining portion of the prostate in all patients. No blood flow should be detected centrally in the hypoechoic area.

TRUS is also used for transrectal aspiration when deemed necessary. This has a success rate of over 80% in curing the abscess, in combination with intravenous antibiotics.

DIFFERENTIAL DIAGNOSIS

Clinical Differential

- Benign prostatic hypertrophy with urinary retention
- Cystitis
- Prostate cancer
- Prostatic abscess
- Seminal vesiculitis
- Urethritis
- Urinary tract infection in men

Imaging Differential

Prostate cancer:

- Size: Prostate carcinoma usually appears small and is more easily distinguishable from the surrounding gland, whereas PA occupies a large area of one or both glands.
- Location: Carcinoma is found more frequently in the peripheral zone of the prostate, whereas PA is usually located in the central gland.
- Echogenicity: PA generally appears as a larger hypoechoic area and is less easily definable during its initial phase.
- Color and power Doppler: High perilesional vascularity is seen in PA but absent within the tumor.

REFERENCES AND SUGGESTED READING

1. Oliveira P, Andrade JA, Porto HC, Filho JE, Vinhaes AF. Diagnosis and treatment of prostatic abscess. *Int Braz J Urol.* 2003;29(1):30-34.
2. Granados EA, Riley G, Salvador J, Vincente J. Prostatic abscess: diagnosis and treatment. *J Urol.* 1992;148(1):80-82.
3. Kalra O, Agrawal N, Sharma S, Sakhuja V, Chugh K. Acute bacterial prostatitis with giant prostatic abscess. *Indian J Nephrol.* 2002;12(3):88.
4. Lim JW, Ko YT, Lee DH, et al. Treatment of prostatic abscess: value of transrectal ultrasonographically guided needle aspiration. *J Ultrasound Med.* 2000;19(9):609-617.

CASE 22: VARICOCELE

PATIENT PRESENTATION

A 37-year-old man presents with a 2-month history of a nonpainful left testicular mass and oligospermia. Palpation of the mass feels like a bag of worms.

CLINICAL SUSPICION

Varicocele

IMAGING MODALITY OF CHOICE

Sonography with color Doppler

FINDINGS

The testis is an elliptical structure that lies within the scrotum. It is surrounded by a tough fibrous layer called the tunica albuginea. From the tunica albuginea, several fibrous septae extend inward toward the hilum, dividing the testes into lobules. Each lobule contain from 1 to 4 seminiferous tubules. The seminiferous tubules converge at the hilum to form an anastomotic network called the Rete testis. The Rete testis gives rise to efferent ductile that penetrate the tunica albuginea to form the head of the epididymis. The epididymis is located on the posterior surface of the testis and is formed from a single highly convoluted tubule that exits the epididymis as the vas deference. The vas deference runs through the inguinal canal and joins the seminal vesicles to form the ejaculatory duct, which pass through the prostate and opens into the urethra (Fig. C22.1).

The testicular artery arises from the front of the aorta below the origin of the renal arteries and descends in the retroperitoneum, passing through the inguinal canal to enter the scrotum. Inside the scrotum it becomes tortuous and gives multiple branches supplying the epididymis, the vas deference, and the testis. Numerous small veins come out from the back of the testis as well as from the epididymis.

These veins merge with each other forming a plexus of vein within the spermatic cord called pampiniform plexus. The plexus end just below the superficial inguinal ring by giving rise to 3 or 4 veins that pass through the inguinal canal to enter the abdomen where they unite forming 2 veins. These veins again unite forming the testicular vein that ascends in the retroperitoneum to end in the IVC on the right side and in the left renal vein on the left side.

Normal vessels in the pampiniform plexus are often not visualized because of their size (up to 1.5 mm in diameter). A diagnosis of varicocele is made when the caliber of these vessels reaches 2 to 3 mm.

On gray-scale sonography, varicoceles appear as multiple serpiginous, anechoic structures superior and posterior to the testis (Fig. C22.2A).

Use of color Doppler imaging greatly aids in diagnosis. Although flow may be too slow to reveal obvious color enhancement during rest, using the Valsalva maneuver and scanning the patient in the upright position may improve detection (Fig. C22.2B).

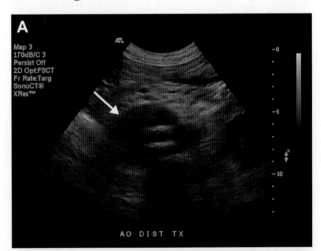

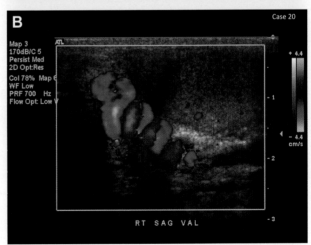

Fig. C22.2 (A) Sonography and (B) color duplex images of the testicular region of a patient with varicocele reveal serpiginous anechoic vascular structures superior and posterior to the testis (arrow).

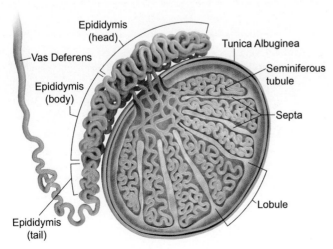

Fig. C22.1 Anatomy of the testis.

Idiopathic varicoceles are generally thought to occur more often on the left side, as the left spermatic vein drains at the left renal vein at a right angle, whereas the right spermatic vein drains directly into the inferior vena cava at an obtuse angle. Therefore, the presence of right varicoceles should prompt for a search for a cause of obstruction, such as retroperitoneal lymphadenopathy or RCC.

DIFFERENTIAL DIAGNOSIS

Extratesticular scrotal masses are categorized as nonneoplastic or neoplastic.

Nonneoplastic

- Cystic masses: hydroceles, epididymal cysts.
- Epididymitis: a common extratesticular lesion that can be complicated by epididymo-orchitis or scrotal abscess.
- Sarcoidosis: a noninfectious granulomatous disorder.
- Fibrous pseudotumors: nodular, possibly reactive proliferation of fibrous tissue and inflammatory cells, most commonly involving the tunica vaginalis.
- Polyorchidism.

Neoplastic

Lipoma, adenomatoid tumors (most often found in the epididymis), rhabdomyosarcoma, liposarcoma, leiomyosarcoma, malignant fibrous histiocytoma, mesothelioma of the tunica vaginalis, and lymphoma.

REFERENCES AND SUGGESTED READING

1. Woodward PJ, Schwab CM, Sesterhenn IA. From the archives of the AFIP: extratesticular scrotal masses: radiologic-pathologic correlation. *RadioGraphics*. 2003;23(1):215-240.

2. Bhosale PR, Patnana M, Viswanathan C, Szklaruk J. The inguinal canal: anatomy and imaging features of common and uncommon masses. *RadioGraphics*. 2008;28(3):819-835; quiz 91.

3. Evers JL, Collins JA. Assessment of efficacy of varicocele repair for male subfertility: a systematic review. *Lancet*. 2003; 361(9372):1849-1852.

CASE 23: TESTICULAR TORSION

PATIENT PRESENTATION

A 10-year-old boy presents with severe acute scrotal pain.

CLINICAL SUSPICION

Testicular torsion

IMAGING MODALITY OF CHOICE

Color Doppler sonography, which is quick, available in an emergency, simultaneously able to assess the structure and vascularity of the testis, and involves no ionizing radiation.

FINDINGS

Diagnosis is based on the appearance of the affected testicle compared with that of the unaffected one.

Gray-Scale Sonography

- Homogenous echotexture: early finding, prior to necrosis (Fig. C23.1A).

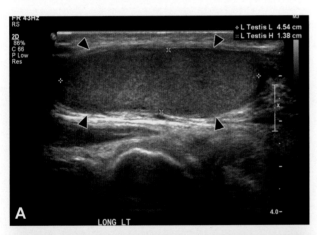

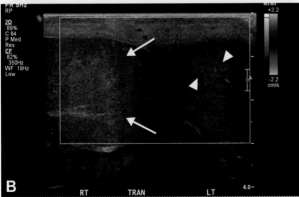

Fig. C23.1 (A) Sonographic study of a patient with testicular torsion reveals slight enlargement of the right testicle, with uniform echogenicity (arrowheads). (B) Color duplex sonography reveals absence of intratesticular vasculature (arrows) as compared to the normal side (arrowheads).

- Heterogenous echotexture: a late finding (after 24 hours), implies necrosis.
- Hypoechoic regions represent necrosis.
- Hyperechoic regions represent hemorrhage (if testis is reperfused).
- Increase in size of the testis and epididymis.
- Twisted spermatic cord may be visible.
- Reactive hydrocele and reactive thickening of the scrotal skin with hyperemia.

Color Doppler Sonography

- Altered blood flow depends on the degree of torsion.
- Incomplete torsion: the resistive index, which is a quantitative indirect measurement of resistance to blood flow, is elevated (RI > 0.75) and to and fro flow. There may be absence of flow in the vein but identifiable flow in the artery.
- Complete torsion: absence of blood flow in the testis and epididymis (Fig. C23.1B).
- Testicular viability is suggested by gray-scale and color Doppler findings.
- Normal echogenicity with mild testicular enlargement is a good sign of viability. Marked enlargement, heterogeneous echotexture, and scrotal wall hypervascularity are signs of testicular infarction and necrosis.

DIFFERENTIAL DIAGNOSIS

Differentiating between testicular torsion and epididymo-orchitis is of utmost clinical importance because both conditions present with scrotal pain, swelling, and redness or tenderness. Both conditions are managed differently. While medical treatment with antibiotics can be sufficient for the treatment of epididymo-orchitis, surgical detorsion and orchipexy should be emergently performed (most testicles can be saved within 6 hours of onset of symptoms).

Clinical Differential

1. The onset of pain is sudden in torsion and more gradual in epididymo-orchitis, but this is not specific.
2. Prehn's sign can be used clinically to help differentiating torsion from epididymo-orchitis. A positive Prehn's sign is the relief of pain when the affected testicle is elevated, which makes epididymo-orchitis more likely. On the other hand, a negative Prehn's sign is failure to relive pain by testicular elevation, and the pain may even get worse, which makes testicular torsion more likely. However, the sign is not reliable, and further evaluation by Doppler sonography is mandatory to reach definitive diagnosis.

Imaging Differential

Color Doppler sonography is used to differentiate torsion from epididymo-orchitis, with high sensitivity and specificity. Normal arterial flow is typically low resistance and high flow.

1. Orchitis: increased vascularity of the affected testicle compared with the contralateral normal side. Normally, venous flow is difficult to detect in the testicle; therefore, brisk venous flow may suggest orchitis.

2. Testicular torsion: flow is absent.

REFERENCES AND SUGGESTED READING

1. Bhatt S, Dogra VS. Role of US in testicular and scrotal trauma. *RadioGraphics*. 2008;28(6):1617-1629.

2. Aso C, Enriquez G, Fite M, et al. Gray-scale and color Doppler sonography of scrotal disorders in children: an update. *RadioGraphics*. 2005;25(5):1197-1214.

CASE 24: EPIDIDYMO-ORCHITIS

PATIENT PRESENTATION

A 35-year-old man presents with acute scrotal pain.

CLINICAL SUSPICION

Epididymo-orchitis, which can be defined as inflammation of the epididymis and /or testis usually secondary to infection.

IMAGING MODALITY OF CHOICE

Doppler sonography of the scrotum

FINDINGS

Ultrasound

- The most affected region is the epididymal head.
- Increased size and decreased, increased, or heterogeneous echogenicity of the affected organ is usually observed depending on the time of evolution (Fig. C24.1A).
- Reactive hydrocele and wall thickening are frequently present.

Color Doppler Sonography

- Inflammation produces increased blood flow in the epididymis, testis, or both (Fig. C24.1B).
- An analysis of the epididymal waveform may reveal a low-resistance pattern compared with a normal pattern.

Complications

- Vascular compromise due to increased intratesticular pressure, resulting in testicular ischemia and even infarction
- Epididymal abscess
- Testicular abscess

DIFFERENTIAL DIAGNOSIS

Testicular torsion is the main differential diagnosis. Pain onset, Prehn`s sign, and color Doppler criteria are used in differentiation (see case 23).

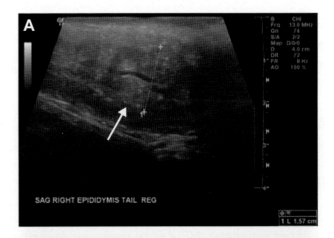

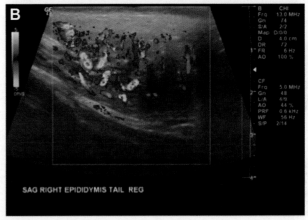

Fig. C24.1 (A) Sonogram of a patient with epididymo-orchitis reveals an enlarged heterogeneously hypoechoic epididymal body and tail (arrow). (B) Color duplex sonography reveals increased vascularity.

REFERENCES AND SUGGESTED READING

1. Chen P, John S. Ultrasound of the acute scrotum. *Appl Radiol.* 2006;35(3):8.
2. Woodward PJ, Schwab CM, Sesterhenn IA. From the archives of the AFIP: extratesticular scrotal masses: radiologic-pathologic correlation. *RadioGraphics.* 2003;23(1):215-240.
3. Muttarak M, Lojanapiwat B. The painful scrotum: an ultrasonographical approach to diagnosis. *Singapore Med J.* 2005; 46(7):352-357; quiz 358.
4. http://www.uptodate.com/contents/evaluation-of-the-acute-scrotum-in-adults. H671410222 B.

CASE 25: TESTICULAR TUMOR

PATIENT PRESENTATION

A 35-year-old man presents with painless, firm testicular swelling. The transillumination test is negative.

CLINICAL SUSPICION

Testicular tumor (such as seminoma)

IMAGING MODALITY OF CHOICE

Ultrasound is used to assess the testicular lesion. CT of the abdomen and pelvis is used for staging to detect any nodal or distant metastases. MRI can be rarely used for further characterization of testicular mass.

Ultrasound of the Scrotum

Whenever a testicular mass is noticed, ultrasound is used to determine the solid or cystic nature of the mass as well as its exact location. Seminoma appears as a hypoechoic, well-defined, solid mass without cystic areas, calcification, or invasion (Fig. C25.1). Nonseminomatous tumors appear more heterogeneous in echotexture, with areas of cystic degeneration. Unfortunately, the sonographic appearance cannot significantly differentiate between tumor types. Color Doppler ultrasound reveals variable vascularity; disorganized flow is typical.

MRI of the Scrotum

Seminomas usually have homogeneous signal intensity (hypointense to normal testis on T2-weighted images). Fibrovascular septa may be detected as bandlike areas of low signal intensity on T1 and T2-weighted images that enhance to a greater degree than the tumor.

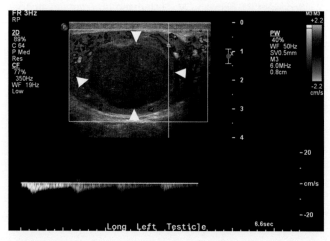

Fig. C25.1 Testicular sonogram with color Doppler interrogation of a patient with a seminoma reveals a large well-defined hypoechoic intratesticular mass (arrowheads).

Nonseminomatous germ cell tumors have heterogeneous signal intensity characteristics and enhancement indicative of necrosis and hemorrhage.

CT of the Abdomen and Pelvis

CT is performed mainly for staging, as the primary site of the nodal metastasis is the para-aortic lymph nodes, especially in seminoma. The affected lymph nodes may appear low in attenuation. Even nodes smaller than 1 cm are suspicious if they are low in attenuation or located in typical drainage areas, including the left renal hilus and retrocaval location.

CT is also used to detect distant metastasis, including liver and lung deposits.

DIFFERENTIAL DIAGNOSIS

Clinical Differential

Testicular malignancies should be differentiated from other causes of painless scrotal mass including hydrocele, varicocele, spermatocele, and scrotal hernia.

Imaging Differential

Unilateral testicular lesions can be classified into common, uncommon neoplastic, or nonneoplastic.

- Neoplastic causes:

    1. Seminoma: The commonest germ cell tumor (40%-45% of all germ cell tumors)
    2. Nonseminomatous germ cell tumors: Such as testicular teratoma, epidermoid, and choriocarcinoma
    3. Lymphoma (4%)
    4. Stromal tumours including Lyedig and Sertoli cell tumors: Rare (2%)
    5. Metastases

- Nonneoplastic causes: Such as testicular cyst, focal infection, or hemorrhage, intratesticular varicocele, and intratesticular AV malformation

REFERENCES AND SUGGESTED READING

1. Woodward PJ, Sohaey R, O'Donoghue MJ, Green DE. From the archives of the AFIP: tumors and tumorlike lesions of the testis: radiologic-pathologic correlation. *RadioGraphics*. 2002;22(1):189-216.
2. Krohmer SJ, McNulty NJ, Schned AR. Best cases from the AFIP: testicular seminoma with lymph node metastases. *RadioGraphics*. 2009;29(7):2177-2183.
3. Cassidy FH, Ishioka KM, McMahon CJ, et al. MR imaging of scrotal tumors and pseudotumors. *RadioGraphics*. 2010;30(3):665-683.

CASE 26: RETROPERITONEAL FIBROSIS

PATIENT PRESENTATION

A 50-year-old woman presents with oliguria and bilateral lower limb swelling and chronic dull aching pain in the abdomen and the flanks that has increased over time. The patient history is significant for chronic use of methysergide as a preventive treatment for migraine headache. Abdominal ultrasound showed bilateral hydronephrosis as well as paraaortic hypoechoic soft tissue mass.

CLINICAL SUSPICION

Retroperitoneal fibrosis

IMAGING MODALITY OF CHOICE

Contrast-enhanced CT (CECT) with excretory or CT urography is the most appropriate study because it provides a comprehensive evaluation of the location, extent, and effect on adjacent organs and vascular structures of the retroperitoneum and helps in the detection of the underlying cause, such as abdominal aortic aneurysm or inflammation relating to pancreatitis or mesenteric lymphadenopathy. MRI has same advantages as CT but with higher tissue characterization resolution. It may be preferred over the CT if the patient shows deterioration of the renal function due to the lack of use of iodinated contrast material.

Retroperitoneal fibrosis (RPF) is characterized by the development of extensive fibrosis throughout the retroperitoneum that can encircle the great vessels as well as the ureters.

On cross-sectional imaging (CT/ MRI), a rind of soft tissue around the vessels (aorta, inferior vena cava) is seen extending from the renal level to the sacrum. It spreads to involve the ureters, with a variable degree of obstruction, and has a variable degree of enhancement, depending on disease stage (Fig. C26.1C). The signal intensity in MRI is similar to the signal of fibrous tissue on T1-weighted image showing low signal. However, on T2-weighted image the signal intensity will vary according to the activity of the disease process. Active inflammation will shows high T2 signal due to edema while inactive disease will show low T2 signal due to fibrosis (Fig. C26.1A and B).

On CT urography or IVP, there is medial deviation of the ureters at L3 or L4, tapering of the distal ureter, and a variable degree of dilation of the proximal ureter (Fig. C26.1D).

Clinical Differential

Two types of retroperitoneal fibrosis exist, differentiated by etiology.

- Primary (idiopathic): two-thirds of cases
  - Probably autoimmune, with antibodies stimulating desmoplastic reaction.
  - Ormond speculation: idiopathic retroperitoneal fibrosis that is similar to collagen vascular disease, which is supported by its coexistence with other inflammatory processes.
- Secondary: one-third of cases
  - Drugs: Methysergide, beta-blockers, hydralazine, ergotamine, LSD.
  - Diseases that stimulate desmoplastic reaction: Malignant tumors, metastases, Hodgkin's, carcinoid tumor, hematoma, radiation, retroperitoneal injury, surgery, infection, and urinary extravasation.

Imaging Differential

Retroperitoneal neoplasm and lymph nodes:

- The mass in retroperitoneal fibrosis is less bulky than are tumors.

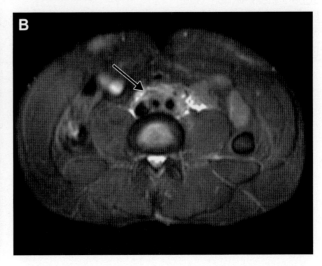

Fig. C26.1 MRI: (A) axial T1WI, (B) axial T2WI, (*continued*)

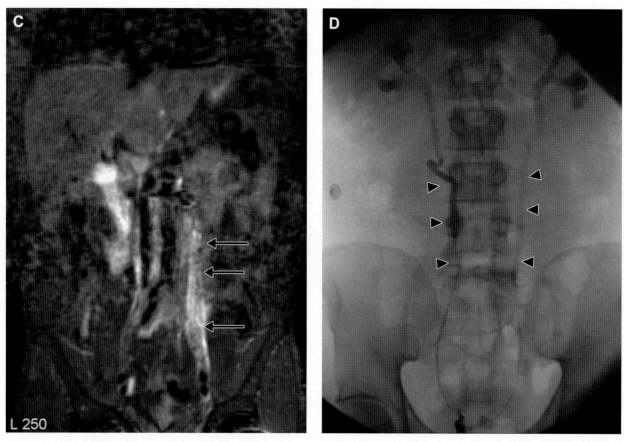

Fig. C26.1 (*continued*) MRI: (C) coronal T2WI, and (D) retrograde pyelography of a patient with retroperitoneal fibrosis reveal a rind of soft tissue surrounding the abdominal vessels (aorta and IVC) that exhibits a hypointense T1WI signal (white arrow, A) and an hyperintense T2WI signal (black arrow, B and C) denoting edema. Medial deviation of both ureters is demonstrated by retrograde pyelography (arrowheads, D).

- RPF does not displace the aorta anteriorly.
- RPF causes medial deviation of the ureters, whereas tumors typically cause lateral deviation.

Retroperitoneal hemorrhage:
- RPF is not hyperdense on unenhanced CT, whereas acute hemorrhage is.
- RPF does not infiltrate the fat planes.

REFERENCES AND SUGGESTED READING

1. Cronin CG, Lohan DG, Blake MA, Roche C, McCarthy P, Murphy JM. Retroperitoneal fibrosis: a review of clinical features and imaging findings. *AJR.* 2008;191(2):423-431.

2. Vivas I, Nicolas AI, Velazquez P, Elduayen B, Fernandez-Villa T, Martinez-Cuesta A. Retroperitoneal fibrosis: typical and atypical manifestations. *Br J Radiol.* 2000;73(866):214-222.

CASE 27: RETROPERITONEAL HEMORRHAGE

PATIENT PRESENTATION

A 60-year-old man with a history of chronic use of anticoagulant therapy for AF presents with severe sudden abdominal pain, pallor, nausea, and dizziness. Routine labs show low hematocrit.

CLINICAL SUSPICION

Intraperitoneal or retroperitoneal hemorrhage

IMAGING MODALITY OF CHOICE

Precontrast and postcontrast CT, which is an accurate, noninvasive method for directly imaging disorders of the retroperitoneal space, quantifying hemorrhage, and determining the site of origin of hemorrhage.

FINDINGS

- Noncontrast CT: Hyperdense (+70 to +90 HU) lesion at the retroperitoneal region (Fig. C27.1B).
- Contrast-enhanced CT: Puddling of contrast in hematoma or growing enhancing focus is a sign of active bleeding.

DIFFERENTIAL DIAGNOSIS

Clinical Differential

Acute abdominal pain is a common symptom among a wide spectrum of diseases. The pathology can be in an abdominal or extra-abdominal location. Abdominal causes are due to inflammatory process such as acute cholecystitis and acute pancreatitis, vascular causes such as acute mesenteric ischemia and ruptured aortic aneurysm, mechanical causes such as intestinal obstruction, and tubal pregnancy. The presence of Grey Turner's sign is more specific for considering retroperitoneal hemorrhage as a cause of acute abdominal pain.

Extra-abdominal causes should always be in mind as it may be life threatening as in myocardial infarction (MI). Other causes include lower lobe pneumonia and esophagitis.

Imaging Differential

Ruptured aneurysm:

- Most abdominal aortic aneurysms (AAA) rupture into the left retroperitoneum. Most patients present with the classic triad of hypotension, a pulsating mass, and back pain.

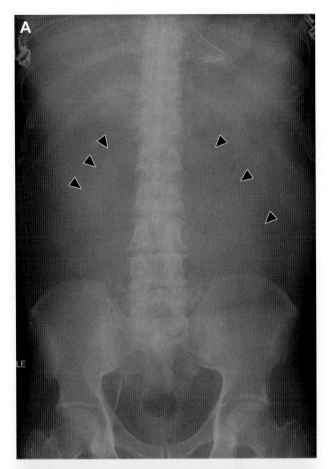

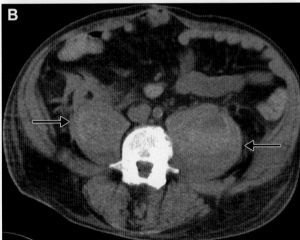

Fig. C27.1 (A) Plain radiography and (B) noncontrast axial CT study of a patient with retroperitoneal hematoma reveal a dense opaque shadow at the paravertebral regions of the abdominal cavity, overlying the psoas muscle (arrowheads). On unenhanced CT, the lesion appears heterogeneous, with hyperdense areas denoting a hemorrhagic component (arrows).

- Bleeding from a ruptured AAA never involves the rectus sheath, uncommonly involves the iliopsoas compartment, and almost always involves multiple retroperitoneal spaces.

Other causes of abdominal hemorrhage:

Intra-abdominal hemorrhage can result from trauma, iatrogenic causes such as postoperative complications, and spontaneous bleeding of retroperitoneal tumors such as angiomyolipoma, myelolipoma, and RCC. CT can be used to detect the source of bleeding and to measure the blood volume. Diagnosis is usually easy as the patient presents with a history of accident, recent operation, or intra-abdominal neoplasm.

REFERENCE AND SUGGESTED READING

1. Federle MP, Pan KT, Pealer KM. CT criteria for differentiating abdominal hemorrhage: anticoagulation or aortic aneurysm rupture? *AJR*. 2007;188(5):1324-1330.

CASE 28: NEUROGENIC BLADDER

PATIENT PRESENTATION

A 52-year-old diabetic man comes to the office complaining of urgency, frequency, and incontinence.

CLINICAL SUSPICION

Neurogenic bladder

IMAGING MODALITY OF CHOICE

Urodynamic studies, ultrasound, and voiding cystourethrography

FINDINGS

Neurogenic bladder can develop due to any lesion affecting the signaling controlling the process of micturition including the brain, spinal cord, and peripheral nerves innervating the bladder. It can be classified according to the bladder muscle tone into flaccid neurogenic bladder, spastic neurogenic bladder, or a mixed pattern.

The spastic type occurs with lesions involving the brain or the spinal cord above the level of S2. There is detrusor muscle hyperreflexia. In the supra pontine lesions, the cystourethrography will show a rounded bladder with small or normal volume. The bladder wall will be thickened and may show trabeculation. The detrusor muscle contractions may lead to a serrated appearance of the mucosa above the trigone. Complete transection of the spinal cord above

S2 will lead to detrusor hyperreflexia as well as detrusor sphincter dyssynergia, where the bladder muscles attempt to void against a closed sphincter. The bladder will acquire the configuration known as Christmas tree shape where it is elongated and pointed (Fig. C28.1). In addition, the contrast will fill the opened posterior urethra. The patient usually presents with frequency and urge incontinence.

The flaccid type occurs with lesions involving the spinal cord at S2-4 or the peripheral nerves supplying the bladder. There is areflexia of the detrusor muscle. The bladder will be atonic, acquiring large volume with no evidence of detrusor contractions. The patient usually presents with retention and overflow incontinence.

Imaging is also important to detect complications of neurogenic bladder and follow-up therapy. The voiding cystourethrography is useful in detection of vesicoureteral reflux. The ultrasound is an easy and effective way to detect secondary hydronephrosis. It also can be used to measure the postvoiding residual urine to monitor therapy response.

DIFFERENTIAL DIAGNOSIS

Bladder outlet obstruction: May include BPH and posterior urethral valve. The innervation to the urinary bladder is still intact, and retention will be relieved once the cause of obstruction is treated

Pelvic mass: Ultrasound or CT can be used to detect the origin of the mass and differentiate it from the urinary bladder

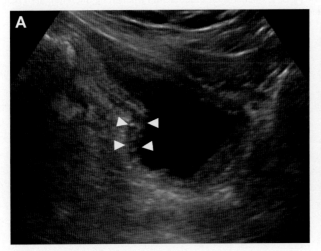
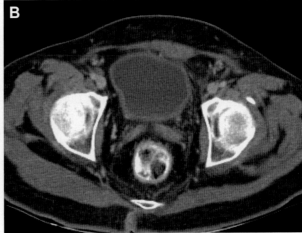

Fig. C28.1 Neurogenic bladder on US and CT. (A) Longitudinal US image demonstrates bladder wall thickening (arrowheads) and elongated apex. (B) Axial, (*continued*)

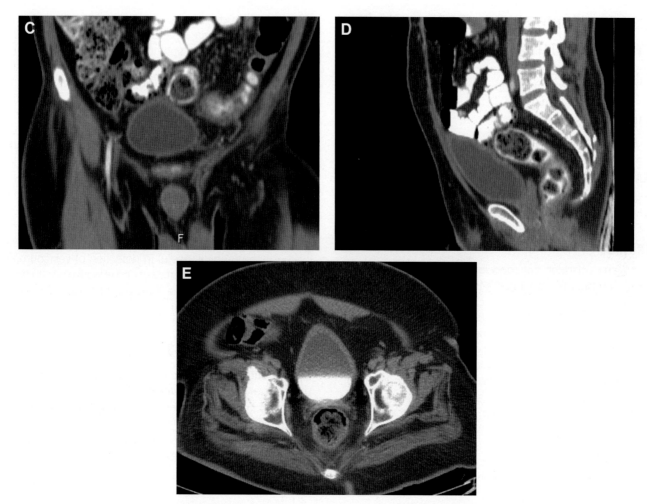

Fig. C28.1 (C) coronal, and (D) sagittal images of a contrast-enhanced CT also demonstrated bladder wall thickening and elongated bladder shape. (E) Axial delayed CT images demonstrate a neurogenic bladder in the excretory phase.

REFERENCES AND SUGGESTED READING

1. Federle MP, Anne VS, Chen JJ-S. Neurogenic bladder. In: Federle MP, ed. *Diagnostic Imaging: Abdomen*. Utah: Amirsys; 2004:III-5-16.

2. Friedenberg RM, Ney C. The radiographic findings in neurogenic bladder. *Radiology*. 1961;76:795-800.

3. Fowler CJ. Investigation of the neurogenic bladder. *J Neurol Neurosurg Psychiatry*. 1996;60(1):6-13.

CASE 29: URETHRAL DIVERTICULUM

PATIENT PRESENTATION

A 46-year-old woman with history of repeated lower urinary tract infection comes to the office complaining of urethral pain and postvoiding dribbling. Pelvic examination reveals tender cystic lesion in the anterior vaginal wall and pus oozing from the urethral orifice.

CLINICAL SUSPICION

Urethral diverticulum

IMAGING MODALITY OF CHOICE

MRI is the modality of choice for diagnosis and localization of the diverticulum.

FINDINGS

The diverticulum appears as an outpouching from the mid-portion of the urethra. It commonly arises from the posterolateral urethral wall (Fig. C29.1). Females are affected more than males. It is formed as a result of obstruction of the ducts of the paraurethral glands, which become dilated and infected with subsequent abscess formation. The abscess ruptures into the urethra leading to diverticulum formation. Stagnation of urine in the diverticulum can lead to various complications including infection, stone formation, and diverticular malignancy.

MRI is superior to other imaging modalities due to its superior tissue characterization and multiplanar imaging. It can visualize the diverticulum, define its location, and detect complications. Image acquisition can be done using torso coil or endoluminal coil, which is a coil inserted inside a hollow organ such as endovaginal or endourethral coil. The endoluminal coil provides better signal to noise

ratio, higher sensitivity to detect smaller diverticulum, and better visualization of the paraurethral region. The imaging protocol includes T2-weighted images in the axial, sagittal, and coronal planes as well as T1-weighted images in the axial plane. Administration of IV gadolinium is required if complication is suspected.

The diverticulum appears as a periurethral unilocular or septated cystic structure exhibiting low signal in T1-weighted images and high signal in T-2 weighted images (Fig. C29.2). Infected diverticulum will demonstrate thick wall and increase signal intensity of the diverticular fluid on T1-weighted images, fluid-fluid levels on T2-weighted images, and enhancement of the diverticular wall and septations after gadolinium administration (Fig. C29.3). A stone formed in the diverticulum will appear as a dependent focus of low signal intensity in T1- and T2-weighted images.

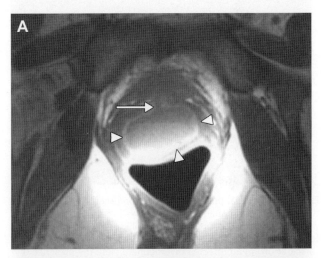
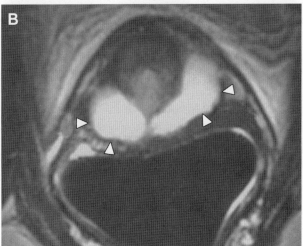

Fig. C29.2 (A) Axial postcontrast T1WI with endovaginal coil reveals low signal intensity unilocular diverticulum (arrowheads) communicating with the urethra (arrow). (B) Axial T2WI in another patient reveals high signal intensity septated diverticulum (arrowheads). Reproduced after copyright permission from *RadioGraphics* (Chou et al, 2008). Copyright RSNA, Radiological Society of North America.

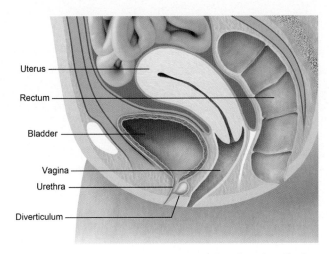

Fig. C29.1 Illustration showing the common location of urethral diverticulum in females.

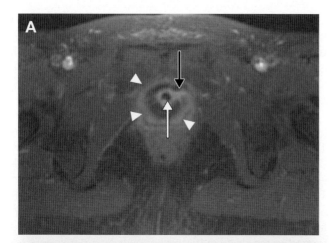

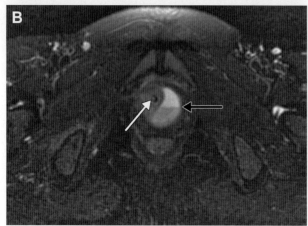

Fig. C29.3 (A) Axial postcontrast fat-suppressed T1WI reveals diverticulum with enhancement of its wall (arrowheads) as well as its connection to the urethra (black arrow). (B) Axial fat-suppressed T2WI in another patient reveals fluid-fluid level (black arrow) in an infected diverticulum. Note the presence of Foley catheter inside the urethra (white arrow). Reproduced after copyright permission from *RadioGraphics* (Chou et al, 2008). Copyright RSNA, Radiological Society of North America.

Diverticular neoplasm will appear as an enhancing soft tissue mass within the diverticulum lumen.

Clinical Differential

Patient is usually asymptomatic and diagnosed incidentally. However, when symptoms occur, they can mimic the clinical presentation of cystitis.

Imaging Differential

Urethral neoplasm: The lesion appears as a soft tissue signal within the urethra.

Bartholin gland cyst: The cyst is posterolateral to the vagina not the urethra.

REFERENCES AND SUGGESTED READING

1. Chou CP, Levenson RB, Elsayes KM, et al. Imaging of female urethral diverticulum: an update. *RadioGraphics*. 2008;28(7): 1917-1930.
2. Elsayes KM, Mukundan G, Narra VR, Abou El Abbass HA, Prasad SR, Brown JJ. Endovaginal magnetic resonance imaging of the female urethra. *J Comput Assist Tomogr*. 2006; 30(1):1-6.

CASE 30: URETHRAL STRICTURE

PATIENT PRESENTATION

A 34-year-old man with a recent history of gonorrhea presents with increased urinary frequency and a sensation of incomplete voiding.

CLINICAL SUSPICION

Urethral stricture secondary to infection

IMAGING MODALITY OF CHOICE

The most commonly used methods of urethral imaging include retrograde urethrography (RUG) and voiding cystourethrography (VCUG). These techniques are generally adequate for evaluating urethral strictures, including stricture characteristics such as their location and length. However, urethrography is limited in its assessment of periurethral processes.

RUG is most useful in assessing the anterior urethra, as the posterior urethra may not be adequately distended. To perform this technique, contrast is injected into the meatus through a Foley catheter, whose balloon is inflated in the fossa navicularis in the glans (Fig. C30.1). Fluoroscopy is then used to visualize the urethra.

VCUG may be performed with RUG, as it is better able to demonstrate the anatomy of the posterior urethra. VCUG is generally performed by filling the bladder with contrast through a Foley catheter. As the patient voids, fluoroscopy captures images of the urethra (Fig. C30.2). Like RUG, VCUG is a widely available and cost-effective procedure.

The male urethra (Fig. C30.3) can be divided into anterior and posterior segments, each of which is further divided into two subsegments. The posterior urethra is composed of the prostatic and membranous segments.

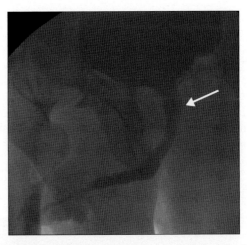

Fig. C30.2 Normal voiding cystourethrogram (VCUG). The filling defect in the prostatic urethra (arrow) is due to the seminal colliculus, or verumontanum, found near the entrance of the seminal vesicles.

The prostatic portion descends approximately 2.5 cm from the bladder and traverses the prostate. The membranous portion continues until the bulbar portion of the penis. This portion is surrounded by the external urethral sphincter.

The anterior urethra can be divided into the bulbar and pendulous urethra. The bulbar urethra lies within the corpus spongiosum proximal to the penoscrotal junction, a bend in the urethra caused by the suspensory ligament of the penis. The penile urethra is found within the corpus spongiosum of the penile portion of the penis. The distal urethra widens to form the fossa navicularis proximal to the meatus.

Urethral strictures are generally the result of trauma (often iatrogenic) and infection. These processes lead to scarring of the tissues surrounding the urethra, and the resulting contraction of the scar results in strictures. Strictures

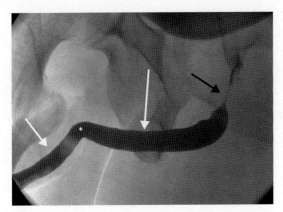

Fig. C30.1 Retrograde urethogram (RUG), demonstrating penile (short white arrow), the penoscrotal junction (*), bulbar urethra (long white arrow), and the membranous urethra (black arrow). The prostatic urethra is poorly visualized in this image, but lies superior to the membranous urethra.

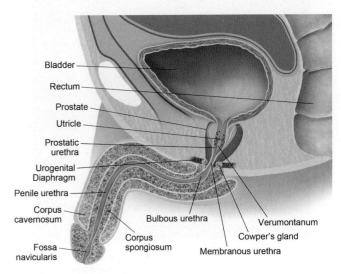

Fig. C30.3 Anatomy of the male urethra.

due to instrumentation most commonly involve the bulbo-membranous region, but may less commonly involve the penoscrotal junction as well (Fig. C30.4). Posterior strictures often result from processes such as trauma or surgery that displace the urethral axis, and subsequent scarring then obliterates the urethra (Fig. C30.5). A common iatrogenic cause of posterior strictures is transurethral resection of the prostate. Infectious etiologies most commonly include gonorrhea and chlamydia, which can cause irregular strictures several centimeters in length (Fig. C30.6). Other causes of urethral obstruction may include neoplasms and congenital malformations.

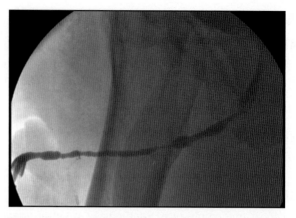

Fig. C30.6 RUG demonstrating stricture of the anterior urethra. Elongated strictures of the anterior urethra are most commonly due to infectious etiologies.

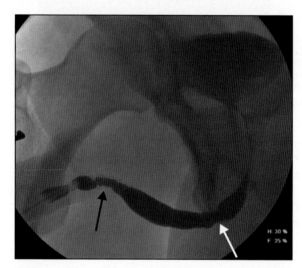

Fig. C30.4 Anterior urethral strictures on RUG in the penile (black arrow) and bulbar urethra (white arrow). Focal strictures in the penoscrotal and bulbomembranous regions, as seen here, are commonly due to prior instrumentation.

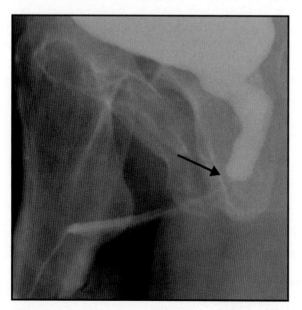

Fig. C30.5 Posterior stricture on VCUG in the membranous urethra (arrow). Common causes of posterior strictures are trauma or transurethral resection of the process, in which the urethral axis may be displaced.

DIFFERENTIAL DIAGNOSIS

Urinary retention may be due to a number of causes:

- Urethral stricture
- Iatrogenic
- Catheterization, instrumentation, transurethral resection of the prostate
- Traumatic
- Pelvic fracture, straddle injury
- Infectious
- Gonorrhea, chlamydia, tuberculosis
- Inflammatory
- Xerotica obliterans
- Urethral obstruction due to neoplasm
- Congenital urethral obstruction
- Neurogenic bladder
- Bladder outlet obstruction
- Bladder neck stenosis
- Posterior urethral valves
- Prostatic enlargement

REFERENCES AND SUGGESTED READING

1. Kawashima A, Sandler CM, Wasserman NF, LeRoy AJ, King BF Jr, Goldman SM. Imaging of urethral disease: a pictorial review. *RadioGraphics*. 2004;24(suppl 1):S195-216.
2. Kim B, Kawashima A, LeRoy AJ. Imaging of the male urethra. *Semin Ultrasound CT MR*. 2007;28(4):258-273.

CASE 31: RETROPERITONEAL SARCOMA

PATIENT PRESENTATION

A 64-year-old woman presents with abdominal pain and on exam is found to have a large left upper quadrant abdominal mass.

CLINICAL SUSPICION

Abdominal mass

IMAGING MODALITY OF CHOICE

CT is the modality of choice for evaluation of abdominal pain and mass. Both CT and MRI can be used to characterize abnormalities of the abdomen and retroperitoneum, including location, size, and shape of any masses. CT scan is superior for assessing calcifications. MRI is better able to characterize soft tissue. Both CT and MRI are useful for detecting metastases or vascular invasion as well as assessing fat content of a lesion.

The retroperitoneum stretches from the diaphragm to the pelvis, and is located between parietal peritoneum anteriorly and transversalis fascia posteriorly. It is bound by the transversus abdominis musculature laterally. It contains structures including the aorta, IVC, kidneys, adrenal glands, ureters, pancreas, and portions of the digestive tract including parts of the duodenum and the ascending and descending colon. Within the retroperitoneum are three compartments, separated by the renal fascia. These include the anterior pararenal space, perirenal space, and posterior pararenal space (Fig. C31.1). On imaging, a retroperitoneal mass is likely if the normal structures of the retroperitoneum are displaced.

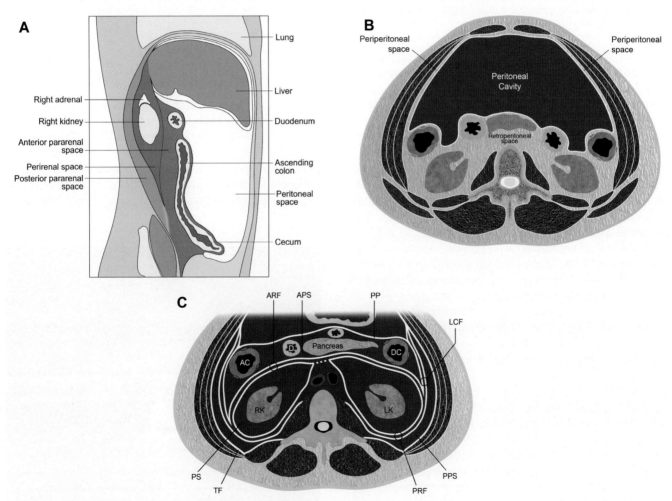

Fig. C31.1 (A) Sagittal view of the three compartments of the retroperitoneum include the anterior pararenal space, the perirenal space, and the posterior pararenal space. (B) Axial view demonstrating the retroperitoneal space posterior to the peritoneal cavity. (C) Axial view demonstrating the compartments of the retroperitoneal space. The three compartments include the anterior pararenal space (APS), perirenal space (PS), and posterior pararenal space (PPS). The retroperitoneum lies between the parietal peritoneum (PP) anteriorly, and the transversalis fascia (TF) posteriorly. The anterior renal fascia (ARF) separates the APS and PS, while the posterior renal fascia (PRF) lies between the PS and PPS. The lateroconal fascia (LCF) separates the APS from the PPS. Retroperitoneal structures in the APS include the pancreas, duodenum (D), ascending and descending colon (AC and DC). In the PS lie the left and right kidneys (LK and RK). In the PPS lie blood vessels and lymphatics but no major organs.

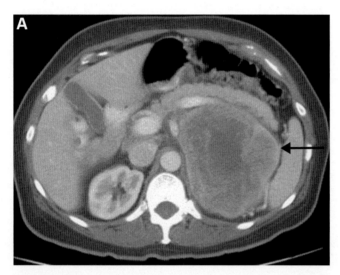
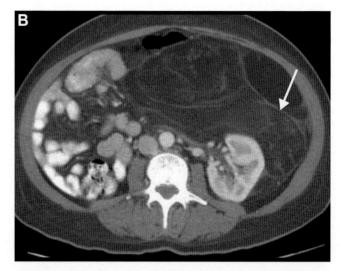

Fig. C31.2 Axial contrast-enhanced CT of the abdomen at two different levels demonstrating large left retroperitoneal infiltrative mass with a soft tissue enhancing component (black arrow, A) with enlargement and stranding of fat at the lower level (white arrow, B), compatible with retroperitoneal liposarcoma.

Retroperitoneal masses can be caused by a variety of processes and may be grouped broadly into solid or cystic masses. Both of these include neoplastic and nonneoplastic causes. Common solid neoplastic diagnoses include lymphoma, soft-tissue sarcoma, neurogenic tumors, germ-cell tumors, and metastases.

Lymphomas are the most common malignant retroperitoneal masses, and they generally are seen as on CT as homogenous masses that grow between retroperitoneal structures but generally do not compress them. The liver, spleen, and paraaortic lymph nodes are commonly enlarged as well. On MRI, lymphomas are isointense on T1, either isointense or hypointense on T2, and generally have homogenous enhancement with contrast. Heterogeneous lymphomas are difficult to distinguish from other retroperitoneal tumors.

The most common sarcomas in the retroperitoneum are liposarcomas (Fig. C31.2). These are generally large, slow-growing tumors that, if well differentiated, will have the appearance of fatty tissue on imaging, with negative attenuation on CT, high signal intensity on non-fat-suppressed T1-weighted with drop of signal on fat-suppressed T1-weighted images, and intermediate intensity on T2 with MRI. These can be differentiated from lipomas by their thick, irregular septa. Less differentiated liposarcomas may have solid components as well as calcifications, and these tumors are generally more aggressive. Leiomyosarcoma is a less common tumor that arises from the smooth muscle tissue within the retroperitoneum, and it may contain areas of necrosis and cystic degeneration (Fig. C31.3).

Neurogenic tumors may arise from either the nerve sheath (as in schwannoma or neurofibroma), sympathetic nerves (as in ganglioneuroma), or from the chromaffin tissue

(as in paraganglioma). These tumors are generally found in younger patients and are often benign.

Germ cell tumors most commonly include teratomas, which are tumors arising from multiple germ layers. These tumors often contain calcifications and fat, and they can be either mature or immature based on the differentiation of the tissue, and may rarely be malignant. Mature teratomas generally appear as a cystic mass. Primary extragonadal germ cell tumors, including both seminomas and nonseminomatous

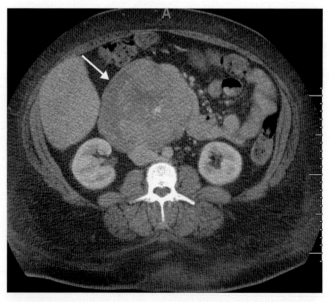

Fig. C31.3 Axial contrast-enhanced CT demonstrating a large lobulated soft tissue density mass (arrow) compatible with retroperitoneal leiomyosarcoma arising from smooth muscle tissue of the retroperitoneum.

germ cell tumors, may also arise in the retroperitoneum, possibly from a defect in migration during embryonal development. Seminomas may also metastasize to the retroperitoneum, so it is important to perform a testicular exam in a young male patient with a retroperitoneal mass (Fig. C31.4).

Nonneoplastic solid masses may be due to pseudotumoral lipomatosis, a benign metaplastic growth of fat cells, or retroperitoneal fibrosis, a likely autoimmune collagen vascular disease. Extramedullary hematopoiesis, found in diseases such as lymphoma, leukemia, and hemoglobinopathies, can also present as a solid retroperitoneal mass.

Neoplastic cystic masses are commonly due to paraganglioma (in which cystic change is seen in a solid neoplasm) and mucinous cystadenoma or adenocarcinoma. Nonneoplastic cysts may be seen with hematoma, urinoma, pseudocysts in the pancreatitis, or lymphocele.

DIFFERENTIAL DIAGNOSIS

Retroperitoneal masses have a wide differential diagnosis:

Solid

- Neoplastic
  - Lymphoma
  - Sarcoma
  - Neurogenic tumors
  - Germ cell tumors
  - Metastases
- Nonneoplastic
  - Pseudotumoral lipomatosis
  - Extramedullary hematopoiesis
  - Retroperitoneal fibrosis

Cystic

- Neoplastic
  - Mature cystic teratoma
  - Paraganglioma
  - Mucinous cystadenoma/cystadenocarcinoma
- Nonneoplastic
  - Hematoma
  - Urinoma
  - Pseudocyst
  - Lymphocele

REFERENCES AND SUGGESTED READING

1. Rajiah P, Sinha R, Cuevas C, Dubinsky TJ, Bush WH Jr, Kolokythas O. Imaging of uncommon retroperitoneal masses. *RadioGraphics.* 2011;31(4):949-76. doi:10.1148/rg.314095132.

2. Nishino M, Hayakawa K, Minami M, Yamamoto A, Ueda H, Takasu K. Primary retroperitoneal neoplasms: CT and MR imaging findings with anatomic and pathologic diagnostic clues. *RadioGraphics.* 2003;23(1):45-57.

3. Sanyal R, Remer EM. Radiology of the retroperitoneum: case-based review. *AJR.* 2009;192(6)(suppl):S112-7 (Quiz S118-21). doi:10.2214/AJR.07.7064.

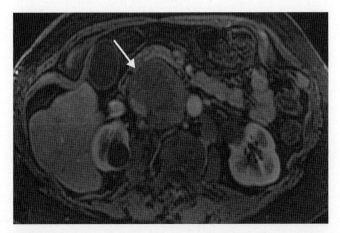

Fig. C31.4 Axial postcontrast T1-weighted image, demonstrating retroperitoneal heterogeneously-enhancing mass in 20-year-old male patient (arrow), most compatible with pathologically proven seminoma.

CASE 32: RENAL INJURY

PATIENT PRESENTATION

An 18-year-old man presents to the emergency room with hematuria after being kicked in the abdomen during a soccer game.

CLINICAL SUSPICION

Renal injury

IMAGING MODALITY OF CHOICE

Contrast-enhanced CT is the preferred imaging modality of choice in settings of suspected renal trauma, replacing older techniques such as intravenous urography. It can accurately detect lacerations, arterial and urinary extravasation, devascularization, and injuries in adjacent organs such as liver and spleen. CT is performed with contrast, and both early and delayed scans are utilized. The early scan, approximately 80 seconds after the administration of contrast, will demonstrate peak vascular enhancement. The delayed scan, after three or more minutes, will allow excretion of the contrast by the kidneys and evaluation for injury in the collecting system.

Renal injury can occur due to either blunt trauma or penetrating injury. Blunt trauma is associated with the large majority of cases. With either mechanism of injury, multiorgan involvement is common, especially with higher-grade renal lesions. Microscopic hematuria is present in the vast majority of cases of renal trauma. The severity of the renal injury can be graded by findings on CT scan. Below is one system of grading from the American Association for the Surgery of Trauma (AAST):

Grade I: Renal contusion or nonexpanding subcapsular hematoma; no parenchymal laceration

Grade II: Nonexpanding perirenal hematoma; renal cortical laceration less than 1 cm without involving collecting system; no extravasation of urine

Grade III: Cortical laceration greater than1 cm without involving collecting system; no extravasation of urine

Grade IV: Laceration extends into collecting system or urine extravasation; main renal artery or vein injury with contained hemorrhage

Grade V: Shattered kidney, avulsion of pedicle, thrombosis of the main renal artery

Grading of the injury in combination with the clinical findings guides management in cases of renal injury. Because of improvements in the grading of renal injuries, there is a trend toward expectant management and away from

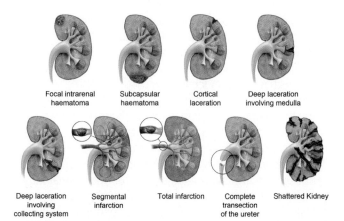

Fig. C32.1 Common renal injuries.

surgical exploration in all but the most severe renal injuries. Generally, grade I and II injuries can be managed expectantly. Grade III, IV, and V injuries are more controversial in their management and may depend on hemodynamic stability. Unstable patients may require surgical repair of the kidney or even nephrectomy.

Common renal injuries include renal contusions, hematomas, lacerations, and infarcts (Fig. C32.1). Renal contusions can be seen as small, poorly defined, hypodense lesions in the cortex (Fig. C32.2). Subcapsular hematomas are nonenhancing collections of fluid at the margin of the kidney that generally appear hyperdense on CT but may vary with the age of the hematoma (Fig. C32.3). Lacerations are linear defects in the renal parenchyma. Minor lacerations are small and do not involve the collecting system, while more severe lacerations involve the collecting system (Fig. C32.4), injure renal vascular structure (Fig. C32.5) or it can cause a "shattered kidney" appearance, in which multiple lacerations create devitalized fragments. These are generally associated with hemorrhage and active bleeding (Fig. C32.6).

Cortical infarcts appear as wedge-shaped areas of decreased enhancement. Smaller infarcts may be due to injuries of smaller vessels such as the accessory renal artery. Damage to the larger arteries can cause segmental infarcts. Global infarct can be secondary to a thrombosis of the main renal artery, which may appear to abruptly terminate on CT. Within several days of infarction the cortical rim sign may appear, with enhancement of the outer cortex. Renal pedicle avulsion, in which the renal artery and vein are completely lacerated, will also present with global infarction as well as medial perirenal hematoma. The ureter, also contained within the pedicle, may be damaged as well, leading to urinary extravasation.

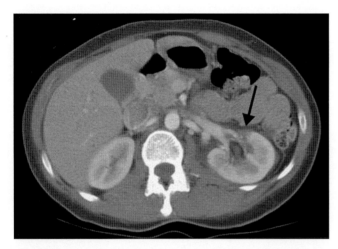

Fig. C32.2 CT scan demonstrating poorly defined hypodensity consistent with renal contusion (arrow) in the left kidney.

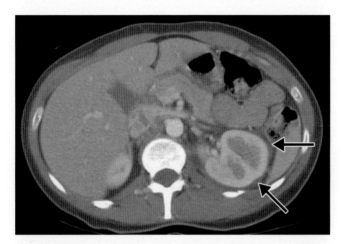

Fig. C32.3 CT scan demonstrating minor left renal injury consisting of nonenhancing subcapsular hematomas (arrows).

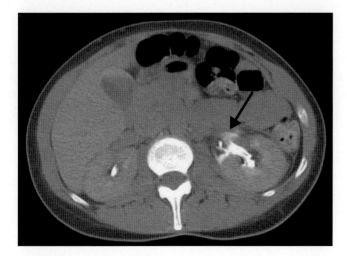

Fig. C32.4 Delayed CT demonstrating urine extravasation from the collecting system (arrow).

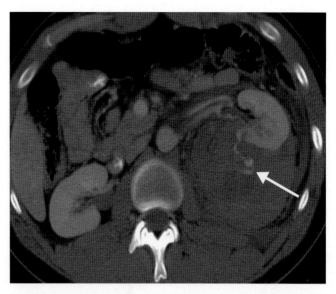

Fig. C32.5 Contrast-enhanced CT showing arterial extravasation following a renal injury (arrow).

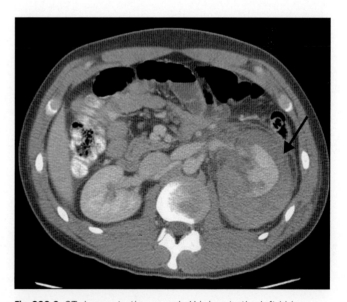

Fig. C32.6 CT demonstrating a grade V injury to the left kidney with shattered kidney and large hematoma (arrow).

DIFFERENTIAL DIAGNOSIS

Hematuria can be due to a number of diagnoses:

- Renal trauma
- Urolithiasis
- Urinary tract infection
- Nephritic syndrome
- Poststreptococcal glomerulonephritis
- Lupus nephritis
- IgA nephropathy
- Henoch-Schönlein purpura
- Goodpasture's disease

REFERENCES AND SUGGESTED READING

1. Alonso RC, Nacenta SB, Martinez PD, Guerrero AS, Fuentes CG. Kidney in danger: CT findings of blunt and penetrating renal trauma. *RadioGraphics*. 2009;29(7):2033-2053. doi:10.1148/rg.297095071.

2. Kawashima A, Sandler CM, Corl FM, et al. Imaging of renal trauma: a comprehensive review. *RadioGraphics*. 2001;21(3):557-574.

3. Sandler CM, Amis ES Jr, Bigongiari LR, et al. Diagnostic approach to renal trauma. American College of Radiology. ACR Appropriateness Criteria. *Radiology*. 2000;215(suppl):727-731.

4. Moore EE, Shackford SR, Pachter HL, et al. Organ injury scaling: spleen, liver, and kidney. *J Trauma*. 1989;29(12):1664-1666.

Chapter 7

Musculoskeletal

By Behrang Amini and Zeyad A. Metwalli

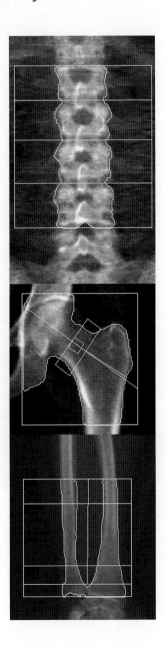

CASE 1

PATIENT PRESENTATION

A 65-year-old postmenopausal woman presents for prescription refill.

CLINICAL SUSPICION

Osteoporosis

IMAGING MODALITY OF CHOICE

Dual-energy x-ray absorptiometry (DXA)

BACKGROUND

Bone is made up of a variety of cells (eg, osteoblasts, osteoclasts, and osteocytes), an organic matrix (predominantly type I collagen), and an inorganic matrix (predominantly calcium hydroxyapatite). Osteoporosis is the most common metabolic disease of bone. It is due to disturbances in bone remodeling that result in less bone tissue (matrix and mineral) per unit volume. Bone mineral density (BMD), the average concentration of mineral in a defined section of bone, is used to diagnose osteoporosis, estimate the risk of insufficiency fractures, and select and monitor treatment. BMD is estimated by a DXA scanner, a low-dose x-ray tube with two energies. The low-energy and high-energy photons are attenuated differently in bone and soft tissue, allowing BMD to be estimated.

FINDINGS

DXA devices are used to calculate BMD in g/cm^2 and to compare the values to a reference database. The comparison is quantified as a T-score, which represents the standard deviation by which the BMD of the patient differs from the mean BMD of a young adult reference population of the same ethnicity and sex, and a Z-score, which represents the standard deviation by which the BMD of the patient differs from the mean BMD of an age-matched reference population of the same ethnicity and sex.

Box C1.1 – TERMINOLOGY

The WHO definition of *osteopenia* conflicts with the way the word has been used by radiologists. Radiologists have used *osteopenia* as a nonspecific and descriptive term for increased lucency of bone as seen on radiographs. This rarefaction could be due to a variety of causes, such as osteoporosis or osteomalacia. Other words, such as *demineralization*, *undermineralization*, and *deossification*, were used incorrectly as synonyms for osteoporosis and osteopenia and added to the confusion.

According to the World Health Organization, osteoporosis is "a systemic skeletal disease characterized by low bone density and microarchitectural deterioration of bone tissue with a consequent increase in bone fragility" and corresponds to a T-score of –2.5 or lower. Patients with *osteopenia* (see Box C1.1), defined as T-scores between –1 and –2.5, have less bone density loss than do those with osteoporosis. A T-score higher than –1 is considered normal.

Typically, the lumbar spine and proximal femur are scanned (Fig. C1.1A,B). The forearm (Fig. C1.1C) can be scanned as an alternative to the hip and lumbar spine

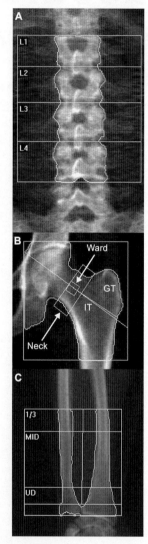

Fig. C1.1 Normal DXA images. (A) In the lumbar spine, regions of interest are drawn around the individual vertebral bodies and individual and combined BMD values are estimated. (B) In the proximal femur, regions of interest are drawn around the femoral neck, greater trochanter (GT), intertrochanteric region (IT), and Ward's triangle. Individual and combined BMD values are estimated. (C) In the forearm, the distal one-third of the radius (excluding the ultradistal [UD] portion) is a good site for estimation of cortical bone mineral loss, whereas the ultradistal portion of the radius is a good indicator of trabecular bone loss.

when these parts cannot be scanned due to artifacts (read further) or when the patient is too heavy for the table. In patients with hyperparathyroidism, the nondominant forearm is scanned in addition to the hip and lumbar spine. This is because BMD loss in hyperparathyroidism is greater in structures with predominantly cortical bone, such as the distal radius.

Interpreting DXA scans requires more than just reading BMD estimates from a computer-generated report. As in other areas of radiology, the images should be assessed for quality and the presence of artifacts related to patient movement and appropriate field-of-view. Various artifacts of can result in a falsely elevated BMD estimate (see Box C1.2 and Fig. C1.2).

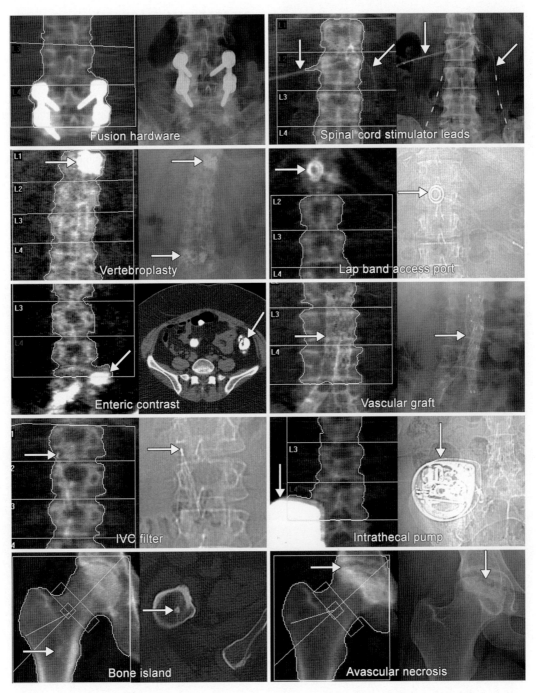

Fig. C1.2 Potpourri of artifacts and incidental findings in DXA. For each case, the DXA image is shown on the left, and the corresponding radiograph on the right. IVC, inferior vena cava.

Box C1.2 – COMMONLY ENCOUNTERED ARTIFACTS

Catheters, pacemaker leads

Vascular grafts, inferior vena cava filters

Surgical hardware, clips

Piercings

Retained enteric contrast

Vertebroplasty cement

Atherosclerotic calcifications

Osteophytes, endplate sclerosis

Compression fracture

Bone island

Paget disease

Neoplasm

In the spine, the vertebral body heights should be assessed and compared with prior DXA studies (when available) to assess for progressive height loss. Finally, the rest of the image should be evaluated for the presence of incidental findings such as calcified leiomyomata, ureteral stones, and avascular necrosis of the femoral head. Figure C1.2 illustrates some common artifacts and incidental findings in DXA.

DIFFERENTIAL DIAGNOSIS

None

REFERENCES AND SUGGESTED READING

1. Jacobson JA, Jamadar DA, Hayes CW. Dual X-ray absorptiometry: recognizing image artifacts and pathology. *AJR.* 2000;174(6):1699-1705.
2. Lorente-Ramos R, Azpeitia-Armán J, Muñoz-Hernández A, García-Gómez JM, Díez-Martínez P, Grande-Bárez M. Dual-energy x-ray absorptiometry in the diagnosis of osteoporosis: a practical guide. *AJR.* 2011;196(4):897-904.

CASE 2

PATIENT PRESENTATION

A 55-year-old woman with chronic knee pain that is worse with activity. The patient reports no morning stiffness. Physical examination reveals crepitus, restricted range of motion, and no joint effusion.

CLINICAL SUSPICION

Osteoarthritis (OA, degenerative joint disease)

IMAGING MODALITY OF CHOICE

Radiographs of the knee that include axial and standing flexion views. Although radiography is often the imaging modality of choice for suspected OA, a confident diagnosis of knee OA can often be made clinically without radiographic examination or even with normal radiographs in adults older than 40 years of age who present with usage-related knee pain, only short-lived morning stiffness (< 30 minutes), functional limitation, and one or more typical physical examination findings (see Box C2.1).

When imaging is indicated, radiographs can provide an estimate of cartilage loss as manifested by joint space narrowing and associated abnormalities of the subchondral bone (read further). The preferred method of imaging the knees, the Rosenberg view, is illustrated in Fig. C2.1. Standard supine (non-weight-bearing) anteroposterior (AP) views can underestimate joint space narrowing, a shortcoming that can be addressed by having the patient stand during radiography. The routine standing view, however, may also underestimate joint space narrowing, although for different reasons. For example, because the maximum stresses in the knee occur between 30 and 60 degrees of flexion, standard weight-bearing radiographs taken with an extended knee are not ideal for evaluation of cartilage loss in these areas. The Rosenberg view addresses this and other issues related to radiographic estimation of cartilage loss.

Box C2.1 – PHYSICAL EXAMINATION FINDINGS OF OSTEOARTHRITIS AT THE KNEE

Crepitus

Painful and/or restricted range of motion

Bony enlargement

Absent or only modest joint effusion

Deformity (fixed flexion, varus or valgus)

Instability

Periarticular or joint-line tenderness

Pain on patellofemoral compression

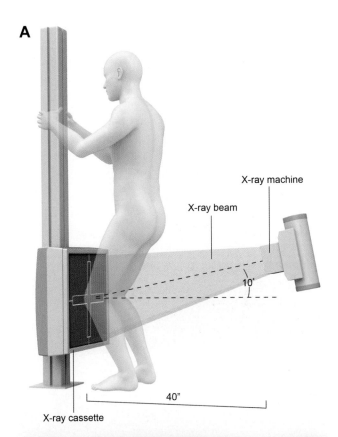

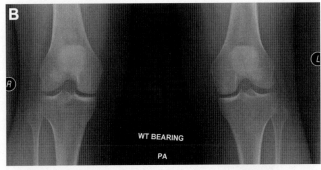

Fig. C2.1 (A) The Rosenberg view: The Rosenberg view is a 45-degree flexion, posteroanterior (PA), weight-bearing view of both knees with the patellae touching the x-ray cassette or image receptor. The x-ray tube is 40 inches from the image receptor, centered at the patellae, and pointing caudad (down) 10 degrees. The Rosenberg view is more sensitive and specific for joint space narrowing than are conventional extension weight-bearing anteroposterior views and is useful for the assessment of knees with early degenerative change. *(Modified from Rosenberg, et al. J Bone Joint Surg Am. 1988;70(10):1479-1483.)* (B) Normal Rosenberg view. Note that the anterior and posterior margins of the tibial plateaus are superimposed. A minimal joint space width of less than 3 mm is considered narrowed.

Axial views of the knee should also be obtained to assess the patellofemoral compartment. Two commonly encountered choices for the axial view of the knee are the sunrise (skyline) and Merchant views. Figure C2.2 details the differences. Because of institutional inertia, most axial views

A

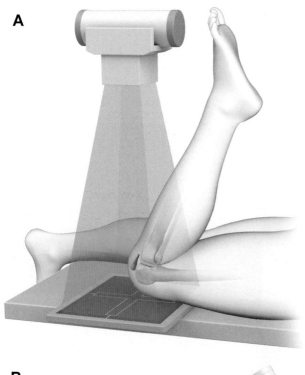

B

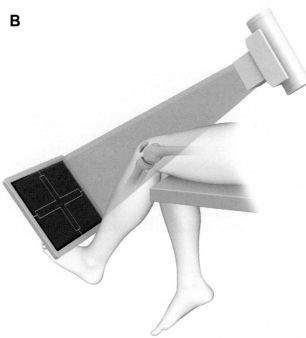

Fig. C2.2 Axial views of the knee. (A) The sunrise view is taken with the knee in flexion and gives an assessment of patellofemoral joint space narrowing; however, the beam is not tangential to the patellofemoral joint space. (B) The Merchant view, also called the Mountain View, because Drs Merchant, et al, were from Mountain View, CA, is more comfortable for patients with knee pain, provides a better assessment of the articulating surfaces of the femur and the patella, and is better for detection of patellar subluxation. *(Modified from MacNab I. J Bone Joint Surg Am. 1952;34A(4):957-967.)*

of the knee are still labeled as sunrise views. A familiarity with your institution's protocols is vital to ensure accurate assessment of knee radiographs.

Additional imaging studies are not indicated in patients for whom radiographs are diagnostic of degenerative joint disease unless treatment depends on additional findings, or when symptoms are not explained by the radiographic findings. Magnetic resonance imaging (MRI) can be obtained when radiographs are nondiagnostic or incongruent with clinical findings (eg, suspected internal derangement, insufficiency fracture, or inflammatory arthropathy) or when pain persists despite normal radiographs. As the meniscus also contributes to the joint space, meniscal degeneration and extrusion can account for a significant amount of joint space narrowing seen on radiographs.

FINDINGS

While early joint space narrowing is best assessed radiographically using Rosenberg views, advanced OA can be appreciated on standard AP views. Radiographic findings of OA of the knee (Fig. C2.3A-C) include joint space narrowing, osteophyte formation, subchondral sclerosis and cyst formation, and bone attrition (flattening). Narrowing of the medial compartment is more common and can lead to varus deformity of the knee ("bowlegged") and widening of the lateral compartment. Mineralized intra-articular bodies can also be appreciated on radiographs. The term "loose body" is avoided by some radiologists because the intra-articular fragments may be adherent to synovial surfaces and therefore not "loose."

MRI provides a direct assessment of the articular cartilage (Fig. C2.3D-F). Cartilage abnormalities in OA include focal signal changes, thinning, and partial-thickness to full-thickness defects (sometimes with exposure of the subchondral bone). Associated subchondral sclerosis manifests on MRI as thickening of the cortical signal void (T1 and T2 hypointensity). Bone marrow signal abnormalities (T1 hypointensity and T2 hyperintensity) are often focal and seen in the presence of cartilage defects. Subchondral cysts appear as well-defined areas of fluid signal (T1 hypointensity and T2 hyperintensity) that may or may not communicate with a synovial space. The sclerotic margin that is often seen around cysts is more apparent on radiographs.

Attrition, the flattening and depression of the articular surfaces of bones, is associated with severe OA. This is best assessed on MR images by noting deviation from the normally convex surfaces of the medial and lateral femoral condyles, the medial facet of the patella, and the flat to slightly convex surface of the lateral tibial plateau.

MRI is also sensitive for meniscal abnormalities ranging from mucoid degeneration to maceration and extrusion.

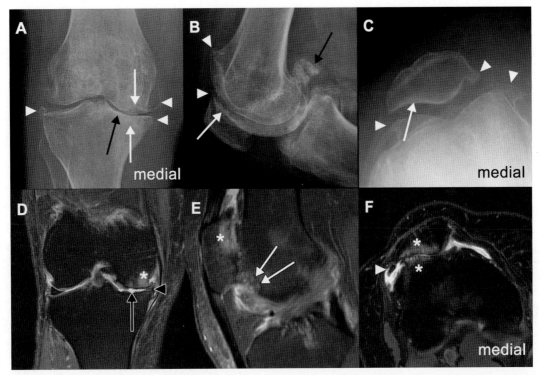

Fig. C2.3 Tricompartmental osteoarthritis in different patients. (A) Anteroposterior view of the knee reveals severe medial compartment joint space narrowing causing mild varus deformity of the knee. Mild subchondral sclerosis (black arrow), subchondral cysts (white arrows), and marginal osteophytes (white arrowheads) are also seen. (B) The lateral view from the same patient reveals similar findings at the patellofemoral compartment and an intra-articular body (long black arrow). (C) Merchant view in another patient reveals osteophytes (white arrowheads) both medially and laterally at the patellofemoral articulation, as well as subchondral sclerosis (white arrow) along the lateral patellar facet. (D) Coronal fluid-sensitive image in another patient reveals a macerated and extruded medial meniscus (black arrowhead), subchondral edema (*), and focal cartilage loss (black arrow). (E) Sagittal fluid-sensitive image reveals subchondral edema (*) and subchondral cysts (white arrows). (F) Fluid-sensitive axial image reveals severe loss of articular cartilage at the lateral patellofemoral compartment associated with subchondral edema (*). An osteophyte (white arrowhead) is also seen.

Mild synovial inflammation and thickening are frequently seen in or near the intercondylar notch, the infrapatellar fat, and the posterior joint. Moderate or large effusions are more frequently seen in patients with pain than in those without pain, and the prevalence of effusions increases with increasing radiographic severity of OA.

Intra-articular bodies may also be present and appear as hypointense structures in the joint capsule or in a Baker cyst.

DIFFERENTIAL DIAGNOSIS
Imaging Differential Diagnosis

Calcium pyrophosphate dehydrate deposition arthropathy (Fig. C2.4) can present as isolated or disproportionate patellofemoral joint space narrowing and should be considered when seen in conjunction with chondrocalcinosis (calcification along fibrocartilage menisci and hyaline cartilage) and calcium deposition in the gastrocnemius tendon origin.

Clinical Differential Diagnosis

OA is the most common cause of chronic atraumatic knee pain in elderly patients. Other considerations for atraumatic knee pain in adults include meniscal and ligament tears, stress fracture (see case 9), transient osteoporosis, and chronic regional pain syndrome. MRI is the imaging modality of choice for evaluation of these conditions.

The presence of severe local inflammation, erythema, and progressive pain unrelated to usage should raise concern for infectious or inflammatory arthropathies.

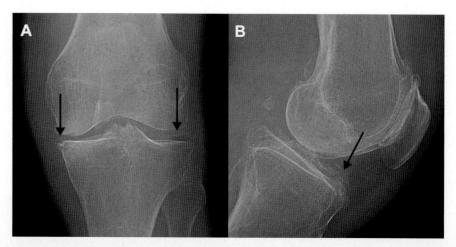

Fig. C2.4 Calcium pyrophosphate dehydrate deposition (CPDD) arthropathy has an appearance similar to that of osteoarthritis and requires joint aspiration for definitive diagnosis. (A) Frontal and (B) lateral views of the knee show the characteristic appearance of CPDD arthropathy: isolated or disproportionate patellofemoral osteoarthritis in conjunction with chondrocalcinosis (black arrows).

REFERENCES AND SUGGESTED READING

1. Bennett DL, Daffner RH, Weissman BN, et al. Expert Panel on Musculoskeletal Imaging. ACR Appropriateness Criteria. Nontraumatic knee pain (online publication). Reston, VA: American College of Radiology (ACR); 2008.

2. Boegård T, Jonsson K. Radiography in osteoarthritis of the knee. *Skeletal Radiol.* 1999;28(11):605-615.

3. Bradley WG, Ominsky SH. Mountain view of the patella. *AJR.* 1981;136(1):53-58.

4. Guermazi A, Zaim S, Taouli B, Miaux Y, Peterfy CG, Genant HG. MR findings in knee osteoarthritis. *Eur Radiol.* 2003;13(6):1370-1386.

5. Jordan KM, Arden NK, Doherty M, et al. Standing Committee for International Clinical Studies Including Therapeutic Trials ESCISIT. EULAR recommendations 2003: an evidence based approach to the management of knee osteoarthritis: report of a task force of the Standing Committee for International Clinical Studies Including Therapeutic Trials (ESCISIT). *Ann Rheum Dis.* 2003;62(12):1145-1155.

6. Rosenberg TD, Paulos LE, Parker RD, Coward DB, Scott SM. The forty-five-degree posteroanterior flexion weight-bearing radiograph of the knee. *J Bone Joint Surg Am.* 1988;70(10):1479-1483.

7. Zhang W, Doherty M, Peat G, et al. EULAR evidence-based recommendations for the diagnosis of knee osteoarthritis. *Ann Rheum Dis.* 2010;69(3):483-489.

CASE 3

PATIENT PRESENTATION

A 55-year-old woman with morning stiffness of the hands and swelling at metacarpophalangeal joints.

CLINICAL SUSPICION

Early rheumatoid arthritis

IMAGING MODALITY OF CHOICE

MRI or ultrasound. Radiographs are insensitive for the diagnosis of early rheumatoid arthritis (~70% of patients in the early stages have normal radiographs) but are used to exclude other causes of joint pain (eg, osteoarthritis and chronic calcium pyrophosphate crystal inflammatory arthritis) and to assess structural damage in established cases of rheumatoid arthritis.

MRI and ultrasound are both sensitive for the detection of synovial proliferation, which is one of the earliest detectable changes in rheumatoid arthritis. They can also assess disease activity and are useful in differentiating active disease from remission. Finally, MRI and ultrasound are used to evaluate suspected soft tissue complications of rheumatoid arthritis, such as ruptured tendons.

The choice between MRI and ultrasound depends on several factors. Ultrasound is relatively inexpensive, readily available, and allows for assessment of multiple joints, but can be time consuming and does not allow for visualization of bone edema or internal bone structure. It also depends on operator experience and radiologist expertise. MRI provides a more global view of a joint and is not operator-dependent, but is expensive, not globally available, requires more time to image a single joint, often requires the use of intravenous contrast, is susceptible to motion artifact, and has lower spatial resolution than ultrasound. The choice often depends on local expertise and the cost and availability of equipment. In most cases, however, MRI will not be cost-effective for monitoring treatment response.

BACKGROUND

Rheumatoid arthritis is an immune-mediated inflammatory disease that results in a symmetric polyarthritis that usually involves the small joints of the hands and feet. Rheumatoid arthritis is the most common of the inflammatory joint diseases, a group that also includes erosive, psoriatic, and reactive arthritis. Early treatment with disease-modifying antirheumatic drugs (DMARDs) such as methotrexate and newer biological agents improves clinical outcomes and reduces the progression of joint damage and disability. Early treatment requires early diagnosis, a task that is beyond the capability of radiography. Indeed, recent

guidelines of the American College of Rheumatology and European League Against Rheumatism rely on physical examination findings and laboratory data (eg, autoantibodies such as rheumatoid factor and anti-citrullinated protein antibody) for diagnosis, and suggest the use of MRI or ultrasound if additional evidence of joint activity is needed for confirmation of the clinical findings.

FINDINGS

Recognition of synovitis is the key to early detection of rheumatoid arthritis by MRI and ultrasound (Fig. C3.1). On ultrasound, synovitis appears as abnormal tissue that is nondisplaceable and poorly compressible. It is usually hypoechoic relative to subcutaneous fat but can sometimes be isoechoic or hyperechoic. A joint effusion is frequently present, and can be differentiated from synovitis by being displaceable. Power Doppler ultrasound is more sensitive than color Doppler for detecting synovial inflammation and has been shown to correlate well with clinical disease activity. While it may be difficult to differentiate synovium from the adjacent cartilage on ultrasound, this can be readily achieved on MRI.

On MRI, synovitis appears as thickened synovium with greater than normal contrast enhancement. T2-weighted sequences can sometimes reveal synovitis as areas of signal that is less intense than joint fluid, but the distinction may be difficult.

Ultrasound and MRI are more sensitive than radiographs for detection of bony erosions. Although computed tomography (CT) is even more sensitive, radiation concerns make it less useful for serial monitoring of disease. On ultrasound, an erosion appears as an intra-articular discontinuity of the bone surface that is visible in two perpendicular planes. Ultrasound, however, is limited by its inability to visualize all parts of a joint (eg, the radial and ulnar aspects of all metacarpophalangeal joints) and can lead to incorrect characterization of normal anatomic variants (eg, normal depressions on the dorsal surfaces of the metacarpal heads) as erosions.

On MRI, an erosion appears as a sharply marginated bone lesion in a juxta-articular location that is visible in at least two planes and has a cortical break that is seen in at least one plane. On T1-weighted images, there is loss of the normal low signal intensity of cortical bone and loss of the normal high signal intensity of trabecular bone. The erosion generally contains inflammatory tissue or fluid, both of which are T2 hyperintense on T2-weighted images. In contrast to fluid, the inflammatory tissue will usually enhance.

In the early phase of disease, radiographs are either normal or reveal periarticular soft tissue swelling, a potentially subtle finding that is better appreciated on physical examination. Late radiographic findings of rheumatoid arthritis include periarticular osteopenia, marginal erosions,

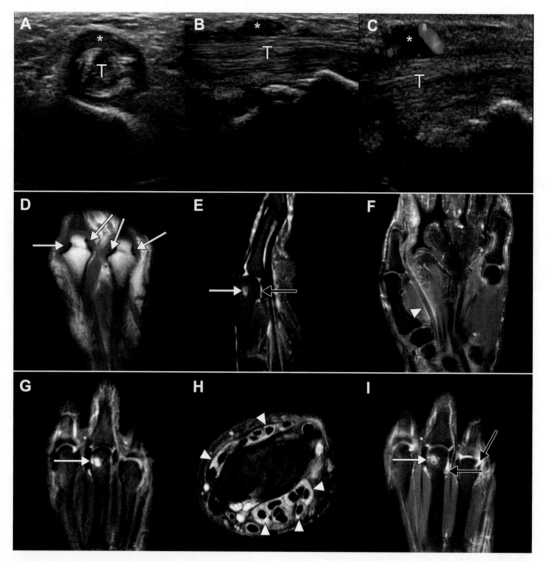

Fig. C3.1 Ultrasound and MRI findings in rheumatoid arthritis in three patients. (A-C) 65-year-old woman with rheumatoid arthritis and trigger finger. Transverse (A) and longitudinal (B,C) images show a thickened and heterogeneous flexor tendon (T) with hypoechoic thickening (*). (C) Color Doppler image shows hyperemia surrounding the tendon. (Ultrasound images used with permission from Dr Frank Malara, Austin Hospital, Melbourne, Australia). (D-I) MR images in two different patients depicting erosions (white arrows), synovitis (black arrows), and tenosynovitis (white arrowheads).

and joint deformity (Fig. C3.2). Joint deformities include ulnar deviation at the metacarpophalangeal joints; radial deviation of the radiocarpal articulation; swan-neck, boutonnière, and hitchhiker's thumb deformities; and telescoping of the fingers.

DIFFERENTIAL DIAGNOSIS
Imaging Differential Diagnosis

Psoriatic arthritis, juvenile idiopathic arthritis, and chronic calcium pyrophosphate crystal inflammatory arthritis can produce similar imaging findings and present an imaging diagnostic challenge. Knowledge of the distribution of various arthritides in the hands (Fig. C3.3) can be helpful in some cases. Typical imaging findings in these conditions are shown in Fig. C3.4.

Clinical Differential Diagnosis

Osteoarthritis and other inflammatory arthritides such as psoriatic arthritis and chronic calcium pyrophosphate crystal inflammatory arthritis.

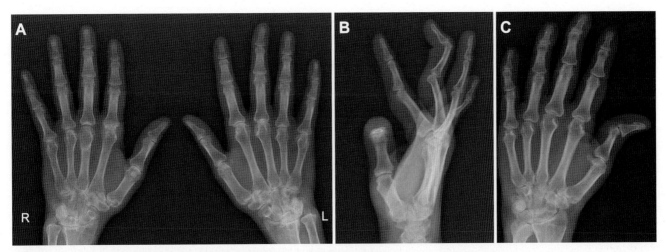

Fig. C3.2 Late radiographic findings in rheumatoid arthritis in the hands of three patients. (A) Radiographs of the hands reveal a symmetric polyarthropathy involving the distal radioulnar, radiocarpal, intercarpal, carpometacarpal, and metacarpophalangeal articulations, with joint space narrowing, periarticular osteopenia, and erosions at multiple sites. There is radial deviation at the radiocarpal articulation, but no obvious ulnar deviation at the metacarpophalangeal joints. Note that the distal interphalangeal joints are spared. (B) Lateral radiograph of the hand in another patient shows a swan-neck deformity of the middle finger: flexion of the metacarpophalangeal and distal interphalangeal joints and hyperextension of the proximal interphalangeal joint. While not pathognomonic, swan-neck and boutonnière deformities (not shown) are more often seen in rheumatoid arthritis than in the other inflammatory arthritides. (C) Frontal view of the hand reveals joint space narrowing and erosions at the radioulnar, radiocarpal, intercarpal, carpometacarpal, and metacarpophalangeal articulations. There is also dorsal subluxation at the interphalangeal joint of the thumb, giving the so-called hitchhiker's thumb deformity.

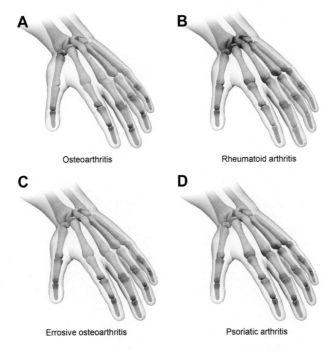

Fig. C3.3 Distribution of the arthritides in the hands. (A) Osteoarthritis is characterized by joint space narrowing, osteophyte formation, and subchondral sclerosis at the proximal and distal interphalangeal joints, as well as the carpometacarpal and interphalangeal joints of the thumb. Calcium pyrophosphate crystal inflammatory arthritis has a similar distribution, but with chondrocalcinosis characteristically seen at the wrist. (B) Rheumatoid arthritis is characterized by involvement of the radiocarpal, intercarpal, carpometacarpal, metacarpophalangeal, and proximal interphalangeal joints, central and marginal erosions, periarticular osteopenia, and joint deformities. Juvenile idiopathic arthritis (formerly juvenile rheumatoid arthritis) has a distribution similar to that of rheumatoid arthritis. (C) Erosive osteoarthritis is characterized by involvement of the proximal and distal interphalangeal joints, erosions with "gull-wing" deformities, and joint ankylosis. (D) Psoriatic arthritis is characterized by involvement of distal interphalangeal joints, erosion of the terminal tufts, "mouse-ear erosions," pencil-in-cup deformities, "sausage digit," joint ankylosis, and fluffy periosteal reaction.

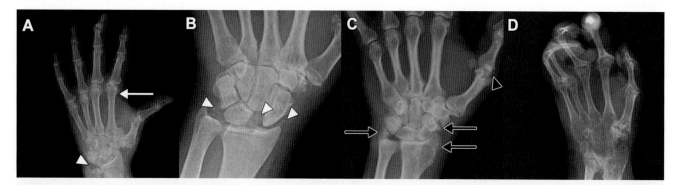

Fig. C3.4 Imaging differential diagnosis for rheumatoid arthritis. (A) Chronic calcium pyrophosphate crystal inflammatory arthritis with radiocarpal, intercarpal, metacarpophalangeal, and interphalangeal joint space narrowing. Changes of osteoarthritis are seen at the distal interphalangeal joints and at the carpometacarpal and interphalangeal joints of the thumb. Chondrocalcinosis is present at the triangular fibrocartilage complex (white arrowhead). A hooklike osteophyte is seen at the index finger metacarpal head (white arrow). No erosion is seen. (B) Chronic calcium pyrophosphate crystal inflammatory arthritis in another patient showing chondrocalcinosis at the wrist (white arrowheads) and widening of the scapholunate interval. (C) Psoriatic arthritis with erosion at the thumb metacarpal head (black arrowhead) as well as several areas of proliferative bone formation (black arrows). (Case used with permission from Dr Hansel Otero, Tufts Medical Center, Boston, MA.) (D) Juvenile idiopathic arthritis with advanced destruction of multiple joints, ankylosis (joint fusion) at the wrist, and overgrowth of the metacarpal heads.

REFERENCES AND SUGGESTED READING

1. Aletaha D, Neogi T, Silman AJ, et al. 2010 rheumatoid arthritis classification criteria: an American College of Rheumatology/European League Against Rheumatism collaborative initiative. *Ann Rheum Dis.* 2010;69(9):1580-1588. Erratum in: *Ann Rheum Dis.* 2010;69(10):1892.

2. Rowbotham EL, Grainger AJ. Rheumatoid arthritis: ultrasound versus MRI. *AJR.* 2011;197(3):541-546.

3. Tan YK, Conaghan PG. Imaging in rheumatoid arthritis. *Best Pract Res Clin Rheumatol.* 2011;25(4):569-584.

CASE 4

PATIENT PRESENTATION

A 50-year-old man with acute-onset pain and swelling of the right first metatarsophalangeal joint. He has had similar episodes in the past that have responded to over-the-counter analgesics.

CLINICAL SUSPICION

Gout

IMAGING MODALITY OF CHOICE

Radiography

BACKGROUND

Gout is the most common crystalline arthropathy. It occurs as a result of longstanding hyperuricemia, which leads to monosodium urate crystal deposition within joints and soft tissues. Precipitation of monosodium urate crystals within the joint space leads to an intense inflammatory reaction, which manifests clinically as gout. Acute gouty arthritis is characterized by excruciating pain and warmth about the joint. The symptoms may be accompanied by fever and leukocytosis and can persist for several days. Gout affects the lower extremities more frequently than the upper extremities and the smaller joints more frequently than the larger joints. The first metatarsophalangeal joint is the most commonly involved joint on first clinical presentation. The distribution is asymmetric, and clinical presentation is typically monoarticular.

FINDINGS

The most common early radiographic feature of gout is soft tissue swelling about the involved joint (Figs. C4.1 and C4.2), which occurs as a result of synovitis, joint capsule distention, and periarticular soft tissue edema. Intermediate-stage and late-stage radiographic features of gout develop 5 to 10 years after onset of clinical symptoms and include:

- Faint soft tissue calcifications about involved joints
- Soft tissue or intraosseous masses representing tophi
- Cortical erosions and irregularity
- Well-defined juxta-articular erosions with sclerotic rims and overhanging margins
- Preservation of bone mineralization and joint space

Secondary degenerative changes with loss of the joint space or even ankylosis may occur at more advanced stages of gout. However, this is rarely seen in the modern era.

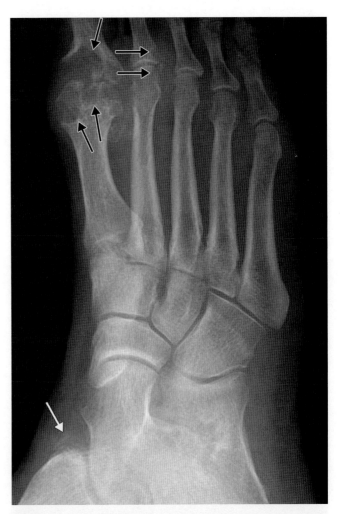

Fig. C4.1 Frontal radiograph of the foot shows large erosions of the first and second metatarsophalangeal joints (black arrows). Small ill-defined soft-tissue mineralization is seen at the tibiotalar joint (white arrow), representing tophi. Diagnosis was confirmed with aspiration of the first metatarsophalangeal joint. Negatively bire-fringent needle-shaped monosodium urate crystals were identified under polarized microscopic examination.

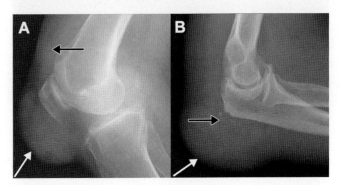

Fig. C4.2 Gout in the larger joints. Although gout most commonly affects the first metatarsophalangeal joint, involvement of larger joints is frequently encountered. (A) Lateral radiograph of the knee shows a large mass in the prepatellar soft tissues with small tophaceous deposits (white arrow) related to gout. A moderate joint effusion is present (black arrow). (B) Lateral radiograph of the elbow shows a large mass in the olecranon bursa (white arrow) with small tophaceous deposits (black arrow).

Although radiographs are preferred in initial evaluation of gout, MRI (Fig. C4.3A,B) may be performed to detect smaller tophi and earlier-stage disease. Tophi characteristically have low to intermediate signal intensity on both T1- and T2-weighted MR images. Enhancement is typically encountered after administration of intravenous gadolinium due to proliferative synovitis, granulation tissue surrounding the tophus, and inflammatory reaction within adjacent soft tissues.

CT is increasingly used for visualization of tophi (Fig. C4.3C,D). The strength of CT in evaluation of gout lies in its capability to detect subtle bony erosions and to measure attenuation of tophi (150 to 200 Hounsfield units, which is lower than that of calcifications and higher than that of soft tissues). Developments in dual-energy CT currently allow quantification of monosodium urate deposits.

DIFFERENTIAL DIAGNOSIS

Imaging Differential Diagnosis

- Septic arthritis: Microbiological examination and culture of synovial fluid is necessary to exclude septic arthritis, which may coexist with gout.

- Acute calcium pyrophosphate crystal arthritis: Formerly known as pseudogout. Cartilage calcification or chondrocalcinosis is a more dominant feature. Synovial fluid analysis may reveal positively birefringent rhomboid crystals.

- Osteoarthritis: Early loss of joint space and lack of erosions differentiate this entity from gout. In gout, joint space loss tends to occur in later stages of the disease.

- Rheumatoid arthritis: Bilateral, symmetrical joint involvement and juxta-articular osteopenia differentiate this from gout, which tends to be asymmetric and without osteopenia.

Clinical Differential Diagnosis

The main clinical differential consideration is acute calcium pyrophosphate crystal arthritis, formerly known as pseudogout. This is an acute-onset, self-limiting synovitis associated with deposition of calcium pyrophosphate crystals. Patients typically present with severe, rapid-onset joint pain, tenderness, swelling, and overlying erythema. The symptoms peak within 6 to 24 hours.

REFERENCES AND SUGGESTED READING

1. Dalbeth N, Doyle A, McQueen FM. Imaging in gout: insights into the pathological features of disease. *Curr Opin Rheumatol.* 2012;24:132-138.

2. Perez-Ruiz F, Dalbeth N, Urresola A, de Miguel E, Schlesinger N. Imaging of gout: findings and utility. *Arthritis Res Ther.* 2009;11:232.

3. Richette P, Bardin T. Gout. *Lancet.* 2010;375:318-328.

4. Tian QS, Dhanda S, Jagmohan P. A re-look at an old disease: a multimodality review on gout. *Clin Radiol.* 2011;66:984-992.

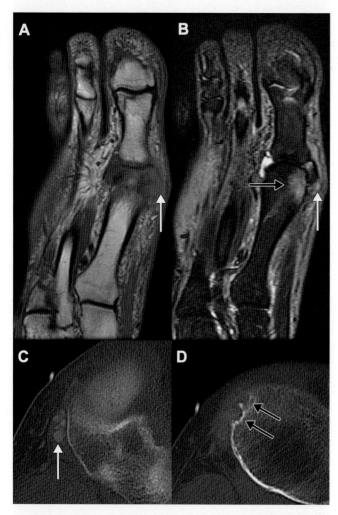

Fig. C4.3 (A,B) Coronal MR images of the foot reveal a small tophus (white arrow) in the soft tissues adjacent to the first metatarsophalangeal joint. The tophus has homogeneous low signal intensity on the T1-weighted image (A) and heterogeneous intermediate to low signal intensity on the T2-weighted image (B). The T2-weighted image also reveals increased signal within the distal metatarsal consistent with edema (black arrow). Small tophaceous deposits such as this are difficult to detect on radiographs. (C,D) Axial CT images in a different patient reveal small tophi adjacent to the proximal tibia (C, white arrow) and small erosions more inferiorly (D, black arrows).

CASE 5

PATIENT PRESENTATION

A 55-year-old man with diabetes mellitus presents with a swollen foot. There is a skin ulcer along the dorsolateral aspect of the fifth metatarsophalangeal joint.

CLINICAL SUSPICION

Osteomyelitis

IMAGING MODALITY OF CHOICE

Radiographs in conjunction with MRI with intravenous contrast (Fig. C5.1). Radiographs have low sensitivity and specificity, with an overall accuracy of about 50% for diagnosis of osteomyelitis, but should be obtained as an adjunct to MRI for their superior visualization of cortical bone. Contrast is useful for the evaluation of soft-tissue complications such as sinus tract formation, development of associated abscesses, and necrosis, and provides information for operative planning for limited limb resection. Noncontrast CT and three-phase bone scintigraphy can be obtained in cases in which clinical suspicion for infection is low or if MRI is contraindicated.

BACKGROUND

Foot infections are common in patients with diabetes mellitus and range from superficial infections and cellulitis to deep infections and osteomyelitis. Osteomyelitis (infection of the bone marrow) is the dreaded complication, and delayed diagnosis can increase the risk of amputation. Physical examination can be unreliable because the clinical findings of osteomyelitis may be masked or blunted in patients with diabetes mellitus. In addition, neuropathic (Charcot) arthropathy, which is present in up to 7.5% of patients with diabetes mellitus, can present with erythema, edema, and elevated temperature of the foot and mimic clinical findings of infection. Ulceration, neuropathy, and exposed bone increase the pretest probability for osteomyelitis.

FINDINGS

Radiography has low sensitivity for osteomyelitis, especially early in the course of the disease. After about 2 weeks, radiographs may reveal demineralization, periosteal reaction, and bony destruction, often in proximity to a pedal ulcer.

The primary MRI finding of osteomyelitis in the foot of a diabetic patient is low bone marrow signal on T1-weighted images at the end of a sinus tract. Secondary signs of osteomyelitis on MRI include skin callus, skin ulcer, sinus tract, cellulitis, abscess, foreign object, and periosteal reaction.

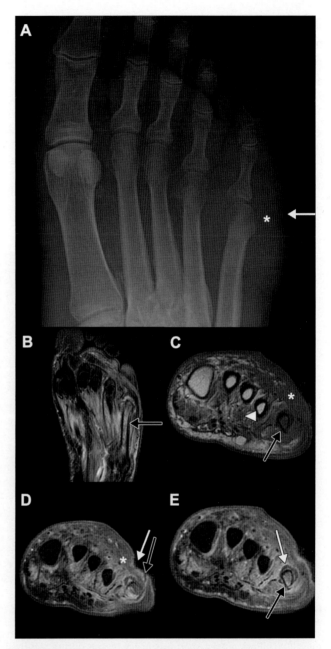

Fig. C5.1 Osteomyelitis in a patient with diabetes mellitus. (A) Radiograph shows a soft tissue defect along the lateral aspect of the foot (white arrow) with associated soft tissue swelling (*) but no bony abnormality. (B) Fluid-sensitive long-axis image of the foot shows bone marrow edema within the fifth metatarsal (black arrow) and soft tissue edema. (C) Short-axis T1-weighted image reveals decreased bone marrow signal (black arrow) that is the same or lower than that of muscle (white arrowhead), consistent with osteomyelitis. Soft tissue edema (*) manifests as decreased signal on T1-weighted images. (D) Postcontrast short-axis image showing the ulcer (white arrow) and a sinus tract (black arrow) extending to the fifth metatarsal. Enhancement (*) is seen in the inflamed soft tissues. (E) A postcontrast short-axis image at the same level as C shows that the bone marrow enhances (black arrow), indicating viable bone. Periosteal elevation (white arrow) is seen as a hypointense line that is lifted off the underlying bone by an enhancing layer of inflammatory tissue.

DIFFERENTIAL DIAGNOSIS

Imaging Differential Diagnosis

Differential considerations include cellulitis (Fig. C5.2A-D) and neuropathic arthropathy (Fig. C5.2E-H). Cellulitis will present on MRI as soft tissue edema and enhancement. There may be adjacent marrow signal abnormalities; however, marrow T2 hyperintensity without corresponding T1 hypointensity is more likely indicative of osteitis (inflammation of the bone marrow). Osteitis in this setting is a reaction to adjacent soft-tissue infection.

Neuropathic arthropathy can also demonstrate soft tissue edema and bone marrow signal abnormalities. The bone marrow changes in neuropathic joints are periarticular in location, whereas those seen in osteomyelitis are typically diffuse and found adjacent to the ulcer or a sinus tract.

Clinical Differential Diagnosis

Neuropathic joint, fracture, and septic arthritis are clinical considerations. In septic arthritis, MRI will reveal a complex joint effusion in the involved joint, intense and usually thick synovial enhancement, and T2 hyperintensity in the adjacent bone marrow without corresponding T1 hypointensity.

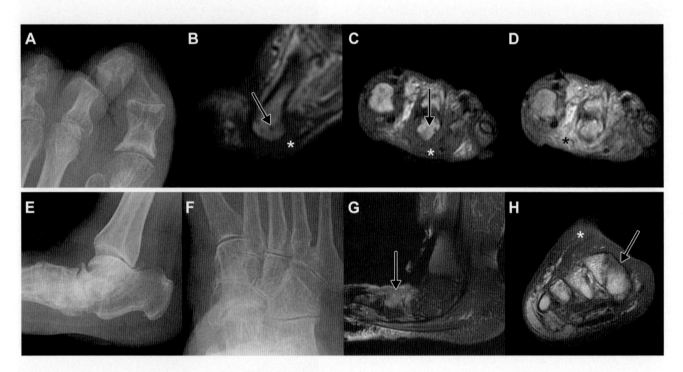

Fig. C5.2 Differential considerations in two patients with diabetes mellitus. (A-D) Cellulitis. (A) Coned-down radiograph in a patient with a pedal ulcer at the second metatarsal head reveals degenerative changes, but no bony destruction. T1-weighted sagittal (B) and short-axis (C) images reveal soft tissue edema (*) and mild bone marrow hypointensity (long black arrows) that is not as hypointense as muscle. (D) Postcontrast short-axis image reveals diffuse soft tissue enhancement (*). (E-H) Neuropathic joint. Coned-down lateral (E) and oblique (F) views of the ankle and midfoot show the typical findings of neuropathic joint, the so-called 6 Ds: increased density (subchondral sclerosis), destruction, intra-articular debris, dislocation, joint distension, and disorganization. (G) Sagittal T2-weighted image reveals bone marrow edema (long black arrow) in a periarticular distribution that is not as dark as muscle on the short-axis T1-weighted image (H), consistent with reactive marrow inflammation (osteitis).

REFERENCES AND SUGGESTED READING

1. Bader MS. Diabetic foot infection. *Am Fam Physician.* 2008; 78(1):71-79.

2. Donovan A, Schweitzer ME. Use of MR imaging in diagnosing diabetes-related pedal osteomyelitis. *RadioGraphics.* 2010; 30(3):723-736.

3. Tomas MB, Patel M, Marwin SE, Palestro CJ. The diabetic foot. *Br J Radiol.* 2000;73(868):443-450.

CASE 6

PATIENT PRESENTATION

A 35-year-old man presents to his primary care physician with increasing right knee pain and swelling over the past several weeks. He denies fevers or recent trauma.

CLINICAL SUSPICION

Inflammatory or neoplastic process in the joint

IMAGING MODALITY OF CHOICE

Knee radiographs are preferred in initial evaluation of knee pain. However, magnetic resonance imaging (MRI) is required to assess soft tissue structures.

BACKGROUND

Pigmented villonodular synovitis (PVNS) is a rare disorder characterized by synovial proliferation in the joint, tendon sheath, and bursa. It is believed to be a neoplastic disorder by most authors, whereas others suspect that it is caused by chronic inflammation. PVNS can be classified as localized or diffuse. Distinction between the two is important, since the former can be treated by simple excision with negligible risk of recurrence, whereas the latter requires extensive synovectomy and possibly chemotherapy because of its risk of recurrence.

Symptoms are nonspecific, but primarily consist of painful joint swelling and decreased motion, most commonly in the knee. The underlying effusion is typically hemorrhagic in appearance. Histologically, PVNS is characterized by diffuse hemosiderin staining related to recurrent hemorrhage of the friable villi of proliferative synovium.

FINDINGS

Radiographic findings (Fig. C6.1A) include a large joint effusion or intra-articular soft tissue mass and well-defined erosions with preservation of the joint space.

MRI findings (Fig. C6.1B-D) include a typically large joint effusion, heterogeneous synovial thickening, areas of "blooming artifact" on gradient-echo imaging due to hemosiderin deposition, prominent synovial enhancement, and subtle bony erosions with preservation of the joint space.

DIFFERENTIAL DIAGNOSIS

Imaging Differential Diagnosis

- Synovial hemangioma (Fig. C6.2A,B) can have similar MRI findings due to repetitive intra-articular hemorrhage and synovial hemosiderin deposition. Serpentine vessels seen with synovial hemangioma will not be seen with PVNS.

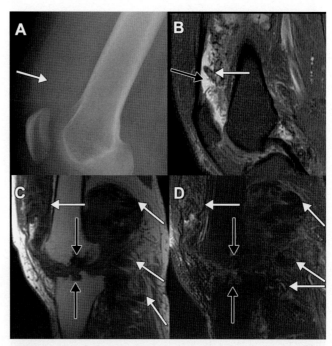

Fig. C6.1 Pigmented villonodular synovitis (PVNS) in two patients. (A) Lateral radiograph of the knee shows a soft tissue density mass (white arrow) in the suprapatellar recess of the joint. (B) T2-weighted image in the same patient reveals low intensity nodular synovial proliferation (white arrow), as well as a moderate joint effusion (black arrow). The nodular appearance of the synovial proliferative tissue is characteristic of PVNS. No bony erosion was identified in this patient. Sagittal T1 (C) and T2 (D) weighted images in another patient show a large amount of hypointense nodular synovial tissue throughout the joint (white arrows), as well as bony erosions within the femur and tibia (black arrows).

- Synovial chondromatosis (Fig. C6.2C,D): The small, round, ossified bodies of synovial osteochondromatosis are generally apparent on radiographs and allow for easy differentiation from PVNS, whereas the nonossified bodies of synovial chondromatosis can occasionally present as a soft tissue mass on radiographs and MRI.

- Gout (Fig. C6.2E,F) and amyloid may have an appearance similar to that of PVNS, with low-intensity nodular lesions on T1- and T2-weighted images. However, no blooming is present on gradient-echo images.

- Hemophilic arthropathy: The proliferative synovium and juxta-articular erosions encountered in hemophilic arthropathy are similar to those seen in PVNS. A history of hemophilia and the presence of epiphyseal and metaphyseal overgrowth on radiographs are helpful in differentiating the two.

Clinical Differential Diagnosis

Internal derangement, septic arthritis, and gout can have similar clinical presentations.

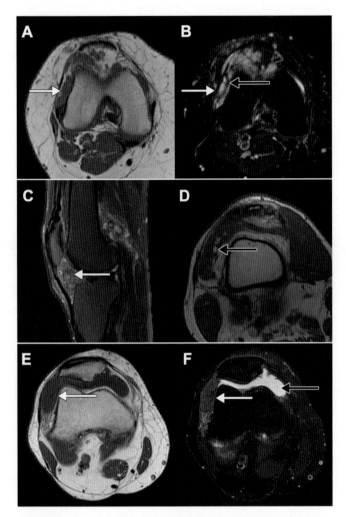

REFERENCES AND SUGGESTED READING

1. Al-Nakshabandi NA, Ryan AG, Choudur H, Torreggiani W, Nicoloau S, Munk PL, Al-Ismail K. Pigmented villonodular synovitis. *Clin Radiol.* 2004;59:414-420.

2. Llauger J, Palmer J, Monill JM, Franquet T, Bagué S, Rosón N. MR imaging of benign soft-tissue masses of the foot and ankle. *RadioGraphics.* 1998;18:1481-1498.

3. Murphey MD, Rhee JH, Lewis RB, Fanburg-Smith JC, Flemming DJ, Walker EA. Pigmented villonodular synovitis: radiologic-pathologic correlation. *RadioGraphics.* 2008; 28(5):1493-1518.

4. Ottaviani S, Ayral X, Dougados M, Gossec L. Pigmented villonodular synovitis: a retrospective single-center study of 122 cases and review of the literature. *Semin Arthritis Rheum.* 2011;40:539-546.

5. Walker EA, Fenton ME, Salesky JS, Murphey MD. Magnetic resonance imaging of benign soft tissue neoplasms in adults. *Radiol Clin North Am.* 2011;49:1197-1217.

Fig. C6.2 Imaging differential considerations. (A,B) Synovial hemangioma. A soft tissue mass (white arrow) that is intermediate in signal intensity can be seen on the T1-weighted image (A) and is hyperintense on the T2-weighted image (B). Hypointense bands are seen within the lesion (black arrow). Serpentine surrounding vessels could be appreciated on contiguous axial images. (C,D) Synovial chondromatosis. (C) T2-weighted sagittal image reveals nodular and hypointense proliferation of the synovium (white arrow), without blooming to suggest hemosiderin deposition. (D) T1-weighted axial image reveals several well-defined hyperintense nodules (one is indicated by the black arrow), consistent with early ossification in the continuum of synovial chondromatosis to synovial osteochondromatosis. These ossified nodules were not apparent radiographically. (E,F) Gout mimicking PVNS. Axial T1-weighted (E) and T2-weighted (F) images reveal a hypointense soft tissue mass in the lateral aspect of the joint. Biopsy showed this to represent a gouty tophus. A small joint effusion (black arrow) was also present.

CASE 7

PATIENT PRESENTATION

A 30-year-old man with pain and deformity of the ring finger metacarpal after punching a wall (Fig. C7.1).

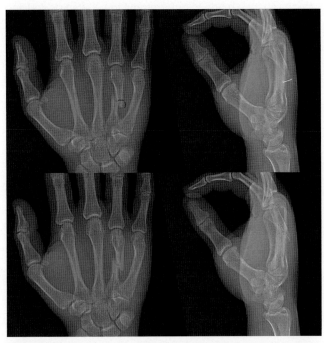

Fig. C7.1 Oblique fracture of the mid diaphysis of the ring finger metacarpal. There is ulnar (medial) displacement by one-half the bone width (black square bracket), dorsal displacement by nearly the full bone width (white square bracket), approximately 5 mm of overlap (black bracket), approximately 20° of volar (toward the palm) angulation, and approximately 5° of radial (lateral, toward the radius) angulation.

CLINICAL SUSPICION

Fracture

IMAGING MODALITY OF CHOICE

Radiographs. Noncontrast CT may be needed for operative planning, and contrast-enhanced CT arteriogram is indicated if there is concern for vascular injury.

FINDINGS

A systematic and standardized approach to fractures will ensure complete evaluation of the patient and proper communication of findings among healthcare professionals. Fractures are classified as open (formerly compound) if a break in the skin and underlying soft tissue communicates directly with the fracture and its hematoma. This is best assessed by direct examination of the patient; however, subcutaneous gas or an obvious soft tissue defect extending to the fracture is a suggestive finding on imaging.

The next step is to describe the location of the fracture (eg, proximal metaphysis of the femur, mid-diaphysis of the humerus). Fractures of the ends of bones must be carefully assessed for extension to the articular surface, since this can have important ramifications for treatment and prognosis. CT is used to fully define the intra-articular extension of fracture planes.

Fracture classification is the next step and involves assessment of the underlying bone, the extent of the fracture, and the plane (or planes) of fracture. A classification scheme is presented in Fig. C7.2.

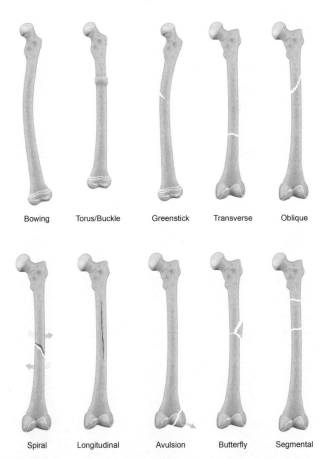

Bowing   Torus/Buckle   Greenstick   Transverse   Oblique

Spiral   Longitudinal   Avulsion   Butterfly   Segmental

Fig. C7.2 Fracture classification. Moving inward, we first assess the underlying bone. A fracture through a bone lesion is called a pathologic fracture. An insufficiency fracture is a type of stress fracture that occurs with normal activity on abnormal (eg, osteoporotic) bone. We next assess whether the fracture is complete or incomplete. Complete fractures extend across the whole width of the bone, while incomplete fractures have a single cortical break. Bowing, torus, and greenstick fractures are incomplete fractures that are frequently seen in children. Fractures may have a single plane (transverse, oblique, etc) or can be comminuted. Segmental fractures are comminuted fractures that divide a long bone into successive pieces by consecutive transverse fractures. Butterfly fractures have a wedge-shaped fragment that is split from the dominant fracture fragments.

Next we assess the relationship of the fracture fragments. By convention, we describe the relationship of the distal fragment to the proximal fragment (Fig. C7.3).

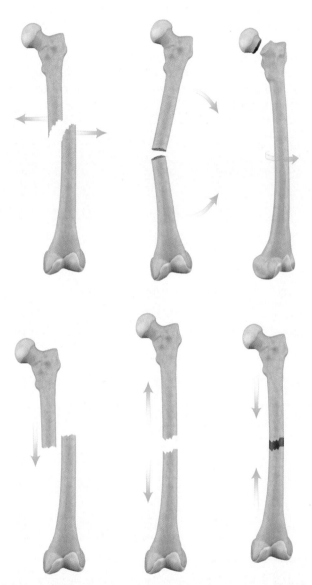

Fig. C7.3 Orientation of fracture fragments. *Displacement* refers to the relationship of fracture fragments along the transverse plane of the long bone, whereas *distraction* and *overlap* describe the relationship of the fracture fragments along the longitudinal axis of the bone. *Impaction* refers to fracture fragments being forcibly driven into each other. *Angulation* refers to the angle the distal fragment forms with the proximal fragment. A laterally angulated distal fragment is said to have valgus angulation, whereas a medially angulated distal fragment is said to have varus angulation. Finally, any rotary component of the fracture is described by noting the relationship of the distal fracture fragment to the proximal fragment as internally or externally rotated.

DIFFERENTIAL DIAGNOSIS

Imaging Differential Diagnosis

Additional fracture planes that upgrade a simple fracture to a comminuted fracture can sometimes be subtle or occult on radiographs. CT can be helpful in such cases. A careful search must be made to determine if there is an underlying bone lesion, since this will dramatically impact immediate and long-term patient management.

Clinical Differential Diagnosis

The clinical differential diagnosis for fractures varies according to site. Some fractures can mimic soft tissue injuries such as muscle strains or ligament tears.

REFERENCES AND SUGGESTED READING

1. Koval K, Zuckerman J. *Handbook of Fractures.* 3rd ed. Lippincott; 2006.

CASE 8

PATIENT PRESENTATION

A 12-year-old runner with 2 months of pain in her right proximal tibia. She wants to know when she can return to running. Imaging workup is initiated (Fig. C8.1).

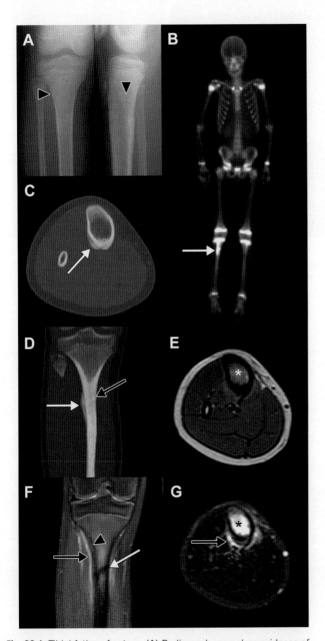

Fig. C8.1 Tibial fatigue fracture. (A) Radiographs reveal no evidence of fracture. An incidental benign lesion (a nonossifying fibroma) is seen (black arrowhead). (B) Whole-body Tc-99m MDP scan reveals increased uptake at the right proximal tibia (white arrow). (C) Axial CT image reveals periosteal reaction (white arrow). (D) Coronal reformation reveals periosteal reaction (white arrow) and a sclerotic line (black arrow) representing the fracture. (E) Axial T1-weighted image reveals loss of normal fat signal of the marrow (*). (F) Coronal fluid-sensitive sequence reveals the nonossifying fibroma (black arrowhead), the fracture (white arrow), and periosteal edema (black arrow). (G) Axial fluid-sensitive sequence reveals marrow (*) and periosteal (black arrow) edema.

CLINICAL SUSPICION

Stress injury

IMAGING MODALITY OF CHOICE

Radiographs are obtained mainly to exclude other causes of pain. In competitive athletes with tight training schedules, MRI can provide prognostic information.

BACKGROUND

Shin splints and tibial fatigue fractures are in the spectrum of soft-tissue and bony abnormalities that develop in response to chronic repetitive stress and can be difficult to differentiate clinically (Fig. C8.2).

Shin splints (also known as medial tibial stress syndrome) refers to pain on the medial aspect of the tibia, often in the mid or distal diaphysis. It is thought to be caused by a combination of traction on the periosteum by the calf muscles and repetitive bending loads across the tibia that result in inflammatory changes of the periosteum followed by periosteal reaction and adaptive changes of the tibial cortex.

Stress fractures occur as the result of repeated loading of bone with forces less than that required for an acute traumatic fracture. Stress fractures due to abnormal activity (eg, excessive running) on normal bone are called *fatigue fractures*, and stress fractures due to normal activity on abnormal (eg, osteoporotic) bone are called *insufficiency fractures*.

Recreational runners presenting with symptoms suggestive of a tibial stress injury can be treated conservatively with rest and analgesics, with follow-up imaging if symptoms persist. However, when faced with a competitive runner with tibial pain, the question is often "when can my patient return to full-impact activity?" Fredericson et al. (1995) have proposed an MRI grading system for tibial stress reactions that can be used to plan how long an athlete should rest before returning to full-impact exercise (Table C8.1 and Fig. C8.2).

FINDINGS

Radiographs can be normal in the early stages. Three-phase bone scintigraphy (commonly, technetium Tc-99m methylene diphosphonate [Tc-99m MDP]) is more sensitive than radiography. Early-phase (arterial and blood pool) images are typically normal. Delayed phase images reveal uptake along the tibia that ranges from a small focus of mild cortical uptake to intense and extensive transcortical uptake. However, differentiation between medial tibial stress syndrome and stress fracture can be difficult with scintigraphy. MRI can depict the full spectrum of stress reactions (Table C8.1 and Fig. C8.2).

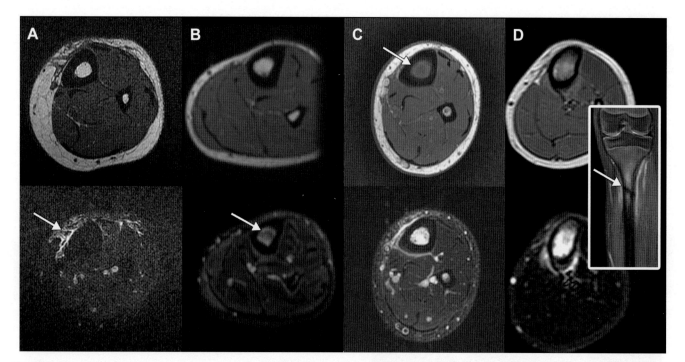

Fig. C8.2 Spectrum of tibial stress injuries as graded by Fredericson et al (1995) (see Table C8.1). T1-weighted images are on the top, and T2-weighted images are on the bottom. Arrows point to changes that elevate the grade. (A) Grade 1, mild to moderate increased T2 signal in the periosteal soft tissues. (B) Grade 2, T2 hyperintensity in the marrow. (C) Grade 3, T1 hypointensity in the marrow. (D) Fracture plane.

Table C8.1 Fredericson Grading of Tibia Stress Reactions

Grade	Scintigraphy	Periosteum MRI	Marrow	Time to Full-Impact Activity
1	Small ill-defined cortical area of mildly increased activity	Mild to moderate increased T2 signal	Normal	2-3 weeks
2	Larger well-defined elongated cortical area of moderately increased activity	Moderate to marked increased T2 signal	Increased T2 signal	4-6 weeks
3	Wide fusiform cortico-medullary area of highly increased activity	Moderate to marked increased T2 signal	Decreased T1 and increased T2 signal	6-9 weeks
4	Extensive transcortical area of intensely increased activity	Moderate to marked increased T2 signal	Decreased T1 and increased T2 signal plus clear fracture plane	6 weeks in a cast followed by 6 weeks of nonimpact activity

DIFFERENTIAL DIAGNOSIS

Imaging Differential Diagnosis

Although imaging findings in *symptomatic* runners are characteristic of various stress injuries, it should be noted that *asymptomatic* runners can have many of the same imaging findings. Therefore, images cannot provide a diagnosis of a tibial stress reaction without the benefit of clinical information, necessitating the inclusion of the dreaded phrase "clinical correlation recommended" in the report.

Rarely, tibial stress fractures can lead to a more extensive edema pattern and can mimic a neoplastic or infectious process.

Clinical Differential Diagnosis

In addition to medial tibial stress syndrome and fatigue fracture, the clinician must consider pathologic fracture by a neoplasm, exertional compartment syndrome, tendinitis, fascial defect, musculotendinous junction disruption, popliteal artery entrapment, effort-induced venous thrombosis, and nerve entrapment.

REFERENCES AND SUGGESTED READING

1. Fredericson M, Bergman AG, Hoffman KL, Dillingham MS. Tibial stress reaction in runners: correlation of clinical symptoms and scintigraphy with a new magnetic resonance imaging grading system. *Am J Sports Med.* 1995;23(4):472-481.

2. Gaeta M, Minutoli F, Vinci S, Salamone I, D'Andrea L, Bitto L, Magaudda L, Blandino A. High-resolution CT grading of tibial stress reactions in distance runners. *AJR.* 2006;187(3): 789-793.

3. Reshef N, Guelich DR. Medial tibial stress syndrome. *Clin Sports Med.* 2012;31(2):273-290.

CASE 9

PATIENT PRESENTATION

A 65-year-old woman with sudden onset of severe, non-traumatic left knee pain. The patient is otherwise healthy.

CLINICAL SUSPICION

Insufficiency fracture, formerly (and incorrectly) known as spontaneous osteonecrosis of the knee (SONK).

IMAGING MODALITY OF CHOICE

Radiography to start. If radiographs are negative or show a joint effusion, MRI should be obtained.

BACKGROUND

Stress fractures are fractures that occur as the result of repeated loading of bone with forces less than that required for an acute traumatic fracture. Stress fractures due to abnormal activity (eg, excessive running) on normal bone are called *fatigue fractures*, and stress fractures due to normal activity on abnormal (eg, osteoporotic) bone are called *insufficiency fractures*. Whereas many stress fractures heal without ever being diagnosed, some may progress to complete fractures and subsequent degenerative changes.

FINDINGS

Initial radiographs may be normal. A careful assessment of the contours of the femoral condyles can reveal a subtle impression along the medial femoral condyle (involvement of the lateral femoral condyle and medial tibial plateau is uncommon, and the lateral tibial plateau is rarely affected). Delayed radiographs (Fig. C9.1A) reveal a subchondral lucency that can progress to flattening and collapse of the articular surface, and finally to degenerative changes.

On MRI (Fig. C9.1B,C), there is extensive bone marrow edema, usually located in the medial femoral condyle extending to the intercondylar notch, out of proportion to degenerative changes that may be present in patients in this age group. When located in the tibia, the bone marrow edema can extend to the tibial tuberosity. A hypointense subchondral crescent or linear focus, either of which indicates the presence of a subchondral fracture, is usually present and is best seen on T1-weighted images. Meniscal tears, particularly large radial meniscal root tears, are often present. Cartilage injuries are also commonly seen in these patients.

The presence of a subchondral fracture and/or articular flattening can suggest progression to collapse of the articular surface and subsequent degenerative changes.

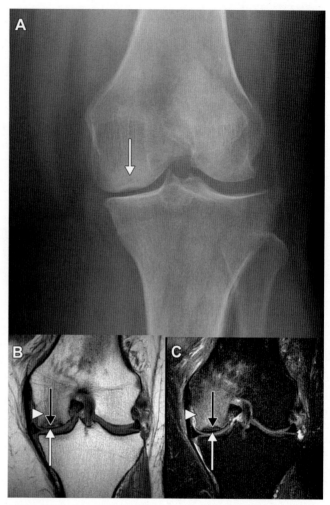

Fig. C9.1 Insufficiency fracture of the medial femoral condyle. (A) Fontal radiograph of the knee reveals lucency and cortical contour deformity of the left medial femoral condyle (white arrow). Fat-sensitive (B) and fluid-sensitive (C) MR sequences reveal a hypointense subchondral crescent (black arrows) and extensive bone marrow edema manifesting as T1 hypointensity (B) and T2 hyperintensity (arrowheads). Note the preserved contour of the medial femoral condyle (white arrow). The radiograph (A) was obtained several months after the MR, by which time articular surface collapse had occurred. Early radiographs were normal.

DIFFERENTIAL DIAGNOSIS

Imaging Differential Diagnosis

Bone marrow signal abnormalities (Fig. C9.2) can be seen with osteoarthritis, osteochondral contusion and fracture, osteochondritis dissecans, and bone infarction.

Clinical Differential Diagnosis

Osteoarthritis, fracture, infection, neuropathy, infarction, and tumor (metastases in this age group).

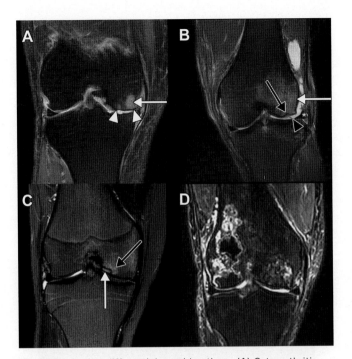

Fig. C9.2 Imaging differential considerations. (A) Osteoarthritis can also result in marrow signal abnormality (white arrow), and can be considered when focal subchondral marrow signal abnormalities are seen in the presence of cartilage defects (between white arrowheads) and osteophytes. The bone marrow edema in osteoarthritis tends to be more focal compared with the diffuse edema seen in insufficiency fractures. (B) Osteochondral injury (contusion or fracture) can be considered in the setting of acute knee pain after trauma and usually has associated findings of cruciate and collateral ligament injury and traumatic meniscal tears (*). This case is from a patient with an anterior cruciate ligament tear (not shown), who also has bone marrow edema (white arrow), a small peeled-off chondral fragment (black arrowhead), and a small cortical step-off of the lateral femoral condyle (black arrow). (C) Osteochondritis dissecans is typically seen in children and young adults, and tends to affect males more frequently than females. The osteochondral lesion is usually on the non-weight-bearing surface of the condyle (white arrow), closer to the notch, and is usually less extensive than in insufficiency fractures. The lesion has a characteristic ovoid appearance with sharply marginated borders. Bone marrow edema is indicated by the black arrow. (D) Infarction (classic osteonecrosis) has a characteristic serpentine configuration and is often bilateral and diffuse. Patients typically have a systemic disorder or a history of steroid use or alcoholism.

REFERENCES AND SUGGESTED READING

1. Gil HC, Levine SM, Zoga AC. MRI findings in the subchondral bone marrow: a discussion of conditions including transient osteoporosis, transient bone marrow edema syndrome, SONK, and shifting bone marrow edema of the knee. *Semin Musculoskelet Radiol.* 2006;10(3):177-186.

2. Moosikasuwan JB, Miller TT, Math K, Schultz E. Shifting bone marrow edema of the knee. *Skeletal Radiol.* 2004;33(7): 380-385.

3. Ramnath RR, Kattapuram SV. MR appearance of SONK-like subchondral abnormalities in the adult knee: SONK redefined. *Skeletal Radiol.* 2004;33(10):575-581. Epub 2004 Jul 13.

4. Sokoloff RM, Farooki S, Resnick D. Spontaneous osteonecrosis of the knee associated with ipsilateral tibial plateau stress fracture: report of two patients and review of the literature. *Skeletal Radiol.* 2001;30(1):53-56.

5. Yamamoto T, Bullough PG. Spontaneous osteonecrosis of the knee: the result of subchondral insufficiency fracture. *J Bone Joint Surg Am.* 2000;82(6):858-866.

CASE 10

PATIENT PRESENTATION

A 65-year-old woman with sudden-onset right hip pain after getting out of bed this morning.

CLINICAL SUSPICION

Insufficiency fracture of the pelvis

IMAGING MODALITY OF CHOICE

Radiographs followed by MRI or bone scintigraphy ("bone scan") as needed for diagnosis or CT if needed for operative planning.

BACKGROUND

Stress fractures can be classified as fatigue (abnormal force on normal bone) or insufficiency (normal force on abnormal bone). In elderly persons, insufficiency fractures of the pelvis and proximal femur are usually due to osteoporosis, but other factors can lead to weakening of bone in this patient population, including radiation therapy, rheumatoid arthritis, prolonged corticosteroid therapy, vitamin D deficiency, and renal failure. Patients with pelvic and proximal femoral insufficiency fractures have prolonged hospital stays and increased morbidity and mortality.

FINDINGS

Radiographs may not depict the fracture plane (Fig. C10.1A), especially in the sacrum and ilium, where overlapping bony structures and bowel contents abound. Parasymphyseal and pubic ramus fractures are usually more readily apparent, and radiographic findings may include cortical disruption, sclerotic lines, and a lucent fracture plane.

Bone scintigraphy (Fig. C10.1B) is sensitive for detection of pelvic insufficiency fractures. The typical butterfly or H-shaped pattern of radiotracer uptake is formed by vertical fractures of the sacral ala joined by a horizontal component. Incomplete H patterns can also be seen, depending on the specific fractures.

CT findings can range from subtle cortical irregularity to irregular sclerosis to obvious fracture planes (Fig. C10.1C). MRI typically reveals bone marrow edema and a fracture plane (Fig. C10.1D,E), although each may be seen in isolation. Associated soft tissue abnormalities are also common, and consist of muscle edema and loss of normal fat planes. Compared with other pelvic and proximal femoral fractures, sacral insufficiency fractures are more likely to present with marrow edema without a clear fracture plane and are less likely to have associated soft tissue changes.

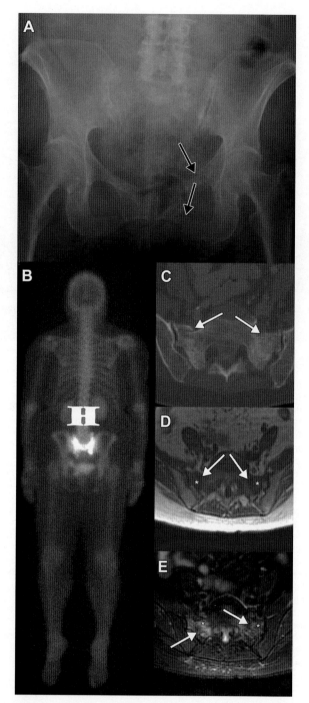

Fig. C10.1 Insufficiency fractures of the pelvis. (A) 65-year-old woman with prior radiation therapy to the pelvis. (A) No sacral fracture was seen on radiography of the pelvis. There are old insufficiency fractures of the inferior and superior pubic rami (black arrows). (B) Tc-99m MDP bone scintigraphy reveals radiotracer uptake in the characteristic H or Honda pattern. (B) CT reveals fracture planes through both sacral ala (white arrows). The underlying bone has a patchy sclerotic appearance due to prior radiation therapy. (D) T1-weighted MR image reveals the fracture planes as hypointense lines (white arrows) superimposed on a background of decreased signal due to marrow edema (*). (E) T2-weighted image reveals the marrow edema (*) as high signal areas. The fracture planes (white arrows) can also be seen. (Case courtesy of Dr John E. Madewell, MD Anderson Cancer Center.)

DIFFERENTIAL DIAGNOSIS

Imaging Differential Diagnosis

The fracture plane may not always be visible on MRI, and the bone marrow edema can be similar to that seen with neoplasm and osteomyelitis. CT can help differentiate these entities from fracture. In a fracture, the trabeculae on either side of the fracture plane are intact, and are not destroyed as in tumor or infection.

Clinical Differential Diagnosis

Avascular necrosis of the femoral head, insufficiency fracture elsewhere in the pelvis, and neoplasm with or without pathological fracture can have similar clinical presentations.

REFERENCES AND SUGGESTED READING

1. Cabarrus MC, Ambekar A, Lu Y, Link TM. MRI and CT of insufficiency fractures of the pelvis and the proximal femur. *AJR*. 2008;191(4):995-1001.
2. Peh WC, Khong PL, Yin Y, et al. Imaging of pelvic insufficiency fractures. *RadioGraphics*. 1996;16(2):335-348.

CASE 11

PATIENT PRESENTATION

A 25-year-old man with suspected splinter in hand.

CLINICAL SUSPICION

Soft tissue foreign object

IMAGING MODALITY OF CHOICE

In the extremities, ultrasound should be used as the initial imaging modality of choice for detection of foreign objects. High frequency (> 7.5 MHz) linear-array transducers are used. Radiography is limited to visualization of radiopaque foreign objects such as metal and glass.

FINDINGS

All soft tissue foreign objects are hyperechoic on ultrasound and will usually have posterior acoustic shadowing (Fig. C11.1A). A surrounding hypoechoic halo of granulation tissue, edema, or hemorrhage can assist in detection of smaller foreign objects. Ultrasound can also be used to identify complications such as abscess formation and vascular injury.

Plastic and wooden foreign objects can be subtle or invisible on radiographs. Secondary signs of laceration such as a skin defect, soft tissue swelling, and subcutaneous gas should be sought to narrow the area of investigation. Radiography can be used to detect metal and glass. The former is well demonstrated on radiographs (Fig. C11.1B,C). The radiopacity of glass is variable and depends on its density and effective atomic number (ie, its ability to attenuate x-ray beams) compared with those of the surrounding soft tissues (Fig. C11.1D). The lead content of glass is often incorrectly cited as the primary factor determining visibility on radiographs.

MRI does not reliably depict most foreign objects. Metallic objects (Fig. C11.1E) can be detected by noting the artifacts associated with their presence, namely loss of signal, geometric distortion, and failure of fat suppression.

Regardless of the imaging modality used, complications of soft tissue foreign objects should be actively investigated. These include vascular injury, infection, and bone injury.

DIFFERENTIAL DIAGNOSIS

Imaging Differential Diagnosis

In the absence of clinical information, avulsion fragments (Fig. C11.2A) and soft tissue calcifications (Fig. C11.2B) can mimic foreign objects.

Clinical Differential Diagnosis

None

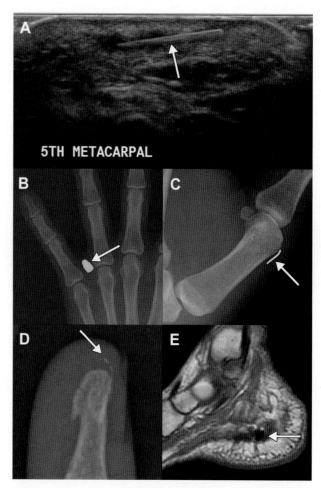

Fig. C11.1 Gallery of soft tissue foreign objects. (A) Wooden splinter on ultrasound of the hand. (B) Bullet. (C) Wire. (D) Two small glass fragments. (E) Metallic clip on a T1-weighted sagittal image of the ankle manifests as loss of signal.

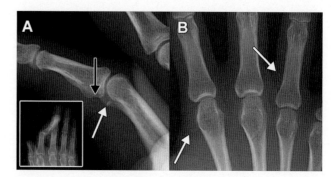

Fig. C11.2 Differential considerations. (A) Avulsion fragment (white arrow) from prior trauma (inset). A donor site (black arrow) for the fragment is identified in the volar base of the middle phalanx. (B) Soft tissue calcifications (white arrows) in a patient with calcinosis cutis.

REFERENCES AND SUGGESTED READING

1. Horton LK, Jacobson JA, Powell A, Fessell DP, Hayes CW. Sonography and radiography of soft-tissue foreign bodies. *AJR.* 2001;176(5):1155-1159.

CASE 12

PATIENT PRESENTATION

A 35-year-old man with wrist pain after a fall on an outstretched hand. On physical examination, there is tenderness over the anatomic snuffbox.

CLINICAL SUSPICION

Scaphoid fracture

IMAGING MODALITY OF CHOICE

Strart with 4-view wrist radiography. Standard frontal and lateral radiographs of the wrist are often inadequate for diagnosis of scaphoid fractures, and specialized views are used (Fig. C12.1). The choice of these views, however, varies according to local preferences.

The blood supply of the scaphoid (Fig. C12.2) leaves it susceptible to avascular necrosis and nonunion after fracture. The risk of avascular necrosis varies according to the location of the fracture. Fractures of the middle third of the scaphoid are associated with avascular necrosis in about one-third of cases, whereas fractures of the proximal fifth are associated with avascular necrosis in nearly all cases.

This concern results in a rather aggressive management approach: In patients with normal radiographs in whom a scaphoid fracture is suspected, the wrist is either further assessed with noncontrast MRI or immobilized with a cast, and radiography is repeated in 10 to 14 days. The choice depends on patient factors (age, hand dominance, activity level, insurance), as well as local preferences and availability of equipment.

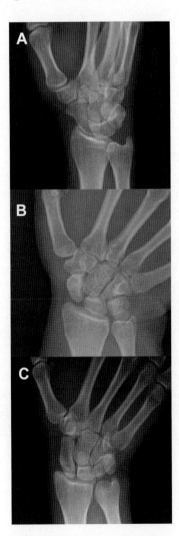

Fig. C12.1 Some of the additional views used for diagnosis of scaphoid fractures. (A) Semipronated view: a 45° ulnar oblique posteroanterior projection (to detect oblique sulcal, waist, and tubercle fractures). (B) Ulnar-deviated posteroanterior view (to detect proximal pole fractures). (C) Ziter's "banana" view (to detect fractures of the waist of the scaphoid).

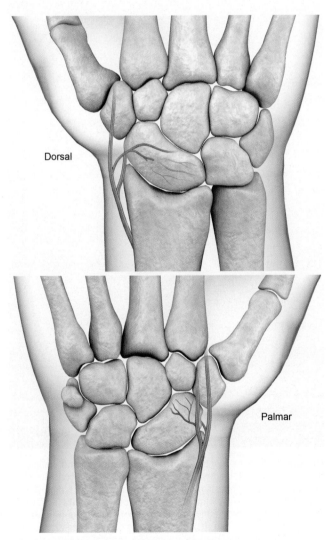

Fig. C12.2 The vascular supply of the scaphoid is distal-to-proximal from two sources: a group of vessels entering the dorsal aspect of the distal pole, and a group of vessels entering the palmar aspect of the distal pole. The dorsal group supplies the proximal two-thirds of the bone, and the palmar group contributes largely to the vascularity of the distal one-third.

FINDINGS

Scaphoid fractures can be subtle on radiography. A fracture plane with separated fragments (Fig. C12.3A) is easy to detect, but a lucent line with at least one disrupted cortex (Fig. C12.3B) is sufficient for diagnosis.

Secondary signs can be sought for detection of scaphoid fractures. The scaphoid fat stripe (fat between the radial collateral ligament and the abductor pollicis longus and extensor pollicis brevis tendons) may be effaced in scaphoid fractures. It must be noted that it is not visualized in about 10% of normal subjects and may be obscured if the wrist is radially deviated. A normal fat stripe, however, virtually excludes a scaphoid fracture.

CT can be obtained if there is continued concern for fracture in the setting of normal radiographs. Axial images and sagittal and coronal reformations should be inspected (Fig. C12.3C). MRI (Fig. C12.3D) characteristically reveals a hypointense line on all pulse sequences with surrounding marrow edema (low signal on T1-weighted and high signal on T2-weighted images).

Delayed diagnosis and treatment can lead to avascular necrosis (Fig. C12.3E), which manifests radiographically as collapse and increased sclerosis of the devitalized segment.

DIFFERENTIAL DIAGNOSIS

Imaging Differential Diagnosis

On radiographs, normal variations in the shape of the scaphoid and differences in angulation can mimic a fracture. The interested reader is referred to Dr Keats' wonderful atlas of normal variants. On MRI, a bone contusion can be mistaken for a fracture and can result in overdiagnosis and overtreatment. A bone contusion presents as marrow edema alone; a fracture presents as bone marrow edema plus a line of low signal intensity on all pulse sequences.

Clinical Differential Diagnosis

In the setting of acute trauma, differential considerations include other fractures (distal radius, carpal bone, etc), bone contusion, and ligamentous injury.

REFERENCES AND SUGGESTED READING

1. American College of Radiology. Expert panel on musculoskeletal imaging. ACR Appropriateness Criteria. In: Reston VA, ed. Acute hand and wrist trauma. Philadelphia: American College of Radiology; 2001:1-7.

2. Duckworth AD, Ring D, McQueen MM. Assessment of the suspected fracture of the scaphoid. *J Bone Joint Surg Br.* 2011;93(6):713-719.

3. Keats TE, Anderson MW. *Atlas of Normal Roentgen Variants That May Simulate Disease.* 8th ed. Mosby; 2004:603-612.

4. Mann FA, Wilson AJ, Gilula LA. Radiographic evaluation of the wrist: what does the hand surgeon want to know? *Radiology.* 1992;184(1):15-24.

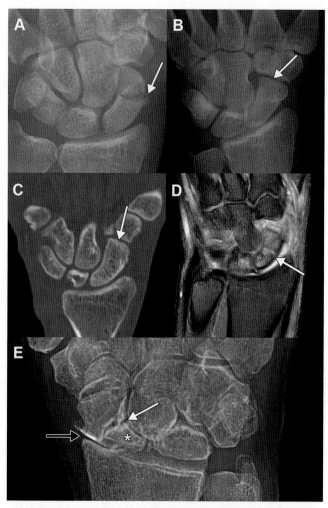

Fig. C12.3 Various scaphoid fractures. (A) Angulated and displaced fracture of the scaphoid waist. A scaphoid fracture is considered unstable if the fragments are displaced by more than 1 mm, are angulated, or are associated with ligamentous instability (eg, scapholunate dissociation). (B) Distal pole fracture with intra-articular extension (white arrow). (C) Distal pole fracture (white arrow) seen on CT. (D) Fluid-sensitive MR image of a scaphoid waist fracture showing the fracture plane (white arrow), as well as bone marrow edema in the scaphoid, lunate, and hamate. (E) Old scaphoid fracture (white arrow), with nonunion and secondary osteoarthritis (black arrow). Avascular necrosis of the proximal fragment (*) manifests radiographically as collapse and increased sclerosis.

CASE 13

PATIENT PRESENTATION

A 10-year-old boy, a restrained passenger involved in a low-speed motor vehicle collision, presented to an outside emergency department. Radiographs of the cervical spine were obtained (Fig. C13.1), and the patient was referred for evaluation of cervical spine injury.

CLINICAL SUSPICION

Pseudosubluxation

IMAGING MODALITY OF CHOICE

Radiography

FINDINGS

Pseudosubluxation refers to an anatomic variant in children due to increased ligamentous laxity, causing apparent anterior malalignment of the C2 vertebral body relative to the C3 vertebral body on lateral radiographs. This apparent malalignment may be accentuated with flexion.

Evaluation of cervical alignment on lateral radiographs involves assessment of at least 3 lines (Fig. C13.2A): the anterior and posterior spinal lines and the spinolaminar line. Each point on the spinolaminar line is formed by the shadows of both laminae joining the base of the spinous

process. A diagnosis of pseudosubluxation can be considered when the spinolaminar line of C1-C3 is normal (Fig. C13.2B,C).

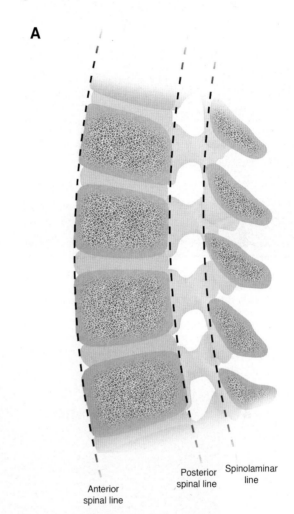

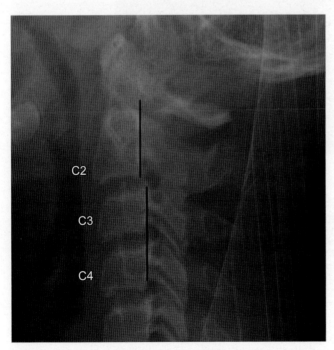

Fig. C13.1 Pseudosubluxation. Lateral radiograph of the cervical spine reveals apparent anterior subluxation of C2 on C3, which is appreciated by comparing a line drawn along the posterior margins of C3 and C4 to a line drawn along the posterior margin of C2.

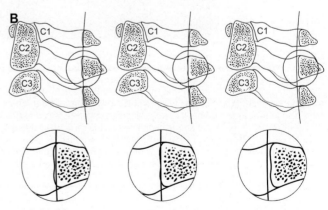

Fig. C13.2 The cervical lines and normal variation. (A) The three spinal lines. (B) The spinolaminar line of C1, C2, and C3 is normal if it (1) passes through, or just behind the anterior cortex of the posterior arch of C2; (2) touches the anterior aspect of the cortex of the posterior arch of C2; or (3) comes within 1 mm of the anterior cortex of the posterior arch of C2. (*continued*)

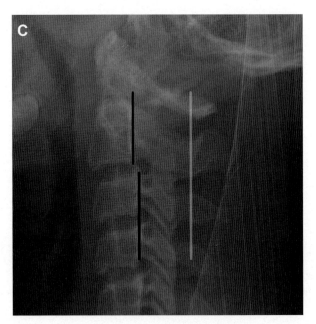

Fig. C13.2 (*continued*) (C) Same image as Fig. C13.1, but with the spinolaminar line of C1-C3 (white line) showing normal alignment. Pseudosubluxation has been attributed to the ligamentous laxity and the more horizontal orientation of the facet joints in children.

DIFFERENTIAL DIAGNOSIS

Imaging Differential Diagnosis

Differentiating pseudosubluxation from true subluxation due to cervical spine injury can be difficult. The presence of soft tissue swelling can suggest true subluxation; however, this can be difficult to assess in younger children, especially when images are obtained in flexion. CT or MRI can be obtained in challenging cases.

This case highlights the importance of being aware of anatomic variants in order to avoid overdiagnosis and overtreatment. The term *anatomic variant* is favored over *normal variant* and *congenital variant* since the former suggests that the finding is of no clinical significance and the latter suggests *in utero* development of the finding. Examples of common and well-known anatomic variants are shown in Fig. C13.3.

Clinical Differential Diagnosis

Fracture, ligamentous injury

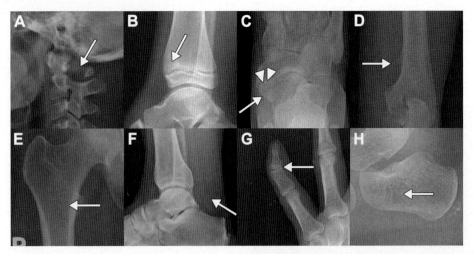

Fig. C13.3 Common and well-known anatomic variants. (A) Congenital absence of the C1 laminae (white arrow). Isolated cases may be asymptomatic; however, intermittent quadriparesis has been reported. In addition, absence of the posterior arch may be associated with atlantoaxial instability, predisposing the patient to osteoarthritis later in life. (Case used with permission from Dr Jason Tsai, Children's National Medical Center, Washington, DC.) (B) Kump's hump (named after the radiologist Warren Kump) is an undulation of the anteromedial aspect of the distal tibial physis. It represents the site of first closure of the physis and should not be mistaken for a fracture. (C) Type II accessory navicular (white arrow) in the foot, also known as the prehallux, is a triangular or heart-shaped ossicle that measures from 2 to 12 mm. It arises from the secondary ossification center of the navicular bone and is connected to the navicular tuberosity by fibrocartilage or hyaline cartilage. Occasionally degenerative changes develop between the accessory navicular and the navicular, as seen here (white arrowheads, cystic changes). (D) The supracondylar process ("avian spur") of the humerus is a bony projection from the anteromedial aspect of the distal humeral diaphysis that can be shaped as a spine or a tubercle. It is often connected to the medial epicondyle by a fibrous band (ligament of Struthers), creating a foramen that transmits the median nerve and brachial artery. Impingement of these structures can occur, leading to ischemia or median nerve neuropathy. (E) Trabecular bars are struts of normal trabecular bone at right angles to the long axis of the diaphysis and are more apparent in patients with osteoporosis. They are most commonly seen in the intertrochanteric region of the femur and can give the appearance of a calcified chondroid matrix on frontal radiographs. Inspection of the lateral radiograph reveals trabecular bars perpendicular to the long axis of the bone. (F) Accessory muscle in the Kager's fat pad (white arrow). This is most commonly an accessory soleus muscle, which descends anterior or anteromedial to the Achilles tendon. Increased mass of the muscle may be associated with exertional pain, possibly related to increasedfascial pressure, inadequate blood supply, or compression of the adjacent posterior tibial nerve. (G) Brachymesophalangia (short middle finger) is the most common hereditary anomaly of the middle phalanges and is more common in the small finger (brachymesophalangia-5). About two-thirds of patients with Down syndrome have brachymesophalangia. Clinodactyly ("bent finger"), a general term for radioulnar deviation of the finger, is most commonly caused by brachymesophalangia. (H) Pseudolesion of the calcaneus (white arrow), a triangle of relative lucency bounded by the normal trabeculae of the calcaneus, can be mistaken for a lesion.

REFERENCES AND SUGGESTED READING

1. Keats TE, Anderson MW. *Atlas of Normal Roentgen Variants That May Simulate Disease*. 8th ed. Philadelphia, PA: Mosby; 2004.

2. Lustrin ES, Karakas SP, Ortiz AO, et al. Pediatric cervical spine: normal anatomy, variants, and trauma. *RadioGraphics*. 2003;23(3):539-560.

3. McIntosh A, Pollock AN. Pseudosubluxation. *Pediatr Emerg Care*. 2010;26(9):691-692.

4. Swischuk LE. Anterior displacement of C2 in children: physiologic or pathologic. *Radiology*. 1977;122(3):759-763.

CASE 14

PATIENT PRESENTATION

A 25-year-old man with anterior knee pain and swelling following blunt trauma.

CLINICAL SUSPICION

Patellar fracture

IMAGING MODALITY OF CHOICE

Four-view radiography of the knee to include anteroposterior, lateral, Merchant, and oblique views. Fractures of the margins of the patella can be occult on anteroposterior views. CT and MRI are reserved for problem solving.

FINDINGS

Patellar fracture classification is descriptive (Fig. C14.1A). Transverse fractures and fractures of the upper and lower poles are best seen on the lateral view (Fig. C14.1B,C). Vertical fractures are usually nondisplaced and often require axial (sunrise or Merchant) views for detection. Osteochondral fractures are associated with acute dislocation of the patella and are typically located on the medial patellar facet. Osteochondral fractures are best seen on axial or internal oblique radiographs, but may require CT or MRI for complete assessment.

DIFFERENTIAL DIAGNOSIS

Imaging Differential Diagnosis

Bipartite or multipartite patella (Fig. C14.2A-D), both anatomic variants, can simulate a marginal fracture of the patella. Because the individual components of a bipartite or multipartite patella mature separately, they will not fit together like pieces in a jigsaw puzzle, whereas the components of a patellar fracture will.

A vascular channel through the patella (Fig. C14.2E) can simulate a vertical fracture on axial views. Finally, the dorsal defect of the patella (Fig. C14.2F), an anatomical variant present in about 1% of the population, can simulate an osteochondral fracture on radiographs. It is typically a large (1-2 cm), round lucency located at the superolateral aspect of the patella. MRI will usually (but not always) reveal intact articular cartilage over the defect (Fig. C14.2F, inset). The defect itself is low to intermediate in signal intensity on T1- and T2-weighted images.

Clinical Differential Diagnosis

Patellar tendon rupture, quadriceps tendon rupture (Fig. C14.2G,H), and bone contusion.

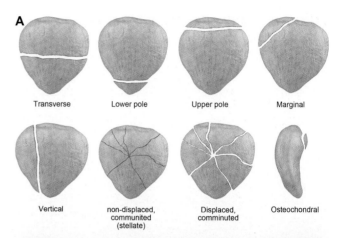

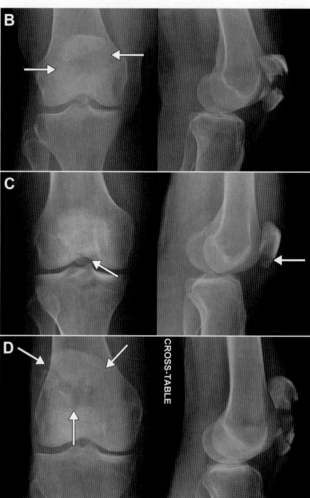

Fig. C14.1 Patellar fractures. (A) Classification scheme. (B) Transverse patellar fracture. (C) Lower pole fracture. (D) Comminuted fracture.

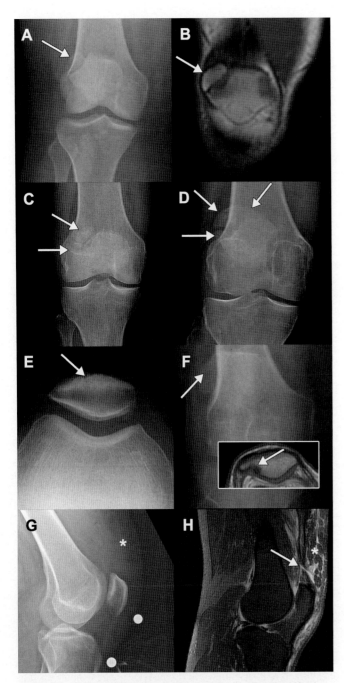

Fig. C14.2 Imaging and clinical differential considerations for patellar fracture. (A) Bipartite patella on radiography. (B) MR image of a bipartite patella. (C) Tripartite patella. (D) Multipartite patella. (E) Vascular channel simulating a vertical fracture. (F) Dorsal defect of the patella. (G,H) Partial quadriceps tendon rupture on a lateral radiograph and fluid-sensitive sagittal MR image. The radiograph reveals anterior soft tissue swelling (*), which is seen on the MRI as subcutaneous T2 hyperintensity. The MRI also shows the tear in the quadriceps tendon (white arrow).

REFERENCES AND SUGGESTED READING

1. Capps GW, Hayes CW. Easily missed injuries around the knee. *RadioGraphics.* 1994;14(6):1191-1210.
2. Johnson JF, Brogdon BG. Dorsal effect of the patella: incidence and distribution. *AJR.* 1982;139(2):339-340.

CASE 15

PATIENT PRESENTATION

A 35-year-old man presents with severe knee pain and in-ability to bear weight after being hit by a car. He has a large knee joint effusion and is diffusely tender about the lateral aspect of the knee.

CLINICAL SUSPICION

Tibial plateau fracture

IMAGING MODALITY OF CHOICE

Radiographs of the knee (Fig. C15.1) are preferred for initial evaluation. Standard anteroposterior and lateral radiographs, however, are suboptimal for assessment of tibial plateau frac-tures. Subtle tibial plateau fractures may be better depicted on internal oblique views, and lipohemarthrosis (blood and fat in a joint effusion) is best seen on a cross-table lateral view. Radiography may still underestimate the extent of bony injury, and further evaluation with CT is often helpful. MRI, which is even more sensitive for detection of fractures, can also depict injuries to menisci, ligaments, and cartilage. The routine use of MRI in assessment of tibial plateau fractures, however, is controversial because of unresolved questions about the clinical significance of preoperative diagnosis of meniscal and ligamentous injuries.

BACKGROUND

Tibial plateau fractures are common knee injuries and often require surgical management. A high prevalence of associ-ated intra-articular soft tissue injuries is also reported. The Schatzker classification system (Fig. C15.2) is commonly used to assess the initial injury, plan the surgical approach, and predict prognosis of the fracture. Higher grades of injury generally imply increasing severity of injury, worse prognosis, and higher incidence of soft tissue injury. The primary morbidity associated with tibial plateau fractures is irreversible damage to articular cartilage and menisci and subsequent development of premature osteoarthritis and long-term disability.

FINDINGS

Radiographs may reveal cortical discontinuity, which is sometimes depicted only on oblique views. Lipohemarthro-sis is a specific sign of intra-articular fracture and manifests radiographically as layering of fat (from bone marrow) and blood within the joint cavity on a cross-table lateral view.

Because appropriate Schatzker classification can be critical to surgical planning, CT is often called upon to iden-tify radiographically occult fractures and better character-ize complex fractures. CT also more accurately depicts the degree of fragment depression.

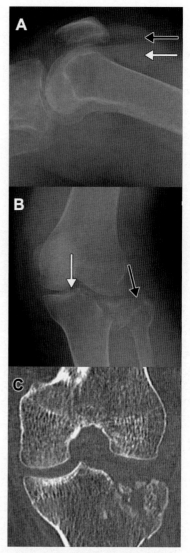

Fig. C15.1 Tibial plateau fractures. (A) Cross-table lateral view of the knee reveals lipohemarthrosis, with fat (black arrow) and blood (white arrow), indicative of an intra-articular fracture. (B) Oblique view reveals a comminuted and depressed fracture of the lateral tibial plateau. The lateral tibial plateau fragment is depressed and displaced laterally. Note subtle extension of the fracture plane to the medial tibial plateau (white arrow) consistent with a Schatzker type IV fracture. Also note the associated fibular head fracture (black arrow). (C) Coronal CT image in another patient shows a comminuted cleavage fracture of the lateral tibial plateau with depression, consistent with a Schatzker type II fracture.

DIFFERENTIAL DIAGNOSIS

Imaging Differential Diagnosis

None

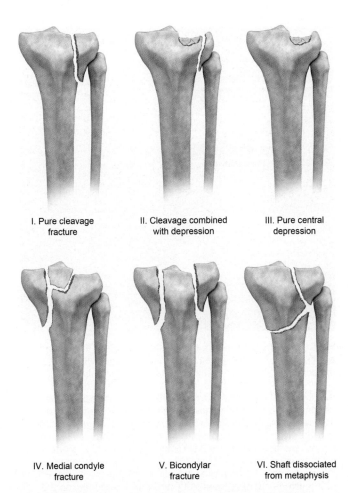

I. Pure cleavage
fracture

II. Cleavage combined
with depression

III. Pure central
depression

IV. Medial condyle
fracture

V. Bicondylar
fracture

VI. Shaft dissociated
from metaphysis

Fig. C15.2 Schatzker classification of tibial plateau fractures. Type I fractures have a single fracture plane across the lateral tibial plateau and condyle. Type II fractures have combined split and compression components. Type III fractures only have a compression component. In type IV fractures, the medial condyle is either split off as a wedge (type A, illustrated in this figure) or crumbled and depressed (type B). Type V fractures are bicondylar without disruption of the metaphysis. Type VI fractures are characterized by a fracture plane that dissociates the metaphysis from the diaphysis. One or both condyles may also be involved. Note that the original report by Schatzker does not define cutoff values for what constitutes depression and that the classification scheme does not depend on the amount of displacement or depression.

Clinical Differential Diagnosis

Posttraumatic knee joint effusions may be attributed to either intra-articular fracture and associated hemarthrosis or internal derangement such as ligamentous or meniscal injury. Intra-articular fractures may affect the tibia, femur, or patella and are often associated with lipohemarthrosis. Cruciate ligament injury (more commonly anterior cruciate ligament) or meniscal tears may also occur in the setting of trauma and may result in joint effusion and inability to bear weight. Typically, joint effusions associated with intra-articular fractures or cruciate ligament injury are larger than those seen with meniscal pathology.

REFERENCES AND SUGGESTED READING

1. Mui LW, Engelsohn E, Umans H. Comparison of CT and MRI in patients with tibial plateau fracture: can CT findings predict ligament tear or meniscal injury? *Skeletal Radiol.* 2007;36: 145-151.

2. Mustonen AO, Koivikko MP, Kiuru MJ, Salo J, Koskinen SK. Postoperative MDCT of tibial plateau fractures. *AJR.* 2009; 193:1354-1360.

3. Schatzker J, McBroom R, Bruce D. The tibial plateau fracture: the Toronto experience 1968–1975. *Clin Orthop Relat Res.* 1979;138:94-104.

CASE 16

PATIENT PRESENTATION

A 30-year-old man presents to the emergency department with back and heel pain after jumping from a second-story window.

CLINICAL SUSPICION

Calcaneus fracture

IMAGING MODALITY OF CHOICE

Four views of the foot, including anteroposterior, oblique, lateral, and axial (Harris) views. Radiographs are best used as a screening tool, with thin slice CT reserved for suspected radiographically occult fracture and for surgical planning.

BACKGROUND

The calcaneus is a complex bone with articular facets with the talus superiorly and an articulation with the cuboid anteriorly. Calcaneal fractures account for the majority of tarsal injuries and typically occur as a result of a fall from a height (axial loading). The majority of calcaneal fractures are intra-articular, and open reduction is necessary in most calcaneal fractures. Because the axial load needed to cause a calcaneal fracture is also transmitted proximally and cephalad, it is important to seek out associated fractures of the tibia, femur, and spine, by either physical examination or imaging. About 10% of patients with calcaneal fractures have associated vertebral body compression fractures, most commonly in the thoracolumbar region.

FINDINGS

Radiographs may reveal a lucent line representing the fracture plane, loss of height in the central portion of the calcaneus, a more vertical orientation of the articular surfaces of the calcaneus, a decrease in Böhler's angle (Fig. C16.1A), and an increase in the critical angle of Gissane (Fig. C16.1A).

Approximately 25% to 30% of calcaneal fractures are extra-articular and do not extend to the many articular facets of the calcaneus. Frontal and lateral radiographs may be normal with extra-articular fractures. Extra-articular fractures are classified as anterior process fractures, mid-calcaneal fractures, and fractures of the posterior calcaneus.

Several classification systems exist for intra-articular calcaneal fractures (Fig. C16.2), including the Hannover, Sanders, Essex-Lopresti, and Crosby classification

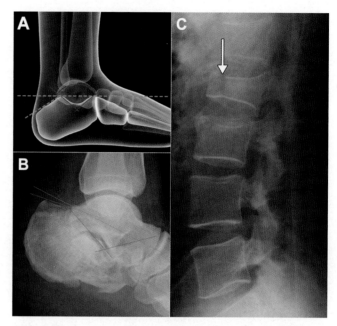

Fig. C16.1 (A) Diagram of the ankle shows Böhler's and Gissane's angles. Böhler's angle (green) is formed by a line connecting the posterior tuberosity of the calcaneus and the apex of the posterior facet of the calcaneus and a line between the apex of the posterior facet and the apex of the anterior process of the calcaneus. Normal values have been reported between 20° and 45° depending on the source. A decrease in the angle indicates that the weight-bearing posterior facet of the calcaneus has collapsed. Gissane's angle (red) is formed by two cortical struts. One extends along the lateral border of the posterior facet, and the other extends anterior to the beak of the calcaneus. Normal values have been reported between 100° and 145° depending on the source. (B) Lateral radiograph of the ankle shows a comminuted intra-articular fracture through the body of the calcaneus. Note the loss of height in the central portion of the calcaneus, flattening of Böhler's angle to about 10°, and no widening of Gissane's angle (about 120° in this case). (C) Lateral radiograph of the spine shows an acute compression fracture of the second lumbar vertebral body (white arrow) in a patient with bilateral calcaneal fractures.

schemes. No single classification scheme includes all types of calcaneal fractures. The Sanders classification (Table C16.1), the most commonly used system, is based on the number of fracture planes extending through the articular surface of the posterior subtalar joint on coronal CT reformations.

In general, extra-articular and intra-articular Sanders Type I fractures are managed nonsurgically. Displaced intra-articular fractures (Sanders Types II-IV) are managed with open reduction and internal fixation within the first 3 weeks after injury.

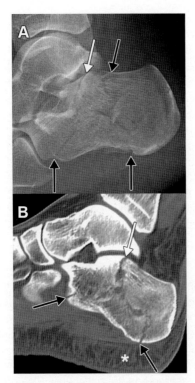

Fig. C16.2 Comminuted intra-articular calcaneal fracture in a 33-year-old man after a motorcycle accident. (A) Lateral radiograph of the ankle shows a comminuted calcaneal fracture with extension of a fracture plane to the posterior facet (white arrow), making this an intra-articular fracture. Additional fractures are annotated (black arrows). The fracture fragments are not significantly displaced, consistent with a Sanders Type I fracture. Note preservation of Böhler's angle. (B) Sagittal CT image better delineates the fracture planes and clearly shows extension of one to the posterior facet (white arrow). Increased attenuation of the subcutaneous fat (*) indicates edema in the plantar soft tissues. Because the fracture fragments were not significantly displaced, this patient was treated conservatively with immobilization.

Table C16.1 Sanders Classification of Intra-Articular Fractures

Type I	Nondisplaced (<2 mm displacement)
Type II	Single displaced fracture plane
Type III	Two displaced fracture planes
Type IV	Highly comminuted

DIFFERENTIAL DIAGNOSIS

Imaging Differential Diagnosis

A pathologic fracture of the calcaneus can have a similar appearance but will be accompanied by disruption of trabeculae surrounding the fracture.

Clinical Differential Diagnosis

Other ankle fractures can have a similar clinical presentation.

REFERENCES AND SUGGESTED READING

1. Badillo K, Pacheco JA, Padua SO, Gomez AA, Colon E, Vidal JA. Multidetector CT evaluation of calcaneal fractures. *RadioGraphics*. 2011;31:81-92.

2. Barei DP, Bellabarba C, Sangeorzan BJ, Benirschke SK. Fractures of the calcaneus. *Orthop Clin North Am*. 2002; 33:263-285.

3. Daftary A, Haims AH, Baumgaertner MR. Fractures of the calcaneus: a review with emphasis on CT. *RadioGraphics*. 2005;25:1215-1226.

4. Matherne TH, Tivorsak T, Monu JU. Calcaneal fractures: what the surgeon needs to know. *Curr Probl Diagn Radiol*. 2007;36:1-10.

CASE 17

PATIENT PRESENTATION

A 50-year-old man presents with persistent shoulder pain and weakness despite symptomatic treatment. The pain is worse with overhead activities and persists at night.

CLINICAL SUSPICION

Acute rotator cuff tear

IMAGING MODALITY OF CHOICE

Radiography to be followed by MRI or ultrasound as needed. External impingement on the rotator cuff (read further) can be assessed on supraspinatus outlet views of the shoulder (Fig. C17.1). MR arthrography is not generally used for rotator cuff pathology, but is reserved for special cases (inconclusive standard MR, some preoperative cases, and suspected labral tears).

BACKGROUND

The rotator cuff, composed of 4 muscles and their tendons (Fig. C17.2A), allows for shoulder movement and stability. Rotator cuff disease is one of the most common musculoskeletal disorders, with an incidence that increases with age. Not all rotator cuff tears, however, are associated with symptoms, with about 20% of subjects older than 50 years of age and as many as 50% of subjects older than 80 years of age having asymptomatic, full-thickness rotator cuff tears.

Unlike the knee, physical examination of the shoulder can be unreliable, making MRI a vital part of patient assessment. In addition, young patients with rotator cuff tears that are not repaired early tend to have poor functional outcomes, making early and accurate diagnosis essential.

External (subacromial) impingement is caused by compression of the rotator cuff, the long head of the biceps tendon, and/or the subacromial-subdeltoid bursa between the humeral head and the coracoacromial arch and is thought to contribute to rotator cuff tears (Fig. C17.2B-E).

FINDINGS

The supraspinatus outlet view is assessed for acromial shape, subacromial excrescences, and inferior osteophytes at the acromioclavicular joint. Curved and especially hooked acromion shapes have been associated with external impingement.

The density and contour of the supraspinatus muscle can also be assessed on the outlet view. The normal supraspinatus muscle has homogeneous soft-tissue density and a bulging superior contour (Fig. C17.1B). Findings suggestive

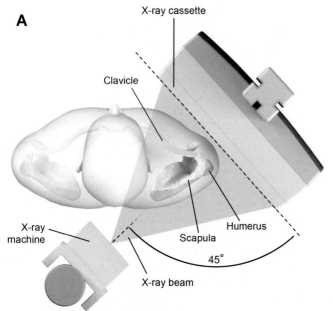

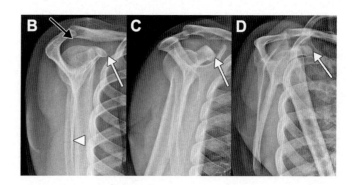

Fig. C17.1 The supraspinatus outlet view. (A) The radiograph is typically taken in a standing patient with her arm resting at her side. The patient is rotated until the body of the scapula is perpendicular to the radiographic plate. The shoulder is placed directly against the radiographic plate and the x-ray beam is directed posteroanteriorly and angled 10° to 15° caudally. (B) On an appropriately positioned radiograph, the scapular body should be seen in profile as a narrow stripe (white arrowhead); the coracoid process (white arrow) should project anteriorly; the supraspinatus fossa and scapular body should form a Y shape; and a clear space (the supraspinatus outlet) should exist between the acromion and the humeral head. The normal supraspinatus muscle should have a bulging superior contour (black arrow). A widened scapular body indicates suboptimal rotation of the patient. (C) If the coracoid process (white arrow) projects over the widened scapular body, the patient was rotated too far anteriorly. (D) If the coracoid process (white arrow) projects anterior to the widened scapular body, the patient was rotated too far posteriorly.

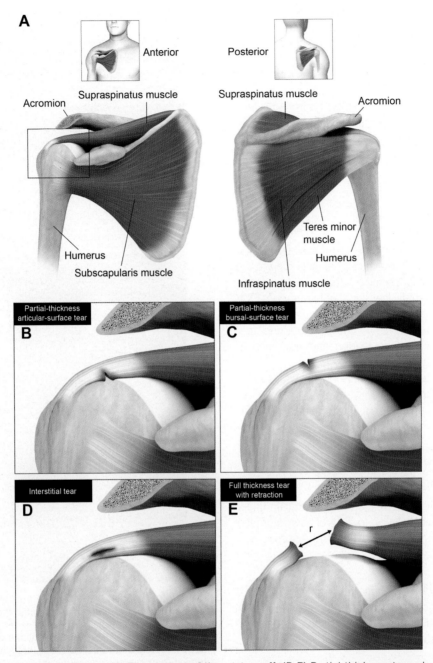

Fig. C17.2 Rotator cuff and rotator cuff tears. (A) The anatomy of the rotator cuff. (B-E) Partial-thickness tears do not extend through the whole thickness of the tendon and are classified as articular-surface (B), bursal-surface (C), and interstitial (D) tears. Low-grade partial thickness tears involve less than 50% of the tendon, moderate-grade partial thickness tears involve about 50% of the tendon thickness, and high-grade partial thickness tears involve more than 50% of the tendon thickness. (E) Full-thickness tears extend from the bursal surface to the articular surface of the tendon and can be complete (involving the whole width of the tendon) or incomplete. Full-thickness tears that involve more than one tendon are called massive tears. The degree of tendon retraction (r) is quantified by how far the torn tendon is from its normal attachment.

of a chronic tear include a flattened or ill-defined superior contour and a heterogeneous appearance of the muscle due to low-density fat infiltration.

Cephalad migration of the humeral head can be seen in complete supraspinatus tears due to the unopposed action of the deltoid muscle. This results in narrowing of the acromiohumeral distance, which can also be appreciated on anteroposterior radiographs of the shoulder. Repetitive contact between the humeral head and the acromion ensues, resulting in sclerosis, subchondral cysts, and osteolysis at the greater tuberosity and inferolateral aspect of the acromion.

Ultrasound and MRI can provide direct evidence of tendon tears (Fig. C17.3). Tears are classified as full-thickness or partial-thickness depending on how much of the tendon is torn.

On ultrasound (Fig. C17.3A,B), full-thickness rotator cuff tears are usually fluid-filled hypoechoic or anechoic defects. This fluid can result in increased through-transmission, which accentuates the appearance of the underlying cartilage, creating the "cartilage interface" or "double cortex" (cartilage plus cortex) sign. Partial-thickness tears have a similar appearance but involve only the bursal or articular surface.

Real-time compression over the defect will displace the fluid and lead to a loss of the normally convex shape of the hyperechoic peribursal fat.

On fluid-sensitive MR sequences (Fig. C17.3C,D), partial-thickness tears appear as increased signal extending to the articular and/or bursal surfaces of the rotator cuff that stands out in contrast to the normally low signal of the tendon. Full-thickness rotator cuff tears extend from the glenohumeral joint to the subacromial bursa. A complete tendon tear involves the entire width of the tendon and may lead to muscle atrophy and fatty infiltration.

CT arthrography (Fig. C17.3E,F) is not in widespread use due to the requirement for intra-articular injection of contrast, but provides an alternative when MRI or ultrasound is not possible.

DIFFERENTIAL DIAGNOSIS

Imaging Differential Diagnosis

Imaging findings have to be correlated with clinical findings, especially in older patients, as up to 40% of asymptomatic controls over 50 years of age old have full-thickness rotator cuff tears.

Clinical Differential Diagnosis

- Tendinosis: Mucoid degeneration of a tendon without inflammation. On MRI and ultrasound, the tendon is thickened and heterogeneous without a discrete defect.

- Calcific tendinitis (Fig. C17.4A,B): Deposition of calcium hydroxyapatite within the tendon. Radiographs will reveal calcific deposits in the tendon or adjacent bursa. Ultrasound shows discrete, linear hyperechoic foci within the tendon with posterior acoustic shadowing.

- Adhesive capsulitis (Fig. C17.4C,D): Clinical syndrome of shoulder pain at rest and with movement that is caused by progressive thickening, fibrosis, and retraction of the joint capsule.

- Subacromial/subdeltoid bursitis: Fluid superficial to the supraspinatus tendon.

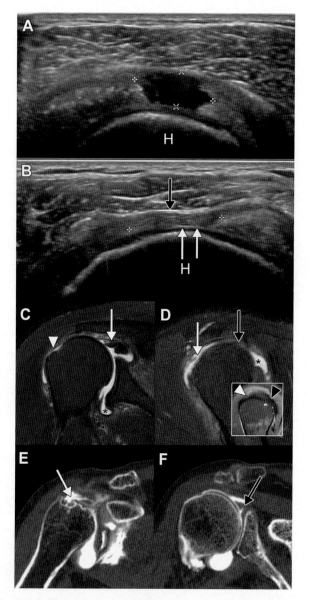

Fig. C17.3 Ultrasound, MRI, and CT findings in rotator cuff tear. (A) Transverse ultrasound image through the rotator cuff reveals a full-thickness tear of the supraspinatus tendon (between cursors) filled with fluid. (B) Transverse ultrasound image in another patient reveals a full-thickness tear through the supraspinatus tendon (between cursors) with sagging of the normally convex contour of the cuff (black arrow) and the cartilage interface sign (white arrows). (Ultrasound images used with permission from Dr Frank Malara, Austin Hospital, Melbourne, Australia.) (C) Coronal oblique fluid-sensitive sequence reveals a moderate joint effusion (*) with a retracted supraspinatus tendon (white arrow). The normal insertion is indicated by the white arrowhead. (D) Sagittal oblique image in the same patient reveals a "bald" humeral head with absent supraspinatus (white arrow) and infraspinatus (black arrow) tendons. Inset shows the normal amount of "hair" for the humeral head with the supraspinatus (white arrowhead) and infraspinatus (black arrowhead) tendons. (E,F) Coronal reformations from a CT arthrogram reveals a high-grade tear at the anterior supraspinatus insertion (white arrow) and a superior labral tear (black arrow).

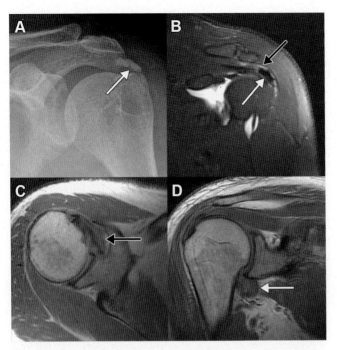

Fig. C17.4 (A,B) Calcific tendinitis. (A) Anteroposterior radiograph reveals globular calcification in the region of the distal supraspinatus tendon (white arrow). (B) Oblique coronal proton density image depicts the calcifications as low-intensity structures along the bursal aspect of the anterior to mid supraspinatus tendon insertion (white arrow). There is associated mild surrounding T2-hyperintensity representing active inflammation. (C,D) Adhesive capsulitis. (C) Axial proton density image reveals scarring in the rotator interval (black arrow). (D) Oblique coronal proton density image reveals a thickened and hypointense inferior capsule (white arrow).

- Greater tuberosity fracture: Can mimic a rotator cuff tear clinically. If displaced, the fracture fragment usually moves posteriorly and superiorly. Displacement of greater than 5 mm is usually associated with a rotator cuff tear.

- Neoplasm: Pain may be nonspecific.

REFERENCES AND SUGGESTED READING

1. Duralde XA, Gauntt SJ. Troubleshooting the supraspinatus outlet view. *J Shoulder Elbow Surg.* 1999;8(4):314-319.

2. Moosikasuwan JB, Miller TT, Burke BJ. Rotator cuff tears: clinical, radiographic, and US findings. *RadioGraphics.* 2005; 25(6):1591-1607.

3. Tuite MJ. Magnetic resonance imaging of rotator cuff disease and external impingement. *Magn Reson Imaging Clin N Am.* 2012;20(2):187-200.

CASE 18

PATIENT PRESENTATION

A 25-year-old man presents to his primary care physician with knee pain, joint swelling, and instability with ambulation following a knee injury while playing football.

CLINICAL SUSPICION

Anterior cruciate ligament (ACL) tear

IMAGING MODALITY OF CHOICE

Radiographs are preferred for the initial evaluation of patients with traumatic knee pain to exclude acute fracture. Soft tissue injuries such as tear of the ACL may be diagnosed by physical examination and history and sometimes by characteristic radiographic findings. However, MRI is often necessary to evaluate associated ligamentous, tendinous, and meniscal injuries that will also need to be treated. Intravenous and intra-articular contrast is not generally used.

BACKGROUND

The ACL acts as an important stabilizer of the knee joint by preventing anterior translation and internal rotation of the tibia in relation to the femur (Fig. C18.1). Injury to the ACL and loss of these functions allow for progressive dam-age to the menisci and articular cartilage and can lead to premature osteoarthritis. The ACL is the most commonly disrupted knee ligament, primarily during actions involving deceleration, twisting, or jumping.

FINDINGS

Radiographic findings associated with ACL injury include joint effusion, Segond fracture and the deep lateral femoral notch sign.

A joint effusion (Fig. C18.2A) is universally present in the setting of acute ACL injury. However, this finding is non-specific and may be present with a wide variety of intra-articular abnormalities.

A Segond fracture is an avulsion fracture of the lateral capsular ligament from the lateral tibial rim (Fig. C18.2B) and has a near 100% association with ACL disruption.

The deep lateral femoral notch sign refers to deepening of the sulcus of the lateral femoral condyle (the condylo-patellar sulcus) and suggests an impacted osteochondral fracture of the lateral femoral condyle.

MRI can directly depict ACL tears (Fig. C18.2C,D), and more important, the associated soft tissue injuries that may need to be simultaneously treated. A disrupted ACL with increased signal on T2-weighted or PD sequences is diagnostic of ACL injury. Partial tears are often better visualized on the axial plane.

Associated injuries include bone contusions and fractures, meniscal tears, and other ligamentous injuries. The well-known O'Donoghue triad of ACL tear, medial meniscal tear, and medial collateral ligament injury is rarely encountered.

The "kissing contusions" of an ACL tear are typically seen at the lateral femoral condyle and posterior lateral tibial plateau (Fig. C18.2C). An avulsion fracture of the tibial attachment of the ACL is more common before skeletal maturity. An avulsion fracture of the lateral tibial condyle (Segond fracture, Fig. C18.2B) may be subtle due to the mild associated bone marrow edema. Meniscal tears usually involve the posterior horns of the medial or lateral menisci. The medial collateral ligament and posterolateral corner of the joint capsule can also be injured. The latter is important to note preoperatively, as failure to address posterolateral corner injuries can predispose the patient to failure of cruciate reconstruction and early osteoarthritis.

DIFFERENTIAL DIAGNOSIS

Imaging Differential Diagnosis

MR imaging plays a crucial role in determining the extent of ACL injury, since complete tears are typically managed surgically whereas partial tears may be treated more conservatively. Although the MR imaging features of ACL

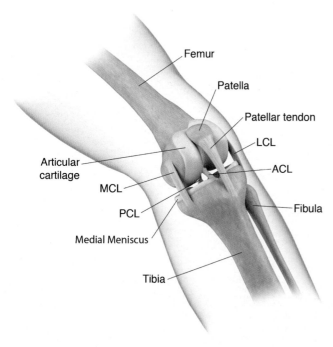

Fig. C18.1 Internal anatomy of the knee and major stabilizers.

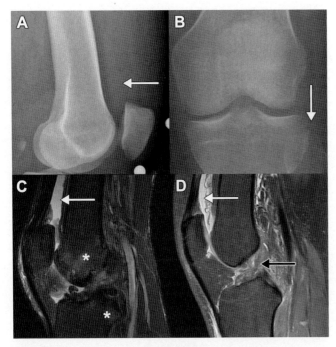

Fig. C18.2 Indirect and direct signs of anterior cruciate ligament tears. (A) Lateral view of the knee shows a joint effusion (white arrow). (B) Frontal radiograph of the knee shows a small bone fragment lateral to the lateral tibial condyle (white arrow) consistent with an avulsion fracture (Segond fracture). (C) Sagittal fluid-sensitive MR image of the knee in a different patient reveals patchy areas of increased signal (*) throughout the lateral femoral condyle and lateral tibial plateau. These represent the "kissing contusions" frequently encountered with ACL tears and the anterior translation of the tibia in relation to the femur. (D) Another sagittal fluid-sensitive MR image of the same knee shows heterogeneously increased signal within and lack of continuity of the ACL fibers (black arrow) consistent with complete disruption. Note the associated joint effusion (white arrows in C and D).

disruption are fairly characteristic, mucoid degeneration of the ACL (Fig. C18.3) must be considered in a patient with previous partial tear and without a history of acute trauma to the knee. An absent or hypoplastic ACL is an uncommon variant that can mimic an ACL tear.

Clinical Differential Diagnosis

A wide variety of intra-articular pathology can be encountered in the setting of trauma and knee pain, including tears of the menisci, cruciate ligaments and collateral ligaments.

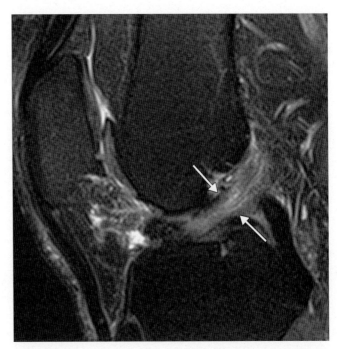

Fig. C18.3 Mucoid degeneration of the ACL. Hyperintense bands interposed between the fibers of a normally oriented anterior cruciate ligament (between white arrows) correspond to amorphous mucoid matrix coll.

REFERENCES AND SUGGESTED READING

1. Ho-Fung VM, Jaimes C, Jaramillo D. MR imaging of ACL injuries in pediatric and adolescent patients. *Clin Sports Med.* 2011;30:707-726.

2. Miller TT. MR imaging of the knee. *Sports Med Arthrosc.* 2009;17:56-67.

3. Remer EM, Fitzgerald SW, Friedman H, Rogers LF, Hendrix RW, Schafer MF. Anterior cruciate ligament injury: MR imaging diagnosis and patterns of injury. *RadioGraphics.* 1992;12: 901-915.

4. Schub D, Saluan P. Anterior cruciate ligament injuries in the young athlete: evaluation and treatment. *Sports Med Arthrosc.* 2011;19:34-43.

5. Stevens KJ, Dragoo JL. Anterior cruciate ligament tears and associated injuries. *Top Magn Reson Imaging.* 2006;17: 347-362.

6. Tuite MJ, Daffner RH, Weissman BN, et al. ACR Appropriateness Criteria: Acute trauma to the knee. *J Am Coll Radiol.* 2012;9(2):96-103.

CASE 19

PATIENT PRESENTATION

A 45-year-old man with left heel pain that occurs on the first steps of the morning and after prolonged sitting. Physical examination reveals sharp pain with palpation of the medial plantar calcaneal region and discomfort in the proximal plantar heel on passive ankle dorsiflexion.

CLINICAL SUSPICION

Plantar fasciitis

IMAGING MODALITY OF CHOICE

Imaging is rarely needed for initial diagnosis of plantar fasciitis; however, radiographs of the foot are often obtained to exclude other causes for heel pain (see Clinical Differential Diagnosis). Ultrasound and MRI are reserved for recalcitrant cases or to exclude other heel pathology (see Clinical Differential Diagnosis).

BACKGROUND

The plantar aponeurosis (Fig. C19.1) is a tendinous (not fascial) band of fibers that runs along the plantar aspect of the foot and provides dynamic longitudinal arch support. Plantar fasciitis is a self-limiting, low-grade inflammation involving the plantar aponeurosis and surrounding structures and typically manifests clinically as chronic pain along the medial aspect of the heel. It has been associated with obesity, excessive foot pronation, excessive running, and prolonged standing.

FINDINGS

Radiographs are usually normal. Chronic inflammation at the calcaneal insertion can rarely lead to erosions of the calcaneus. Plantar calcaneal spurs (Fig. C19.2A), which have been associated with plantar fasciitis in the past, can also be seen in asymptomatic adults, and their significance in plantar fasciitis is controversial.

MRI findings (Fig. C19.2B-D) include thickening of the plantar aponeurosis, typically proximally, extending to the calcaneal attachment. The thickened plantar aponeurosis will have intermediate signal intensity on T1-weighted and proton-density-weighted images and high signal intensity on T2-weighted images. There may also be edema of the adjacent fat pad and soft tissues and limited marrow edema within the medial calcaneal tuberosity.

DIFFERENTIAL DIAGNOSIS

Imaging Differential Diagnosis

MRI should be carefully evaluated to exclude other causes of heel pain (see Clinical Differential Diagnosis). Some

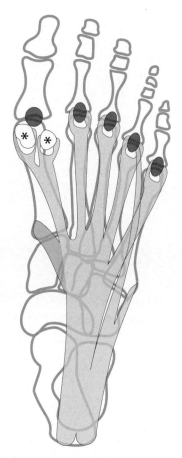

Fig. C19.1 The plantar aponeurosis is composed of central, medial, and lateral segments. The base is attached to the calcaneus and has fibers continuous with those of the Achilles tendon. The central segment (tan) is the thickest component. Its proximal attachment is to the posterior aspect of the medial calcaneal tuberosity. Its distal attachments are at the level of the metatarsophalangeal joints, dividing into five pairs of superficial and deep fascicles. The deep branches (not shown) insert onto the metatarsophalangeal joints. The superficial branches bifurcate into sagittal septa, which attach onto the plantar plates (red), interosseous ligament, and deep transverse metatarsal ligaments of the second through fifth digits and the plantar plate and sesamoid bones (*) of the great toe. The medial segment (purple) arises from the central segment and attaches to the inferior portion of the abductor hallucis muscle. The lateral segment (green) attaches proximally to the lateral aspect of the medial process of the calcaneal tuberosity and is continuous medially with the central segment. Distally, it has a medial band that inserts onto the plantar plate of the fourth and sometimes third metatarsophalangeal joints, and a lateral band that attaches to the base of the fifth metatarsal.

entities can have imaging findings that are similar to those of plantar fasciitis. Xanthomatous deposits in various tendons and ligaments, including the plantar aponeurosis, can occur in the setting of familial hypercholesterolemia. Plantar xanthomatosis can present as fusiform thickening of the plantar aponeurosis, but there is typically a characteristic

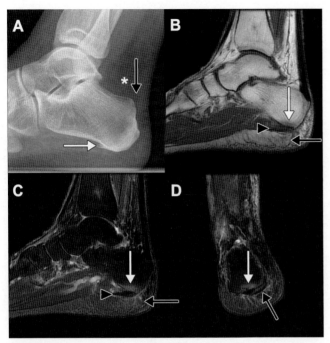

Fig. C19.2 Plantar fasciitis. (A) Lateral radiograph of the ankle reveals a tiny plantar calcaneal spur (white arrow). No fracture is seen. The retrocalcaneal bursa (black arrow) and Kager's fat pad (*) are clear. (B) Sagittal T1-weighted image reveals mild thickening of and intermediate signal intensity in the proximal plantar aponeurosis (black arrowhead). There is subtle loss of fat signal in the adjacent marrow (white arrow) and heel fat pad (black arrow). (C) Sagittal T2-weighted image reveals mild thickening of the plantar aponeurosis (black arrowhead) with some increased signal proximally, as well as adjacent bone marrow edema (white arrow). Mild edema is also seen in the adjacent fat pad of the heel (black arrow). (D) Coronal T2-weighted image reveals mild thickening of and increased signal in the plantar aponeurosis (black arrow) and adjacent bone marrow edema (white arrow).

speckled or reticulated appearance on both T1- and T2-weighted images corresponding to xanthomatous deposits.

Plantar fasciitis can be associated with seronegative spondyloarthropathies, such as rheumatoid arthritis. In such cases, abnormalities are usually bilateral and often associated with Achilles tendinitis and retrocalcaneal bursitis.

Because entrapment of the first branch of the inferior calcaneal nerve (Baxter neuropathy) has been associated with plantar fasciitis and calcaneal spurs, the abductor digiti minimi muscle (supplied by the inferior calcaneal nerve) should be assessed for isolated atrophy. When isolated abductor digiti minimi atrophy is present, the surgeon may decide to perform a surgical release of the inferior calcaneal nerve in addition to plantar fasciotomy.

Clinical Differential Diagnosis

- Plantar fibromatosis (Fig. C19.3A)
- Haglund syndrome (insertional tendinopathy of the Achilles tendon, retrocalcaneal bursitis, and bursitis behind the Achilles tendon)
- Baxter neuropathy (compression of the inferior calcaneal nerve)
- Stress fracture (Fig. C19.3B)

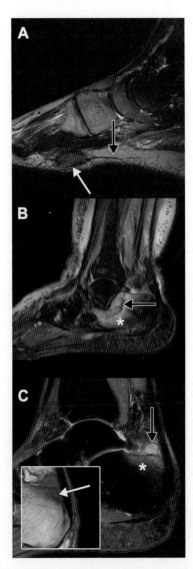

Fig. C19.3 Clinical differential considerations in plantar fasciitis. (A) Plantar (superficial) fibromatosis. Soft tissue mass (white arrow) along the mid-to-distal plantar aponeurosis (black arrow). (B) Stress fracture of the calcaneus. The fracture plane is seen as a hypointense serpiginous line (black arrow) with surrounding marrow edema (*). (C) Rheumatoid arthritis. Retrocalcaneal bursitis and soft tissue pannus (black arrow) with erosion in the calcaneus (inset, white arrow). The plantar aponeurosis was normal.

- Tarsal tunnel syndrome,
- Inflammatory arthritis (eg, rheumatoid arthritis, Fig. C19.3C)
- Tendinitis and tenosynovitis (eg, Achilles)
- Fat pad inflammation
- Infection (soft tissue or bony)
- Neoplasm

REFERENCES AND SUGGESTED READING

1. Goff JD, Crawford R. Diagnosis and treatment of plantar fasciitis. *Am Fam Physician*. 2011;84(6):676-682.
2. Narváez JA, Narváez J, Ortega R, Aguilera C, Sánchez A, Andía E. Painful heel: MR imaging findings. *RadioGraphics*. 2000;20(2):333-352.

CASE 20

PATIENT PRESENTATION

A 55-year-old man, with a left total knee arthroplasty placed 5 years ago, presents with left knee pain.

CLINICAL SUSPICION

Aseptic loosening

IMAGING MODALITY OF CHOICE

Radiography to start; however, aseptic and septic loosening usually cannot be differentiated with radiographs, and sequential imaging with Tc-99m sulfur colloid scintigraphy and labeled white blood cells or joint aspiration may be necessary.

BACKGROUND

Knee arthroplasty (Fig. C20.1A) is primarily performed to relieve pain caused by severe arthritis. The hardware has a finite lifespan and is ideally placed in older patients with moderate levels of activity. Hardware failure can be due to complications in and around any of the components. The most common causes of failure before 2 years (early failure) are infection and instability. The most common causes of failure after 2 years (late failure) are polyethylene wear and aseptic loosening.

FINDINGS

Tibial components (Fig. C20.1B,C) can normally have a thin (< 1 mm) lucency around the baseplate and stem. Increase in the width of the lucency, development of focal lucencies greater than 2 mm, or component migration indicate loosening (Fig. C20.2).

Polyethylene wear (Fig. C20.3A) not only can lead to instability (through loss of ligament tension/balance), but can also lead to histiocytic osteolysis, a reaction of bone to polyethylene debris. Knees with a particle-induced histiocytic response typically have joint effusions due to synovitis.

Radiography is often hampered by suboptimal positioning on an individual study and by differences in positioning between studies. The x-ray beam should be tangential to the base plate of the tibial plateau for assessment of the tibial component and for accurate and reproducible measurements of the polyethylene. Radiographs should be carefully assessed for the presence of other complications, such as subluxation (Fig. C20.3B), subsidence, fracture, and displacement of the polyethylene disc or patellar component.

Bone scintigraphy (commonly, Tc-99m MDP) is often called upon to determine whether loosening is septic (infectious) or aseptic. When periprosthetic uptake is the

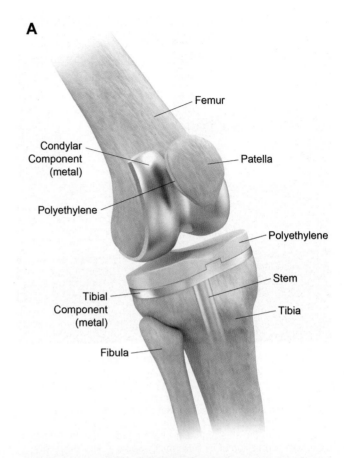

A

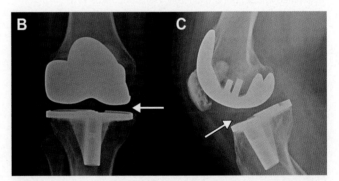

Fig. C20.1 Total knee arthroplasty. (A) Diagram of a total knee arthroplasty. The metal condylar component can be cemented or not. The metal tibial component is usually cemented. A slab of polyethylene articulates with the condylar component and may be fixed to the tibial tray or allow some motion between the polyethylene and the tray. The patella may or may not be resurfaced (a resurfaced patella is illustrated). A resurfaced patella consists of a cemented polyethylene component usually without a metal backing. (B) Frontal and (C) lateral radiographs of a normal total knee arthroplasty. The polyethylene thickness (white arrow) is normal (> 8 mm) as evaluated on standing anteroposterior and lateral views.

same as that of surrounding nonarticular bone, a prosthetic abnormality is very unlikely. The presence of increased uptake, however, is not helpful, since marked increase in

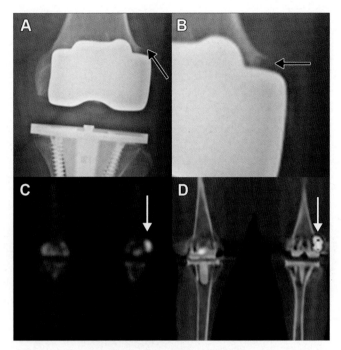

Fig. C20.2 Aseptic Loosening. (A,B) Frontal radiograph of the knee shows lucency (black arrow) along the superolateral aspect of the femoral component of a total knee arthroplasty. (C) Planar image from a Tc-99m MDP bone scintigraphy shows increased uptake in the superolateral aspect of the femoral component. (D) SPECT/CT fusion shows that the focus of increased uptake corresponds to the area of lucency seen on radiographs. (Images used with permission of Dr Susanna C. Spence, The University of Texas Medical School at Houston, Houston, Texas.)

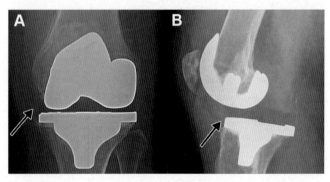

Fig. C20.3 Other complications. (A) Frontal radiograph of the knee shows thinning of the polyethylene disk (black arrow) to about 3 mm. (B) Lateral radiograph of the knee in a different patient reveals posterior dislocation of the tibia (black arrow) across a knee arthroplasty.

uptake can be noted for up to 1 year after surgery and mild to moderate uptake for as long as 4 years. In such cases, joint aspiration may be needed for definitive diagnosis.

Sequential imaging with Tc-99m sulfur colloid scintigraphy and labeled white blood cells is the best way of differentiating septic from aseptic loosening; however, it is rarely performed. Sulfur colloid and leukocytes both accumulate within bone marrow, but only leukocytes accumulate at sites of infection. Visualization of Tc-99m sulfur colloid and labeled leukocytes in the same location indicates the presence of marrow, whereas leukocyte activity without corresponding accumulation of sulfur colloid indicates infection.

DIFFERENTIAL DIAGNOSIS

Imaging Differential Diagnosis

Aseptic and septic loosening can be difficult to differentiate on radiography.

Clinical Differential Diagnosis

Infection may be difficult to differentiate from other complications because patients may not have fever and chills or leukocytosis. Aspiration is highly sensitive and specific in patients who are not being empirically treated with antibiotics. Sensitivity of aspiration decreases with antibiotic treatment.

REFERENCES AND SUGGESTED READING

1. Love C, Tomas MB, Marwin SE, Pugliese PV, Palestro CJ. Role of nuclear medicine in diagnosis of the infected joint replacement. *RadioGraphics.* 2001;21(5):1229-1238.
2. Miller TT. Imaging of knee arthroplasty. *Eur J Radiol.* 2005; 54(2):164-177.

CASE 21

PATIENT PRESENTATION

A 30-year-old man with right shoulder deformity after a fall. The patient's upper arm is abducted and held in external rotation.

CLINICAL SUSPICION

Glenohumeral dislocation

IMAGING MODALITY OF CHOICE

Radiography. Axillary or scapular "Y" views should be obtained in addition to standard anteroposterior views to evaluate the position of the humeral head in relation to the glenoid fossa. Anterior glenohumeral dislocations account for more than 95% of all shoulder dislocations. Posterior shoulder dislocations may be occult on routine frontal views and are more apparent on axillary or scapular "Y" views. Postreduction shoulder radiographs should be performed to evaluate for the presence of associated fractures. CT can also be used to better depict bony abnormalities. Postreduction MRI may be needed to assess associated soft tissue injuries that can cause shoulder instability.

Box C21.1 – TERMINOLOGY

Glenohumeral subluxation: Excessive translation of the humeral head in relation to the glenoid without a complete separation of the articular surfaces. Spontaneous reduction to anatomic position will occur when the distracting force is no longer present.

Glenohumeral dislocation: Excessive translation of the humeral head in relation to the glenoid that results in complete separation of the articular surfaces. Spontaneous reduction will not occur even when the distracting force is no longer present.

BACKGROUND

The glenohumeral joint is the most commonly dislocated joint in the human body. A complex web of soft-tissue structures maintains the stability of this "ball-in-socket" joint. Disruption of these structures is common after traumatic shoulder dislocation and may lead to recurrent dislocation and chronic instability. The bony glenoid fossa or "socket" is augmented by a soft tissue labrum that effectively deepens the socket and improves stability of the joint.

Anterior glenohumeral dislocation often results from a fall on the outstretched hand with the arm in abduction and external rotation. This may result in impaction injury of the posterosuperior aspect of the humeral head into the anteroinferior glenoid rim (Bankart lesion) and an impaction fracture of the humeral head (Hill-Sachs lesion). Bankart lesions may involve the bony glenoid rim (bony Bankart lesion or fracture) or result in a wide variety of soft tissue injuries (fibrous Bankart lesion).

Conversely, posterior glenohumeral dislocation may result in an impaction fracture of the anteromedial aspect of the humeral head (reverse Hill-Sachs lesion) and injury to the posterior glenoid rim (reverse Bankart lesion).

FINDINGS

Anterior glenohumeral dislocation can manifest radiographically by a humeral head that is displaced medially and inferiorly in relation to the glenoid fossa and is typically inferior to the coracoid process (Fig. C21.1A,B). An impaction fracture of the posterosuperior humeral head (Hill-Sachs lesion) is identified in up to 90% of patients (Fig. C21.1C,D). A fracture of the anterioinferior glenoid

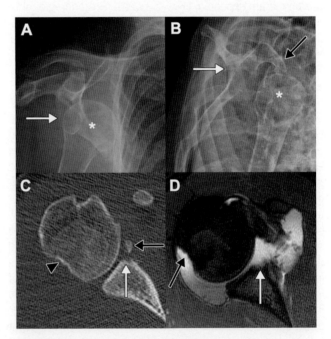

Fig. C21.1 Anterior glenohumeral dislocation. (A) Frontal radiograph of the right shoulder shows displacement of the humeral head (*) medially and inferiorly in relation to the glenoid (white arrow), consistent with anterior glenohumeral dislocation. Note associated minimally displaced right-sided rib fractures. (B) A transthoracic lateral view of the same shoulder confirms that the humeral head is dislocated anteriorly in relation to the glenoid fossa and lies inferior to the coracoid process (black arrow). (C) Axial CT image in another patient shows fracture fragments (black arrow) and a bony defect in the anteroinferior glenoid (white arrow) related to a prior Bankart fracture. A bony defect is also seen in the posterolateral humeral head, consistent with an old Hill-Sachs fracture. (D) Axial fluid-sensitive MR arthrogram image of the right shoulder in the same patient depicts an old Hill-Sachs fracture of the posterolateral aspect of the humeral head (black arrow) related to prior glenohumeral dislocation. Irregularity of the anteroinferior glenoid (white arrow) is also seen, related to old bony Bankart lesion. This patient developed recurrent shoulder dislocation attributed to these prior injuries.

rim (bony Bankart lesion) can be identified on radiographs but is best seen on CT (Fig. C21.1C) and MRI (Fig. C21.1D).

Posterior glenohumeral dislocation, which is classically associated with seizure or electrocution injury, presents with more subtle radiographic findings. The anteroposterior radiograph of the shoulder may appear nearly normal, although the addition of appropriately positioned axillary views may improve the rate of radiographic detection to 100%. A scapular "Y" view is also acceptable if the axillary view cannot be obtained due to patient pain. This view projects the scapula as the letter Y: the long stem of the Y is the body of the scapula, and the upper arms of the Y are the coracoid process anteriorly and the spine of the scapula and the acromion posteriorly. The humeral head should be centered at the junction of the arms with the stem.

On the anteroposterior radiograph, the humeral head is typically fixed in internal rotation and more superior in position than expected (Fig. C21.2A). Posterior glenohumeral dislocation may be associated with a reverse Hill-Sachs lesion related to impaction of the anterior humeral head against the posterior glenoid rim ("trough sign," Fig. C21.2). An associated injury of the posterior glenoid rim constitutes a reverse Bankart lesion.

Luxatio erecta is an uncommon condition characterized by inferior or subglenoid humeral dislocation. Luxatio erecta is typically associated with hyperabduction and extension during a fall or with overhead shots in racquet sports. On radiographs, the humeral head will be dislocated inferior to the glenoid with the humerus locked in abduction. Luxatio erecta is associated with a high rate of greater tuberosity fracture, rotator cuff tear, and axillary nerve injury.

Noncontrast MRI can depict a wide variety of bony and soft tissue abnormalities associated with glenohumeral dislocation that can lead to instability of the glenohumeral joint and contribute to recurrent dislocation. Injection of intra-articular gadolinium contrast (MR arthrography) may increase sensitivity for detection of intra-articular pathology (Figs. C21.1D and C21.2C). Please note, however, that MR arthrography is an off-label (but common) use of gadolinium.

MRI may depict the bony abnormalities associated with anterior and posterior glenohumeral dislocation. Hill-Sachs and reverse Hill-Sachs lesions manifest as deformities of the posterolateral and anteromedial humeral head, respectively.

Fibrous Bankart and reverse Bankart lesions typically involve injury to the glenoid labrum, which presents as a focal contour or size abnormality. Insinuation of intra-articular contrast or joint fluid between the torn labrum and glenoid rim depicts a tear, but may not always be present. Labral lesions can result in recurrent glenohumeral dislocation and instability of the shoulder joint and are important to proper treatment of the patient. A detailed discussion of labral lesions, however, is beyond the scope of this text.

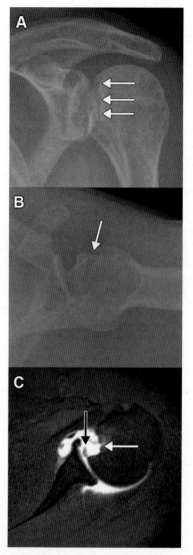

Fig. C21.2 Posterior glenohumeral dislocation in a 51-year-old man with shoulder pain and the humeral head fixed in internal rotation. (A) Anteroposterior radiograph of the shoulder shows the trough line sign (white arrows), representing the margin of an impaction fracture of the anteromedial aspect of the humeral head (reverse Hill-Sachs fracture). Note that the glenohumeral alignment is near-normal on the anteroposterior radiograph. (B) Axillary view shows posterior translation of the humeral head in relation to the glenoid fossa. Note the impaction fracture of the anteromedial aspect of the humeral head (reverse Hill-Sachs fracture, white arrow). (C) Axial T1-weighted, fat-suppressed MR arthrogram after reduction shows the large reverse Hill-Sachs fracture (white arrow). The posterior labrum (not shown) was completely disrupted (reverse Bankart lesion). Note the intra-articular fragment (black arrow).

DIFFERENTIAL DIAGNOSIS
Imaging Differential Diagnosis

None

Clinical Differential Diagnosis

The clinical differential diagnosis of shoulder deformity is typically narrowed by the clinical history. In the setting of trauma, visible deformity of the shoulder may be related to either fracture or dislocation or a combination of the two. Anterior glenohumeral dislocation is statistically more likely, and the patient's arm will often be held in external rotation. In contrast, the humerus is typically fixed in internal rotation in the setting of posterior glenohumeral dislocation. Associated bony injuries may range from small impaction fractures to more dramatic intra-articular displaced fractures of the greater tuberosity or proximal humeral diaphysis.

REFERENCES AND SUGGESTED READING

1. Emery KH. Imaging of sports injuries of the upper extremity in children. *Clin Sports Med*. 2006;25:543-568.

2. Goud A, Segal D, Hedayati P, Pan JJ, Weissman BN. Radiographic evaluation of the shoulder. *Eur J Radiol*. 2008;68:2-15.

3. Omoumi P, Teixeira P, Lecouvet F, Chung CB. Glenohumeral joint instability. *J Magn Reson Imaging*. 2011;33:2-16.

4. Sanders TG, Zlatkin M, Montgomery J. Imaging of glenohumeral instability. *Semin Roentgenol*. 2010;45:160-179.

CASE 22

PATIENT PRESENTATION

A 17-year-old adolescent boy presents with swelling of the right thigh that started 3 weeks ago, followed by the development of dull aching pain.

CLINICAL SUSPICION

Bone or soft tissue sarcoma

IMAGING MODALITY OF CHOICE

Radiography. Findings suspicious for a primary bone malignancy should prompt contrast-enhanced MRI for assessment of local disease extent and staging studies such as a chest CT (to look for lung metastases) and bone scintigraphy or F-18 FDG PET (to look for remote bone metastases). F-18 FDG PET is more sensitive than bone scintigraphy for detection of systemic metastases in a wide-range of soft tissue and bone sarcomas.

BACKGROUND

Musculoskeletal complaints in children can be due to a variety of conditions, including traumatic, neoplastic, and rheumatological. Radiography is the initial imaging modality of choice. The job of the radiologist when confronted with "rule out fracture" (more commonly "r/o fx") is not to simply exclude fracture, but to carefully evaluate the radiograph for more ominous causes of pain. If a lesion is found, attempts should be made to characterize it as benign or aggressive (aggressive lesions include benign lesions such as osteomyelitis, as well as malignant lesions such as osteosarcoma).

An outside-in approach starts with an evaluation of the skin and soft tissues for mass or distortion.

An assessment of the periosteum should follow. Periosteal reactions (Fig. C22.1) can be subtle and suggest a bone or soft tissue abnormality. Periosteal reaction can be described as solid, lamellated (single or multiple), spiculated, buttressed, or Codman triangle. Aggressive types of periosteal reaction are spiculated, lamellated, and Codman triangle.

The cortex is assessed next. The normal cortex should be smooth along its periosteal and endosteal surfaces. Loss of the inner margin of the cortex (endosteal scalloping) can suggest the presence of tumor in the medullary cavity of the bone.

The pattern of bone destruction is assessed next, and can be defined as geographic, moth-eaten, or permeative (Fig. C22.2). For the geographic pattern of destruction, the margin of the lesion is further characterized as well defined with sclerosis (IA), well defined without sclerosis (IB), and ill defined (IC). The worst feature is taken as representative of the worst biological activity lesion.

Finally, we look inside the lesion and assess the radiographic density as lytic, sclerotic, or mixed and determine whether we can discern the matrix of the lesion. The matrix

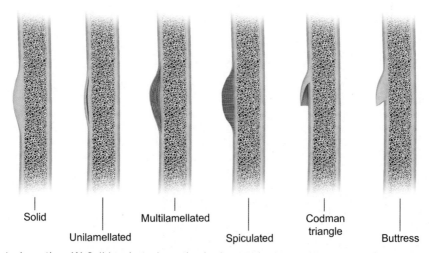

| Solid | Unilamellated | Multilamellated | Spiculated | Codman triangle | Buttress |

Fig. C22.1 Types of periosteal reaction. (A) Solid periosteal reaction is characterized by an intact underlying cortex with solid and continuous overlying bone formation. (B) Unilamellated periosteal reaction indicates a slowly growing lesion that allows enough time for the bone to contain it. (C) A multilamellated (onionskin) periosteal reaction indicates a waxing and waning process, with the bone continually trying and failing to contain the lesion. It suggests a lesion of intermediate aggressivity. (D) The spiculated periosteal reaction is the most aggressive type and is highly suggestive of malignancy. This type of periosteal reaction is also known as "hair-on-end" or "sunburst," although some authors make a distinction between "hair-on-end" (perpendicular to the cortex) and "sunburst" (radiating outward in a curved fashion). (E) Codman triangle (perhaps more correctly referred to as Codman angle) refers to elevation of the periosteum away from the cortex, forming an angle where the elevated periosteum and bone join. (F) Buttress or buttressed periosteal reaction refers to beaklike solid periosteal new bone formation and is the interrupted version of the solid periosteal reaction. It should be distinguished from Codman triangle.

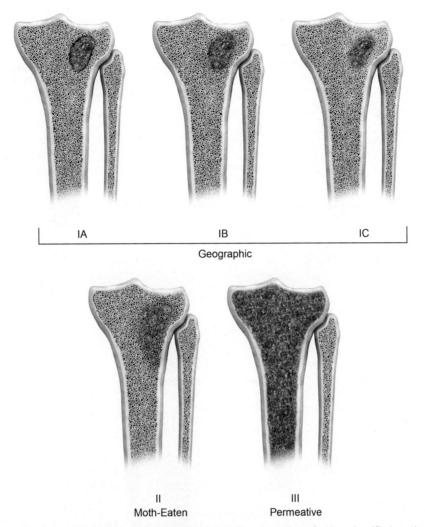

IA   IB   IC
Geographic

II   III
Moth-Eaten   Permeative

Fig. C22.2 Patterns of bone destruction. Geographic lesions are focal and discrete and are further classified on the basis of their margin as type IA (well defined with sclerosis), IB (well defined without sclerosis), and IC (ill defined). IA and IB lesions have an abrupt transition between the lesion and the adjacent unaffected bone (narrow zone of transition). IC lesions have a somewhat wider zone of transition. Infiltrative lesions have ill-defined margins and a broad zone of transition and may be classified as moth-eaten (II) or permeative (III; small, patchy, ill-defined areas of lytic bone destruction).

of a lesion is the acellular, intercellular material produced by mesenchymal cells and can be osteoid (osteoblasts), chondroid (chondroblasts), collagen (fibroblasts), or myxoid.

Mineralization of the matrix can suggest the type of matrix. Calcification in chondroid lesions often manifests as punctate, flocculent, comma-shaped, or arclike or ringlike mineralization (see case 24). Osteoid lesions have fluffy, amorphous, and cloudlike mineralization that manifests as radiographic opacity.

The age of the patient and location of the tumor can help narrow differential considerations (Fig. C22.3).

FINDINGS

The patient in the case presentation had conventional osteosarcoma (Fig. C22.4A-C). Radiography is usually

adequate for diagnosis in the setting of characteristic findings of conventional (intramedullary) osteosarcoma, which include medullary and cortical bone destruction, aggressive periosteal reaction, soft tissue mass, and bone formation by the tumor. Radiography usually underestimates the soft tissue component of the tumor, the medullary extent of the disease, and the presence of skip lesions (lesions elsewhere in the same bone).

Bone scintigraphy will reveal increased uptake associated with the primary lesion (Fig. C22.4D), as well as local and remote metastases.

MRI is more sensitive for detection of lesions but has a limited field of view. The mineralized components of osteosarcoma are low signal intensity on all pulse sequences, whereas the solid, nonmineralized portions of the tumor usually are hypointense on T1-weighted images,

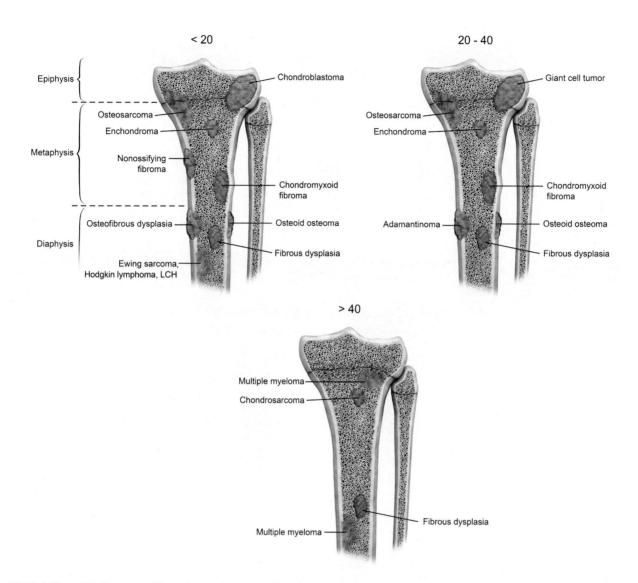

Fig. C22.3 Differential diagnosis of bone tumors by age and location.

hyperintense on T2-weighted images, and enhance on postcontrast images. Necrotic and liquefied components of the lesion appear as nonenhancing, T1-hypointense, and T2-hyperintense areas.

DIFFERENTIAL DIAGNOSIS

Imaging Differential Diagnosis

The main radiographic differential consideration for conventional osteosarcoma in young patients is Ewing sarcoma. Although the permeative or moth-eaten pattern of bone destruction and lamellated periosteal reaction of Ewing sarcoma are easily differentiated from conventional

osteosarcoma, occasionally Ewing sarcoma can have areas of ossification and a sunburst periosteal reaction and can resemble osteosarcoma.

Other forms of intramedullary osteosarcoma, such as small cell and telangiectatic osteosarcoma (Fig. C22.5A), may not have radiographically evident osteoid production and can mimic other aggressive lytic lesions of bone (Fig. C22.5B,C).

Clinical Differential Diagnosis

Musculoskeletal complaints in children can be due to a variety of conditions, including traumatic, neoplastic, and rheumatological.

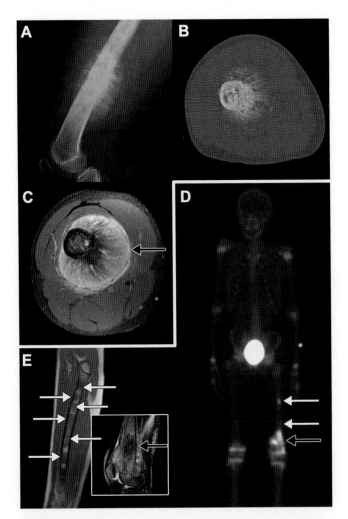

Fig. C22.4 Imaging findings in conventional osteosarcoma. (A) Lateral radiograph of the femur reveals intramedullary sclerosis and a spiculated periosteal reaction. (B) Axial CT image in the same patient reveals intramedullary sclerosis and the mineralized spicules of the periosteal reaction. (C) Postcontrast axial T1-weighted image shows elevation of the periosteum (black arrow) with enhancement of the underlying mass. The hypointense subperiosteal lines represent the mineralized spicules of the periosteal reaction. (D) Bone scintigraphy in another patient with osteosarcoma reveals increased uptake associated with the primary lesion in the left distal femur (black arrow) and at least two skip lesion (white arrows). The injection site was in the left forearm. (E) Sagittal T1-weighted image of the femur in the same patient shows the primary lesion in the distal femur (inset, black arrow) and multiple skip lesions (white arrows) throughout the proximal and mid femoral diaphysis.

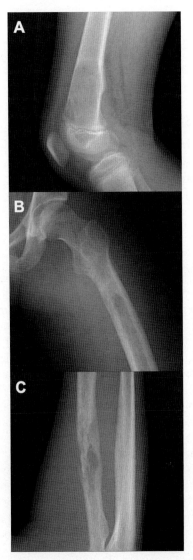

Fig. C22.5 Imaging differential considerations in osteosarcoma in children. (A) Telangiectatic osteosarcoma without significant matrix osteoid production. (B) Ewing sarcoma must be in the differential diagnosis for bone tumors in children. (C) Osteomyelitis can have an aggressive appearance.

REFERENCES AND SUGGESTED READING

1. Moser RP Jr, Madewell JE. An approach to primary bone tumors. *Radiol Clin North Am.* 1987;25(6):1049-1093.

CASE 23

PATIENT PRESENTATION

A 22-year-old woman with gradual onset of wrist pain, swelling, and tenderness.

CLINICAL SUSPICION

Bone or soft tissue neoplasm, inflammatory arthropathy

IMAGING MODALITY OF CHOICE

Radiography to start. CT or contrast-enhanced MRI as needed for further characterization.

FINDINGS

Giant cell tumors of bone are purely lytic lesions with a geographic type of bone destruction, typically with well-defined margins (Fig. C23.1). Marginal sclerosis is rare, and the lesions typically have the IB or IC patterns of bone destruction (see case 22, Fig. C22.2). Giant cell tumors of bone are frequently expansile and eccentrically located in the metaphysis with extension to the epiphysis. Some giant cell tumors can have an aggressive imaging appearance with cortical destruction and a soft tissue mass. CT shows the same findings to better advantage and can better define any soft tissue extension.

MRI reveals intermediate signal intensity on T1-weighted images, variable signal on T2-weighted images (due to hemorrhage), and heterogeneous enhancement. Giant cell tumors can cause secondary aneurysmal bone cyst formation that manifests as fluid-fluid levels on MRI.

Scintigraphy can reveal intense uptake around the periphery of the lesion corresponding to reactive bone formation or hyperemia and central photopenia corresponding to the tumor itself.

DIFFERENTIAL DIAGNOSIS

Imaging Differential Diagnosis

The differential diagnosis for epiphyseal lesions includes giant cell tumor, chondroblastoma, subchondral cyst, Langerhans cell histiocytosis, osteomyelitis, lymphoma, metastasis, and clear cell variant of chondrosarcoma (Fig. C23.2A-C).

The differential diagnosis for fluid-fluid levels on MRI or CT includes primary aneurysmal bone cyst, giant cell tumor with secondary aneurysmal bone cyst formation, and telangiectatic osteosarcoma (Fig. C23.2D-F).

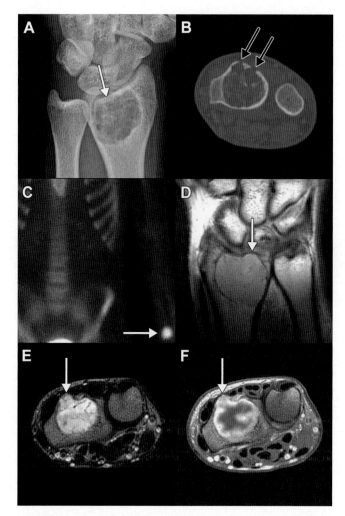

Fig. C23.1 Imaging findings in giant cell tumor of bone. (A) Oblique radiograph of the wrist shows an eccentric lucent lesion located in the distal radius. The lesion has a narrow zone of transition and extends to the articular surface (white arrow). (B) Axial CT shows that the lesion is slightly expansile and has two areas of cortical breakthrough dorsally (black arrows). (C) Bone scintigraphy shows radiotracer localization to the lesion. (D-F) MR images show the dorsal soft tissue extension of the lesion (white arrows) to better advantage. The lesion has intermediate signal intensity on the T1-weighted image (D) and high signal intensity on the T2-weighted image (E) and has thick, peripheral enhancement.

Clinical Differential Diagnosis

Other soft tissue or bone neoplasms, fracture, and arthritis

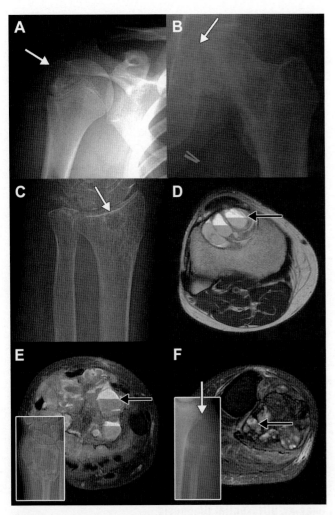

Fig. C23.2 Differential considerations for giant cell tumor. A variety of lesions can present as isolated epiphyseal lesions, including chondroblastoma (A), clear cell variant of chondrosarcoma (B), and subchondral cyst (C), among others. Fluid-fluid levels (arrows) can be seen in primary aneurysmal bone cyst (D), in giant cell tumor with secondary aneurysmal bone cyst formation (E), and in telangiectatic osteosarcoma (F).

REFERENCE AND SUGGESTED READING

1. Manaster BJ, Doyle AJ. Giant cell tumors of bone. *Radiol Clin North Am.* 1993;31(2):299-323.

CASE 24

PATIENT PRESENTATION

A 60-year-old woman with shortness of breath. Chest radiography in the emergency department revealed a lesion in the left proximal humerus that prompted dedicated radiography of the left shoulder (Fig. C24.1A). She denies symptoms related to her left upper arm.

CLINICAL SUSPICION

Enchondroma

IMAGING MODALITY OF CHOICE

Follow-up radiography or MRI

FINDINGS

An enchondroma in the long bones typically has flocculent internal mineralization that assumes the form of dots, rings, and arcs (Fig. C24.1A).

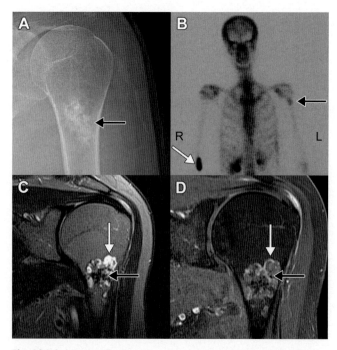

Fig. C24.1 Imaging findings in enchondroma. (A) Frontal radiograph of the left shoulder reveals a lesion in the proximal left humeral diaphysis with flocculent mineralization (black arrow). (B) Bone scintigraphy reveals mild uptake associated with the lesion (black arrow). The injection site on the right arm is indicated (white arrow). (C) Fluid-sensitive coronal image shows a lobulated, hyperintense lesion in the proximal humerus (white arrow). Mineralization is seen as foci of low signal intensity (black arrow). (D) Postcontrast image reveals heterogeneous, predominantly peripheral, enhancement and small hypointense foci (black arrow) corresponding to calcifications.

Enchondromas have a variable appearance on bone scintigraphy depending on their level of activity, but will usually have some uptake. On MRI, enchondromas have lobulated margins, low to intermediate signal intensity on T1-weighted images, high signal intensity on T2-weighted images (Fig. C24.1C), and enhancement on postcontrast images (Fig. C24.1D). Internal calcifications manifest as signal voids or as low signal-intensity foci.

Enchondromas can be entirely radiolucent in short tubular bones (eg, hands and feet) (Fig. C24.2A). If enchondromas are large enough, they can cause thinning and expansion of the cortex, often with scalloped inner cortical margins (endosteal scalloping, Fig. C24.2B,D). CT and MRI (Fig. C24.2C,D) can further define the extent of the tumor and give a better appreciation of cortical thinning.

Two related entities are Ollier disease (multiple enchondromas, Fig. C24.2E) and Maffucci syndrome (multiple enchondromas with soft tissue hemangiomas or lymphangiomas, Fig. C24.2F).

The most important complication is malignant transformation to chondrosarcoma, which occurs predominantly in a long or flat bone and is rare in the tubular bones of the hands and feet (Fig. C24.2G,H). New pain at the site of the lesion in the absence of a fracture should raise suspicion for malignant transformation. Sarcomatous transformation in patients with Ollier disease and Maffucci syndrome is many times more common than in patients with solitary enchondromas.

DIFFERENTIAL DIAGNOSIS

Imaging Differential Diagnosis

Well-differentiated chondrosarcomas can be difficult to differentiate from enchondromas, both by imaging and by pathology (due to sampling error with biopsy). Localized thickening of the cortex, deep endosteal scalloping (greater than two-thirds of cortical thickness) and large size (longer than 4 cm) are suggestive of malignancy. Cortical destruction, aggressive periosteal reaction, and a soft tissue mass indicate a malignant lesion. Recently, Parlier-Cuau et al. (2011) proposed criteria for management of solitary central cartilaginous tumors of long bones (Box C24.1). These criteria have not been validated but can serve as a reasonable guide to management of these common lesions.

Bone infarctions (Fig. C24.3A,B) can resemble heavily calcified enchondromas. Lobulated margins, punctate or annular matrix calcifications, and absence of peripheral sclerosis point to a diagnosis of enchondroma.

Enchondromas in the short tubular bones that extend to the articular surface can mimic giant cell tumors (Fig. C24.3C). Peripheral sclerosis and matrix calcification (may be absent in the hands and feet) can suggest a diagnosis of enchondroma.

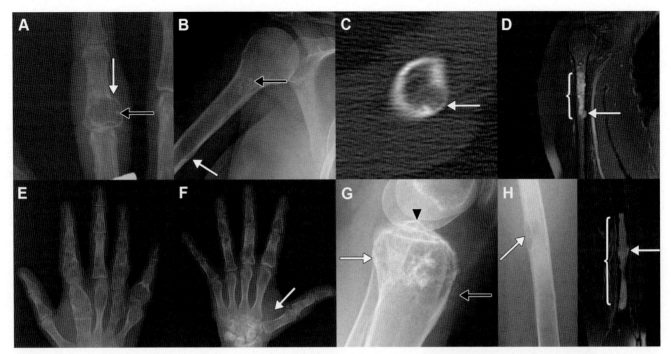

Fig. C24.2 More imaging findings related to enchondromas. (A) Enchondromas in the short tubular bones of the hands and feet are usually entirely lucent, although this lesion has small internal calcifications (black arrow). The most common complication in the hands and feet is pathological fracture (white arrow). Malignant transformation is rare in the hands and feet. (B) An enchondroma in the proximal humeral diaphysis has flocculent calcifications proximally (black arrow) and a focus of thinning of the inner margin of the cortex (endosteal scalloping) distally (white arrow). Note that only the proximal aspect of the lesion has the characteristic calcifications. (C) CT in the same patient shows endosteal scalloping (white arrow), which reflects the lobular growth pattern of cartilage. Endosteal scalloping and the lobular growth pattern is better seen on MRI (D), which is also better at delineating the extent of the lesion (bracket). (E) Ollier disease is a nonhereditary condition characterized by the presence of multiple enchondromas that are asymmetrically distributed and usually unilateral. (F) Maffucci syndrome is a nonhereditary condition characterized by multiple enchondromas and hemangiomas or lymphangiomas (less common). The phleboliths associated with a hemangioma are indicated by the arrow. (G) Chondrosarcoma. Lateral radiograph of the knee reveals a lesion with a chondroid matrix in the proximal tibia with cortical expansion anteromedially (black arrow), lobulated extension into the tibial spines proximally (black arrowhead), and endosteal scalloping posteriorly (white arrow). (H) Chondrosarcoma in another patient. Lateral radiograph of the femur reveals a predominantly lytic lesion in the mid diaphysis that results in endosteal scalloping (white arrows). Mineralization may be absent in higher-grade chondrosarcomas. T2-weighted coronal image in the same patient shows the extent of the lesion (bracket).

BOX C24.1 – ENCHONDROMA VERSUS LOW-GRADE CHONDROSARCOMA

Aggressive Features (Consider Excision)

Any one of the following:

- Cortical destruction
- Moth-eaten or permeative bone destruction
- Spontaneous pathologic fracture
- Periosteal reaction
- Peritumoral edema on MR
- Soft tissue mass

Active Features (Consider Biopsy or Excision)

Two of the following:

- Pain related to the tumor
- Endosteal scalloping > 2/3 of cortical thickness
- Extent of endosteal scalloping > 2/3 lesion length
- Cortical thickening
- Enlargement of the medullary cavity

Possibly Active Features (Consider Further Imaging)

- Only one active feature present

Quiescent Features (Consider Follow-Up)

- No active or aggressive feature present

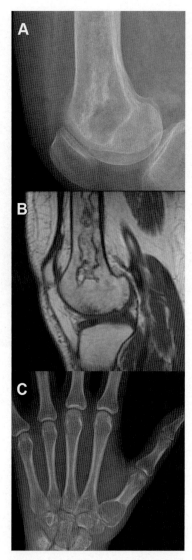

Fig. C24.3 Imaging differential considerations for enchondroma. (A) Bone infarction in the distal femur has a smoky appearance with a serpentine margin. (B) Sagittal T1-weighted image in the same patient reveals a distinct serpentine hypointensity surrounding an area of fat signal. (C) Giant cell tumor of the base of the thumb metacarpal with secondary aneurysmal bone cyst formation.

Clinical Differential Diagnosis

Fracture, tumor

REFERENCES AND SUGGESTED READING

1. Parlier-Cuau C, Bousson V, Ogilvie CM, Lackman RD, Laredo JD. When should we biopsy a solitary central cartilaginous tumor of long bones? Literature review and management proposal. *Eur J Radiol.* 2011;77(1):6-12.

2. Murphey MD, Flemming DJ, Boyea SR, Bojescul JA, Sweet DE, Temple HT. Enchondroma versus chondrosarcoma in the appendicular skeleton: differentiating features. *RadioGraphics.* 1998;18(5):1213-1237.

CASE 25

PATIENT PRESENTATION

A 17-year-old adolescent girl, a competitive dancer in her school, presents with right knee pain. Radiographs reveal a distal femoral lesion (Fig. C25.1A).

CLINICAL SUSPICION

Incidental cystic bone lesion (nonossifying fibroma in this case)

IMAGING MODALITY OF CHOICE

Radiographs are preferred in the initial evaluation of any bone lesion and allow for adequate characterization of a wide variety of cystic bone lesions. Further evaluation may be unnecessary in the presence of characteristic radiographic findings.

BACKGROUND

Benign cystic bone lesions are most reliably differentiated from malignant lesions on the basis of the pattern of bone destruction (see case 22). The interface between a typically

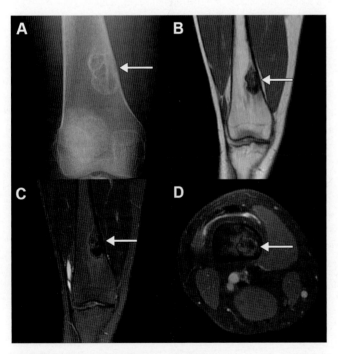

Fig. C25.1 Nonossifying fibroma. (A) Radiograph reveals an eccentric, cortically based lucent lesion with a well-defined, lobulated, sclerotic border in the medial, distal femoral metadiaphysis. (B) T1-weighted image reveals a low-signal intensity rim and low to intermediate internal signal. (C) T2-weighted image with fat suppression reveals heterogeneous, predominantly low signal intensity, which is more common than T2- hyperintensity. (D) Postcontrast image reveals mild peripheral enhancement.

benign lesion and the adjacent normal bone is so well defined ("narrow zone of transition") that it may be drawn with a fine-point pen. Malignant lesions, on the other hand, tend to have a gradual transition between lesion and normal bone ("broad zone of transition"). Occasionally, further evaluation with CT or MRI may be indicated.

Nonossifying fibromas (see Box C25.1) are benign fibrous lesions composed of spindle cells in a collagenous matrix. Nonossifying fibromas are extremely common, occurring in up to 20% of children. However, they typically regress and are rarely seen after age 30. Recognizing nonossifying fibromas as benign "don't touch" lesions is important, since the radiologic diagnosis precludes biopsy in the large majority of cases.

FINDINGS

On radiographs, nonossifying fibromas typically present as elliptic, slightly expansile, cortically based, lucent lesions with a thin, sclerotic border. They are eccentrically located and arise near the physis (Fig. C25.1). Periosteal reaction is typically absent, unless the lesion is complicated by fracture (Fig. C25.2A).

Because they are common incidental lesions on MR imaging performed for internal derangement of joints, familiarity with their signal characteristics is important. MRI (Fig. C25.1B-D) reveals low signal intensity on T1-weighted images and variable T2 signal based on the amount of fibrous tissue: High T2 signal is seen during the development of these lesions, and low signal intensity is seen as the lesions mature and heal. Thin peripheral enhancement is typical.

DIFFERENTIAL DIAGNOSIS

Imaging Differential Diagnosis

The radiographic appearance of a nonossifying fibroma is usually sufficient for diagnosis. However, if a unicameral bone cyst or an aneurysmal bone cyst arises in a small tubular bone such as the fibula (Fig. C25.2B), it may resemble a nonossifying fibroma occupying the entire diameter of the bone. Unicameral bone cysts typically occur in the proximal humerus or proximal femur and are typically asymptomatic unless fractured. They may appear multiloculated

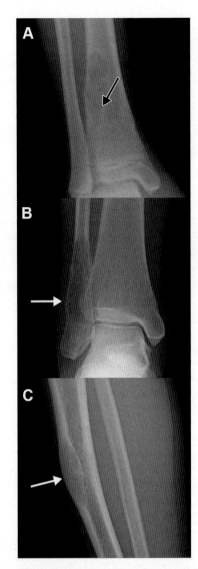

Fig. C25.2 Complications of and differential considerations for nonossifying fibroma. (A) Pathologic fracture. Frontal view of the distal lower leg reveals a spiral fracture (black arrow) through a nonossifying fibroma in the distal tibial diaphysis. (B) Aneurysmal bone cyst in the fibula (white arrow). (C) Osteofibrous dysplasia in the anterior tibia (white arrow).

on MRI. The fallen fragment sign is a classic radiographic finding associated with this lesion and occurs when a piece of fractured cortical bone sinks to the gravity-dependent portion of the lesion. Aneurysmal bone cysts are benign lesions that are typically expansile in appearance. Fluid-fluid levels are characteristically identified on CT or MRI.

When a lesion with imaging characteristics similar to those of nonossifying fibroma or fibrous dysplasia arises in the anterior tibia in a young patient, osteofibrous dysplasia should be considered in the differential diagnosis (Fig. C25.2C). These lesions have lobulated sclerotic margins and are usually confined to the cortex. Unlike nonossifying fibromas, osteofibrous dysplasias can result in cortical destruction and invasion of the medullary cavity.

Clinical Differential Diagnosis

None

REFERENCES AND SUGGESTED READING

1. Biermann JS. Common benign lesions of bone in children and adolescents. *J Pediatr Orthop.* 2002;22:268-273.

2. Levine SM, Lambiase RE, Petchprapa CN. Cortical lesions of the tibia: characteristic appearances at conventional radiography. *RadioGraphics.* 2003;23:157-177.

3. Miller SL, Hoffer FA. Malignant and benign bone tumors. *Radiol Clin North Am.* 2001;39:673-699.

4. Motamedi K, Seeger, LL. Benign bone tumors. *Radiol Clin N Am.* 2011;49:1115-1134.

5. Subhas N, Bui KL, Sundaram M, Ilaslan H, Recht MP. Incidental tumor and tumor-like lesions around the knee. *Semin Musculoskelet Radiol.* 2009;13:353-370.

CASE 26

PATIENT PRESENTATION

A 19-year-old man with a 3-month history of left hip pain. The pain wakes him up at night and improves with over-the-counter analgesics.

CLINICAL SUSPICION

Osteoid osteoma

IMAGING MODALITY OF CHOICE

Radiography to start. CT is the imaging modality of choice.

BACKGROUND

Osteoid osteoma is a relatively common benign bone tumor. Patients classically complain of nocturnal pain (sometimes severe enough to disrupt sleep) that is relieved with aspirin. This classic clinical presentation is present in more than 75% of patients with osteoid osteoma. Symptomatic patients can be treated with medication, surgery, or percutaneous ablation.

Histologically, osteoid osteoma is a benign, bone-producing tumor that is characterized by a nidus of cellular, highly vascularized tissue. Central calcification may or may not be present within the nidus. The nidus is often surrounded by a zone of reactive bone formation.

Three subtypes of osteoid osteoma can be defined on the basis of the location in bone: cortical (most common), medullary, and subperiosteal.

FINDINGS

Cortical osteoid osteomas (Fig. C26.1) are the most common type and typically present as a small cortical lucency surrounded by fusiform sclerosis involving one side of the diaphysis. The nidus may not be obvious if the surrounding reactive sclerosis is severe enough.

Medullary osteoid osteomas typically do not result in as much reactive sclerosis, and subperiosteal osteoid osteomas often do not result in any reactive sclerosis. Subperiosteal osteoid osteomas can present as soft-tissue masses that result in irregular bony resorption along the periosteal surface.

CT can be helpful if a nidus is suspected to be obscured by surrounding sclerosis on radiographs. CT reveals a well-defined soft-tissue attenuation lesion surrounded by variable amounts of sclerosis. Punctate, amorphous, or ringlike calcification(s) can often be seen within the nidus (Fig. C26.1G).

Bone scintigraphy is very sensitive for detection of osteoid osteomas and classically reveals the double-density sign (Fig. C26.1F): a central focus of very high uptake (nidus) surrounded by a larger area of less-intense uptake (reactive bone).

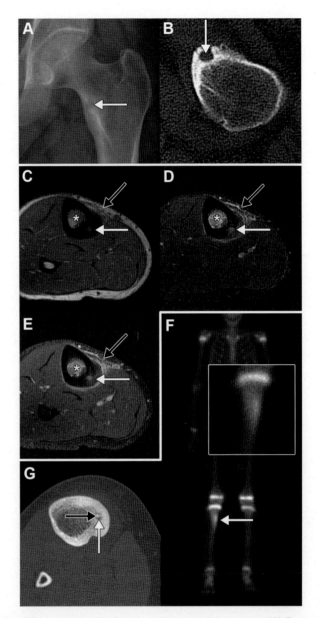

Fig. C26.1 Imaging findings in cortical osteoid osteoma. (A) Frontal radiograph of the left femur reveals a lucent lesion (white arrow), corresponding to the nidus, with surrounding fusiform sclerosis. (B) CT in the same patient reveals the intracortical nidus (white arrow) located centrally within the area of cortical thickening. The nidus can also be eccentrically oriented toward the periosteal or endosteal surfaces. (C-E) MRI in a different patient reveals cortical thickening with a central nidus (white arrow) that is intermediate signal intensity on the T1- and T2-weighted images (C and D, respectively) and has mild enhancement (E). There is also edema within the bone marrow (*) and surrounding soft tissues (black arrow). (F) Bone scintigraphy in another patient reveals focal increased uptake in the right proximal tibia (white arrow). The inset shows the double density sign to better advantage. (G) CT in this patient reveals the nidus (white arrow) with a central calcification (black arrow).

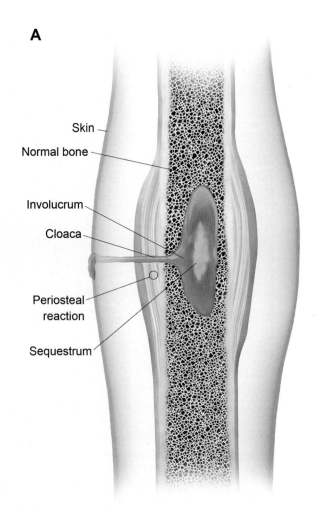

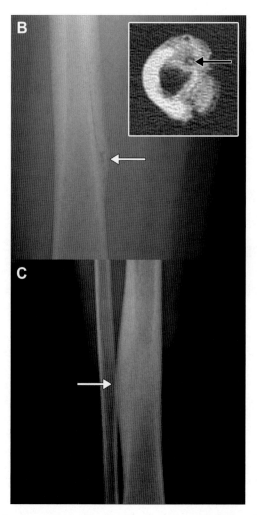

Fig. C26.2 Imaging differential diagnosis for osteoid osteoma. (A) Diagram of chronic osteomyelitis. The involucrum, or abscess cavity, forms inside normal bone, isolating a piece of devitalized bone, the sequestrum. The drainage tract from the involucrum to the surface of bone is called the cloaca. Periosteal reaction is often present. (B) Chronic osteomyelitis in the mid femoral diaphysis. There is cortical thickening surrounding the involucrum (white arrow). Inset shows the CT at this level with a small sequestrum (black arrow) inside the involucrum. (C) Stress fracture in the mid tibial diaphysis with cortical thickening.

On MRI, the nidus has low to intermediate signal on T1-weighted images, heterogeneously high signal on T2-weighted images, and variable enhancement. Central calcifications, when present, have low signal on both T1- and T2-weighted images. The nidus is surrounded by fusiform low signal on both T1- and T2-weighted sequences, corresponding to the surrounding sclerosis, and peritumoral edema both within the bone marrow and surrounding soft tissues.

DIFFERENTIAL DIAGNOSIS
Imaging Differential Diagnosis

Chronic osteomyelitis (Fig. C26.2A,B), can result in cortical thickening, which tends to be irregular and associated with a periosteal reaction. The abscess cavity can mimic

the nidus, and the sequestrum can mimic mineralization within the nidus.

Stress fracture (Fig. C26.2C) can result in cortical thickening without an obvious fracture plane and can mimic the appearance of osteoid osteoma.

Clinical Differential Diagnosis

Neoplasm (benign and malignant), trauma (fracture or stress reaction).

REFERENCE AND SUGGESTED READING

1. Iyer RS, Chapman T, Chew FS. Pediatric bone imaging: diagnostic imaging of osteoid osteoma. *AJR.* 2012;198(5): 1039-1052.

CASE 27

PATIENT PRESENTATION

A 72-year-old man with renal cell carcinoma presents with insidious onset of left hip pain that is incompletely relieved by rest.

CLINICAL SUSPICION

Metastatic disease to bone

IMAGING MODALITY OF CHOICE

Bone scintigraphy ("bone scan"), followed by radiography or MRI as needed to clarify findings on bone scintigraphy. Bone scintigraphy allows for a survey of the whole body and is very sensitive for bone metastases but is not very specific, and other imaging modalities may be needed for clarification of equivocal findings.

FINDINGS

Bone scintigraphy (box C27.1) typically reveals areas of focal increased uptake (Fig. C27.1A). Radiographs can be normal or reveal sclerotic (Fig. C27.1B), lytic (Fig. C27.1C), or mixed lesions. Table C27.1 lists the common radiographic appearance of various metastases.

The dreaded complication of spinal metastases is spinal cord compression, which may require surgical intervention or urgent radiotherapy.

Metastases can also lead to weakening of bone and subsequent pathological fracture. Patients with metastases to the long bones can be risk stratified to determine if they would benefit from prophylactic fixation. The Mirels classification (Tables C27.2 and C27.3) classifies the risk of pathologic fracture based on scoring four variables on a scale of 1 to 3: location of lesion, radiographic appearance, size, and pain. An overall score is calculated, and a recommendation for or against prophylactic fixation is made (Fig. C27.1C,D).

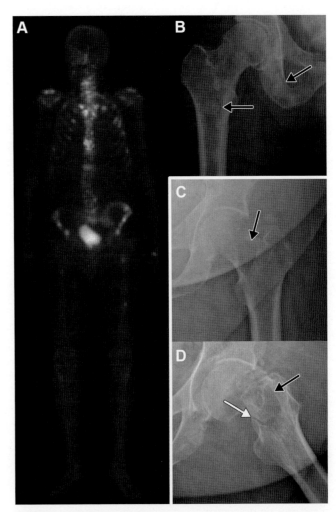

Fig. C27.1 Metastatic disease and pathological fracture. (A) Bone scintigraphy reveals widespread bone metastases. (B) Radiography reveals multiple sclerotic lesions (black arrows) in this patient with prostate cancer. (C) Single metastatic lesion of renal cell carcinoma in a 70-year-old man (black arrow). Scoring the lesion according to the Mirels classification (Tables C27.2 and C27.3), we note that the lesion is lytic (+3), located in the nonintertrochanteric lower extremity (+2), and results in thinning of greater than two-thirds of the cortex (+3). The patient reportedly had functional pain associated with the lesion (+3). The total Mirels score of 11 places the patient at high risk of pathologic fracture. (D) Pathological fracture (white arrow) that developed in this patient during transport. The underlying lytic lesion (black arrow) can be seen on either side of the fracture plane.

BOX C27.1 – TERMINOLOGY

The terms *bone scan* and *bone survey* are often confused with one another.

- *Bone scan* refers to nuclear medicine bone scintigraphy (see chapter 1).
- *Bone survey* is a series of radiographs of multiple bones.

DIFFERENTIAL DIAGNOSIS

Imaging Differential Diagnosis

A single focus of increased uptake on scintigraphy in patients with known malignancy is nonspecific and can present a diagnostic challenge (Fig. C27.2). In the spine, the probability of a solitary focus of uptake representing a metastasis depends on location (Fig. C27.2E-H). Uptake in the body that is contiguous with the pedicle most likely represents a metastasis, whereas uptake in the facet joints, body only,

Table C27.1 Typical Radiographic Appearance of Metastases

Typically Lytic	Typically Mixed	Typically Sclerotic
• Lung carcinoma	• Lung carcinoma	• Prostate
• Breast carcinoma	• Breast carcinoma	• Bronchial carcinoid tumor
• Hepatocellular carcinoma	• Cervical carcinoma	• Bladder carcinoma involving prostate
• Melanoma	• Ovarian carcinoma	• Nasopharyngeal carcinoma
• Squamous cell carcinoma, skin	• Testicular tumors	• Gastric carcinoma
• Pheochromocytoma		• Medulloblastoma
• Ewing tumor		• Neuroblastoma
• Wilms' tumor		
• Gastrointestinal tract carcinomas		
• Uterine carcinoma		
• Adrenal carcinoma		
• Thyroid carcinoma		
• Renal cell carcinoma		

Table C27.2 Mirels Classification

	1	2	3
Location	Upper extremity	Lower extremity	Intertrochanteric
Radiography	Blastic	Mixed	Lytic
Size[a]	<1/3	1/3-2/3	>2/3
Pain	Mild	Moderate	Functional[b]

[a]Size is determined as a fraction of the cortical thickness.
[b]Functional pain is defined as severe pain or pain aggravated by limb function.

Table C27.3 Fracture Risk

Score	Fracture Risk	Recommendation
≥9	33%-100%	Prophylactic fixation is recommended.
=8	15%	Clinical judgment should be used.
≤7	<4%	Observation and radiation therapy can be used.

and both body and posterior elements with sparing of the pedicles most likely represent benign processes.

A potential pitfall of bone scintigraphy is in the setting of diffuse metastatic disease, which can result in diffuse skeletal uptake of radiotracer. This appearance, the so-called super scan (Fig. C27.3), can obscure focal lesions in the skeleton. The key to avoiding this pitfall is recognizing the greater contrast between bone and soft tissue and an absence or considerable reduction of activity in the kidneys. Metabolic disease (eg, renal osteodystrophy) can have a similar appearance but is said to have a homogeneous appearance compared to the more heterogeneous appearance of diffuse metastatic disease. Reliable differentiation between the two, however, is often not possible.

Although multiple myeloma (see case 28) can be similar on radiographs, lesions of myeloma are frequently photopenic or occult on bone scintigraphy.

Clinical Differential Diagnosis

Insufficiency fractures, degenerative changes of the spine, and muscle strains can have a similar presentation.

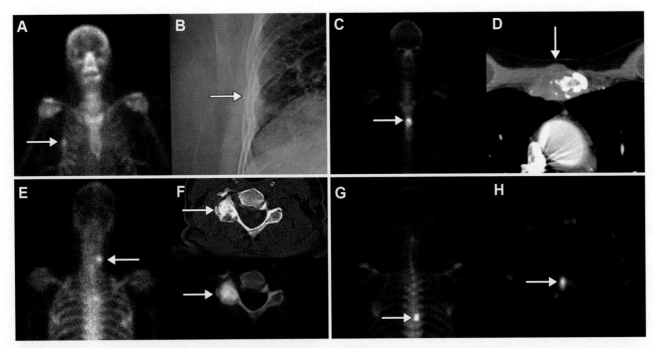

Fig. C27.2 Imaging differential diagnosis and pitfalls. (A,B) In patients with known carcinoma, 90% of solitary rib lesions on bone scintigraphy are due to benign causes. (A) Solitary rib lesion on Tc-99m MDP bone scintigraphy (white arrow) in a patient with renal cell carcinoma corresponds to a healing rib fracture (white arrow), (B). (C,D) A solitary sternal lesion in a patient with breast carcinoma has an 80% probability of representing a metastasis. (C) Solitary sternal lesion (white arrow) on Tc-99m MDP bone scintigraphy in a patient with breast carcinoma is concerning. (D) CT through the sternum in this patient shows a destructive lesion with a soft tissue component (white arrow) in the sternum. (E-H) Solitary lesions in the spine can also present a challenge on planar imaging; however, the location of the focus of uptake can be better evaluated using SPECT and SPECT/CT fusion. Lesions in the facet (apophyseal) joints, lesions beyond the vertebral body surface, lesions involving only the body, and lesions involving the body and posterior elements with sparing of the pedicles are most likely benign, whereas those involving the body and pedicle are likely malignant. (E) Posterior projection from a Tc-99m MDP bone scintigram shows a solitary lesion in the lower cervical spine in a patient with breast cancer. In about 20% of patients with breast cancer, disease relapses with a solitary bone lesion, most commonly in the spine. (F) CT (top) and SPECT-CT fusion (bottom) localizes the lesion to the right facet joint, with CT imaging features characteristic of osteoarthritis. (G) Posterior projection from a bone scintigram shows a solitary lesion in the mid-thoracic spine (white arrow) in a patient with a neuroendocrine carcinoma. (H) SPECT image localizes the lesion to the vertebral body and pedicle. The lesion represented a metastasis.

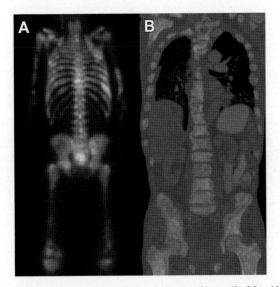

Fig. C27.3 Super scan. (A) Posterior projection from a Tc-99m MDP bone scintigraphy reveals diffuse and lumpy uptake throughout the skeleton with little or no soft tissue or renal uptake. (B) Coronal CT reformation in the same patient reveals widespread and diffuse sclerotic skeletal metastases. The patient had prostate cancer.

REFERENCES AND SUGGESTED READING

1. Roberts CC, Daffner RH, Weissman BN, et al. Expert Panel on Musculoskeletal Imaging. ACR Appropriateness Criteria. Metastatic bone disease. ACR; 2009.

2. Wilner D. *Radiology of Bone Tumors and allied Disorders.* Philadelphia: WB Saunders; 1982:1646.

CASE 28

PATIENT PRESENTATION

A 70-year-old man with persistent low back pain and fatigue despite symptomatic treatment. Initial radiographs revealed degenerative findings in the lumbar spine. Routine laboratory workup revealed elevated total protein and calcium.

CLINICAL SUSPICION

Multiple myeloma

IMAGING MODALITY OF CHOICE

Radiographic skeletal survey. Whole-body low-dose CT and whole-body MRI, although more sensitive, are not routinely used at this time.

BACKGROUND

Monoclonal gammopathies (Box C28.1) are a group of disorders associated with monoclonal proliferation of plasma cells. Multiple myeloma is a neoplastic proliferation of a single clone of plasma cells that produces skeletal destruction and/or soft tissue masses. Patients can present with bone pain, pathological fracture, anemia, hypercalcemia, and renal insufficiency.

The radiologist's job in assessing patients with monoclonal gammopathies includes:

- Verifying the extent of bone and soft tissue involvement (Fig. C28.1)
- Providing information needed for staging (requires familiarity with the staging system used by the referring physicians)
- Assessing for complications (see Box C28.2 and Fig. C28.2)
- Assessing treatment response

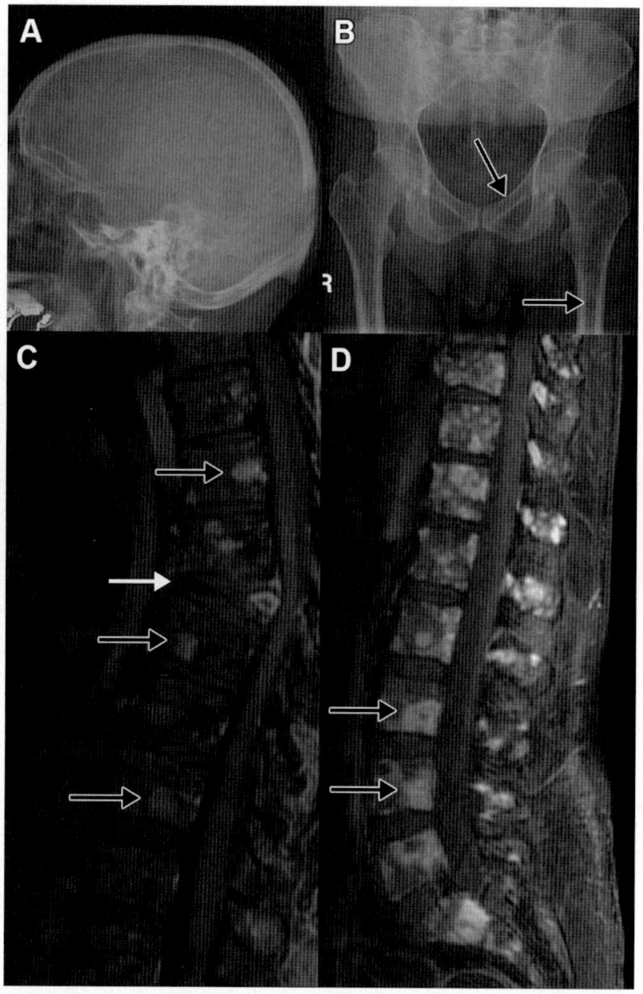

Fig. C28.1 Multiple myeloma in different patients. (A) Multiple lytic lesions in the skull. (B) Lytic lesions in the pelvis (black arrows) can be difficult to detect due to overlying bones and bowel gas. (C) Multiple focal enhancing lesions in the spine (black arrows) and a compression fracture (white arrow). Radiography (not shown) did not depict any of the focal lesions. (D) Micronodular pattern of multiple myeloma on postcontrast sagittal image (salt-and-pepper appearance). Scattered focal lesions (black arrows) can also be seen.

BOX C28.1 – MONOCLONAL GAMMOPATHIES

- Monoclonal gammopathy of undetermined significance (MGUS)
- Smoldering multiple myeloma
- Multiple myeloma
- Nonsecretory multiple myeloma
- Solitary plasmacytoma
- Multiple solitary plasmacytomas
- Plasma cell leukemia

BOX C28.2 – COMPLICATIONS OF MULTIPLE MYELOMA

- Pathological fracture
- Spinal cord compression
- Avascular necrosis (due to steroid therapy)
- Infection (due to cytotoxic drugs and steroid therapy)
- Leptomeningeal spread
- Amyloidosis

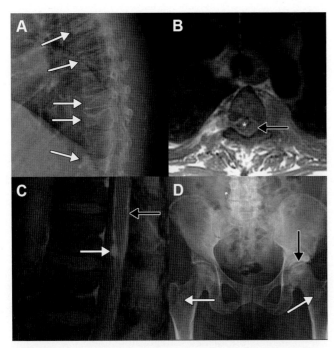

Fig. C28.2 Complications of multiple myeloma and its treatment. (A) Multiple compression fractures (white arrows) in a patient with multiple myeloma. (B) Spinal cord (*) being compressed from epidural spread of disease (black arrow). (C) Leptomeningeal spread (extension of disease through the subarachnoid spaces of the spinal cord and brain) manifests as smooth (black arrow) or nodular (white arrow) enhancement along the spinal cord and along the cauda equina. (D) Avascular necrosis of the left femoral head (black arrow) due to steroid therapy. Presence of sclerotic lesions (white arrows) indicates treated disease (the patient previously had lytic lesions in these locations).

FINDINGS

The most common radiographic presentation of multiple myeloma is as multiple lytic foci. In the skull, this manifests as round, punched-out areas of bone destruction that are usually uniform in size (Fig. C28.1A). Multiple foci of bone destruction can also be seen in the remainder of the axial skeleton (eg, spine, pelvic bones; Fig. C28.1B) and the proximal appendicular skeleton (proximal humeri and femora). Compression fractures are often seen in the spine.

Multiple myeloma can also manifest radiographically as osteoporosis, without definite focal lesions. This is predominantly seen in the spine and may be accompanied by compression fractures of vertebral bodies. Uncommonly, multiple myeloma lesions can be predominantly sclerotic (osteosclerotic myeloma).

Bone scintigraphy is usually normal in multiple myeloma, but increased uptake can be seen on occasion.

CT is superior to radiography in demonstrating the extent of the lesions, presence of cortical destruction, and soft tissue involvement. MRI can show focal (Fig. C28.1C),

micronodular (Fig. C28.1D), or diffuse abnormalities that are hypointense on T1-weighted images and hyperintense on T2-weighted images and enhance on postcontrast images.

Although bone lesions in untreated multiple myeloma are most often lytic, some patients present with sclerotic lesions. For example, patients with POEMS syndrome more commonly have sclerotic or mixed lesions. POEMS syndrome is a paraneoplastic syndrome related to a plasma cell dyscrasia (eg, multiple myeloma). The acronyms POEMS (polyneuropathy, organomegaly, endocrinopathy, M protein, and skin changes) and PEP (plasma cell dyscrasia, endocrinopathy, and polyneuropathy) capture some, but not all, of the associated manifestations. Other manifestations include sclerotic bone lesions, Castleman disease (a lymphoproliferative disorder), papilledema, thrombocytosis, erythrocytosis, pleural effusions, edema, and ascites. The vast majority of patients have radiographic evidence of bone lesions at presentation. Slightly less than half of these lesions are purely sclerotic (well defined or fluffy), approximately half are mixed sclerotic and lytic, and a small number (2%) are purely lytic bone lesions, which tend to have sclerotic margins giving them a unique ring-like appearance.

DIFFERENTIAL DIAGNOSIS

Imaging Differential Diagnosis

In the absence of laboratory findings suggestive of multiple myeloma, one may consider lytic metastases (see case 27).

Clinical Differential Diagnosis

In the setting of persistent bone pain and fatigue despite symptomatic treatment, the differential considerations include metastatic disease, multiple myeloma, vitamin D deficiency, hyperparathyroidism, and polymyalgia rheumatica. A complete blood count, erythrocyte sedimentation rate, chemistry panel, serum and urine protein electrophoresis, radiography, and vitamin D levels can be obtained to initiate the proper workup.

REFERENCES AND SUGGESTED READING

1. Angtuaco EJ, Fassas AB, Walker R, Sethi R, Barlogie B. Multiple myeloma: clinical review and diagnostic imaging. *Radiology.* 2004;231(1):11-23. Epub 2004 Feb 27.

2. Nau KC, Lewis WD. Multiple myeloma: diagnosis and treatment. *Am Fam Physician.* 2008;78(7):853-859.

CASE 29

PATIENT PRESENTATION

A 75-year-old man presents with right hip pain.

CLINICAL SUSPICION

Fracture or neoplasm

IMAGING MODALITY OF CHOICE

Radiographs

BACKGROUND

Paget disease of bone is a chronic skeletal disorder of unknown etiology characterized by intense focal resorption of bone followed by disorderly bone formation that results in abnormal bone remodeling. The disease has three phases:

- Lytic (incipient active): Osteoclastic resorption predominates.
- Mixed (active): Both osteoclastic and osteoblastic hyperplasia with predominant osteoblastic activity.
- Blastic (late inactive): Osteoblastic activity gradually declines.

FINDINGS

Abnormal bony resorption and apposition results in a variety of radiographic appearances, depending on the phase of the disease (Fig. C29.1).

> ### BOX C29.1 – COMPLICATIONS OF PAGET DISEASE
>
> - Osteoarthritis
> - Deformity
> - Fracture
> - Nerve entrapment
> - Secondary neoplasm (rare)

The lytic phase (osteoclastic) presents in the long bones as an advancing wedge of osteolysis that begins in the subchondral bone of the epiphysis and extends peripherally into the metaphysis and diaphysis at a rate of about 1 cm per year. The classic appearance has been likened to a flame or blade of grass (Fig. C29.1E). Marginal sclerosis is typically absent. In the skull, the advancing osteolysis is known as osteoporosis circumscripta (Fig. C29.1A,B) and presents as large lucent areas that are most prominent in the inner table and usually cross suture lines.

Most patients present in the mixed phase, which manifests radiographically as advancing osteolysis, coarsening and thickening of bone trabeculae, cortical thickening, and osseous expansion. In the long bones, the advancing osteolysis toward the diaphysis is accompanied by focal bone sclerosis in the epiphysis and metaphysis (Fig. C29.1F). In the pelvis, there is sclerosis of the iliopectineal and ischiopubic lines and enlargement of the pubic rami and ischium (Fig. C29.1G). Acetabular protrusion can also

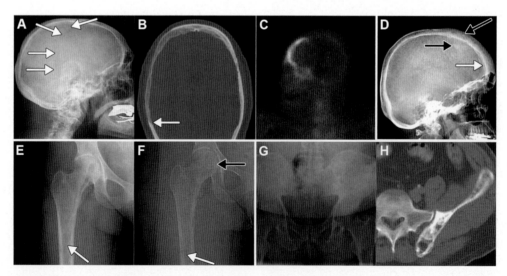

Fig. C29.1 Paget disease of bone. (A) Osteoporosis circumscripta with a well-defined lucency in the frontoparietal skull (white arrows). (B) CT in the same patient shows the osteolysis to better advantage. Note the well-defined posterior margin (white arrow). (C) Tc-99m MDP bone scintigraphy in the same patient shows uptake along the periphery of the lesion. (D) Cotton-wool appearance in another patient. Areas of sclerosis (black arrows) are seen in the frontal bone. Also note mild thickening of the frontal bone (white arrow). (E) Blade of grass appearance in the right femur with a well-defined front of osteolysis (white arrow). (F) Image obtained 3 years later shows osteolysis further down the femur (white arrow) with development of coarsened trabeculae and mild cortical expansion more proximally (black arrow). (G) Later-stage Paget disease with sclerosis, cortical expansion, and coarsened trabeculae involving the left ilium, ischium, and pubis. (H) CT in the same patient shows the sclerosis, cortical expansion, and coarsened trabeculae.

be seen when there is para-acetabular involvement. The characteristic picture-frame appearance in the spine describes the cortical thickening along all four margins of the vertebral body. In the skull, the areas of lucency fill in with globular or fluffy foci of variable density ("cotton-wool appearance"; Fig. C29.1D).

The blastic phase is characterized by osteosclerosis. There is expansion of the bone with coarse trabeculae and cortical thickening. The bones are weak at this point, and radiographs should be carefully evaluated for insufficiency fractures. In the skull, there is sclerosis and thickening of the diploic space, resulting in the "Tam-O'-Shanter" skull (a type of Scottish hat). In the spine, the sclerosis can present as an enlarged vertebral body and posterior elements that may be accompanied by sclerosis (ivory vertebra).

Bone scintigraphy reveals increased radionuclide uptake in affected bone in all three phases of Paget disease, particularly in active disease. Osteoporosis circumscripta is a notable exception, where intense radionuclide uptake is seen only in the margins of the lesion (Fig. C29.1C).

DIFFERENTIAL DIAGNOSIS

Imaging Differential Diagnosis

The differential diagnosis depends on the radiographic appearance and the phase of disease. For example, the lucent lesions in the skull seen in the osteoclastic phase can resemble metastases or multiple myeloma. The diffuse osteosclerosis present in the mixed and osteoblastic phases can also be seen with some bone metastases, myelofibrosis, fluorosis, mastocytosis, and renal osteodystrophy. Calvarial hyperostosis seen in the mixed and osteoblastic phases can also be seen with hyperostosis frontalis interna, fibrous dysplasia, and skeletal metastases.

Clinical Differential Diagnosis

Fracture, osteoarthritis, and neoplasm can present with nonspecific pain.

REFERENCE AND SUGGESTED READING

1. Theodorou DJ, Theodorou SJ, Kakitsubata Y. Imaging of Paget disease of bone and its musculoskeletal complications: review. *AJR.* 2011;196(6)(suppl):S64-S75.

CASE 30
PATIENT PRESENTATION

A 35-year-old man presents with approximately 1 year of hip pain and discomfort that is worse with activity. Two months previously, he began palpating a mass in the right hip that has not grown significantly since it first appeared. On further questioning, the patient reports significant sports trauma approximately a year and half ago but does not re-call direct trauma to the right hip at that time. Physical examination reveals a firm, mobile, nontender soft tissue mass along the anterolateral aspect of the right proximal thigh. Radiographs were obtained (Fig. C30.1A).

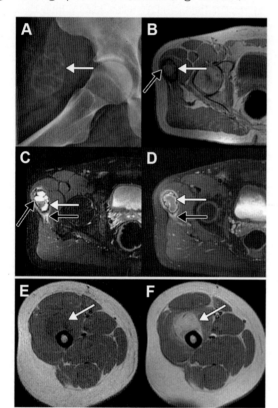

Fig. C30.1 Myositis ossificans (heterotopic ossification). (A) Frog-leg lateral view of the right hip reveals an ovoid mass with peripheral mineralization (white arrow). (B) Axial T1-weighted image reveals a well-defined mass (white arrow) with intermediate internal signal and peripheral hypointensity corresponding to peripheral mineralization. The mass has intermediate signal with an area that is slightly more hyperintense (black arrow). (C) T2-weighted axial image reveals peripheral hypointensity (white arrow), a fluid-fluid level within the mass (black arrowhead), and mild perilesional edema (black arrow). (D) Postcontrast im-age reveals peripheral hypointensity with circumferential internal enhancement (white arrow) and perilesional enhancement (black arrow). (E,F) Early myositis ossificans in another patient. A lesion (white arrow) in the vastus intermedius muscle is T1- hypointense (E), T2- hyperintense (not shown), and heterogeneously enhancing (F). The mass abuts the femoral cortex without erosion or medullary extension. The appearance is nonspecific, and a soft tissue sarcoma cannot be excluded on the basis of imaging findings. The lesion resolved on follow-up MRI.

CLINICAL SUSPICION

Soft tissue neoplasm versus benign soft tissue mass.

IMAGING MODALITY OF CHOICE

Initial imaging may not be necessary when faced with a patient with a soft tissue mass. Although soft tissue sarco-mas are rare, short-term follow-up is imperative to exclude this diagnosis. If the mass persists or enlarges, further work-up should be initiated, keeping in mind that appropriate treatment of sarcoma patients requires the coordinated efforts of medical and surgical oncologists, radiation thera-pists, and diagnostic and interventional radiologists. The community surgeon may not be familiar with principles of modern treatment of sarcomas, leading to an excisional biopsy or an unplanned resection, both of which will leave the patient with surgical margins infiltrated with tumor ("positive margins").

Appropriate imaging in a case of suspected soft tissue neoplasm begins with radiography and is followed with MRI. Suspicious findings should prompt referral to an oncological specialist.

FINDINGS

Some soft tissue masses have characteristic imaging find-ings that allow a diagnosis to be made confidently. Myositis ossificans, perhaps more appropriately called traumatic het-erotopic ossification (Fig. C30.1), is a benign, self-limiting, nonneoplastic response to injury. Mature bone develops in the lesion in about 2 months, and is said to be diag-nostic. Radiography and CT typically reveal a well-defined soft tissue mass with mineralization that is more mature peripherally than centrally. Initial MRI (Fig. C30.1E,F) and even biopsy can suggest a malignant process. MRI at this stage may reveal fluid-fluid levels, enhancement, and per-ilesional edema, an appearance that can mimic that of a hemorrhagic sarcoma. The characteristic mineralized rim may not be apparent on MRI at this stage. Mature hetero-topic ossification, on the other hand, has signal character-istics of bone on MRI: a well-defined, hypointense rim with trabeculae, dense fibrosis, and central fat.

Other soft tissue lesions can also present diagnostic challenges at imaging. Although lipomas have a charac-teristic appearance on MRI (Fig. C30.2A,B), distinguishing them from well-differentiated liposarcomas may not always be possible. On MRI, lipomas have a signal similar to that of fat on all pulse sequences and no enhancement on post-contrast images. Any complexity in a fatty tumor should lead to careful evaluation for signs of malignancy. At the ag-gressive malignant end of the spectrum of fatty tumors are poorly differentiated liposarcomas (Fig. C30.2C,D), which have a heterogeneous appearance on MRI and often little to no fat. In between and on the less aggressive side of

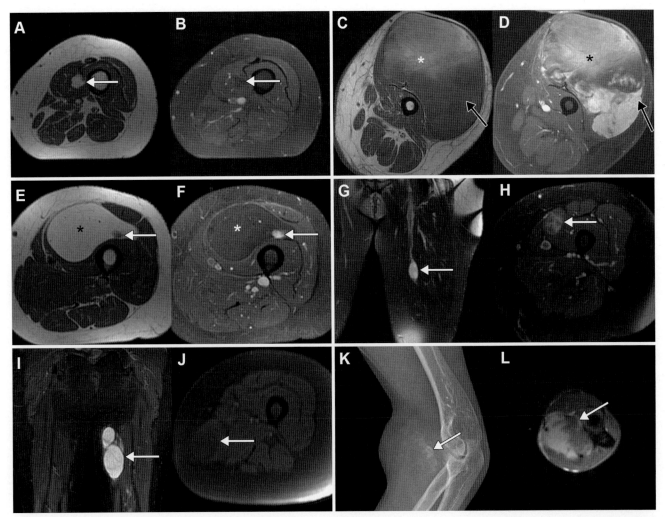

Fig. C30.2 Spectrum of imaging findings in soft tissue lesions. (A) Liopma: Axial T1-weighted image reveals a T1-hyperintense mass in the vastus medialis muscle that loses signal on the fat-saturated postcontrast image (B) and has no significant internal enhancement. (C,D) Liposarcoma: A large heterogeneous, multilobulated mass occupies the entirety of the anterior compartment of the thigh and has enhancing areas (black arrow) corresponding to active tumor. Areas of T1 hyperintensity and nonenhancement (*) are indicative of cystic/ hemorrhagic change. (E,F) Atypical lipomatous tumor: Axial T1-weighted image reveals a tumor in the intermuscular planes of the anterior thigh that is predominantly fatty in nature (*), but which has an enhancing and nonfatty component (F, white arrow). Image-guided biopsy will ideally target this portion of the lesion, as sampling the fatty component may result in a diagnosis of lipoma. (G,H) Intramuscular myxoma: A fusiform, T2- hyperintense lesion is seen in the vastus medialis muscle (G, white arrow). (H) The mass has heterogeneous enhancement on postcontrast imaging. (I,J) Schwannoma: A fusiform lesion in the vastus medialis muscle is predominantly T2-hyperintense (I) with thin septations. No significant enhancement is present on the postcontrast image (J). (K,L) Synovial cell sarcoma: A mass at the elbow is partially calcified but lacks the typical mature mineralization of myositis ossificans. Postcontrast image (L) reveals a heterogeneously enhancing lesion (white arrow).

the spectrum are intermediate-grade malignant neoplasms with a mature lipomatous proliferation (well-differentiated liposarcomas; Fig. C30.2E,F). These are locally aggressive but do not metastasize. In the extremities, one may refer to them as *atypical lipomatous tumors* to convey the good prognosis patients have after complete resection. In the abdomen, where complete resection with negative tumor margins is often impossible, local recurrence is common, and mortality rates approach 80%, the term *well-differentiated liposarcoma* is more appropriate.

Other soft tissue tumors can have nonspecific appearances and usually require biopsy to exclude malignancy. Intramuscular myxomas (Fig. C30.2G,H) can have a wide range of imaging characteristics. Peripheral nerve sheath tumors have a spectrum of biological behavior ranging from benign schwannomas (Fig. C30.2I,J) and neurofibromas to malignant peripheral nerve sheath tumors. Synovial cell sarcomas (Fig. C30.2K,L) are uncommon malignant tumors that can be associated with calcification in 20% to 30% of cases.

DIFFERENTIAL DIAGNOSIS

Imaging Differential Diagnosis

Soft tissue masses often have a nonspecific appearance at imaging, and a wide variety of benign and malignant processes need to be considered.

Clinical Differential Diagnosis

- Benign, nonneoplastic: Hematoma, heterotopic ossification.
- Benign, neoplastic: Lipoma, myxoma.
- Malignant: Sarcoma, soft tissue metastasis.

REFERENCES AND SUGGESTED READING

1. Rosenthal TC, Kraybill W. Soft tissue sarcomas: integrating primary care recognition with tertiary care center treatment. *Am Fam Physician*. 1999;60(2):567-572.
2. Wilson AN, Davis A, Bell RS, et al. Local control of soft tissue sarcoma of the extremity: the experience of a multidisciplinary sarcoma group with definitive surgery and radiotherapy. *Eur J Cancer*. 1994;30A(6):746-751.

CASE 31

PATIENT PRESENTATION

A 4-year-old boy presents with a palpable, hard lump proximal to the knee. On physical examination, a hard mass is palpated along the posterolateral aspect of the distal femur. No associated erythema or tenderness is present. Lateral radiograph of the knee was obtained (Fig. C31.1A).

CLINICAL SUSPICION

Osteochondroma

IMAGING MODALITY OF CHOICE

Radiographs are preferred for initial evaluation of a palpable mass in an extremity to guide further diagnostic evaluation. Radiographs can be performed quickly with minimal cost or radiation to the patient. Suspicious or noncontributory findings should be further assessed by cross-sectional imaging.

BACKGROUND

An osteochondroma is a cartilage-capped bony excrescence, with well-defined marrow and cortex that are contiguous with the underlying bone. An osteochondroma may occasionally result in pain from trauma or nerve impingement. However, pain or rapid enlargement may suggest malignant degeneration to a chondrosarcoma, a rare but dreaded complication. MRI may be performed if malignant degeneration of an osteochondroma is suspected.

FINDINGS

Radiographs typically reveal a bony protrusion whose marrow and cortex are contiguous with those of the normal underlying bone. Osteochondromas can be pedunculated (with a stalk) or have a broad-based connection to the underlying bone (Fig. C31.1A,B).

CT and MRI better depict the contiguity of the cortex and marrow of an osteochondroma with those of the underlying bone. MRI (Fig. C31.1C) is the modality of choice for assessment of the overlying cartilage cap, which should be well defined and less than 1 cm in thickness.

Complications of osteochondromas include fracture (Fig. C31.2A), nerve impingement (Fig. C31.2B,C), and transformation of the cartilage cap into chondrosarcoma (Fig. C31.2D).

DIFFERENTIAL DIAGNOSIS

Imaging Differential Diagnosis

Chondrosarcoma: Rarely (< 1%), an osteochondroma may undergo malignant transformation to a chondrosarcoma (Fig. C31.2D). This may be considered if the

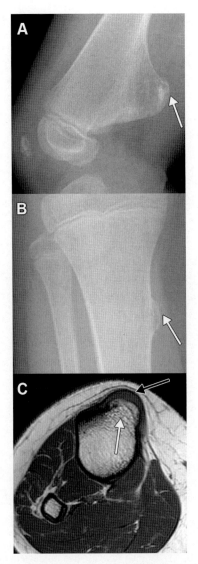

Fig. C31.1 Osteochondroma. (A) Lateral radiograph of the knee in a 4-year-old child shows a large, broad-based structure protruding from the posterior aspect of the distal femur (white arrow). There is contiguity of the bone marrow and cortex of the distal femur with those of lesion. Note that the osteochondroma projects away from the knee joint. (B) Frontal radiograph of the knee in an 11-year-old girl shows a small sessile structure protruding from the medial aspect of the proximal tibial diaphysis (white arrow). There is contiguity of the bone marrow and cortex of the proximal tibia with those of the lesion. (C) Axial T1-weighted image at the level of the proximal tibia and fibula in the same patient reveals contiguity of the marrow and cortex of the tibia with those of the lesion (white arrow). A thin intermediate signal intensity cartilaginous cap is present (black arrow).

lesion continues to grow beyond skeletal maturity or if the patient develops increasing pain. Associated bony destruction or a cartilage cap greater than 1 cm in thickness may also suggest the diagnosis. MRI with contrast can be very helpful in identifying this complication.

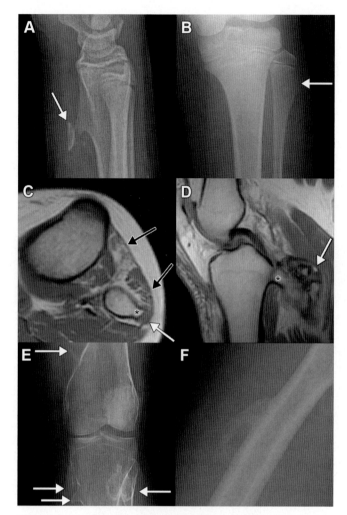

Multiple hereditary exostoses (Fig. C31.2E): Multiple osteochondromas may be seen in patients with this inherited autosomal dominant condition. These patients may have short stature due to early physeal closure, and the lesions have a higher incidence of malignant degeneration.

Heterotopic ossification (myositis ossificans, Fig. C31.2F): This entity is typically posttraumatic and is characterized by mature bone formation. The lesion may secondarily contact nearby bone; however, no connection to the underlying marrow should be seen.

Clinical Differential Diagnosis

- Benign, nonneoplastic: Hematoma, heterotopic ossification.
- Benign, neoplastic: Lipoma, myxoma.
- Malignant: Sarcoma, soft tissue metastasis.

REFERENCES AND SUGGESTED READING

1. Lee KC, Davies AM, Cassar-Pullicino VN. Imaging the complications of osteochondromas. *Clin Radiol.* 2002;57:18-28.
2. Miller SL, Hoffer FA. Malignant and benign bone tumors. *Radiol Clin North Am.* 2001;39:673-699.
3. Murphey MD, Choi JJ, Kransdorf MJ, Flemming DJ, Gannon FH. Imaging of osteochondroma: variants and complications with radiologic-pathologic correlation. *RadioGraphics.* 2000;20:1407-1434.
4. Stieber JR, Dormans JP. Manifestations of hereditary multiple exostoses. *J Am Acad Orthop Surg.* 2005;13:110-120.
5. Wootton-Gorges SL. MR imaging of primary bone tumors and tumor-like conditions in children. *Magn Reson Imaging Clin N Am.* 2009;17:469-487.

Fig. C31.2 Complications and differential considerations in osteochondroma. (A) Lateral radiograph of the distal forearm reveals a fracture (white arrow) through an osteochondroma arising from the distal radius. (B,C) Common fibular nerve impingement. (B) Radiograph shows an osteochondroma arising from the posterolateral aspect of the proximal fibula (white arrow). (C) Axial T1-weighted image reveals the osteochondroma (*) in close proximity to an enlarged common peroneal nerve (white arrow) and associated fatty atrophy of the muscles in the anterior and lateral compartments of the proximal calf (black arrows). (D) Large osteochondroma (*) arising from the posterior proximal tibia with a nodular and thick cartilage cap (white arrow). Biopsy showed chondrosarcoma. (E) Multiple hereditary exostoses (white arrows). (F) Posttraumatic exostosis in the thigh. There is no continuity of the bone marrow of the femur with that of the lesion. This is a follow-up image for the patient shown in Fig. C30.1E and C30.1F of case 30.

CASE 32

PATIENT PRESENTATION

A 13-year-old girl presents with a limp.

CLINICAL SUSPICION

Slipped capital femoral epiphysis

IMAGING MODALITY OF CHOICE

Anterior and lateral radiographs of the hip are preferred in assessment of patients with suspected slipped capital femoral epiphysis (SCFE). Radiographs are generally sufficient in detecting posterior slippage of the femoral epiphysis. However, MRI is more sensitive than radiography and may detect physeal widening characteristic of SCFE before it is readily apparent on radiographs. The lower cost and availability of radiographs frequently preclude evaluation with MRI.

BACKGROUND

SCFE is the most common hip abnormality in adolescents, occurring in approximately 2 of every 100,000 individuals, and affects boys more commonly than girls. SCFE is due to an atraumatic fracture through the proximal femoral physis, which can result in posterior and medial displacement of the proximal femoral epiphysis in relation to the metaphysis. Predisposing factors include obesity, malnutrition, endocrine abnormalities, developmental dysplasia of the hip, and black race. The findings are bilateral in 9% to 18% of cases at initial presentation, and many patients with unilateral involvement will ultimately develop SCFE in the contralateral extremity by maturity.

Slipped capital femoral epiphysis is associated with the growth spurt in adolescence, which results in rapid growth of the physis and alterations in its orientation. The peak age for boys (13-14 years) is approximately one year older than that for girls. Greater body weight, particularly in overweight children, as well as increased physical activity, can increase shear forces on the physis and predispose the child to fracture of the proximal femoral physis and slippage of the proximal epiphysis. Approximately 50% of patients present with hip pain, whereas 25% present with knee pain.

Treatment consists of stabilization of the proximal femoral physis with placement of pins or screws across the site of slippage. Reduction of the slipped epiphysis may be attempted in severe cases. However, this may increase the rate of avascular necrosis. The goal of immobilization is physeal fusion, which typically occurs within 1 year of pin placement. Untreated SCFE can ultimately result in premature osteoarthritis in young adulthood or even late adolescence.

FINDINGS

Radiographs of the hip in patients with SCFE may reveal widening of the physis, which is often the earliest sign of physeal fracture. With progression of posterior and medial slippage, the proximal femoral epiphysis may appear smaller. On the lateral view, there will be medial displacement of the epiphysis (Fig. C32.1A), which is often not evident on the frontal view in mild cases. A line drawn along the superior edge of the femoral neck (line of Klein) that does not intersect the epiphysis is indicative of medial displacement of the femoral head (Fig. C32.2).

MR evaluation may reveal physeal widening at an earlier stage than would be apparent on radiographs. Other less sensitive findings include hyperintensity of the physis on T2-weighted imaging, marrow edema, and synovitis. Avascular necrosis of the femoral head is seen in more advanced cases.

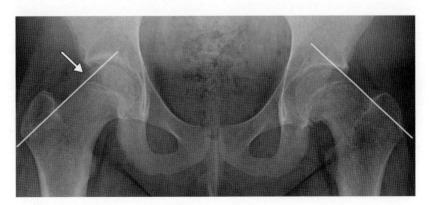

Fig. C32.1 Frontal view of the pelvis in a 13-year-old girl with left hip pain. Lines of Klein (white lines) are drawn along the superior edge of both femoral necks. The line on the right hip intersects the normal femoral epiphysis (arrow), but the line on the left is lateral to the femoral epiphysis. This is indicative of posterior and medial slippage of the left femoral epiphysis or SCFE.

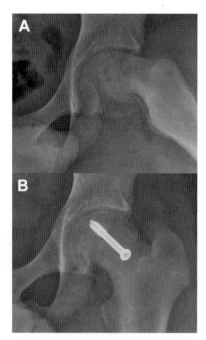

Fig. C32.2 A 13-year-old boy with left hip and knee pain diagnosed as having SCFE. (A) Frog-leg lateral view of the left hip shows posterior and medial displacement of the left femoral epiphysis. (B) Postoperative frontal view of the left hip after percutaneous placement of a screw through the proximal femoral physis. Prophylactic pinning of the normal right femoral physis was also performed in this case (not shown).

DIFFERENTIAL DIAGNOSIS

Imaging Differential Diagnosis

A traumatic Salter-Harris type I fracture of the proximal femoral epiphysis can have an identical appearance to SCFE. However, an unequivocal history of trauma should be present.

Clinical Differential Diagnosis

Children with hip pathology can present with knee pain and vice versa. Osgood-Schlatter disease (Fig. C32.3), typically a chronic avulsion injury of the tibial tuberosity, is an alternative clinical consideration in adolescent patients presenting with knee pain. Patients with muscle strain may also present with hip or knee pain. In younger patients, Legg-Calvé-Perthes (LCP) disease (Fig. C32.4), an idiopathic avascular necrosis of the femoral head, should be considered if hip pain is the presenting complaint. LCP occurs more commonly in boys between the ages of 2 and 14 years with a peak at 5 to 6 years of age. LCP is the result of subchondral fracture of the proximal femoral epiphysis, which leads to fragmentation, sclerosis, and flattening of the femoral head. This can also result in early onset arthritis if untreated or discovered at an advanced stage.

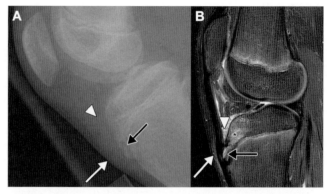

Fig. C32.3 A 13-year-old boy with right knee pain diagnosed with Osgood-Schlatter disease. (A) Lateral radiograph of the knee shows minimal fragmentation of the tibial tuberosity (black arrow), which can be seen normally, subtle thickening of the anterior soft tissues (white arrow), and effacement of the inferior infrapatellar (Hoffa) fat pad (white arrowhead). (B) Sagittal T2-weighted MR image with fat suppression reveals T2-hyperintensity indicative of edema in the anterior tibial epiphysis (*) extending to the tibial tuberosity (black arrow), as well as edema in the inferior infrapatellar (Hoffa) fat pad (white arrowhead) and minimally in the pretibial soft tissues (white arrow).

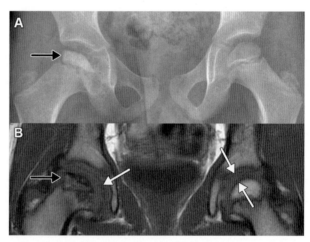

Fig. C32.4 A 6-year-old boy with a limp and right hip pain diagnosed as having Legg-Calvé-Perthes disease. (A) Frontal radiograph of the pelvis shows flattening and fragmentation of the proximal right femoral epiphysis (black arrow). The left femoral head is normal. (B) Coronal T1-weighted MR image of the pelvis shows fragmentation and collapse of the proximal right femoral epiphysis (black arrow). The articular cartilage of the right femoral head (white arrow) is intact and of similar thickness to that of the articular cartilage of the left femoral head (between white arrows).

REFERENCES AND SUGGESTED READING

1. Boles CA, el-Khoury GY. Slipped capital femoral epiphysis. *RadioGraphics.* 1997;17:809-823.

2. Dillman JR, Hernandez RJ. MRI of Legg-Calve-Perthes disease. *AJR.* 2009;193:1394-1407.

3. Gottsegen CJ, Eyer BA, White EA, Learch TJ, Forrester D. Avulsion fractures of the knee: imaging findings and clinical significance. *RadioGraphics.* 2008;28:1755-1770.

Interventional Radiology

By Bilal Anwer

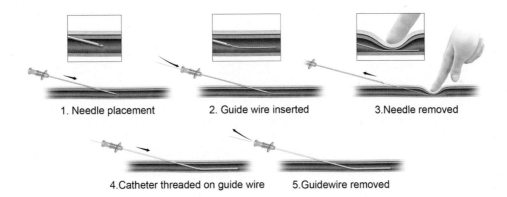

1. Needle placement   2. Guide wire inserted   3.Needle removed

4.Catheter threaded on guide wire   5.Guidewire removed

INTRODUCTION TO INTERVENTIONAL RADIOLOGY

Interventionalist radiologists are trained in performing diagnostic and therapeutic interventions in patients. This requires expertise in imaging, technical skills, pharmacology, sedation/anesthesia, and management of patients preprocedure and postprocedure. A well-rounded interventionalist understands disease processes and how they adversely alter normal physiology. They use this knowledge to work up the patient appropriately, use different imaging modalities to tailor a custom treatment for each patient, skillfully and safely perform the procedure, and follow up the patient to ensure optimal outcome.

This chapter is a basic outline of Interventional Radiology (IR) meant to introduce medical practitioners in other fields to the practice of IR. It contains the most common techniques, tools, and procedures involved in IR today. IR practice is diverse, innovative, and flexible. It is based on the practitioner preferences, training, experience, and ongoing literature review. The procedures covered in this chapter are performed commonly and may vary depending on the institution and interventionalist performing them.

The workup starts with a thorough history and physical, with particular attention to pertinent medical and surgical history, history of allergies, current medications, and a focused physical exam. It is necessary to identify risk factors for contrast allergy, contrast-induced nephropathy, and bleeding.

CONTRAST ALLERGY

Previous reaction to a contrast agent and a history of allergies or asthma place the patient at a higher risk for an allergic reaction to contrast during or after the procedure. Contrast reactions are covered in chapter 1 of this book. Pretreatment with a histamine blocker like diphenhydramine and a steroid such as prednisone can help reduce the risk of contrast reaction during the procedure. Low-osmolar contrast agents and carbon dioxide angiography can be used in patients with a history of moderate to severe contrast reaction. It is important to discuss alternative treatments or risk versus benefit of using contrast during an intervention with the patient prior to starting the procedure.

CONTRAST-INDUCED NEPHROPATHY (CIN)

CIN is defined as an increase in baseline creatinine by either 0.5 mg/dL or 25% after 1 to 3 days following administration of contrast. The renal function generally returns to baseline after a week. Pharmacologic agents such as N-acetylcysteine (Mucomyst), use of a limited volume of low osmolar contrast agents, carbon dioxide as an alternative contrast agent, and preprocedural and postprocedural hydration with saline can lower the risk of CIN.

HEMATOLOGIC PARAMETERS

Routine laboratory tests include prothrombin time (PT), activated partial thromboplastin time (PTT), platelets, and international normalized ratio (INR). Table 8.1 illustrates safety threshold and steps to rectify abnormalities of these parameters.

Antiplatelet agents such as aspirin or clopidogrel are held for 5 to 7 days before the procedure. Hemoglobin and hematocrit level is also documented in patients with an increased chance of bleeding due to a coagulopathy or angiography and biopsy of vascular organs or lesions.

PREPARATION FOR THE PROCEDURE

Prior to any procedure, an informed consent must be obtained. To provide this, the patient must understand the procedure planned, reasons for undergoing the procedure, risks and benefits, and alternative therapies including consequences of refusing the procedure. The consent also includes the risk of CIN and allergic reaction to contrast agents. Sedation and anesthesia are also addressed as part of the consent.

If sedation or anesthesia is planned, the patient is to be NPO (nothing by mouth) for 8 hours prior to the procedure. Medications such as antihypertensives and insulin should not be discontinued prior to the procedure. Antibiotics are given within 2 hours of procedures involving the biliary system, genitourinary system, drainage of abscesses, transjugular intrahepatic portosystemic shunt or endograft placement, and tissue ablative therapies.

INTRAPROCEDURAL CARE

During the procedure, the interventionalist takes steps to reduce radiation exposure to the patients and himself or herself by using techniques such as collimation, reduced fluoroscopy

Table 8.1 Important Preprocedural Hematologic Parameters

Parameter	Safety Threshold	Measures to Correct Abnormalities
PT/INR	< 3 s/1.6-1.8	Withhold coumadin, administer fresh frozen plasma or vitamin K
PTT	< 6 s	Withhold heparin 2-6 h prior to procedure
Platelet	> 50,000	Platelet transfusion
Bleeding time	< 8 s	Administer cryoprecipitate, platelet transfusion

s = second

Chapter 8 Interventional Radiology 487

time, pulsed fluoroscopy, reduced patient to image intensifier distance and increased distance from the radiation source, use of lead shields, and wearing protective gear. Excessive radiation can cause tissue damage in the short term and increase the chance of malignancies in the distant future.

Steps are taken to prevent blood-borne pathogen (hepatitis B or C, HIV) exposure to the interventionalist and patient. Appropriate precautions are taken before, during, and after the procedure to minimize the risk of exposure. The patient's vital signs are monitored by a dedicated nurse throughout the procedure.

Anxiolytics and pain medications are used during the procedure to lessen patient discomfort. A benzodiazepine such as midazolam (anxiolytic and antegrade amnesia) and an opioid narcotic such as fentanyl are most commonly used to establish moderate sedation (patient is responsive to verbal commands and maintains airway protection reflexes). Procedures that are particularly painful or that involve the pediatric population are performed with general anesthesia established by an anesthesiologist.

One should anticipate, understand, and be ready to manage/treat intraprocedural events such as hypotension, respiratory depression with hypoxia, vasovagal reactions (hypotension with bradycardia, nausea, and diaphoresis), hypertension, hemorrhage, and contrast reactions. Interventionalists are also expected to be proficient at advanced cardiovascular life support (ACLS) in the event of a cardiopulmonary arrest.

POSTPROCEDURAL FOLLOW-UP

Postprocedural care is dictated by the type of procedure performed. Needle punctures for biopsies, aspiration of fluid, and venous access can generally be managed by applying manual digital pressure directly on the puncture site for a few minutes to achieve hemostasis, followed by application of a sterile dressing.

Arterial punctures with placement of sheaths require application of digital pressure above, at, and below the arteriotomy site for at least 15 minutes post sheath removal. The site needs to be carefully monitored for enlarging hematoma. The patient should be on bed rest with the ipsilateral extremity immobile for 6 hours. Use of arterial closure devices has the advantage of hemostasis almost immediately following deployment and much shorter bed rest time.

Solid organ biopsies (liver, spleen, and kidney) have a higher chance of bleeding and the patient is monitored for 3 to 4 hours post procedure for signs of bleeding. Lung biopsies are followed by immediate and 3-hour chest x-rays to monitor for a pneumothorax, which may need to be evacuated by chest tube placement in symptomatic patients.

Specific orders regarding activity, diet, pain control, hydration, and monitoring vital signs are also written. Discharge or transfer criteria include tolerance of oral intake, adequate pain control, appropriate mentation, and stable vital signs.

Inpatient and outpatient follow-up should be arranged based on the procedure performed. It is an integral part of being a well-rounded interventionalist. Some treatments are done in a staged fashion, requiring long-term follow-up.

COMMON TECHNIQUES AND INSTRUMENTS
SELDINGER TECHNIQUE

The Seldinger technique (Fig. 8.1) is used on a daily basis for percutaneous arterial catheterization. It involves the use of a needle, guidewire, and catheter. Vascular access is most commonly attained via the common femoral artery. Using the femoral head and inguinal ligament as a landmark under fluoroscopy, an appropriate skin entry site in chosen. Local anesthetic is given using 1% or 2% lidocaine at the beginning of the procedure in an intradermal and subcutaneous fashion. Aspiration prior to injection is used to avoid intravascular injection of lidocaine.

A superficial skin nick is made directly over the arterial pulse. Using a blunt hemostat, subcutaneous dissection is performed. While palpating the femoral artery pulse, an 18 gauge needle (Fig. 8.2) is advanced in a controlled fashion at a 45 degree angle toward the femoral head. Brisk pulsatile bright red blood is encountered upon a successful arterial puncture. A 0.035-inch Bentson wire is advanced through the needle into the common femoral

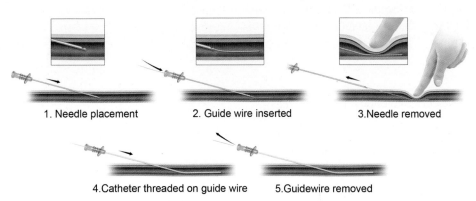

1. Needle placement 2. Guide wire inserted 3. Needle removed

4. Catheter threaded on guide wire 5. Guidewire removed

Fig. 8.1 The steps of the Seldinger technique.

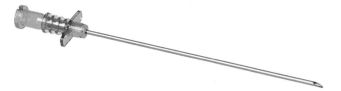

Fig. 8.2 A single-wall needle with a sharp beveled edge for vascular catheterization.

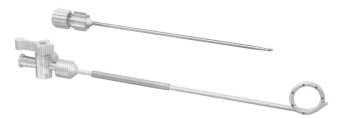

Fig. 8.3 Pigtail catheter with inner metallic component.

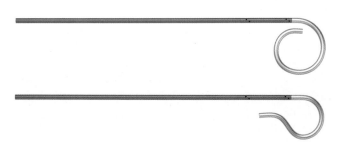

Fig. 8.4 High-flow catheters, including pigtail and modified pigtail.

artery and abdominal aorta under fluoroscopic guidance. While holding pressure at the arteriotomy site, the needle is slowly removed and the wire is cleaned with wet gauze. A sheath or catheter is then advanced over the guidewire into the common femoral artery in a smooth fashion. The guidewire and sheath inner stiffener is removed and the sheath is flushed with normal saline. The sheath can then be used to exchange for different types, sizes, and length of catheters. Catheters are always advanced over a guidewire to prevent arterial injury.

Some practitioners prefer a 21 gauge needle and thinner 0.018-inch wire to access the common femoral artery. This can then be upsized to a 0.035-inch Bentson wire using a 5 French (Fr) sheath (1 Fr = 1/3 mm). Complications of this procedure include:

- Retroperitoneal hemorrhage if the arterial access is too high.

- Low arterial access into the superficial or deep femoral artery increasing the chance of arterial thrombosis, pseudoaneurysm, or arteriovenous fistula formation.

- Arterial injury, dissection, or occlusion. The Seldinger technique is also used for central venous access.

GUIDEWIRES

Guidewires, as the name implies, are used primarily to direct catheters into specific locations within a blood vessel, cavity, or organ. Guidewires mainly differ by length, diameter, stiffness, tip characteristics, and pliability. The exterior may be hydrophobic or hydrophilic. Standard guide wires come in 0.035 or 0.038-inch diameters. Microwires are available for microcatheters or small gauge needles. Choice of guidewire is based on the preference of the interventionalist and procedure being performed.

CATHETERS

There are angiographic and drainage catheters (Figs. 8.3-8.5). Angiographic catheters differ by pliability, external coating, and tip contour.

- Reverse curve catheters are used to access vessels and need to be formed into the correct shape inside the vessel. They can also be shaped by the interventionalist.

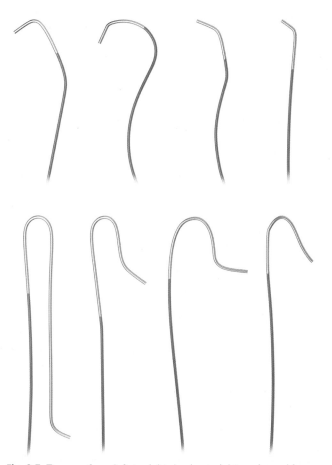

Fig. 8.5 Top row, from left to right: basic straight angiographic catheters—spinal, cobra, headhunter, and angled shapes. Bottom row, from left to right: basic reverse-curve catheters—Bookstein, Simmons (sidewinder), Shetty, and visceral hook.

- Pigtail catheters are used for angiography or venography of large vessels and for drainage of air or fluid. They have multiple side holes along the distal shaft and pigtail loop. Drainage catheters have a string that is pulled to secure the shape of the pigtail loop to prevent dislodgement.
- Guiding catheters have a specific shape that can help cannulate tortuous or angled vessels.
- Microcatheters are used in select small caliber vessels.

SHEATHS

Sheaths (Fig. 8.6) are placed when lengthy vascular interventions and multiple catheter/guidewire exchanges are anticipated. They provide a safe passage of guidewires and catheters into the artery. Sheaths can also be placed to control persistent oozing or hematoma at the arterial access site. Sheaths are composed of an inner stiffener and outer thin wall. The inner stiffener is present to prevent buckling during insertion and is removed once access has been established. They also have a valve at the proximal end to prevent free backflow. A side arm is available for injection of contrast. Some have a peel-away outer component that can be easily removed once a more stable access to a vein, organ, or cavity has been established. Vascular sheaths can also be used for nonvascular procedures.

BALLOONS

Inflatable balloons are used to open stenosis within vessels, or other parts of the body such as the urinary tract, and biliary systems. The procedure is called percutaneous transluminal balloon angioplasty (PTA). Using an inflation device, the balloon can be inflated or deflated to a measurable pressure using air, saline, or contrast. It causes a controlled stretch injury to the lumen, which then scars into place. Balloons differ by diameter, length, shape, burst pressure, surface, and pliability. Balloons are also used to expand stents placed within vessels and channels. They are inflated within the stent to achieve the desired lumen diameter and force the stent to appose the wall of the vessel or channel.

STENTS

Stents are used in a variety of procedures to maintain luminal patency within arteries, veins, bile ducts, bowel, urinary tract, and artificially created channels. Stents are tubular metallic cages that differ by length, longitudinal flexibility, elasticity or plasticity, radial force, composition, radiopacity, shortening with deployment, and compatibility with magnetic resonance imaging (MRI). There are self-expanding, balloon-expandable (Fig. 8.7), drug-eluting, and covered stents. Choice of stent of varies by procedure and comfort level of the interventionalist.

OCCLUSIVE AGENTS

Several options are available to achieve occlusion of vessels, aneurysms, biliary tract, fistulas, ureters, and vascular malformations. The choice of agent used depends on whether temporary versus permanent and proximal versus distal occlusion is desired. It also varies by the type of procedure, availability of materials, comfort level of the interventionalist, and part of the body.

- Coils are used for permanent vascular occlusion (Fig. 8.8). The selection of coil depends on the diameter and length of the vessel.
- Gelfoam is a spongelike agent that expands upon contact with fluid. It is used for temporary vascular occlusion of vessels or bleeding tracts. It can be made into slurry or cut into small pledgets and then injected into the desired location via a catheter.
- Polyvinyl alcohol (PVA) particles cause inflammatory reaction in the vessel wall and are used to occlude small arteries or arterioles.
- Embospheres and PVA microspheres are spherical agents that occlude small vessels to achieve a permanent thrombosis.
- Absolute ethanol is a liquid agent that scleroses the vessels walls and surrounding tissue for permanent occlusion. Small volumes are usually sufficient, and it may cause pain after embolization.

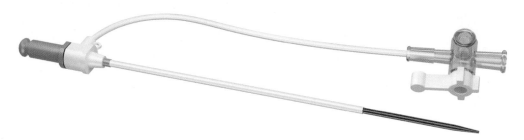

Fig. 8.6 Vascular access catheter consisting of sheath with a side arm and inner dilator.

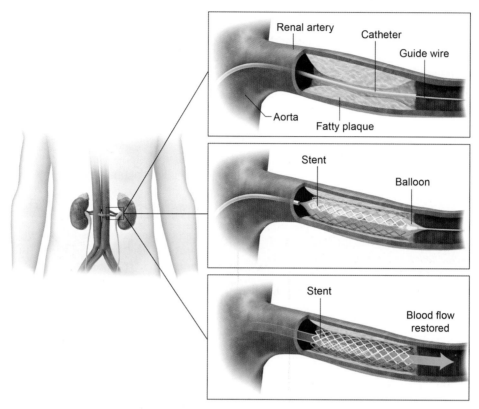

Fig. 8.7 Balloon-expandable stent placement to treat renal artery stenosis.

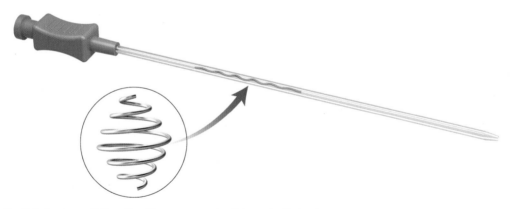

Fig. 8.8 A microcoil (inset), with an unwound coil in a plastic loader.

- Onyx is a liquid agent that is typically used in neurovascular interventions to treat arteriovenous malformations and endoleaks after endovascular aneurysm repair.
- Avitene is fibrils that are suspended in solution and result in an inflammatory reaction that achieves permanent occlusion in vessels.
- Glue is an adhesive liquid agent that achieves permanent occlusion of arteriovenous malformation, fistulas, aneurysms, varicoceles, and gastrointestinal bleeding.
- Detachable balloons can be used to occlude arteries and arteriovenous lesions.

NEEDLES

Needles come in varying lengths, diameters (gauges), and tips. They can be used to access vessels or organs, aspirate fluid from cavities, and biopsy masses. The type of needle used depends on the procedure being performed. References will be made to one-step and two-step needles in this chapter.

One-step needles (Fig. 8.9) consist of an inner hollow metallic needle and outer thin sheath with side holes at the distal end. They can be used to drain or access fluid within the peritoneal or thoracic cavities.

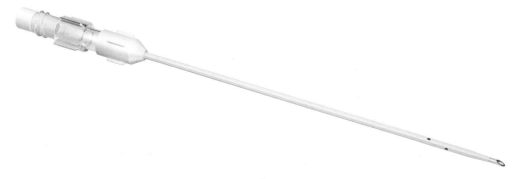

Fig. 8.9 One-step needle also known as the Yueh needle.

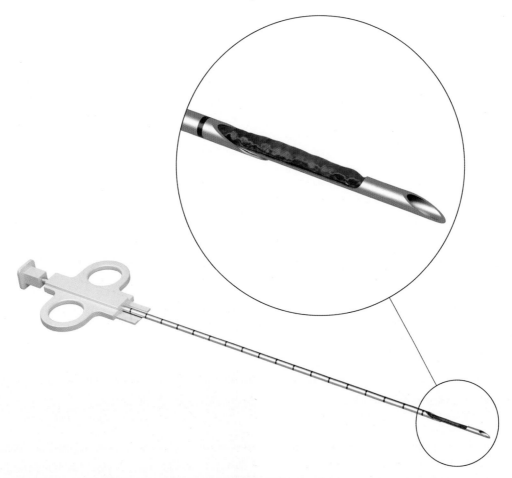

Fig. 8.10 Two-step spring loaded biopsy needle with slotted inner stylet.

Noncutting and cutting needles are typically used for biopsies. A small sample can be aspirated into the needle attached to syringe or automatically pulled into the needle via capillary action or manual aspiration. A two-step needle (Fig. 8.10) is used for soft tissue mass biopsies and typically consists of a slotted inner stylet that catches the specimen and spring-loaded cutting outer cannula. The stylet is advanced into the biopsy target and the cutting outer cannula is manually fired. The outer cannula is then retracted to reveal the specimen within the slot.

REFERENCE AND SUGGESTED READING

1. Valji K. Patient care and evaluation, standard angiographic and interventional techniques. In: *Vascular and Interventional Radiology.* 2nd ed. WB Saunders. 2006.

CASE 1: ARTERIAL ANEURYSMS

PATIENT PRESENTATION

An 80-year-old male presents to the ED with mild abdominal pain and pulsating midline mass on abdominal exam. The patient is hemodynamically stable.

CLINICAL SUSPICION

Abdominal aortic aneurysm (AAA)

IMAGING MODALITY OF CHOICE

CT Angiogram

Advantages: CT angiogram is readily available and accurately demonstrates the size and shape of the AAA and its relationship to branch arteries and aortic bifurcation. It can also assess for aneurysm rupture, impending rupture, or leaking aneurysm, as well as determine the type of aneurysm. This information is essential for surgical or interventional planning. Ultrasound examination can be done at bedside and is an even quicker and cheaper modality without radiation exposure. MRI/MRA is expensive, slow, and not readily available. Noncontrast MRI has the advantage of delineating arterial anatomy better than a noncontrast CT examination in a patient with renal dysfunction.

FINDINGS

CT findings of abdominal aortic aneurysm:

- Abdominal aorta dilated to greater than 3 cm
- Retroperitoneal hematoma that may involve the periaortic, pararenal, or perirenal spaces or psoas muscle with aneurysm rupture.

Treatment of a ruptured aortic aneurysm is typically done surgically in a hemodynamically unstable patient. Endovascular graft repair is ideally performed in stable patients with a nonruptured aortic aneurysm and favorable arterial anatomy, and in patients who are poor candidates for surgery due to comorbidities.

Several subtypes and complications of abdominal aortic aneurysm have been described; some of these have a prognosis that is significantly worse than others:

True aortic aneurysm: This refers to dilatation of the aorta due to weakening of the aortic walls. All three layers of the aortic wall (intima, media, and adventitia) are involved. This is the most common type of aneurysm, and atherosclerosis is the most common cause. Imaging usually shows fusiform dilatation of the aorta with atherosclerotic calcification and eccentric thrombus. Treatment depends on the size of the aneurysm and growth rate, both of which directly correlate with risk of rupture. Aneurysms larger than 5 cm in diameter

in women and 5.5 to 6 cm in size in men have an annual risk of rupture of around 15%. Aneurysms greater than or equal to 8 cm in diameter have an annual rupture rate of up to 50%. A growth rate of 3 to 4 mm/y is typical for aneurysms, and a growth rate of greater than 10 mm/y warrants intervention.

Pseudoaneurysm: This is a false aortic aneurysm, characterized by disruption of the aortic wall layers with blood inside the aorta contained by only a thin layer of adventitia or surrounding soft tissue (Fig. C1.1). This can be caused by an insult to the aorta from trauma, infections, instrumentation, or inflammation. Pseudoaneurysms are at a high risk for rupture regardless of their size. They are usually saccular in shape with a defined neck. These usually require immediate treatment with endovascular stent graft placement or surgical repair.

Dissecting aneurysm: These are considered pseudoaneurysms due to a lack of confinement by all three layers of the vessel wall. The aortic dilatation is caused by splitting or dissection of an arterial wall by blood entering through an intimal tear or by an intramural hematoma; these are more frequent in the thoracic aorta where the dissection starts in the proximal aorta and descends into the abdominal aorta. Patients with an increased risk of dissection include those with a history of connective tissue disorders such as Marfan syndrome, hypertension, or advanced atherosclerotic disease with penetrating aortic ulcers. On imaging, one can see the intimal flap with true lumen and blood/contrast in the false lumen.

Mycotic aneurysm: These are infectious in etiology and are considered pseudoaneurysms (Fig. C1.2). There is usually hematogenous spread of infection from a

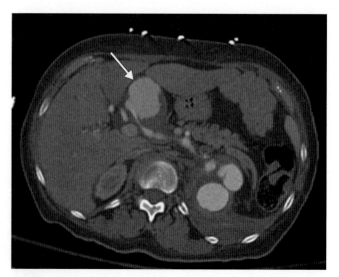

Fig. C1.1 Large hepatic artery saccular aneurysm with eccentric thrombus and wall thickening (arrow).

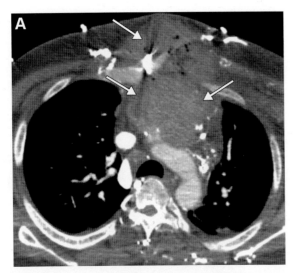 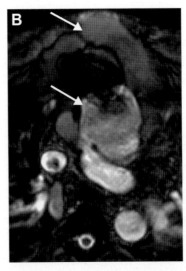

Fig. C1.2 Large mycotic pseudoaneurysm (lower arrows) of a saphenous vein coronary artery bypass graft secondary to sternal dehiscence and abscess (upper arrows). Figure A is a contrast-enhanced axial CT image and Figure B is a T2-weighted axial MRI image at the same level.

source such as endocarditis or a psoas or vertebral body infection. They are more common in the thoracic aorta, suprarenal aorta, or at the branch point. Imaging findings include a saccular shape, lobular contours, and aortic/periaortic inflammation or gas. The risk for rupture is very high.

Aneurysmal dilatation of the aorta can also be seen in people with inflammatory conditions such as periaortic retroperitoneal fibrosis, autoimmune disorders such as rheumatoid arthritis, and arteritis. These are usually symptomatic with patients having fever, weight loss, and hydronephrosis from ureteral involvement. An increased risk of rupture is present irrespective of size.

REFERENCES AND SUGGESTED READING

1. Rakita D, Newatia A, Hines JJ, Siegel DN, Friedman B. Spectrum of CT findings in rupture and impending rupture of abdominal aortic aneurysms. *RadioGraphics.* 2007;27: 497-507.

2. Brown PM, Zelt DT, Sobolev BJ. The risk of rupture in untreated aneurysms: the impact of size, gender, and expansion rate. *Vasc. Surg.* 2003;37(2):280-284.

3. Kaufman JA, Lee MJ. *Vascular and Interventional Radiology, the Requisites.* Mosby Inc.; 2004. ISBN:0815143699.

4. Krishna K, Machan L. Stent grafts for abdominal aortic aneurysms. In: *Handbook of Interventional Radiologic Procedures.* 4th ed. Lippincott Williams & Wilkins. 2010;188.

CASE 2: ARTERITIS

PATIENT PRESENTATION

A 25-year-old Asian female presents to the ED with cold and pulseless upper extremities.

CLINICAL SUSPICION

Takayasu's arteritis

IMAGING MODALITY OF CHOICE

Interventional Angiography

Advantages: Angiography accurately demonstrates the vessels involved and the extent of the disease in large and medium sized vessels. Immediate intervention can be performed if necessary. CT angiogram or MR angiogram is better for small vessels because it can show the effect of the disease on the visceral organs. PET/CT has a limited role and can show areas of active inflammation. Angiographic findings in arteritis include vascular stenosis, obstruction, aneurysmal dilatation, or rupture.

FINDINGS

Several types of arteritis and their complications have been described depending on their characteristics and the vessels involved:

> **Takayasu's arteritis:** This is a large-vessel vasculitis that is a panarteritis. It typically involves the thoracic aorta and its branching vessels but can affect the pulmonary and coronary arteries as well as the abdominal aorta (Figs. C2.1 and C2.2). Aortic branches most commonly

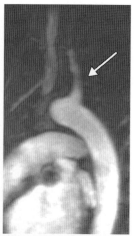
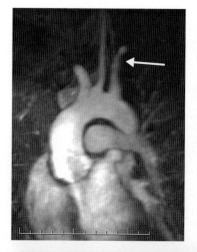
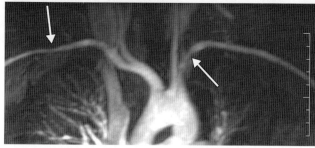

Fig. C2.2 Volume rendering MR angiographic images demonstrate bilateral stenotic areas involving both subclavian arteries (arrows) secondary to Takayasu's arteritis.

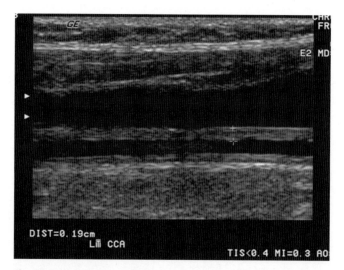

Fig. C2.1 Ultrasound examination of the left common carotid artery demonstrates diffuse wall thickening secondary to Takayasu's arteritis, resulting in stenosis.

involved include left common iliac, carotid, left subclavian, renal, and superior mesenteric arteries. Dilatation of the aorta is due to weakening of the aortic walls. Inflammation of the vessel wall results in wall irregularity, diffuse vessel stenosis, occlusion, and even aneurysms. The typical patient is a young adult, particularly of Asian descent, with upper extremity claudication, fever, malaise, or abdominal pain from mesenteric ischemia.

Giant cell arteritis: This is a large vessel vasculitis also known as temporal arteritis. It is typically seen in adults older than 50 years of age who present with jaw claudication, sensitivity of the scalp, transient ischemic attacks, and visual symptoms. Angiography shows irregularity and stenosis of the superficial temporal artery. Arterial biopsy is usually performed to confirm the diagnosis.

Polyarteritis nodosa: This is a small- to medium-vessel necrotizing vasculitis typically involving the renal and mesenteric vessels. It is seen in middle-aged adults who present with fever, abdominal pain, fibromyalgia, and erythema nodosum. Imaging shows aneurysms up to 1 cm in size typically at vessel bifurcations and pseudoaneurysms of intrarenal arteries. This condition is fatal if not treated.

Kawasaki disease: Also known as mucocutaneous lymph node syndrome, this is a medium-vessel vasculitis that is largely seen in children under 5 years old. They may present with fever, conjunctival inflammation, erythematous lips, "strawberry" tongue, and cervical lymphadenopathy. Patients can also develop coronary artery aneurysms that may thrombose or rupture leading to myocardial infarction. Echocardiography and angiography can be used to detect these aneurysms.

Henoch-Schönlein purpura: This is a hypersensitivity related vasculitis affecting small vessels. It is usually seen in children and young adults who present with skin rash, lower extremity purpura, hematuria, arthritis of large joints, and bowel inflammation. CT of the abdomen may show bowel and mesenteric inflammation, enlarged mesenteric lymph nodes, intussusception, ascites, and renal pelvis suburothelial hemorrhage.

Behcet's disease: This chronic inflammatory disease involves multiple organ systems. It is typically seen in 20- to 40- year-old patients who present with oral and genital aphthous ulcers, uveitis, and arthritis. Abdominal pain and bowel perforation can occur as well. Imaging shows occlusion and aneurysms of the pulmonary artery, aortic arch, subclavian arteries, and coronary arteries. CT of the abdomen may show masslike, polypoid thickening and enhancement of the bowel wall mucosa, bowel perforation, or fistulas.

Wegener's granulomatosis: This is a small-vessel vasculitis. These patients typically present with renal failure, proteinuria, and hematuria, but the disease can affect the nose, lungs, and central nervous system. It is mainly seen in middle-aged adults. Imaging findings include erosions of the bony nasal septum, cavitary lung lesions, microaneurysms, renal scarring/hemorrhage, and bowel ischemia.

Lupus vasculitis: This is a necrotizing small-vessel vasculitis typically seen in young women. The superior mesenteric artery is most commonly affected, but any part of the gastrointestinal tract can be affected. Imaging shows bowel wall inflammation, pneumatosis from ischemia, engorged mesenteric vessels, ascites, mesenteric lymphadenopathy, and mesenteric thrombosis.

Buerger's disease: Also known as thromboangiitis obliterans, it is typically seen in smokers and affects small- and medium-sized vessels in the extremities leading to vascular occlusion and limb claudication. On angiography, there are multiple symmetrical segmental stenoses and occlusions in the distal arteries of the upper and lower extremities. These arteries lack proximal atherosclerosis and have inadequate collateral vessels described as "corkscrew collaterals."

There are other types of vasculitides due to a primary disease or related to inflammatory conditions, infection, malignancy, and drug hypersensitivity, sequelae of which can be seen on imaging. Treatment for vasculitis is based on steroids and immunoregulatory agents such as cyclophosphamide.

REFERENCES AND SUGGESTED READING

1. Gotway MB, Araoz PA, Macede TA, et al. Imaging findings in Takayasu's arteritis. *AJR.* 2005;184:1945-1950.

2. Ha HK, Lee SL, Rha SE, et al. Radiologic features of vasculitis involving the gastrointestinal tract. *RadioGraphics.* 2000;20:779-794.

3. Stanson AW, Friese JL, Johnson CM, et al. Polyarteritis nodosa: spectrum of angiographic findings. *RadioGraphics.* 2001,21:151-159.

CASE 3: ADRENAL VEIN SAMPLING

PATIENT PRESENTATION

A 45-year-old female presents with hypertension and hypo-kalemia. Hyperaldosteronism is suspected.

DIAGNOSIS

An MRI of the abdomen shows a 2-cm right adrenal adenoma (Fig. C3.1).

TREATMENT OPTIONS

- Medical management
- Surgical excision

PROCEDURE INDICATIONS

Adrenal vein sampling is performed prior to surgical excision in a patient with an elevated venous blood aldosterone-renin ratio. A diagnosis of primary hyperaldosteronism due to an adrenal adenoma in a symptomatic patient is necessary prior to adrenalectomy.

PROCEDURE CONTRAINDICATIONS

Absolute contraindications include an unstable patient or coagulopathy. Relative contraindications include renal insufficiency or severe contrast allergy.

PROCEDURE OVERVIEW

The goal of adrenal vein sampling is to determine whether there is autonomous secretion of aldosterone from the adrenal adenoma. In these cases, the tumor can be

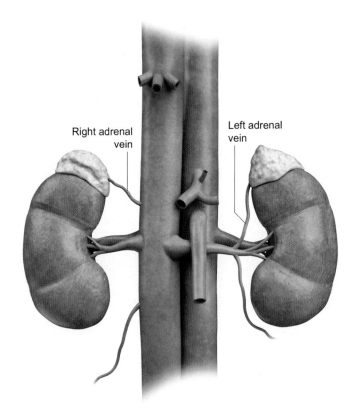

Fig. C3.2 Conventional adrenal vein anatomy.

excised surgically. In some cases, there may be increased secretion bilaterally due to bilateral adrenal cortical hyperplasia, which is managed medically. Samples taken from bilateral adrenal glands compare the aldosterone and cortisol levels from each adrenal gland versus systemic levels (Fig. C3.2). This can help direct the treatment or rule out adrenal gland hypersecretion as a culprit for the patient's symptoms.

Typically, access to the inferior vena cava is achieved via the right femoral vein after cleansing of the skin and local anesthesia of groin with lidocaine. A 5 Fr curved catheter is advanced through a femoral vein access. The right adrenal central draining vein is usually located in the mid posterior IVC above the right renal vein. The left adrenal vein drains into the left renal vein. Contrast injection is used to confirm cannulation of the adrenal vein, which demonstrates a delta or triangular pattern of the adrenal gland (Fig. C3.3). Gentle suction or passive bleeding is then used to obtain blood sample for assay. A peripheral vein sample is also simultaneously obtained to compare the cortisol levels, which should be significantly lower in the peripheral vein than the central adrenal vein.

The left adrenal vein usually drains into the left renal vein. Using a reverse curve catheter, the left adrenal central draining vein is accessed via the left renal vein and samples are obtained (Fig. C3.4).

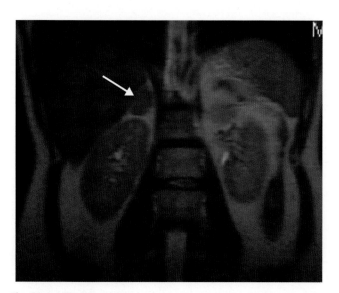

Fig. C3.1 MRI T2-weighted coronal image shows a right adrenal gland mass (arrow).

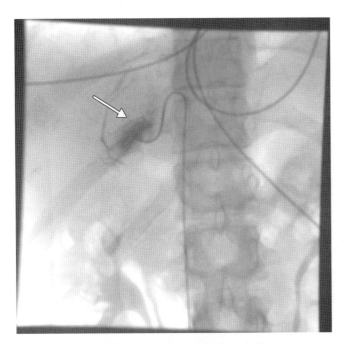

Fig. C3.3 Right adrenal vein contrast injection confirms proper placement of sampling catheter. Notice staning of the right adrenal gland with contrast (arrow). There is also excretion of contrast into the renal collecting systems.

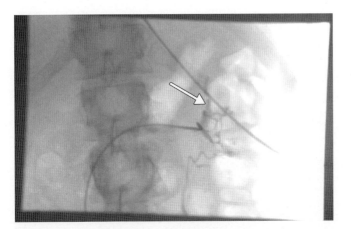

Fig. C3.4 The adrenal vein is accessed via the left renal vein. Contrast injection confirms proper placement of catheter (arrow).

COMPLICATIONS

- Adrenal vein rupture
- Dissection
- Thrombosis
- Adrenal gland hemorrhage or infarction
- Hypertensive crisis
- Groin or retroperitoneal hemorrhage
- Infection

REFERENCE AND SUGGESTED READING

1. Daunt N. Adrenal vein sampling: how to make it quick, easy, and successful. *RadioGraphics.* 2005;25:S143-S158.

CASE 4: ANEURYSM COIL EMBOLIZATION

PATIENT PRESENTATION

A 70-year-old male with right upper quadrant pain.

DIAGNOSIS

A CT of the abdomen demonstrates a large hepatic artery aneurysm (Fig. C4.1).

TREATMENT OPTIONS

- Medical management
- Surgical ligation
- Endovascular coil embolization

PROCEDURE INDICATIONS

Symptomatic aneurysms are always treated. There is controversy over treatment of asymptomatic aneurysms. Generally, solid organ or splanchnic arterial pseudoaneurysms or enlarging true aneurysms are treated due to an increased chance of rupture. Hepatic artery aneurysms are treated preemptively due to increased risk of rupture in women who are pregnant or plan to become pregnant, patients with portal hypertension, or liver transplant candidates.

PROCEDURE CONTRAINDICATIONS

There are no absolute contraindications to embolization of hepatic artery aneurysm, especially in cases of rupture and hemorrhage.

Relative contraindications include:

- Severe allergy to intravenous contrast
- Renal insufficiency
- Coagulopathy
- Pregnancy

PROCEDURE OVERVIEW

The goal is to occlude the aneurysm to prevent hemodynamic forces from enlarging it further or causing it to rupture. This can be achieved by placing a covered stentgraft across the aneurysm neck, embolizing the proximal and distal arteries, or embolizing the aneurysm with multiple coils.

Access to the hepatic artery is typically achieved via the femoral artery or brachial artery approach. Typically, a 5 Fr curved catheter is use to gain a stable access to the celiac axis. An angiogram is performed to map the arterial anatomy (Fig. C4.2). Once the common hepatic artery is identified, the 5 Fr catheter or a microcatheter can be advanced to the hepatic artery aneurysm neck and multiple coils are advanced into the aneurysm using a guidewire (Figs. C4.3 and C4.4). In other cases, based on the arterial anatomy and size of the artery, a stent graft can be placed across the neck of the aneurysm or coils can be used to occlude the proximal or distal feeding vessels to stop the flow of blood into it. Confirmation of complete occlusion is identified via another angiogram.

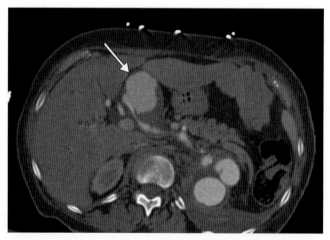

Fig. C4.1 Large hepatic artery saccular aneurysms with eccentric thrombus and wall thickening (arrow). The aorta is also abnormal with evidence of graft repair and surrounding hematoma.

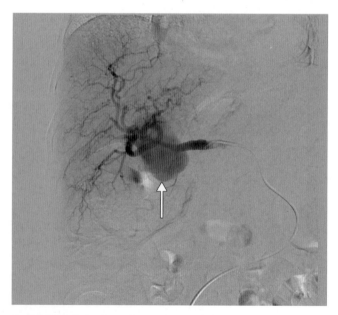

Fig. C4.2 Digital subtraction angiographic images show contrast injection into the right hepatic artery via a 5 Fr catheter. A saccular aneurysm is again demonstrated (arrow).

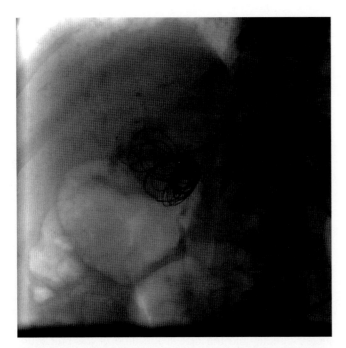

Fig. C4.3 Fluoroscopic guided placement of coils within the right hepatic artery aneurysm

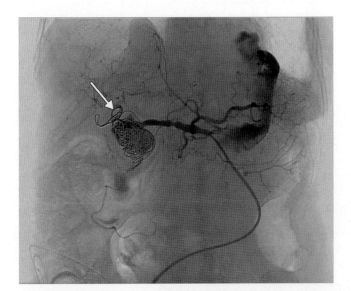

Fig. C4.4 Digital subtraction angiogram following coil embolization of aneurysm shows near complete occlusion of aneurysm sac (arrow). Notice the contrast extravasation that can occur with rupture of the aneurysm during coil placement.

COMPLICATIONS

- Hemorrhage
- Hepatocyte or biliary infarction
- Pseudoaneurysm
- Artery dissection
- Infection
- Nontargeted embolization resulting in infarction of visceral organs

REFERENCES AND SUGGESTED READING

1. Sandhu J. Visceral aneurysms and pseudoaneurysms: when and how to treat. *J Vascular Intervent Radiol.* 2002;13(2)(suppl):P141-P145.
2. Kandarpa K, Machan L. Visceral aneurysms. In: *Handbook of Interventional Radiologic Procedures.* 4th ed. 2010.

CASE 5: ARTERIOVENOUS FISTULA DECLOTTING

PATIENT PRESENTATION

A 35-year-old male with renal failure and a malfunctioning arteriovenous fistula.

DIAGNOSIS

A Doppler ultrasound shows arteriovenous (AV) fistula thrombi with diminished velocities.

TREATMENT OPTIONS

- Surgical thrombectomy
- Endovascular thrombectomy/thrombolysis

PROCEDURE INDICATIONS

Evaluation of the arteriovenous fistula is warranted when it fails to mature, malfunctions, or completely fails.

PROCEDURE CONTRAINDICATIONS

Absolute contraindications include uncorrectable coagulopathy and either systemic or fistula infections. Relative contraindications include:

- Contrast allergy.
- Significant cardiopulmonary disease that may be complicated by pulmonary emboli.

- Ischemia distal to the arteriovenous anastomosis that may worsen following increased flow through the fistula.

PROCEDURE OVERVIEW

The goal of declotting is to restore high flow through the fistula that is optimal for hemodialysis.

Ultrasound is used to evaluate the location of thrombus and the fistula is accessed using a needle pointing toward the anastomosis and another pointing away from the anastomosis. These are then upsized to 6 or 7 Fr sheaths. An angiogram is performed to confirm forward flow in the fistula, which is essential to prevent arterial emboli (Fig. C5.1). A guidewire is passed across the thrombus. Mechanical thrombectomy can then be done using angioplasty and a sweeping motion with a Fogarty balloon (Fig. C5.2), spinning a catheter or using a mechanical thrombectomy device such as a trerotola device. Chemical thrombolysis can also be done with tPA (tissue plasminogen activator) injected directly into the clot at the time of the procedure or over a period of 1 to 2 days using an infusion catheter. Follow-up angiogram is performed down to the right atrium to confirm declotting.

Chemical thrombolysis can also be used to soften clots less than 5 days old, followed by mechanical thrombectomy.

Occasionally, venous or anastomotic stenoses may be encountered. Every stenosis greater than 50% is potentially

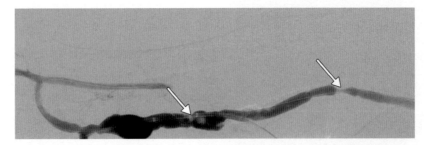

Fig. C5.1 Digital subtraction angiogram of the venous side of an arteriovenous fistula shows multiple small filling defects within aneurysmal venous portion consistent with clots (left arrow). There is also a focal stenosis more medially (right arrow).

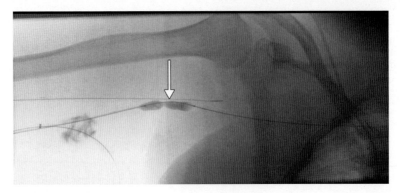

Fig. C5.2 Fluoroscopic image shows balloon angioplasty of the stenotic vein segment. Notice the waist (arrow) on the balloon at the location of the stenosis.

hemodynamically significant. A combination of balloon angioplasty and stents can be used to dilate the stenosis to less than 30%, and the flow is then documented on subsequent angiogram.

COMPLICATIONS

- Venous rupture leading to nonfunctioning fistula
- Sepsis
- Bleeding
- Pulmonary emboli
- Pseudoaneurysm formation

REFERENCES AND SUGGESTED READING

1. Valji K. Hemodialysis access. In: *Vascular and Interventional Radiology*. 2nd ed. WB Saunders. 2006.

2. Kandarpa K, Machan L. Dialysis fistulae. dialysis grafts. In: *Handbook of Interventional Radiologic Procedures*. 4th ed. Lippincott Williams & Wilkins. 2010.

3. Zaleski G. Declotting, maintenance, and avoiding procedural complications of native arteriovenous fistulae. *Semin Intervent Radiol*. 2004;21(2):83-93.

4. Bittl JA. Catheter interventions for hemodialysis fistulas and grafts. *J Am Coll Cardiol Intv*. 2010;3(1):1-11. doi:10.1016/j.jcin.2009.10.021.

CASE 6: PERCUTANEOUS BILIARY DRAINAGE CATHETER

PATIENT PRESENTATION

A 45-year-old male with elevated bilirubin, jaundice, and abdominal pain.

DIAGNOSIS

CT scan of the abdomen and pelvis shows a pancreatic head mass obstructing the common bile duct resulting in biliary dilatation.

TREATMENT OPTIONS

- Whipple procedure with hepaticojejunostomy
- ERCP with biliary stent placement
- Percutaneous biliary drainage catheter

PROCEDURE INDICATIONS

Decompression of the biliary system in patients with biliary obstruction from unresectable tumors, biliary stricture, liver transplant, or primary sclerosing cholangitis. Patients with cholangitis needing biliary diversion prior to surgery or brachytherapy for treatment of cholangiocarcinoma are also appropriate candidates.

PROCEDURE CONTRAINDICATIONS

Relative contraindications include thrombocytopenia and elevated INR.

PROCEDURE OVERVIEW

Percutaneous biliary drainage catheter placement can be performed under ultrasound and fluoroscopy guidance.

Ultrasound and fluoroscopic guidance are fast and effective in placement of percutaneous biliary catheters. The patient is placed in supine position. The overlying skin is cleansed and anesthetized. Using sterile technique, a 20-gauge needle is directed into the liver to access the bile ducts. If the ducts are dilated, ultrasound can be used to directly puncture one of the dilated hepatic ducts. Alternatively, under fluoroscopic guidance the needle can be directed toward the hepatic hilum from the liver periphery under fluoroscopy. Contrast is injected as the needle is advanced to opacify any hepatic ducts that may be encountered (Figs. C6.1 and C6.2). This method includes trial and error. It is not unusual to puncture the hepatic artery/vein or portal vein while looking for the bile ducts. Alternatively, the needle is advanced into a central position and then withdrawn while aspirating for bile or injecting contrast. Once the needle

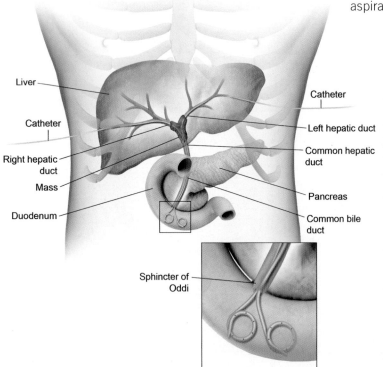

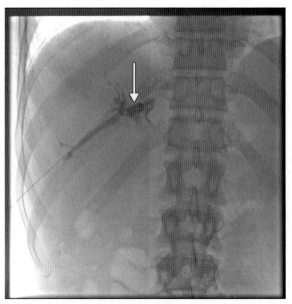

Fig. C6.1 Right transhepatic needle placement into a dilated right hepatic duct (arrow). Contrast injection shows appropriate access of the biliary system.

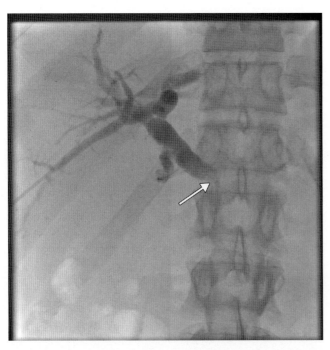

Fig. C6.2 Cholangiogram through a sheath showing dilated hepatic and common bile ducts with narrowing distally (arrow) from an obstructive mass. Notice the dilated cystic duct.

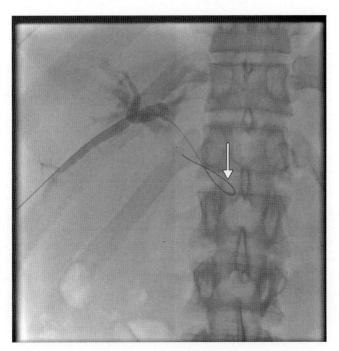

Fig. C6.3 A microwire advanced into the common bile duct to the point of obstruction (arrow).

the biliary anatomy, confirms the point of obstruction, and evaluates communication of the right and left hepatic ducts. The sheath allows a stiffer wire to be advanced into the bile duct to the point of obstruction.

It is preferential to pass the point of biliary obstruction with the wire leading into the duodenum so an internal/external biliary catheter can be placed allowing both natural internal flow of bile into the duodenum and externally into a drainage bag. The biliary catheter should have side holes along an appropriate length to allow this to occur. The eventual goal would be to cap the external drainage portion of the drain and direct bile into the duodenum, allowing the patient not to have a bag attached to his or her body. A hydrophilic guidewire can help cross the point of obstruction. If the point of obstruction cannot be traversed with the wire, a small pigtail catheter can be advanced into the dilated biliary tree over the wire. Ideally, an 8.5 or 10 Fr catheter with extended side holes is advanced over the wire into the duodenum and the pigtail loop formed within the bowel (Fig. C6.4).

Contrast injection confirms appropriate placement. If the dilated right and left hepatic ducts do not communicate, an individual drainage catheter should be placed on each side.

The catheter is secured to the skin with sutures and connected to a bag for gravity drainage. This access can

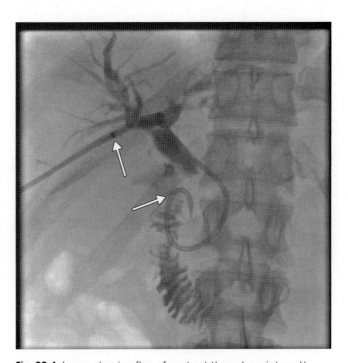

Fig. C6.4 Image showing flow of contrast through an internal/external biliary catheter with the pigtail end within the duodenum. The radiopaque marker (upper arrow) on the tube marks the location of the last side hole, which should be within the biliary duct. The pigtail loop is incompletely formed (lower arrow).

punctures bile ducts, a microwire is advanced into the bile duct (Fig. C6.3). A sheath with stiffener is advanced over the wire and confirmation of appropriate placement is done with contrast injection. The cholangiogram maps be used for future biliary interventions such as opening of biliary strictures, placing biliary stents, and removing stones with a choledochoscope. The bag can be replaced with a cap within a few days depending on how the patient's condition changes. This allows all flow of bile into the duodenum.

COMPLICATIONS

- Catheter obstruction or dislodgement
- Bile leakage
- Cholangitis
- Hemorrhage
- Damage to the biliary system
- Pancreatitis
- Pneumothorax
- Damage to surrounding structures such as vessels and bowel

REFERENCES AND SUGGESTED READING

1. Valji K. Biliary system. In: *Vascular and Interventional Radiology.* 2nd ed. 2006.
2. Kandarpa K, Machan L. Percutaneous biliary interventions. In: *Handbook of Interventional Radiologic Procedures.* 4th ed. 2010;577.

CASE 7: BLAND EMBOLIZATION

PATIENT PRESENTATION

A 25-year-old male presents with pelvic fractures and hemodynamic instability.

DIAGNOSIS

A CT of the pelvis demonstrates a pelvic hematoma and active arterial extravasation (Fig. C7.1).

TREATMENT OPTIONS

- Medical management
- Surgical ligation
- Endovascular embolization

PROCEDURE INDICATIONS

Blunt or penetrating trauma resulting in extraperitoneal or retroperitoneal hemorrhage with hemodynamic instability despite resuscitation and transfusion. Major vascular injury identified on CT with active arterial extravasation of contrast in the absence of hemoperitoneum.

PROCEDURE CONTRAINDICATIONS

Hemoperitoneum in settings of hemodynamic instability usually requires exploratory laparotomy. Pregnancy, contrast allergy, and renal insufficiency are relative contraindications.

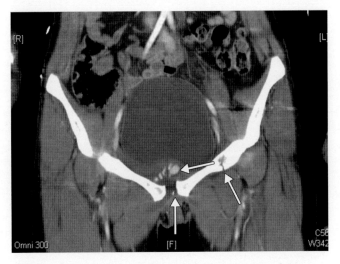

Fig. C7.1 Coronal contrast-enhanced CT coronal image of the pelvis shows active bleeding within a hematoma elevating the base of the urinary bladder (horizontal arrow). Note symphysis pubis diastasis (vertical arrow) and left superior ramus root fracture (right arrow).

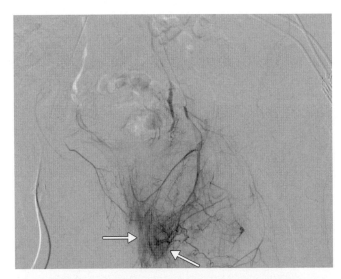

Fig. C7.2 Digital subtraction angiographic image of a left internal iliac artery contrast injection shows active extravasation from the internal pudendal artery. Note the blush of contrast close to midline corresponding to the pelvic hematoma seen on the CT examination (arrows).

PROCEDURE OVERVIEW

The goal is to identify the site of bleeding and achieve hemostasis by occluding the leaking vessel. This can be achieved by injecting gel foam slurry or metallic coils into the target vessel.

Access to the pelvis arterial system is typically achieved via the femoral artery after cleansing of the skin and local anesthesia of groin with lidocaine. Typically, a pigtail flush catheter is advanced into the aorta and an abdominal aortogram is performed to identify solid organ or retroperitoneal arterial injury. A 5 Fr catheter is then advanced into the common iliac arteries to map the arterial anatomy and potentially identify external iliac artery extravasation. The catheter is then advanced into the origin of the internal iliac arteries, which are then evaluated with angiography (Fig. C7.2). If there is a single focus of hemorrhage, targeted embolization can be performed by selecting the leaking artery with a microcatheter and injecting gel foam or deploying coils to stop it. If there are multiple foci of hemorrhage, massive pelvic vascular injury is suspected, requiring the embolization of the proximal internal iliac artery with gelfoam slurry/pledgets or coils (Fig. C7.3).

COMPLICATIONS

- Recurrent or continue hemorrhage
- Infection
- Impotence

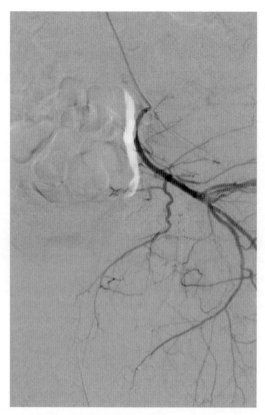

Fig. C7.3 Post gel foam pledget injection shows complete occlusion of the internal pudendal artery and cessation of contrast extravasation.

- Gluteal necrosis
- Nontargeted embolization resulting in infarction of visceral organs or lower extremities

REFERENCES AND SUGGESTED READING

1. Valji K. Pelvic and lower extremity arteries. In: *Vascular and Interventional Radiology.* 2nd ed. 2006.
2. Kandarpa K, Machan L. Trauma management. In: *Handbook of Interventional Radiologic Procedures.* 4th ed. 2010;245.

CASE 8: CHOLECYSTOSTOMY PLACEMENT

PATIENT PRESENTATION

A 74-year-old female with sepsis and multiple comorbidities presents with right upper quadrant (RUQ) pain.

CLINICAL SUSPICION

Acute cholecystitis

DIAGNOSIS

A right upper quadrant ultrasound shows a distended gallbladder with edematous walls, biliary sludge, and positive Murphy's sign consistent with acute cholecystitis (Fig. C8.1).

TREATMENT OPTIONS

- Surgical cholecystectomy
- Medical management
- Percutaneous cholecystostomy tube placement

PROCEDURE INDICATIONS

Urgent decompression of the gallbladder in patients who are poor surgical candidates.

PROCEDURE CONTRAINDICATIONS

Relative contraindications include thrombocytopenia and elevated INR.

PROCEDURE OVERVIEW

Percutaneous cholecystostomy catheter placement can be performed with ultrasound alone or under ultrasound and fluoroscopy guidance. The modality of choice depends on the comfort level of the interventionalist and patient stability. Ultrasound and fluoroscopic guidance are fast and effective in placement of percutaneous cholecystostomy catheters. The patient is placed in supine position. Prophylactic antibiotics should be administered. An ultrasound is used to localize the gallbladder and map the approach. The overlying skin is cleansed and anesthetized with lidocaine. Using sterile technique, an 18-gauge needle is passed into the gallbladder under ultrasound guidance (Fig. C8.2). A transhepatic or transperitoneal approach can be taken, with the latter more feasible for a distended gallbladder. A transperitoneal approach increases the risk of bile peritonitis due to unrestricted leakage of bile into the peritoneum.

When the gallbladder is reached, bile will spontaneously efflux or can be aspirated from the needle. Contrast administration under fluoroscopy will confirm appropriate gallbladder access. A wire can then be passed into the gallbladder and the track is sequentially dilated to accept an 8.5 or 10 Fr drainage catheter. The catheter is locked into place with the pigtail within the gallbladder (Fig. C8.3).

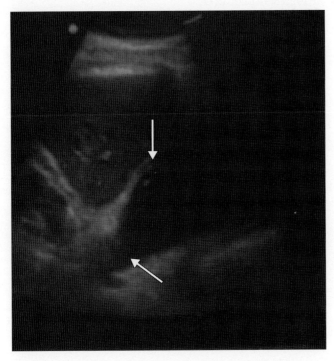

Fig. C8.1 Longitudinal US image shows distended gallbladder with wall edema (upper arrow) and sludge at neck (lower arrow). This shows an optimal placement window through the liver.

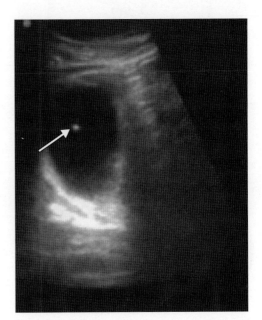

Fig. C8.2 Transverse US image showing echogenic needle tip (arrow) within gallbladder.

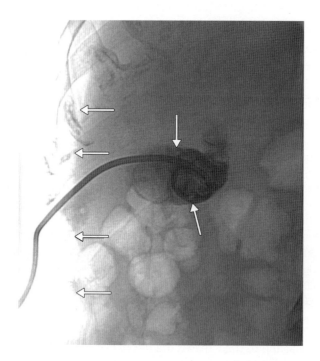

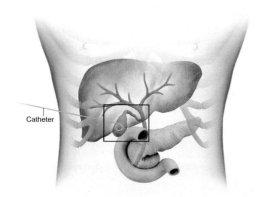

Catheter

Appropriate placement can be confirmed with ultrasound or contrast injection through the catheter under fluoroscopy. The catheter is secured to the skin with sutures and connected to a bag for gravity drainage.

Of note, the catheter should not be removed for at least 6 weeks so the fistula track can mature. This avoids bile spillage into the peritoneum.

COMPLICATIONS

- Catheter obstruction or dislodgement
- Cholangitis
- Bile peritonitis
- Infection
- Hemorrhage

REFERENCES AND SUGGESTED READING

1. Sosna J, Kruskal JB, Copel L, Goldberg, Kane RA. US-guided percutaneous cholecystostomy: features predicting culture-positive bile and clinical outcome. *Radiology.* 2004;230, 785-791.

2. JP McGahan, Lindfors KK. Percutaneous cholecystostomy: an alternative to surgical cholecystostomy for acute cholecystitis? *Radiology.* 1989;173:481-485.

3. Melin MM, Sarr MG, Bender CE, Van Heerden JA. Percutaneous cholecystostomy: a valuable technique in high-risk patients with presumed acute cholecystitis. *Br J Surg.* 1995;8(9):1274-1277.

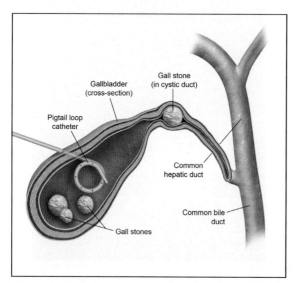

Fig. C8.3 Fluoroscopic image shows cholecystostomy tube transversing the liver shadow (left arrows) with pigtail end within the gallbladder lumen (right arrows). Contrast injection outlines gallbladder confirming optimal placement.

CASE 9: PERCUTANEOUS BIOPSY

PATIENT PRESENTATION

A 53-year-old female with history of hepatitis C and remote history of lymphoma presents with enlarged right axillary lymph nodes.

CLINICAL SUSPICION

Metastasis

DIAGNOSIS

An ultrasound examination of the left axilla shows lymphadenopathy (Fig. C9.1). A staging CT of the chest abdomen and pelvis demonstrates a left liver mass as well.

TREATMENT OPTIONS

- Surgical resection
- Chemotherapy
- Radiation therapy

PROCEDURE INDICATIONS

Prior to treatment, biopsies of the liver mass and axillary lymphadenopathy are done to ascertain a diagnosis and presence of metastatic disease.

PROCEDURE CONTRAINDICATIONS

Relative contraindications include thrombocytopenia and elevated INR. Ascites is an additional relative contraindication to the liver mass biopsy.

PROCEDURE OVERVIEW

Core needle biopsy and fine needle aspiration can be performed under ultrasound or CT guidance depending on the location of the lesion being biopsied. Ultrasound guidance is fast and effective in superficial lymph node biopsies. The overlying skin is cleansed and anesthetized with lidocaine. Using sterile technique, a 21- or 22-gauge needle is advanced into the lymph node (Fig. C9.2). Using agitation and gentle suction, fine needle aspiration is done.

The sample is analyzed by pathology for adequacy. A large gauge two-step needle is then advanced into the enlarged lymph node under real-time ultrasound guidance. Core biopsies are taken. Postprocedure ultrasound is done to evaluate for complications. Hemostasis is achived by direct manual pressure.

A CT-guided biopsy can be performed with either CT fluoroscopy or interval CT scans. An initial CT scan of the region of interest is done with a radiopaque marker or grid on the skin (Fig. C9.3). The biopsy approach and needle tract are planned based on the location of the lesion and adjoining/overlying structures. The skin is then marked, cleansed, and anesthetized. Using interval CT scans or CT

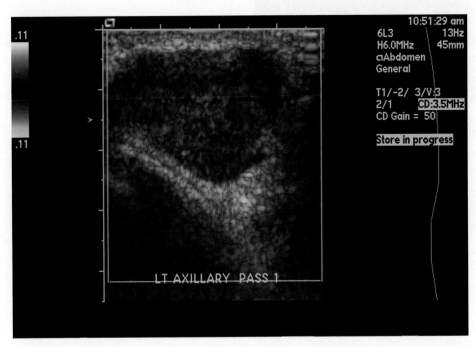

Fig. C9.1 Left axillary ultrasound image shows an enlarged lymph node with diffuse cortical thickening and abnormal hilum.

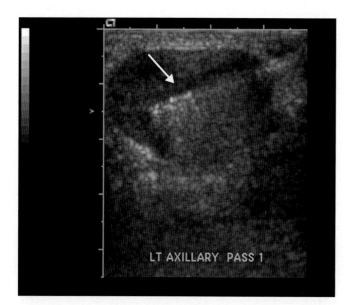

Fig. C9.2 Grey-scale ultrasound image shows an echogenic needle (arrow) within the enlarged lymph node.

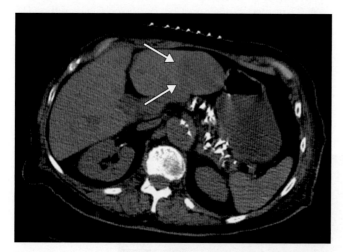

Fig. C9.3 Noncontrast axial CT image of a left liver mass (arrows) with overlying radiopaque skin marker.

fluoroscopy, a guide such as a guide needle is advanced into the lesion using sterile technique (Fig. C9.4). A spring loaded two-step needle is advanced into the guide and

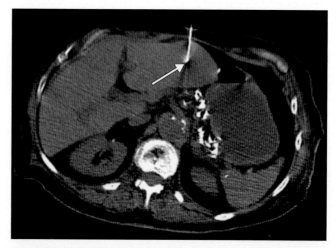

Fig. C9.4 Noncontrast axial CT image shows the biopsy needle (arrow) within the left liver mass.

used to take core biopsies. A postprocedural CT scan is done to evaluate for complications. Hemostasis is achieved by direct manual pressure or injection of gel foam slurry into the biopsy track.

COMPLICATIONS

- Wound infection
- Hemorrhage
- Damage to surrounding structures such as vessels and bowel

REFERENCES AND SUGGESTED READING

1. http://www.sirweb.org/medical-professionals/GR_PDFs/nb.pdf.
2. Uppot RN, Harisinghani MG, Gervais DA. Imaging-guided percutaneous renal biopsy: rationale and approach. *AJR*. 2010; 194(6):1443-1449.
3. Kandarpa K, Machan L. Abdominal biopsies. In: *Handbook of Interventional Radiologic Procedures*. 4th ed. 2010;516.
4. Valji K. Percutaneous biopsy. In: *Vascular and Interventional Radiology*. 2nd ed. 2006.

CASE 10: PERCUTANEOUS GASTROSTOMY PLACEMENT

PATIENT PRESENTATION

A 75-year-old female with recent stroke and hemiparesis presents with dysphagia.

CLINICAL SUSPICION

Swallowing dysfunction

DIAGNOSIS

A swallow study demonstrates frank aspiration with liquid and solids. A consult is placed for gastrostomy tube placement for nutritional support.

TREATMENT OPTIONS

- Surgical gastrostomy tube
- Percutaneous endoscopic gastrostomy tube
- Percutaneous image guided gastrostomy

PROCEDURE INDICATIONS

Nutritional support in patients with stroke or esophageal obstruction, decompression of gastroenteric contents in patients with gastroparesis or gastric outlet obstruction, and diversion in cases of esophageal leaks.

PROCEDURE CONTRAINDICATIONS

Absolute contraindications include inability to access stomach due to overlying colon, spleen, or liver, and uncorrectable coagulopathy. Relative contraindications include large ascites, gastric varices, distorted anatomy from prior surgery, or severe gastroesophageal reflux leading to aspiration of feedings.

PROCEDURE OVERVIEW

The patient is placed in supine position. A nasogastric tube is placed under fluoroscopic guidance. An ultrasound is used to outline the liver border to avoid it during the tube placement. The left subcostal or epigastric region is prepped in sterile fashion, and 1 mg of glucagon is administered to reduce gastic peristalsis. The stomach is insuflated with air via the nasogastric tube until adequate gastric distension is achieved. A puncture site is chosen and infiltrated with lidocaine. A small incision is made and a large gauge needle is used to puncture the stomach. Confirmation of gastric placement is done with aspiration of air and contrast injection under fluoroscopic guidance (Fig. C10.1). Gastropexy device is deployed to

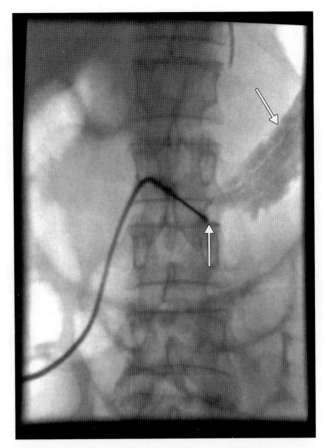

Fig. C10.1 Percutaneous access of a gas distended stomach with a needle (left arrow). Notice opacification of the stomach rugal folds (right arrow) with contrast.

approximate the anterior gastric wall to the abdominal wall. A stiff wire is then looped into the stomach through the needle. The needle is removed and fascial dilators are used to dilate the tract to accept a 12 Fr or large gastrostomy tube. The gastrostomy catheter is advanced into the stomach over the guidewire and the loop is formed in the stomach. Confirmation of placement is done with contrast injection under fluoroscopic guidance (Fig. C10.2). The catheter is secured to the skin with prolene sutures and the site is dressed. The tube can be used for feeding in 24 hours if there are no signs of peritonitis, there are active bowel sounds, and gastric contents can be aspirated from the tube.

COMPLICATIONS

- Peritonitis
- Wound infection
- Hemorrhage
- Gastrointestinal perforation
- Tube displacement

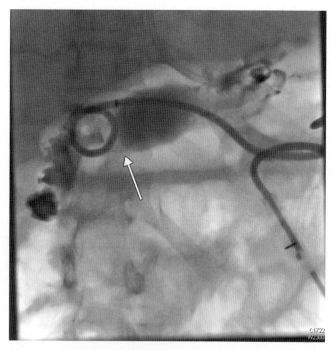

Fig. C10.2 Final image showing pigtail end of gastrostomy catheter in the stomach pylorus (arrow) as confirmed by contrast injection.

- Aspiration of gastric contents
- Tube leakage
- Sepsis

REFERENCES AND SUGGESTED READING

1. Bell SD, Carmody EA, Yeung EY, Thurston WA, Simons ME, Ho CS. Percutaneous gastrostomy and gastrojejunostomy: additional experience in 519 procedures. *Radiology.* 1995;194:817-820.

2. Dewald CL, Hiette PO, Sewall LE, Fredenberg PG, Palestrant AM. Percutaneous gastrostomy and gastrojejunostomy with gastropexy: experience in 701 procedures. *Radiology.* 1999; 211:651-656.

3. Kandarpa K, Machan L. Percutaneous gastrostomy, percutaneous gastrojejunostomy, jejunostomy, and cecostomy. In: *Handbook of Interventional Radiologic Procedures.* 4th ed. 2010;555.

CASE 11: HEMODIALYSIS CATHETER PLACEMENT

PATIENT PRESENTATION

A 48-year-old female presents with elevated creatinine and hyperkalemia.

DIAGNOSIS

Acute renal failure

TREATMENT OPTIONS

- Medical management
- Arteriovenous fistula or graft creation
- Hemodialysis or peritoneal dialysis catheter placement (Fig. C11.1)

PROCEDURE INDICATIONS

A hemodialysis catheter is placed in patients with acute renal failure needing urgent dialysis for electrolyte imbalance, fluid overload, uremia, etc. It is also used in patients with chronic renal failure as a bridge to arteriovenous fistula/graft creation or renal transplant.

PROCEDURE CONTRAINDICATIONS

Coagulopathy, thrombocytopenia, and inability to get central venous access.

PROCEDURE OVERVIEW

The goal of dialysis catheter placement is to provide long-term access for exchanging blood to and from a hemodialysis machine. The catheter has an arterial and venous lumen. The arterial lumen withdraws blood from the patient, and the venous lumen returns blood to the patient from the machine. The flow rates are typically between 200 and 500 mL/min. There are different types of dialysis catheters on the market, but all of them work on the same principle.

Prior to initiating the procedure, patency of the target central vein is established with Doppler ultrasound. Typically, access to a central vein such as the internal jugular vein is achieved using a micropuncture needle under real-time ultrasound guidance after cleansing and anesthetizing the skin. The system is upsized to a 5 Fr sheath over a guidewire. The guidewire can then be used to measure the length of dialysis catheter needed and the desired location of the catheter tip. A 3 to 8 cm long subcutaneous tunnel is created leading to the venotomy. The dialysis catheter is fed through the tunnel to pull the Dacron cuff into the tunnel. The cuff eventually causes fibrosis and creates a barrier to infection. It also anchors the catheter into place. The venotomy is then sequentially dilated to

accept a sheath through which the dialysis catheter will be fed into the vein. The sheath with its stiffener is then advanced over the guidewire into the central vein. The stiffener is then removed and the dialysis catheter is fed through the sheath into the central vein. The sheath is then peeled away while ensuring the catheter remains in place (Fig. C11.2). The arterial and venous lumens are then

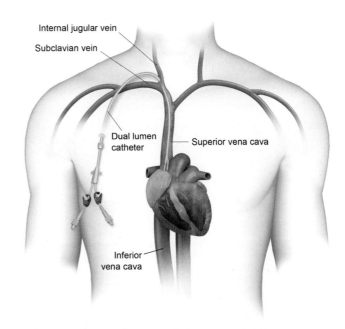

Fig. C11.1 Dual-lumen tunneled hemodialysis catheter placed via the right internal jugular vein.

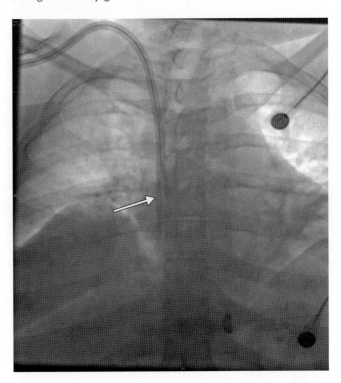

Fig. C11.2 Right internal jugular tunneled hemodialysis catheter (arrow).

locked with predetermined volumes of 1000 units/mL heparin to prevent thrombosis. The venotomy and subcutaneous tunnel defects are then sutured. The hemodialysis catheter is secured with Prolene sutures and dressings are applied.

COMPLICATIONS

- Hemorrhage
- Infection
- Thrombosis or injury of central vein
- Clotting or kinking of catheter

REFERENCES AND SUGGESTED READING

1. Valji K. Vascular access placement and foreign body retrieval. In: *Vascular and Interventional Radiology.* 2nd ed. 2006.
2. Kandarpa K, Machan L. Dialysis catheter management. In: *Handbook of Interventional Radiologic Procedures.* 4th ed. 2010;467.

CASE 12: INFERIOR VENA CAVA FILTER PLACEMENT

PATIENT PRESENTATION

A 68-year-old immobile female with intracranial hemorrhage develops left lower extremity swelling and erythema.

CLINICAL SUSPICION

Deep venous thrombosis

DIAGNOSIS

Duplex venous ultrasound of the left leg shows acute deep venous thrombus extending into the common iliac vein (Figs. C12.1 and C12.2).

TREATMENT OPTIONS

- Compression stockings with anticoagulation
- Mechanical thrombectomy
- Chemical thrombolysis
- Inferior vena cava filter placement

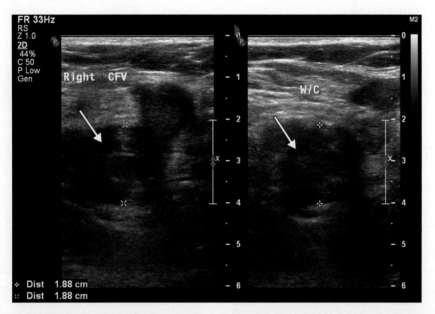

Fig. C12.1 Gray-scale ultrasound image of the right common femoral vein shows a noncompressible vein with an expansile echogenic thrombus (arrows). Image on the left is without manual compression. Image on the right is with manual compression.

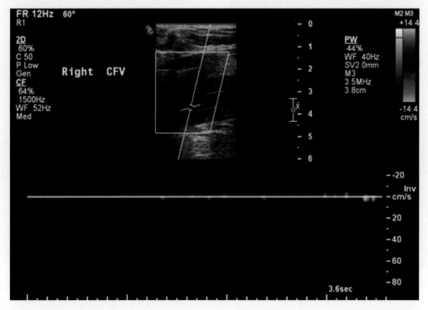

Fig. C12.2 Color Doppler image at the same location in the right common femoral vein shows no venous flow or waveform consistent with complete occlusion of the vein lumen by thrombus.

PROCEDURE INDICATIONS

- Patients with contraindication (such as gastrointestinal or intracranial hemorrhage) to anticoagulation
- Progression of thromboembolism despite anticoagulation
- Planned thrombolysis or thrombectomy
- Subtherapeutic anticoagulation
- Large burden of thrombus
- High risk of deep venous thrombus development due to immobility, surgery, etc.

PROCEDURE CONTRAINDICATIONS

- Total thrombosis of the vena cava
- Inability to gain access to or image the vena cava during filter placement
- Allergy to a filter component
- Severe uncorrectable coagulopathy

PROCEDURE OVERVIEW

The goal of placement of a filter within the vena cava is to catch large emboli that can potentially lead to symptomatic pulmonary emboli and hemodynamic instability. There are three types of filters: permanent filters that are not intended for removal, temporary filters that must be removed, and temporary filters that can be converted into permanent filters. Choice of the type of filter being placed depends on the indication. The filters can be placed in the superior or inferior vena cava depending on the source of emboli. In our case, an inferior vena cava filter is indicated.

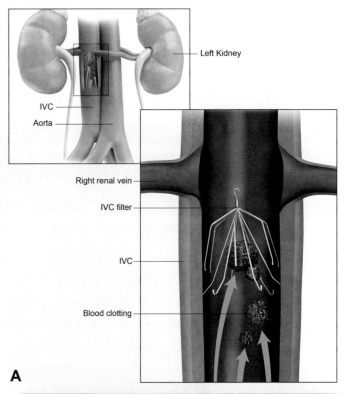

A

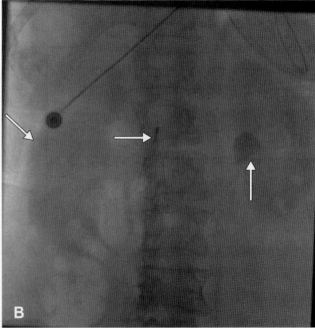

Fig. C12.3 Cavogram by injection of contrast shows a patent inferior vena cava and inflow from bilateral renal veins (upper arrows). Notice the pigtail catheter (lower arrow) used to inject the contrast.

Fig. C12.4 (A) Infrarenal IVC filter catching blood clots. (B) Final image after IVC filter placement shows a metallic filter in upright position (horizontal arrow). Notice contrast opacification of bilateral kidneys and the left renal pelvis (left and right arrows).

Ideally, the right internal jugular or femoral vein is accessed with a micropuncture needle after cleaning and anesthetizing the overlying skin. Using a guide wire and catheter, the inferior vena cava is accessed. A cavogram is then performed to identify variant anatomy and diameter of the vena cava, extent of venous thrombus, and identify the lowest renal vein orifice (Fig. C12.3). A landmark such as the level of vertebral body can be used as a reference point for the lowest renal vein orifice. The catheter is then exchanged for a filter delivery sheath. The filter must be in the correct orientation (jugular or femoral) prior to insertion. After correct positioning of the filter tip, it is deployed per the manufacturer's instructions (Fig. C12.4). Another cavogram is done through the delivery sheath at a high injection rate to document optimal venous blood flow in the IVC and correct positioning of the filter. The sheath is then removed and hemostasis is achieved by manual compression at the puncture site.

COMPLICATIONS

- Vena cava thrombosis or perforation
- Filter fracture, migration, or infection

REFERENCES AND SUGGESTED READING

1. Kandpal H, Sharma R, Gamangatti S, Srivastava DN, Vashisht S. Imaging the inferior vena cava: a road less traveled. *RadioGraphics*. 2008;28:669-689.
2. Kinney TB. Inferior vena cava filters. *Semin Intervent Radiol*. 2006;23(3):230-239.
3. Kandarpa K, Machan L. Vena cava filters. In: *Handbook of Interventional Radiologic Procedures*. 4th ed. 2010;376.

CASE 13: PERCUTANEOUS NEPHROSTOMY PLACEMENT

PATIENT PRESENTATION

A 55-year-old female with history of a large pelvic mass presents with acute abdominal pain and elevated creatinine.

CLINICAL SUSPICION

Obstructive hydroureteronephrosis

DIAGNOSIS

CT abdomen and pelvis shows bilateral hydroureteronephrosis (Fig. C13.1).

TREATMENT OPTIONS

- Surgical resection of obstructing mass
- Retrograde ureteral stent placement
- Percutaneous nephrostomy tube placement

PROCEDURE INDICATIONS

- Acute elevation in creatinine with obstructive hydronephrosis
- Pyonephrosis with sepsis
- Obstructing calculi or tumors
- Preparation for surgical ureteral intervention
- Urinary diversion due to urine leak or fistula

PROCEDURE CONTRAINDICATIONS

Relative contraindications include thrombocytopenia and elevated INR.

PROCEDURE OVERVIEW

Percutaneous nephrostomy catheter placement can be performed under ultrasound, fluoroscopy, or CT guidance. Ultrasound and fluoroscopic guidance are fast and effective in placement of percutaneous nephrostomy catheters. The patient is placed in the prone position. The overlying skin is cleansed and anesthetized with lidocaine. Using sterile technique, a needle is passed from a direct posterior approach into the posterolateral kidney aiming for the most posterior lower renal calyx. This can done using direct ultrasound or using anatomic landmarks fluoroscopic guidance. When the collecting system is reached, urine will spontaneously efflux from the needle in a pressurized system. Contrast administration under fluoroscopy will confirm appropriate renal access (Fig. C13.2). A wire can then be passed into the renal pelvis and ureter. The track is then

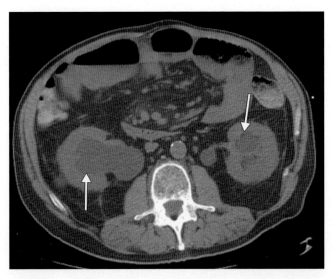

Fig. C13.1 CT abdomen shows bilateral hydronephrosis (arrows) and left hydroureter.

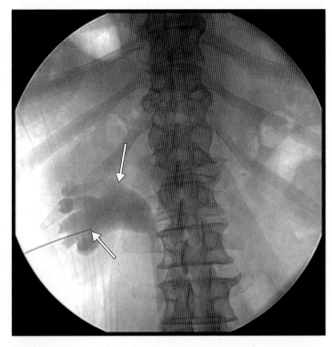

Fig. C13.2 Contrast injection from a percutaneous needle shows appropriate access of a lower pole calyx (lower arrow) and opacification of a dilated renal collecting system (upper arrow).

sequentially dilated to accept an 8 or 10 Fr catheter that is locked into placed with the pigtail within the renal pelvis (Fig. C13.3). Contrast injection under fluoroscopy confirms appropriate placement. Urine should flow freely from the catheter, which is then secured to the skin with sutures and connected to a bag for gravity drainage.

This access can be used in the future for ureteral interventions such as ureteral stent placement, lithotripsy, and

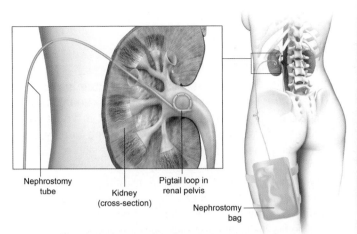

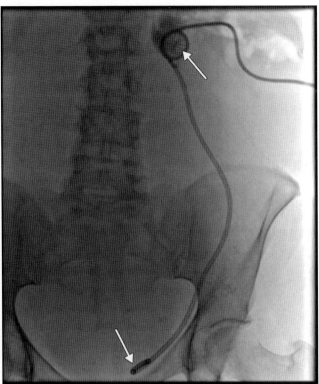

Fig. C13.4 Left nephroureteral stent with lower pigtail formed within the urinary bladder (lower arrow) and the proximal loop in the left renal pelvis. Notice jets of contrast opacifying the left renal pelvis (upper arrow).

COMPLICATIONS

- Catheter obstruction or dislodgement
- Pyonephrosis/nephritis
- Hemorrhage
- Damage to renal pelvis or ureter
- Damage to surrounding structures such a vessels and bowel

REFERENCES AND SUGGESTED READING

1. Dyer RB, Regan JD, Kavanagh PV, Khatod EG, Chen MY, Zagoria RJ. Percutaneous nephrostomy with extensions of the technique: step by step. *RadioGraphics*. 2002;22:503-525.

2. Valji K. Urologic and genital systems. In: *Vascular and Interventional Radiology*. 2nd ed. 2006.

3. Kandarpa K, Machan L. Percutaneous nephrostomy and antegrade ureteral stenting. In: *Handbook of Interventional Radiologic Procedures*. 4th ed. 2010;590.

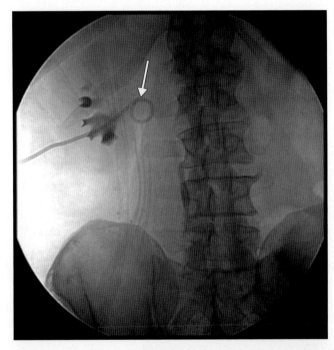

Fig. C13.3 Final image shows placement of a pigtail nephrostomy catheter (arrow) with decompression of the renal collecting system.

dilating of ureteral strictures. The nephrostomy tube can potentially be turned into a nephroureteral stent if the point of obstruction can be traversed with a guidewire to enter the urinary bladder. A nephroureteral stent has an external drainage portion connected to a bag outside. An extension of the external portion extends through the ureter into the urinary bladder where it forms a pigtail loop preventing superior migration (Fig. C13.4). This allows for natural flow of urine into the urinary bladder. In the future, the external portion of the catheter can be capped, eliminating the need for drainage bags and reducing potential complications such as catheter dislodgement and infection.

CASE 14: PARACENTESIS

PATIENT PRESENTATION

A 45-year-old male presents with history of hepatic cirrhosis and abdominal distension.

CLINICAL SUSPICION

Ascites

DIAGNOSIS

An ultrasound examination of the abdomen demonstrates a large amount of ascites (Fig. C14.1).

TREATMENT OPTIONS

- Diuresis
- Paracentesis
- Transjugular intrahepatic portosystemic shunt
- Liver transplant

PROCEDURE INDICATIONS

Paracentesis can serve a dual purpose:

1. Therapeutic: Relieve respiratory compromise or abdominal pain/pressure.
2. Diagnostic: Evaluate for exudative (infectious, malignant) versus transudative (hypoalbuminemia, fluid overload) ascitic fluid.

PROCEDURE CONTRAINDICATIONS

Relative contraindications:
- Thrombocytopenia
- Elevated INR
- Pregnancy
- Intra-abdominal adhesions

PROCEDURE OVERVIEW

Paracentesis is a relatively simple procedure that can be done at the bedside with or without ultrasound guidance. Interventional radiologists use ultrasound to find a large pocket of fluid, away from small bowel and urinary bladder. Using sterile technique, the overlying skin is anesthetized. Using a large gauge one-step needle, the peritoneal cavity is accessed under real-time ultrasound guidance (Fig. C14.2). Color Doppler can be used to identify and avoid vessels such as the inferior epigastric artery.

The needle is then removed and the plastic sheath is left in place. The ascites is drained using a negative pressure source such as vacuum bottles. The procedure is halted when the patient's symptoms improve and most of the ascites has been evacuated (Fig. C14.3). After 5 L of ascites has been evacuated, the patient receives 8 g of intravenous albumin for every additional liter removed in order to counter hemodynamic imbalance.

COMPLICATIONS

- Persistent leak from puncture site
- Wound infection
- Hematoma
- Bowel perforation
- Vascular injury
- Hypotension
- Hepatorenal syndrome

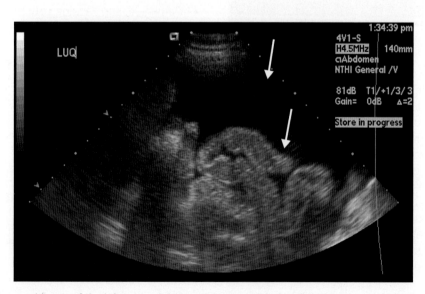

Fig. C14.1 Gray-scale ultrasound image of the left upper abdomen shows anechoic free fluid (upper arrow). Notice loops of (lower arrow) deep to the fluid.

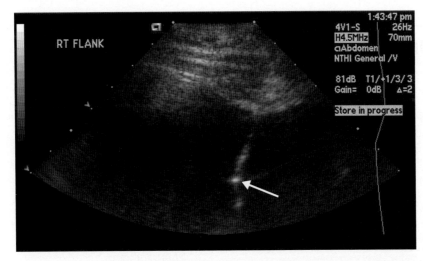

Fig. C14.2 Gray-scale ultrasound image shows echogenic needle (arrow) transversing the peritoneum with its tip in the free fluid.

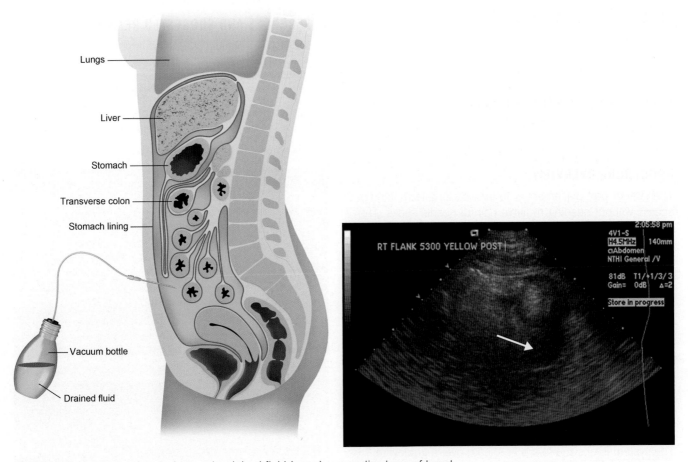

Fig. C14.3 Postprocedure image shows only minimal fluid (arrow) surrounding loops of bowel.

REFERENCE AND SUGGESTED READING

1. Ross GJ, Kessler HB, Clair MR, Gatenby RA, Hartz WH, Ross LV. Sonographically guided paracentesis for palliation of symptomatic malignant ascites. *AJR.* 1989;153(6):1309-1311.

CASE 15: PORT PLACEMENT

PATIENT PRESENTATION

A 50-year-old female presents with metastatic breast cancer.

CLINICAL SUSPICION

Metastatic breast cancer needing chemotherapy

DIAGNOSIS

None

TREATMENT OPTIONS

- Chemotherapy via port
- Surgical resection
- Radiation therapy

PROCEDURE INDICATIONS

A port can be used for administration of chemotherapy, long-term antibiotics, and contrast for CT/MRI examinations. It can also be used for obtaining blood samples.

PROCEDURE CONTRAINDICATIONS

Coagulopathy, thrombocytopenia, and inability to obtain central venous access.

PROCEDURE OVERVIEW

The goal of port placement is to provide long-term venous access without needing multiple painful needle sticks. The port reservoir and catheter are completely internal and placed in the chest. The port catheter delivers the drug directly into the central venous system avoiding potential peripheral vein toxicity. The port reservoir is buried under the skin and can be accessed using a special needle such as the Huber needle, which is a specially designed long, hollow, beveled tip needle that can go through the skin as well as the silicone septum of the implanted port's reservoir. The patient can bathe and go about daily activities without difficulty.

Prior to initiating the procedure, patency of the target central vein is established with Doppler ultrasound. Typically, access to the internal jugular vein is achieved using a micropuncture needle under real-time ultrasound guidance after cleansing and anesthetizing the skin (venotomy site). The system is upsized to a 5 Fr sheath over a guidewire.

The guidewire can then be used to measure the length of catheter needed and the desired location of the catheter tip. An infraclavicular chest pocket is then created under the skin so it is large enough to accept the port reservoir. The pocket can be flushed with an antibiotic solution as prophylaxis against future infection. A 3- to 8-cm long subcutaneous tunnel is created from the pocket to the venotomy over the clavicle. The catheter is connected to the port reservoir. It is then fed through the tunnel to place the reservoir into the pocket in a snug fashion. The catheter is then cut to length based on the prior measurement. A peel away sheath with its stiffener is then advanced over the guidewire into the central vein. The stiffener is removed and the catheter is fed through the sheath into the central vein. The sheath is then peeled away while ensuring the catheter remains in place (Fig. C15.1). The venotomy and reservoir pocket are then closed with meticulous suturing. The port is locked with heparin to prevent occlusion with blood clots.

COMPLICATIONS

- Hemorrhage
- Infection
- Pneumothorax
- Central vein thrombosis or injury
- Catheter embolism, clotting, or kinking

REFERENCES AND SUGGESTED READING

1. http://www.sir.net.au/portacath_pi.html.
2. Struk DW, Bennett JD, Kozak RI. Insertion of subcutaneous central venous infusion ports by interventional radiologists. *Can Assoc Radiol J*. 1995;46:32-36.
3. Valji K. Vascular access placement and foreign body retrieval. In: *Vascular and Interventional Radiology*. 2nd ed. 2006.

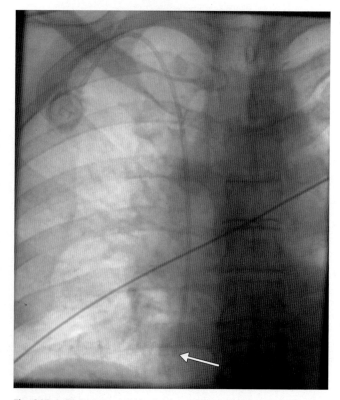

Fig. C15.1 Right internal jugular port with catheter tip (arrow) in the right atrium.

CASE 16: RADIOFREQUENCY ABLATION

PATIENT PRESENTATION

A 70-year-old male presents with history of metastatic melanoma and a small liver lesion.

CLINICAL SUSPICION

Surveillance exam

DIAGNOSIS

An MRI of the abdomen demonstrates an enlarging 1.4 cm liver lesion consistent with metastatic disease (Fig. C16.1).

TREATMENT OPTIONS

- Systemic chemotherapy
- Surgical resection
- Image guided ablation (radiofrequency, microwave, or cryoablation)

PROCEDURE INDICATIONS

Radiofrequency ablation (RFA) induces in situ thermal coagulation necrosis through the delivery of high-frequency alternating current to the tissues. It has been used for many years for treatment of small primary or metastatic lesions (3-4 cm in size) in the liver, kidney, adrenal gland, bone, and lung. It offers a curative treatment without the need for surgical resection in patients who are poor surgical candidates due to comorbid conditions, multiple tumor lesions, or lesions in an inoperable location. Other ablation modalities such as microwave and cryoablation are being

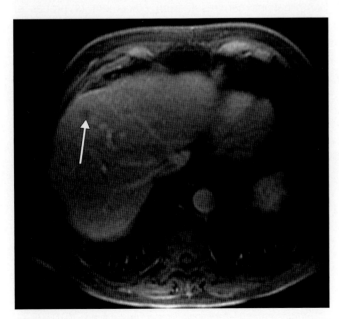

Fig. C16.1 Axial MR image shows a 1.4-cm hypointense lesion in the right liver (arrow).

used in addition to RFA, but interventionalists have more experience with RFA than any other ablation modality.

PROCEDURE CONTRAINDICATIONS

Large lesions may not be adequately treated despite the use of multiple treatment probes. Also, lesions near big vessels may not be heated adequately due to the heat sink effect, in which thermal energy is rapidly dissipated by the flowing blood. Superficial lesions increase the risk of bleeding and damage to surrounding structures such as bowel and adjacent organs. Likewise, lesions that are near bile ducts or the renal collecting system can lead to biliary and urinary complications. Elevated INR or low platelets can increase the chance of hemorrhage during the procedure. The interventionalist needs to carefully review prior available imaging when planning an ablation.

PROCEDURE OVERVIEW

The goal of ablation is to cause necrosis of the entire volume of the targeted tissue for a curative outcome. RFA uses high-frequency alternating current delivered to the tissue via a probe, which acts like an electrode. The electric current agitates the ions in the tissue around the tip of the electrode, creating heat, which leads to localized coagulation necrosis. The patient is part of a closed-loop circuit that includes an RF generator, an electrode needle (probe), and a large dispersive electrode (ground pads).

The ablation can be done with ultrasound, CT, or MR guidance. The patient is usually placed under general anesthesia, though the procedure can be done with intravenous sedation. An initial scan of the liver is done to localize the lesion and confirm the treatment approach planned from prior imaging. Depending on the size and location of the lesion, one or more probes are placed under image guidance with the probe tip inside the lesion (Fig. C16.2). Multiple probes used should ideally be placed in a parallel fashion. To achieve a low rate of tumor recurrence, the target diameter of an ablation cavity must ideally be 1 cm larger than the diameter of the targeted tumor, ensuring abalation of microscopic invasion around the lesion. In order to produce irreversible cellular damage, tissue heating to a temperature of 50 to 55°C for 4 to 6 minutes is required. At temperatures more than 100°C, tissue charring, or carbonization, occurs with gas production, which acts as an insulator to the electromagnetic heating of tissue and hinders current conductivitiy. So ideally, temperatures of 55°C should be achieved during the treatement. Internally cooled electrodes infused by cold saline are available to minimize carbonization, and perfused electrodes with small apertures allowing contact of saline with tissue can achieve higher tissue conductivity of the RF current. Once the probes are placed, the ablation can be done manually or run by an automated program. By monitoring the tissue impedance and probe tip temperatures, one can modulate the RF current to maximize

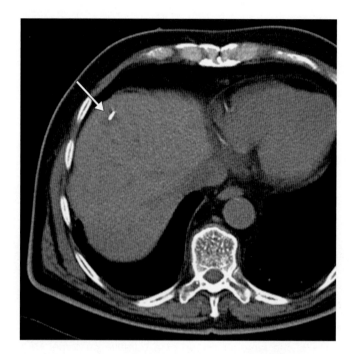

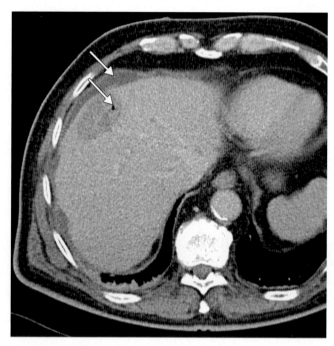

Fig. C16.3 Postablation contrast-enhanced CT shows the ablation cavity with nonenhancing ablated tissue and focus of gas (lower arrow). Perihepatic hypodense fluid (upper arrow) was infused prior to starting the ablation to protect the hemidiaphragm from thermal injury.

A follow-up CT or MRI is typically done 8 to 12 weeks postablation to evaluate for any residual tumor. Subsequent imaging is done to detect tumor recurrence or development of new lesions.

COMPLICATIONS

Complications can result from placement of probes or from thermal damage during treatment. Placement of the probes can result in bleeding, infection, or tumor seeding. During treatment, nontargeted thermal damage can be caused to adjacent organs and bowel, biliary, or urinary systems. Electrical burns can occur at the grounding pad sites if the size or number of grounding pads is inadequate to optimally dissipate the energy. The procedure can also potentially cause failure of the entire organ if there is minimal functional reserve to begin with.

REFERENCES AND SUGGESTED READING

1. Choi H, Loyer EM, DuBrow RA, et al. Radio-frequency ablation of liver tumors: assessment of therapeutic response and complications. *RadioGraphics.* 2001;21:S41-S54.

2. Rhim H, Dodd GD III, Chintapalli KN, et al. Radiofrequency thermal ablation of abdominal tumors: lessons learned from complications. *RadioGraphics.* 2004;24:41-52.

3. Kandarpa K, Machan L. Hepatic tumor ablation. In: *Handbook of Interventional Radiologic Procedures.* 4th ed. 2010;536.

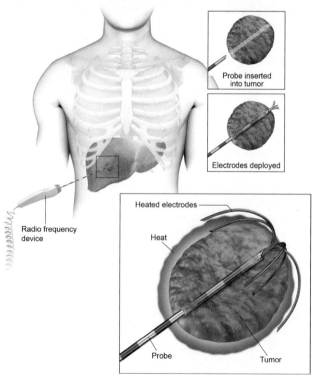

Fig. C16.2 Noncontrast CT image shows part of the RFA probe transversing the liver lesion (arrow).

tissue coagulation and minimize carbonization, thereby achieving an optimal zone of ablation. Intermittent imaging during the ablation is used to monitor the treatment effects on the tissue. A contrast-enhanced CT scan at the end of the procedure may allow evaluation of initial treatment outcome or evaluation for residual tumor (Fig. C16.3).

CASE 17: PERCUTANEOUS CYSTOSTOMY PLACEMENT

PATIENT PRESENTATION

A 25-year-old male presents with pelvic fractures and gross hematuria.

CLINICAL SUSPICION

Urethral trauma

DIAGNOSIS

A retrograde urethrogram shows a complete type II injury of the membranous urethra with contrast extravasation (Fig. C17.1).

TREATMENT OPTIONS

- Surgical repair
- Urinary diversion with suprapubic catheter

PROCEDURE INDICATIONS

Percutaneous nephrostomy placement may be used to relieve urinary retention in patients when transurethral catheterization is contraindicated or unsuccessful. Patients with spinal cord injury, urethral injury, or urinary bladder outlet obstruction due to prostatic hypertrophy or a mass are candidates for this procedure.

PROCEDURE CONTRAINDICATIONS

Relative contraindications:

- Thrombocytopenia
- Elevated INR
- Pregnancy
- Adhesions from prior surgery or radiation

PROCEDURE OVERVIEW

Suprapubic catheter placement is a relatively simple procedure that can be done with fluoroscopic or ultrasound guidance. An ultrasound can be used to identify the urinary bladder and presence of any intervening bowel. Fluoroscopy can outline an adequately distended urinary bladder. Using sterile technique, the overlying skin is anesthetized with lidocaine.

Using a 10-mL syringe connected to a large gauge needle, the urinary bladder is punctured under real-time ultrasound or fluoroscopic guidance while aspirating. When urine is encountered, the syringe is removed. Confirmation of needle placement into the bladder is also done with contrast injection. A guidewire is then passed through the needle into the urinary bladder (Fig. C17.2). The needle is removed and the tract is sequentially dilated to accept the suprapubic catheter. A pigtail catheter is then advanced into the urinary bladder over the wire. The wire is removed

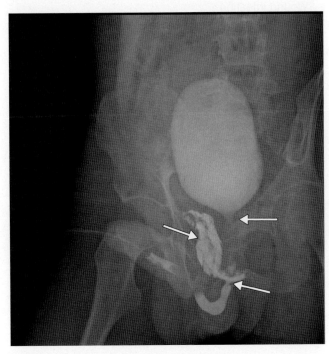

Fig. C17.1 Complete type II injury of the membranous urethra (right lower arrow) with contrast extravasation (left arrow). Note elevation of the urinary bladder (right upper arrow) due to hematomas around pelvic fractures. Contrast in the urinary bladder is from recent contrast-enhanced CT exam.

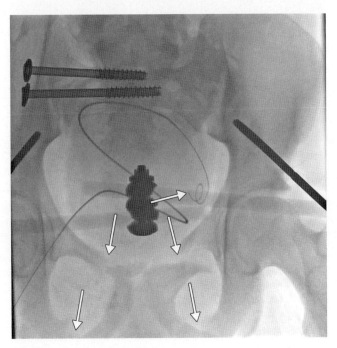

Fig. C17.2 A suprapubic guidewire (upper horizontal arrow) follows the curvature of the urinary bladder through a Kumpe catheter. The patient has pelvic fracture fixation hardware and bilateral pubic rami fractures (vertical arrows).

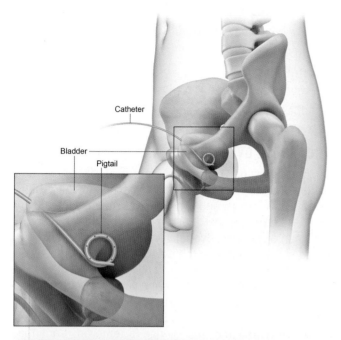

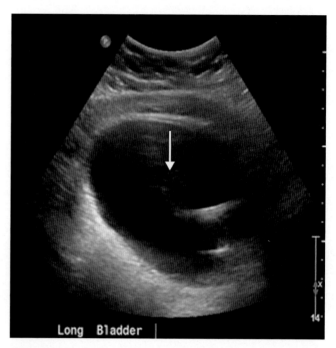

Fig. C17.4 Ultrasound image of the same patient shows the catheter loop (arrow) within the urinary bladder.

COMPLICATIONS

- Persistent leak from puncture site
- Hematuria
- Wound infection
- Hematoma
- Visceral injury

REFERENCE AND SUGGESTED READING

1. Cronin CG, Prakash P, Gervais DA, et al. Imaging-guided suprapubic bladder tube insertion: experience in the care of 549 patients. *AJR.* 2011;196:182-188.

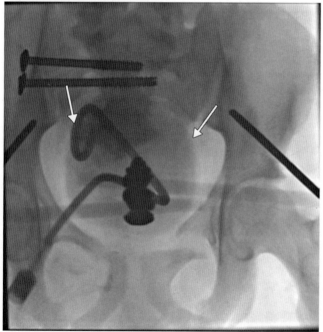

Fig. C17.3 Final fluoroscopic image following contrast injection shows a suprapubic catheter (left arrow) within the urinary bladder (right arrow).

to form the pigtail loop, which is then locked (Figs. C17.3 and C17.4). Appropriate placement is confirmed with contrast injection. The catheter is then secured to the skin with Prolene sutures, and the site is dressed appropriately.

CASE 18: TRANSARTERIAL CHEMOEMBOLIZATION

PATIENT PRESENTATION

A 54-year-old male with hepatitis C presents with abdominal fullness.

CLINICAL SUSPICION

Hepatocellular carcinoma

DIAGNOSIS

A CT of the abdomen demonstrates a large arterially enhancing hepatic mass, which was biopsy-proven hepatocellular carcinoma (Fig. C18.1).

TREATMENT OPTIONS

- Surgical resection
- Systemic chemotherapy or external beam radiation
- Transarterial chemoembolization (TACE) (Fig. C18.2)
- Transarterial Y-90 microsphere radiation treatment or bland embolization

PROCEDURE INDICATIONS

Nonresectable vascular liver tumors such as hepatocellular carcinoma or liver metastasis can be treated with TACE.

PROCEDURE CONTRAINDICATIONS

Liver failure is an absolute contraindications to TACE. Relative contraindications:

- Inability to prevent reflux of particles into the gastroduodenal artery that can cause bowel perforation or ulceration
- Allergy to intravenous contrast
- Renal insufficiency
- Coagulopathy

Consideration should also be given to the patient's life expectancy.

PROCEDURE OVERVIEW

A CT or MRI liver protocol is done in advance for treatment planning. Vascular tumors obtain the majority of their blood supply via the hepatic artery. Using this to advantage, particles containing chemotherapeutic agent are injected into the arterial supply of the tumor achieving both ischemic and cytotoxic injury to the tumor cells by lodging into small arterial feeders.

Access to the hepatic artery is typically achieved via the femoral artery after cleansing the skin and local anesthesia

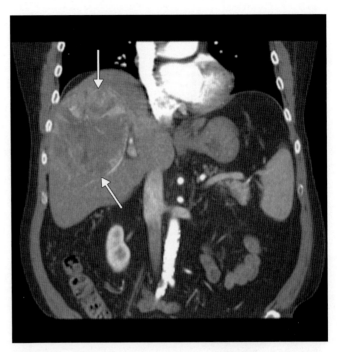

Fig. C18.1 Large right hepatic mass with peripheral arterial enhancement (arrows).

of groin with lidocaine. Typically, an aortogram is done to evaluate for any parasitized vascular supply to the tumor and presence of variant arterial anatomy not seen on by prior imaging. 5 Fr curved catheter is used to gain a stable access to the celiac artery. An angiogram is performed to map the arterial anatomy. It is important to map out all arterial feeders to the liver tumor and identify collateral vessels and nontargeted vessels (Fig. C18.3). Establishing patency of the portal vein and evaluating for arteriovenous fistulas is also an important step achieved during the angiogram. Any potential collateral supply should be embolized to achieve optimal ischemia of the tumor. Additional vessels may need to be embolized to prevent nontargeted chemoembolization. A microcatheter is then advanced into the main artery feeding the tumor using a guidewire. A repeat angiogram is performed to ensure optimal positioning and forward flow. Once the catheter is secured, drug-eluting microspheres containing a calculated dose of chemotherapeutic agent or lipiodol mixed with chemotherapeutic agent can then be infused through the microcatheter. Additional lesions can then be treated in a similar fashion. During the procedure, a C-arm three-dimensional cone beam CT can be used for trouble shooting. Once the complete dose has been infused, the apparatus is removed and hemostasis is achieved via manual pressure applied to the groin or an arterial closure device. A follow-up CT or MRI scan of the liver can be done in 3 months to assess response to the therapy.

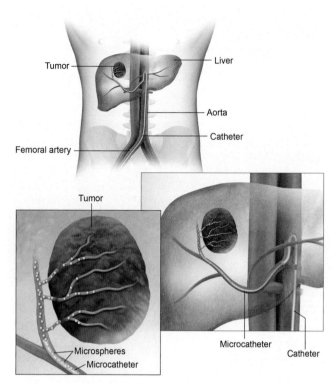

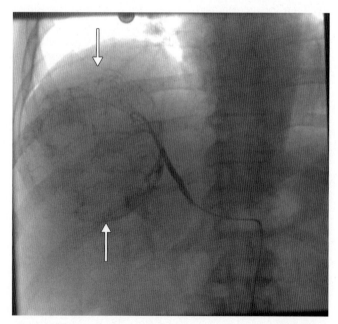

Fig. C18.2 Transarterial chemoembolization of hepatic tumor.

COMPLICATIONS

- Hemorrhage
- Postembolization syndrome
- Pseudoaneurysm
- Artery dissection
- Hepatic abscess
- Nontargeted embolization resulting in infarction of visceral organs

REFERENCES AND SUGGESTED READING

1. Lee KH, Sung KB, Lee DY, et al. Transcatheter arterial chemoembolization for hepatocellular carcinoma: anatomic and hemodynamic considerations in the hepatic artery and portal vein. *RadioGraphics.* 2002:22:1077-1091.

2. Kalva SP, Thabet A, Wicky S, et al. Recent Advances in transarterial therapy of primary and secondary liver malignancies. *RadioGraphics,* 2008;28:101-117.

3. Valji K. Hepatic, splenic, and portal vascular systems. In: *Vascular and Interventional Radiology.* 2nd ed. 2006.

4. Kandarpa K, Machan L. Chemoembolization of hepatocellular carcinoma. In: *Handbook of Interventional Radiologic Procedures.* 4th ed. 2010;262.

Fig. C18.3 Right hepatic artery angiogram outlines the arterial supply (arrows) to the large right hepatic mass without reflux or distal collateral flow.

CASE 19: THORACENTESIS

PATIENT PRESENTATION

A 50-year-old female presents with history of shortness of breath and lung cancer.

CLINICAL SUSPICION

Pleural effusion

IMAGING MODALITY OF CHOICE

Chest x-ray shows a large right pleural effusion (Fig. C19.1).

TREATMENT OPTIONS

- Treating the cause of pleural effusion (eg, antibiotics for infection, diuresis for congestive heart failure)
- Thoracentesis
- Chest tube/ pleural drain placement
- Pleurodesis or pleural decortication

PROCEDURE INDICATIONS

Thoracentesis can serve a dual purpose:

1. Therapeutic: to relieve respiratory compromise.
2. Diagnostic: to evaluate for exudative (infectious, malignant) versus transudative effusions (hypoalbuminemia, fluid overload).

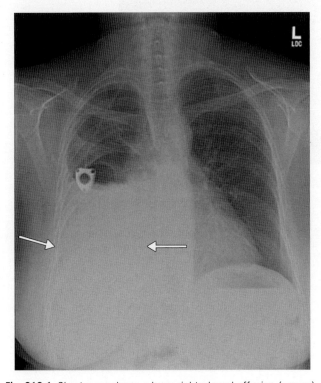

Fig. C19.1 Chest x-ray shows a large right pleural effusion (arrows). A right-sided port is present.

PROCEDURE CONTRAINDICATIONS

There are no absolute contraindications. Relative contra-indications:

- Small pleural effusion
- Chest wall infection
- Positive pressure ventilation
- Single functioning lung
- Bullous emphysema

PROCEDURE OVERVIEW

Thoracentesis is performed with the patient in a sitting position. Ultrasound is used to image the pleural space and plan a safe approach. It also demonstrates the size, location, and other characteristics of the pleural effusion.

If the pleural effusion is large, the patient's skin can be marked and thoracentesis may be performed without real-time ultrasound guidance. For small and loculated pleural effusions, real-time ultrasound guidance is used. After skin cleansing and local anesthetic with lidocaine, a posterior or lateral intercostal approach is used to guide a large bore one-step needle connected to a syringe into the pleural space as negative pressure is manually applied to the syringe (Fig. C19.2). Once fluid is encountered, the plastic sheath is passed over the needle into the pleural space and subsequently connected to a negative pressure source such as a vacuum bottle. For therapeutic thoracentesis, no more than 1 to 1.5 L of fluid is removed to avoid reexpansion pulmonary edema (Fig. C19.3). If a larger amount of fluid needs to be removed, slow drainage with a pleural catheter can be done over 1 to 2 hours. For diagnostic thoracentesis, 100 to 150 mL is sufficient.

The procedure should be stopped if the patient becomes hemodynamically unstable, has worsening dyspnea, or develops coughing. The sheath is removed with the patient performing a Valsalva maneuver to prevent aspiration of air causing pneumothorax. A postprocedure chest x-ray is done as a baseline and to document any complications that may require further intervention.

COMPLICATIONS

- Pneumothorax
- Bleeding
- Reexpansion pulmonary edema
- Vasovagal reaction
- Cough
- Shortness of breath
- Infection
- Organ or diaphragm laceration

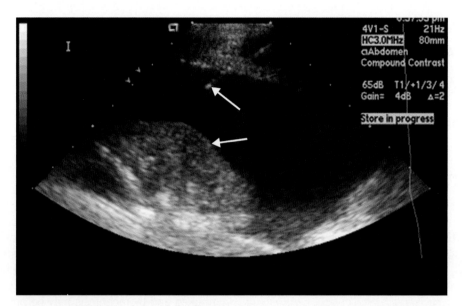

Fig. C19.2 Gray-scale ultrasound image shows needle transversing the pleural space into the effusion (upper arrow). Note the collapsed lung (lower arrow) deep to the needle tip.

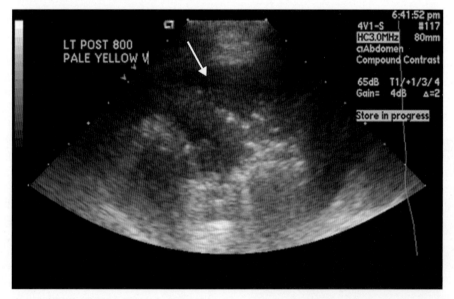

Fig. C19.3 Postprocedure gray-scale ultrasound image shows removal of the majority of the pleural fluid (arrow).

REFERENCES AND SUGGESTED READING

1. Jones PW, Moyers JP, Rogers JT, et al. Ultrasound-guided thoracentesis: is it a safer method? *FCCPCHEST.* 2003;123(2):418-423.

2. Sokolowski JW. Guidelines for thoracentesis and needle biopsy of the pleura. *A J Respir Crit Care Med.* 1989;140(1):257.

CASE 20: TRANSJUGULAR INTRAHEPATIC PORTOSYSTEMIC SHUNT (TIPS) PLACEMENT

PATIENT PRESENTATION

A 50-year-old male presents with history of alcoholic hepatic cirrhosis and persistent hematemesis.

CLINICAL SUSPICION

Bleeding gastroesophageal varices

DIAGNOSIS

A CT shows dilated varices, and bleeding esophageal varices are confirmed on esophagogastroduodenoscopy (Fig. C20.1).

TREATMENT OPTIONS

- Medical management
- Sclerotherapy or banding
- Transjugular intrahepatic portosystemic shunt (TIPS)

PROCEDURE INDICATIONS

Acute or recurrent variceal bleeding that is refractory to sclerotherapy or banding or medical management can be managed successfully by placement of a TIPS. Other indications include refractory ascites or portal decompression in patients with hepatic venous outflow obstruction, hepatic hydrothorax, and hepatorenal syndrome.

PROCEDURE CONTRAINDICATIONS

Absolute contraindications include right-sided heart failure with increased central venous pressure, polycystic liver disease, and severe liver failure.

Relative contraindications:

- Portal vein thrombosis
- Severe hepatic encephalopathy poorly controlled by medications
- Sepsis or hepatic infection
- Hepatic tumors
- Large ascites that can be drained via paracentesis

PROCEDURE OVERVIEW

The goal of placement of an intrahepatic portosystemic shunt is to bypass the vascular resistance in the cirrhotic liver by creating a channel between the portal and hepatic veins, thereby reducing portal pressure/hypertension. This should alleviate variceal bleeding in most cases.

General anesthesia is established. Ideally, the right internal jugular vein is accessed with a micropuncture needle after cleaning and anesthetizing the overlying skin. Using a guide wire, sheath, and multipurpose curved 5 Fr catheter, the right hepatic vein is accessed. The hepatic wedge pressure, free hepatic venous pressure, and right atrial pressures are measures for baseline. With clinically significant cirrhosis, one would expect a gradient of 12 mm Hg or greater between the hepatic wedge and right atrial pressures, signifying portal hypertension. A venogram is done to delineate the hepatic venous anatomy (Fig. C20.2). The 5 Fr catheter is then exchanged for a commercially available transjugular liver access needle. The needle is then directed in an anterior inferior fashion through the hepatic vein wall toward the right portal vein. The needle is retracted and once blood is aspirated, contrast is injected to evaluate portal access. Multiple attempts are sometimes required to access the right portal vein via the right hepatic vein (Fig. C20.3). If

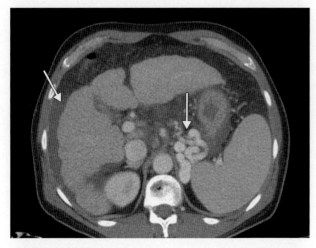

Fig. C20.1 Contrast-enhanced CT of the upper abdomen shows dilated perisplenic varices (right arrow). Note nodular surface of an atrophied liver consistent with cirrhosis. There is also a small amount of ascites (left arrow) and prominence of the spleen, sequelae of portal hypertension.

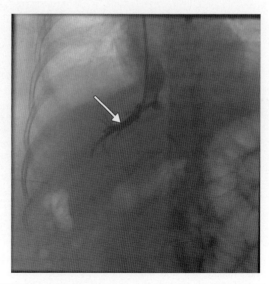

Fig. C20.2 Contrast injection through sheath opacifies a central hepatic vein (arrow) with reflux of contrast into the right atrium.

the access is appropriate, a wire is placed through the needle into the splenic or superior mesenteric vein via the portal vein. A marked pigtail catheter is then inserted over the wire into the splenic vein. This can be used for venography, pressure measurements, and figuring out the length of the stent needed (Fig. C20.4).The tract through the liver parenchyma is dilated using 8 mm balloon so it can accept an 8 to

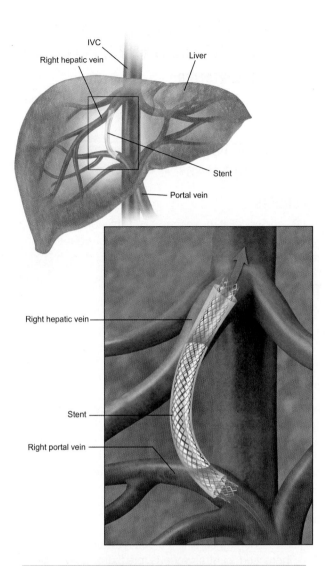

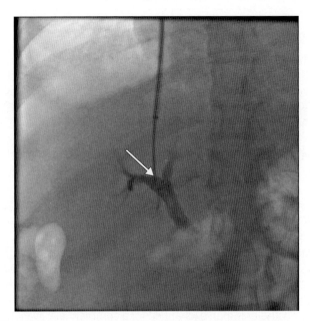

Fig. C20.3 Successful puncture of the right portal vein with needle (arrow). Contrast injection through the needle shows opacification of the right, left, and main portal veins.

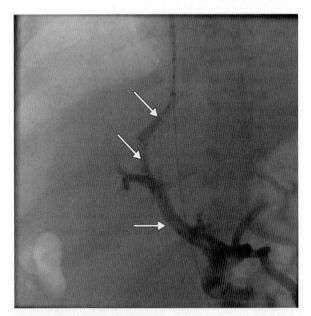

Fig. C20.4 A guidewire and catheter with markings (arrows) advanced through the hepatic vein and dilated intrahepatic tract into the main portal vein. The markings are set 1 cm apart, which can be used to measure the length of stent required. Note the dilated varices.

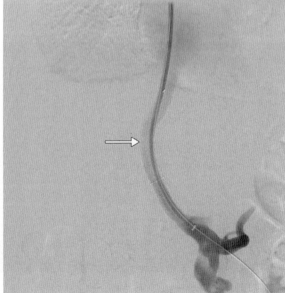

Fig. C20.5 Digital subtraction venogram post stent deployment shows contrast flow through the shunt (arrow) into the right atrium.

10 mm stent graft. Once the stent is deployed, any stenosis may be dilated using high-pressure balloons. Two stents may be required for adequate coverage of the portal and hepatic veins. Patency of the shunt is confirmed by a repeat retrograde venogram that should show free-flowing contrast from the portal vein into the hepatic vein and IVC (Fig. C20.5). Embolization and/or sclerosis of varices depends on the operator, goal of TIPS creation, and size of varices. The pressures are again measured for documentation and should show a drop in the pressure gradient. Ideal pressure gradient is between 5 and 12 mm Hg, depending on the reason for TIPS creation. Hemostasis is achieved by manual compression at the puncture site.

COMPLICATIONS

- Life-threatening hemoperitoneum from laceration of the liver capsule
- Worsening of hepatic encephalopathy
- TIPS occlusion or stenosis
- Congestive heart failure
- Pulmonary edema
- Pneumothorax
- Arteriovenous fistula formation
- Cardiac arrhythmias

REFERENCES AND SUGGESTED READING

1. ACR-SIR-SPR guideline for the creation or a transjugular intrahepatic portosystemic shunt (TIPS). http://www.acr.org/~/media/92F663B169CA46C5AD6DB73E4D6A5D14.pdf.
2. Haskal ZJ, Martin L, Cardella JF, et al, for the Society of Interventional Radiology Standards of Practice Committee. Quality improvement guidelines for transjugular intrahepatic portosystemic shunts. *J Vasc Interv Radiol.* 2003;14:S265-S270.
3. Freedman AM, Sanyal AJ, Tisnado J, et al. Complications of transjugular intrahepatic portosystemic shunt: a comprehensive review. *RadioGraphics.* 1993;13:1185-1210.
4. Valji K. Hepatic, splenic, and portal vascular systems. In: *Vascular and Interventional Radiology.* 2nd ed. 2006.
5. Kandarpa K, Machan L. Transjugular intrahepatic portosystem shunt placement. In: *Handbook of Interventional Radiologic Procedures.* 4th ed. 2010;390.

CASE 21: UTERINE ARTERY EMBOLIZATION

PATIENT PRESENTATION

A 43-year-old female with pelvic pressure, pain, and menorrhagia.

CLINICAL SUSPICION

Uterine fibroids

DIAGNOSIS

Multiple large uterine fibroids are seen with ultrasound and confirmed on MRI of the pelvis (Fig. C21.1).

TREATMENT OPTIONS

- Hormonal treatment
- Hysterectomy or myomectomy
- Uterine artery embolization placement
- Medical management of symptoms
- High intensity focused ultrasound (HIFU) treatment

PROCEDURE INDICATIONS

Uterine fibroids can cause multiple symptoms prompting the patient to seek treatment. These symptoms include menorrhagia, pelvic pain/pressure, abdominal distension, and infertility/miscarriage. Genitourinary problems such as hydronephrosis, urinary bladder compression, constipation, and lower extremity edema from venous compression can also be the result of large uterine fibroids. The uterine arteries may also need to be embolized for uncontrollable or life-threatening uterine hemorrhage. In placenta accreta, temporary occlusion with balloons may be indicated immediately prior to delivery.

PROCEDURE CONTRAINDICATIONS

Absolute contraindications:

- Pregnancy
- Malignancy such as leiomyosarcoma or endometrial cancer
- Active pelvic inflammatory disease

Relative contraindications include renal insufficiency and pedunculated fibroid with a narrow stalk.

PROCEDURE OVERVIEW

Uterine fibroid embolization is achieved by embolizing bilateral feeding uterine arteries and/or a collateral feeder such as the ovarian artery. The goal of the embolization is ischemia and subsequent infarction of the fibroid, resulting in a decrease of its overall volume and potential involution. Access to bilateral uterine arteries is typically achieved via

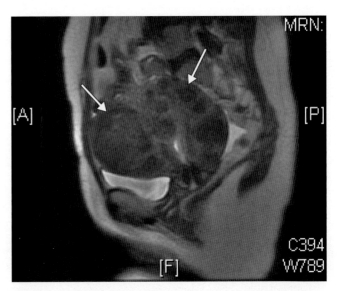

Fig. C21.1 MRI sagittal T2-weighted sagittal images show multiple uterine fibroids in myometrial, submucosal, and subserosal locations (arrows).

the femoral artery after cleansing of the skin and local anesthesia of the groin with lidocaine.

Typically, a 4 Fr or 5 Fr catheter is advanced into the contralateral internal iliac artery, and the arterial anatomy is delineated via the injection of contrast. Upon identification of the uterine artery, the catheter is advanced into its origin (Fig. C21.2). A microcatheter is then advanced into the

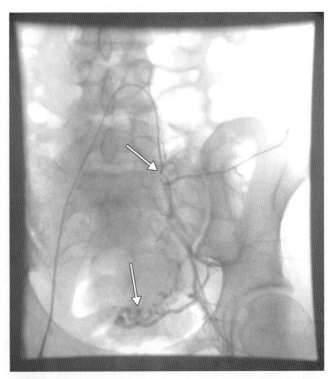

Fig. C21.2 Injection of contrast into the left internal iliac artery (upper arrow) shows the typical corkscrew appearance of the left uterine artery (lower arrow).

uterine artery. Once the arterial anatomy and placement is studied with contrast injection, the uterine artery embolization can begin (Fig. C21.3).

The choice of embolization agent depends on the operator. Embolization agents include gel foam pledgets, polyvinyl alcohol particles, or calibrated microspheres. Coil embolization is avoided due to its permanence and subsequent difficulty of a repeat embolization in case of fibroid recurrence. Contrast along with the embolic agent is then injected into the uterine artery until near-complete stasis of flow is achieved indicating successful embolization of the uterine artery (Fig. C21.4). The agent occludes small peripheral branches of the uterine artery demonstrating an outline and staining of the fibroids with contrast. Using the same catheter or a new catheter from the contralateral groin, the other uterine artery is embolized in a similar fashion.

The catheter is then exchanged for a pigtail catheter, which is used to perform an aortogram to delineate any collateral supply to the fibroids, such as the ovarian artery. If there is substantial blood supply to the fibroids via the collateral, it may be embolized in a similar fashion. Upon conclusion, the catheter is removed and hemostasis is achieved via manual compression of the puncture site or with an arterial closure device.

Success of the procedure is evaluated with a follow-up pelvic MRI or ultrasound in a few months and postprocedure clinic follow-up.

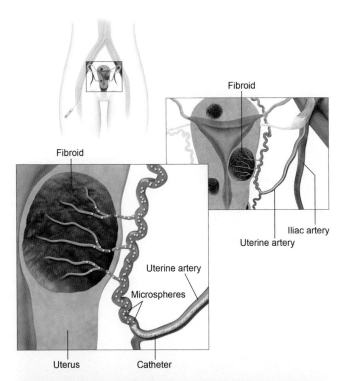

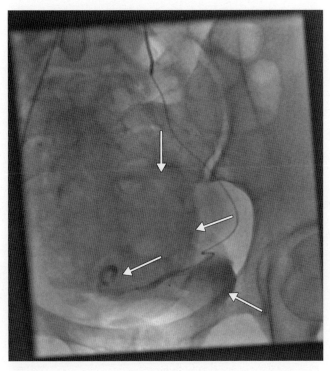

Fig. C21.4 Conclusion of embolization of the left uterine artery shows no flow of contrast into the distal left uterine artery or its branches (left arrow). Notice staining of the large uterus with contrast material (upper right arrows). The urinary bladder is displaced to the left (lower right arrow).

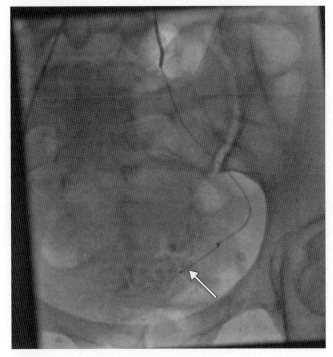

Fig. C21.3 Injection of contrast mixed with embolization agent into the left uterine artery via a microcatheter (arrow).

COMPLICATIONS

- Infection
- Painful expulsion of submucosal fibroid
- Ovarian failure
- Nontargeted embolization of pelvis or lower extremities.
- Hematoma or pseudoaneurysm at arterial puncture site
- Postembolization syndrome (pain, fever, anorexia, leukocytosis)
- Loss of fertility
- Fibroid recurrence particularly with large volume uterine fibroids

REFERENCES AND SUGGESTED READING

1. Sterling KM. UFE: indications/patient selection. *J Vascular Intervent Radiol.* 2002;13(2)(suppl):P235-P239.
2. Goodwin SC. Techniques of UAE. *J Vascular Intervent Radiol.* 2001;12(1)(suppl):P257-P264.
3. Coddington CC. Uterine fibroids: basic concepts and medical management. *J Vascular Intervent Radiol.* 2000;11(2)(suppl):13-23.
4. Shlansky-Goldberg R. Complications with UFE and their management. *J Vascular Intervent Radiol.* 2003;14(2)(suppl): P69-P73.
5. Kandarpa K, Machan L. Uterine fibroid embolization. In: *Handbook of Interventional Radiologic Procedures.* 4th ed. 2010;281.

CASE 22: RADIOEMBOLIZATION OF HEPATIC MALIGNANCY

PATIENT PRESENTATION

A 67-year-old female presents with abdominal pain and history of neuroendocrine tumor.

CLINICAL SUSPICION

Metastasis

DIAGNOSIS

CT of the abdomen demonstrates an arterially enhancing mass consistent with metastatic disease (Fig. C22.1).

TREATMENT OPTIONS

- Surgical resection
- Systemic chemotherapy
- Transarterial chemoembolization (TACE)
- Transarterial Y-90 radioembolization

PROCEDURE INDICATIONS

Nonresectable vascular liver tumors such as hepatocellular carcinoma or liver metastasis are ideal candidates for Y-90 internal radiation therapy.

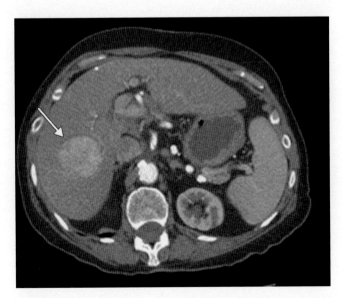

Fig. C22.1 Right hepatic arterially enhancing mass (arrow).

PROCEDURE CONTRAINDICATIONS

Absolute contraindications include liver failure, significant hepatopulmonary shunting and reflux of Y-90 into arteries supplying the gastroduodenal region. Some patients have a shunt between the hepatic and pulmonary circulation. Others may have a gastric or gastroduodenal artery in close proximity or in communication with the hepatic arteries. Therefore, injecting Y-90 into the hepatic artery supplying the tumor may send some of the beads into the gastroduodenal or pulmonary circulation resulting in radiation-induced pneumonitis or bowel ulceration/perforation, respectively. Relative contraindications include allergy to intravenous contrast, renal insufficiency, coagulopathy, and pregnancy. Consideration should also be given to the patient's life expectancy.

PROCEDURE OVERVIEW

A CT or MRI of the liver protocol is done in advance for treatment planning. Vascular tumors receive the majority of their blood supply via the hepatic artery. Using this to advantage, microspheres containing Y-90 (beta-radiation emitting radioisotope) are injected into the arterial supply of the tumor achieving both ischemic and radiation injury to the tumor cells by lodging into small arterial feeders.

Radioembolization is performed as a two-step process. The first part is a preparatory step. It is used to delineate arterial supply to targeted tumors and plan the exact arterial location where the Y-90 spheres or resin will be delivered. The second part is treatment of the tumors by delivering the Y-90. The two steps are typically done as two separate procedures on different days.

Access is typically achieved via the femoral artery after cleansing of the skin and local anesthesia of the groin with lidocaine. Typically, an aortogram is done to evaluate for any parasitized vascular supply to the tumor and presence of variant arterial anatomy not seen on by prior imaging. 5 Fr curved catheter is used to gain a stable access to the celiac artery. An angiogram is performed to map the arterial anatomy (Fig. C22.2). It is important to map out all arterial feeders to the liver tumor and identify collateral vessels and nontargeted vessels. Establishing patency of the portal vein and evaluating for arteriovenous fistulas is also an important step achieved during the angiogram. Any potential collateral supply should be embolized to consolidate the blood supply to the tumor. Arteries, such as the right gastric artery and gastroduodenal artery, supplying bowel should be bypassed or embolized prior to treatment to avoid nontargeted radiation damage. A microcatheter is then advanced into the main artery

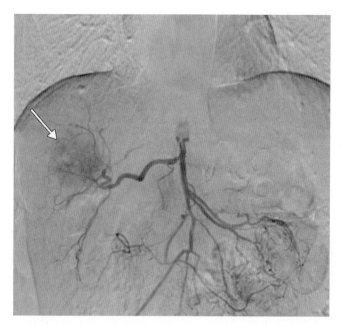

Fig. C22.2 Superior mesenteric artery axis angiogram outlines the arterial supply to the right hepatic mass (arrow). A replaced right hepatic vein is present.

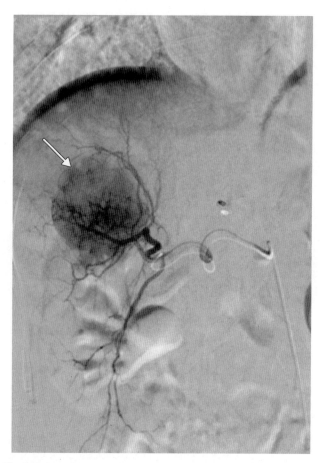

Fig. C22.3 Arteriogram after selective catheterization with a microcatheter prior to Y-90 microsphere injection shows arterial feeders to the liver mass (arrow).

feeding the tumor using a guidewire. A repeat angiogram is performed to ensure optimal positioning and forward flow (Fig. C22.3).

Hepatopulmonary shunting due to arteriovenous fistulas and extrahepatic bowel activity due to arterial reflux can be ruled out by injecting Tc-99 labeled macro aggregated albumin (MAA) into the catheter. Using scintigraphy, hepatopulmonary shunt fraction is calculated (Fig. C22.4). Shunt fractions greater than 20% result in a high absorbed dose by the lung and precludes treatment with Y-90 microspheres. Similarly, extrahepatic bowel radiation can cause severe ulceration and damage to the gastrointestinal tract, and treatment with Y-90 microspheres is contraindicated with arterial reflux into the gastroduodenal region.

The dose is then calculated based on volume of the tumor, volumes of the liver lobes, and shunt fraction.

On the day of treatment, the microcatheter is placed at the previously planned arterial location. Once the catheter is secured, particles containing the Y-90 microspheres are injected into the catheter through a storage delivery port. The port is necessary to prevent radiation contamination of the surrounding environment and to limit the dose to the operator. Once the complete dose is injected, the apparatus is disposed of by the radiation safety officer. A radiation survey is performed of the room, the operators,

equipment, and patient. A follow-up scintigraphic exam can be done after 30 hours to document and confirm appropriate delivery of the radiation dose. A CT or MRI of the liver can be performed in 3 months to assess response to the therapy.

COMPLICATIONS

- Gastroduodenal ulceration
- Radiation pneumonitis
- Bone marrow suppression
- Hepatitis
- Hemorrhage
- Arterial pseudoaneurysm or dissection
- Abscess

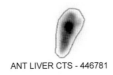

ANT LIVER CTS - 446781

POST LIVER CTS - 430809

1

3% LUNG UPTAKE

ANT LUNG CTS - 11932

POST LUNG CTS - 14489

1

ANT LUNG_SS   1

Fig. C22.4 Planar scintigram obtained after hepatic arterial injection of Tc-99m labeled MAA shows radionuclide activity in the liver, particularly the liver tumor. Only 3% hepatopulmonary shunt fraction was seen. No activity is seen in the gastrointestinal region.

REFERENCES AND SUGGESTED READING

1. Murthy R, Nunez R, Szklaruk J, et al. Yttrium-90 microsphere therapy for hepatic malignancy: devices, indications, technical considerations, and potential complications. *RadioGraphics*, 2005;25:S41-S55.

2. Kandarpa K, Machan L. Radioembolization of hepatic malignancies. In: *Handbook of Interventional Radiologic Procedures.* 4th ed. 2010;267.

Chapter 9

Pediatric Radiology

*By Megan Speer, Michael Mahlmann, Jennifer Caero,
and Ajaykumar C. Morani*

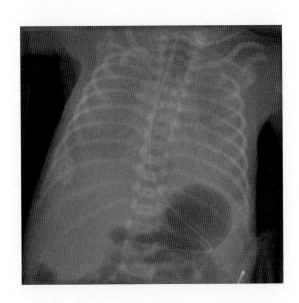

INTRODUCTION

Imaging in the pediatric population is unique, and it is essential for physicians to limit patient exposure to ionizing radiation in the medical workup due to increased risk of cancer development. Children are at higher risk of cancer development because they are more radiosensitive and live more years than adults. The use of nonionizing radiation in children with ultrasound and MRI is recommended when possible. Also, as demonstrated in the case presentations in this chapter, the initial imaging modalities of choice in the evaluation of the majority of pediatric patients include radiographs, which have a low amount of ionizing radiation, and ultrasound. Therefore, it is important to be aware of the imaging modalities and techniques available to promote radiation protection in the imaging of children and to take a conscientious approach to imaging this population.

CASE 1: SURFACTANT DEFICIENCY DISEASE

PATIENT PRESENTATION

Premature infant born at 28 weeks of gestation develops shortness of breath shortly after birth.

CLINICAL SUSPICION

Surfactant deficiency disease

IMAGING MODALITY OF CHOICE

Chest radiograph

FINDINGS

Surfactant deficiency disease, also called respiratory distress syndrome or hyaline membrane disease, is primarily seen in premature infants. It is a lung disease that occurs as a result of surfactant deficiency, resulting in alveolar collapse and decreased pulmonary compliance.

On frontal chest radiograph, there are low lung volumes associated with diffuse haziness or fine reticular granular opacities due to generalized alveolar collapse (Fig. C1.1). Prominent air bronchograms are seen due to patent larger bronchi in the diseased lung. Pleural effusions are an uncommon finding with surfactant deficiency disease.

Treatment with surfactant replacement therapy can lead to clearing of the granular opacities and increased lung volumes. In some cases, there may be asymmetric clearing of lung opacities indicating partial response to treatment. In addition to surfactant replacement therapy, neonates with surfactant deficiency commonly require mechanical ventilation for treatment and respiratory support.

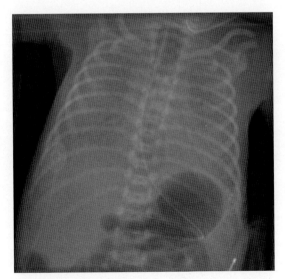

Fig. C1.1 A 32-week-old premature infant with low lung volumes, diffuse hazy pulmonary opacities, and prominent air bronchograms, consistent with surfactant deficiency disease.

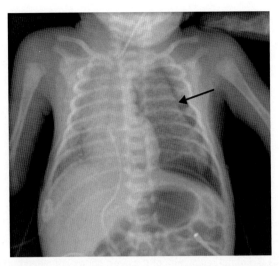

Fig. C1.2 Frontal radiograph of the chest shows a preterm infant with surfactant deficiency disease and a left-sided pneumothorax (arrow), resulting as a complication of mechanical ventilation.

During this time, chest radiograph may show coarse granular opacities and mixed areas of overinflation and atelectasis before returning to normal appearance. Appearance on the chest radiograph may mimic meconium aspiration leading to misdiagnosis if not clinically correlated. Mechanical ventilation can also be associated with several potential complications, including pulmonary interstitial emphysema and air-block complications such as pneumomediastinum, pneumothorax (Fig. C1.2), and pneumopericardium.

Acute pulmonary interstitial emphysema most often occurs in the setting of severe surfactant deficiency and is a result of airway overdistention and subsequent rupture of alveoli with air entering the adjacent pulmonary interstitium. Radiographically, pulmonary interstitial emphysema appears as multiple well-defined cystic or bubblelike lucencies that can be focal or diffuse and often resolve with appropriate timely management (Fig. C1.3). Rarely, pulmonary interstitial emphysema may persist and develop into a localized expansive, multicystic mass on chest radiograph.

DIFFERENTIAL DIAGNOSIS

Clinical Differential

Several other common causes of shortness of breath in newborn infants include meconium aspiration syndrome, transient tachypnea of the newborn, and pneumonia. Meconium aspiration syndrome is respiratory distress due to intrapartum or intrauterine aspiration of meconium in mostly postterm babies. Transient tachypnea of the newborn, also referred to as wet lung disease, is self-limited and results from delayed clearance of fluid from the lungs. Neonatal pneumonia can occur intrauterine, during birth, or thereafter and may be caused by a number of pathogens, most commonly due to beta-hemolytic streptococci.

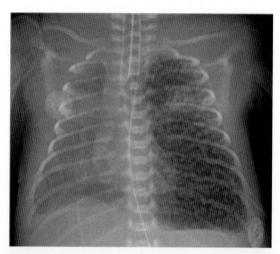

Fig. C1.3 Frontal radiograph of the chest shows left-sided bubble-like lucencies consistent with pulmonary interstitial emphysema, a complication associated with management of surfactant deficiency disease.

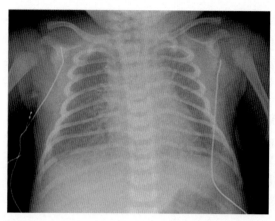

Fig. C1.4 Frontal radiograph of the chest in a full-term infant with transient tachypnea of the newborn shows normal lung volumes with diffuse, bilateral prominent interstitial lung markings.

Imaging Differential

Evaluation of a chest radiograph in a newborn demonstrating diffuse pulmonary disease should begin with assessment of the lung volumes and pulmonary opacities. Low lung volumes are more commonly seen in infants with surfactant deficiency disease and beta-hemolytic streptococcal pneumonia, whereas high lung volumes are more common in meconium aspiration syndrome, transient tachypnea of the newborn, and other types of neonatal pneumonia. The lung volumes with all of these entities, however, may be normal.

Findings of meconium aspiration on chest radiograph include patchy and asymmetric lung opacities. Transient tachypnea of the newborn may demonstrate a combination of airspace opacities, prominent interstitial lung markings, and pleural effusion (Fig. C1.4). Neonatal pneumonia, other than beta-hemolytic pneumonia, is characterized by asymmetric, patchy perihilar opacities and may or may not have pleural effusion. Distinguished from the other types of neonatal pneumonia, the findings of beta-hemolytic pneumonia can be similar to those of surfactant deficiency disease with diffuse fine granular opacities.

REFERENCES AND SUGGESTED READING

1. Agrons GA, Courtney SE, Stocker JT, et al. From the archives of the AFIP: lung disease in premature neonates: radiologic-pathologic correlation. *RadioGraphics.* 25(4):1047-1073.

2. Donnelly L. *Pediatric Imaging: The Fundamentals.* 1st ed. Philadelphia, PA: Saunders; 2009.

CASE 2: CONGENITAL DIAPHRAGMATIC HERNIA

PATIENT PRESENTATION

Term infant presents at birth with severe respiratory distress. Physical examination demonstrates a scaphoid abdomen and auscultation of the lungs reveals poor air entry on the left.

CLINICAL SUSPICION

Congenital diaphragmatic hernia

IMAGING MODALITY OF CHOICE

Frontal chest radiograph

FINDINGS

Congenital diaphragmatic hernia is caused by a defect in the diaphragmatic musculature with herniation of the abdominal contents into the chest, resulting in underdevelopment of the lungs. The lung ipsilateral to the hernia is most commonly affected with hypoplastic changes due to long-standing mass effect from the hernia. The opposite lung may also be affected by mass effect, which results from shift of the mediastinum with subsequent compression. Pulmonary hypoplasia or development is a major factor in determining prognosis of these infants. Three basic types of congenital diaphragmatic hernia exist: (1) posterolateral Bochdalek hernia, (2) anterior Morgagni hernia, and (3) hiatus hernia. Bochdalek hernia is the most common congenital diaphragmatic hernia and most often occurs on the left side because the liver protects the right posterior Bochdalek foramen.

In the prenatal period, ultrasound has a high sensitivity in the detection of congenital diaphragmatic hernia. Ultrasound demonstrates bowel loops undergoing peristalsis in the chest and absence of the abdominal stomach bubble. Fetal MR imaging is useful for determining the degree of pulmonary hypoplasia, which can be useful for predicting neonatal survival.

Associated anomalies, including congenital heart disease, can occur in 25% to 50% of patients with congenital diaphragmatic hernia and contribute to the patient's mortality. Because the bowel herniates into the left side of the thorax, there are varying degrees of left lung hypoplasia, a leading cause of morbidity and mortality in these children. Primary treatment includes respiratory support with mechanical ventilation followed by surgical repair.

Typical findings on chest radiograph in infants with a left-sided posterolateral congenital diaphragmatic hernia include air-filled or fluid-filled loops of bowel in the left hemithorax, mediastinal shift away from the hernia, and paucity of bowel gas in the scaphoid abdomen secondary to bowel loops herniating in the chest (Fig. C2.1). In some cases, abnormal position of support tubes may also be a clue to the diagnosis. Often, the combination of clinical scenario and appearance of the abnormal radiolucency on chest radiograph are diagnostic of diaphragmatic hernia.

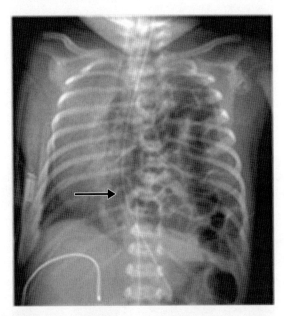

Fig. C2.1 Chest radiograph shows large left congenital diaphragmatic hernia with multiple air-filled loops of bowel in the left chest. The mediastinum and nasogastric tube (arrow) are displaced to the right.

DIFFERENTIAL DIAGNOSIS

Clinical Differential

Infants presenting at birth with severe respiratory distress may be the result of several clinical etiologies. This may be secondary to a diffuse pulmonary lung disease such as neonatal pneumonia and meconium aspiration syndrome, or lung anomalies.

Imaging Differential

Congenital pulmonary airway malformation (CPAM) and congenital lobar emphysema are included in the differential of localized lung radiolucencies seen in neonates.

Congenital pulmonary airway malformation is a congenital adenomatoid proliferation of the bronchioles with lack of normal alveolar development (Figs. C2.2 and C2.3). A single lobe is typically involved and there is no lobar predilection. Three types of CPAMs exist, and they are differentiated based on the size of the cysts at imaging or pathology. Findings on chest radiography and CT differ with the type of malformation. The lesions may appear predominantly cystic, mixed solid and cystic, or solid depending on the size and number of cysts and whether the cysts contain air or fluid.

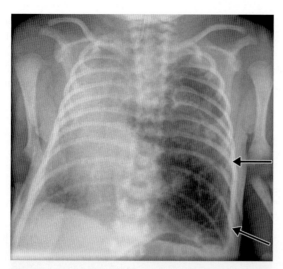

Fig. C2.2 Frontal chest radiograph shows multiple cystic lucencies in the left lower thorax (arrows) with mediastinal shift to the right.

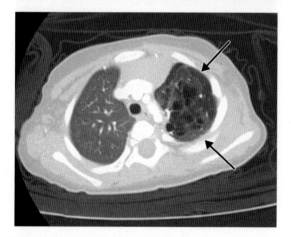

Fig. C2.3 Axial contrast-enhanced CT of the same patient shows multicystic mass in the left chest consistent with a congenital pulmonary airway malformation.

Congenital lobar emphysema is characterized by over-inflation of the alveoli thought to result from a ball-valve type of anomaly in the bronchus that causes progressive air trapping. The most common lobe affected is the left upper lobe, followed by the middle lobe, right upper, and both lower lobes.

Chest radiographs and CT classically demonstrate a hyperinflation of the lobe involved. If seen in the immediate postneonatal period, however, it may mimic a solid masslike lobar lesion as it is completely filled with fluid. Gradually, it gets aerated with progressive although slow clearance of fluid, appearing partially cystic and partially solid; before it appears completely hyperinflated with air.

REFERENCES AND SUGGESTED READING

1. Donnelly LF, Frush DP. Localized radiolucent chest lesions in neonates: causes and differentiation. *AJR.* 1999;172(6): 1651-1658.

2. Daltro P, Werner H, Gasparetto TD, et al. Congenital chest malformations: a multimodality approach with emphasis on fetal MR imaging. *RadioGraphics.* 2010;30:385-395.

3. Chavhan G, Babyn PS, Cohen RA, et al. Multimodality imaging of the pediatric diaphragm: anatomy and pathologic conditions. *RadioGraphics.* 2010;30:1797-1817.

4. Donnelly L. *Pediatric Imaging: The Fundamentals.* 1st ed. Philadelphia, PA: Saunders; 2009.

CASE 3: PNEUMONIA

PATIENT PRESENTATION

A 5-year-old male presents with 3 days of fever and cough.

CLINICAL SUSPICION

Pneumonia

IMAGING MODALITY OF CHOICE

Frontal and lateral chest radiographs should be obtained in children with suspected pneumonia.

FINDINGS

Evaluation of suspected community-acquired pneumonia is one of the most common indications for imaging in children. On chest radiograph, focal air space consolidation with air bronchograms in a lobar or segmental distribution or patchy areas of multifocal consolidation is seen (Fig. C3.1).

In younger children, bacterial pneumonia frequently has a very round, well-defined appearance on chest radiography, simulating a mass (Fig. C3.2). This is referred to as round pneumonia and is most common in children younger than 8 years of age. Round pneumonia is more common in the lower lobes and is most often caused by *Streptococcus pneumoniae* infection. The reason for this appearance in children is thought to be due to underdevelopment of collateral pathways of air circulation. In the appropriate clinical setting in a child with cough and fever, a lung mass seen on chest radiograph should be considered to be round pneumonia, and additional imaging with

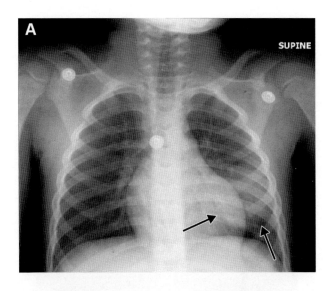

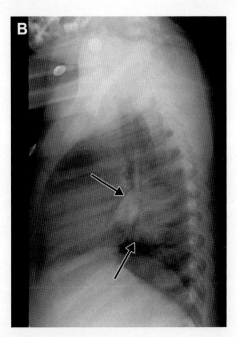

Fig. C3.2 Frontal (A) and lateral (B) radiographs of the chest demonstrates a rounded, masslike opacity in the left lower lobe representing round pneumonia (arrows).

CT is not indicated. Follow-up radiographs should be obtained several weeks after appropriate antibiotic therapy to ensure resolution. After 8 years of age, however, if a round mass is seen on chest radiograph, other pathology should be considered.

Radiographs are frequently requested in pediatric patients with suspected pneumonia to help differentiate between bacterial and viral pneumonia. The cause of viral pneumonia in children varies depending on the child's age, but viral infections are much more common than bacterial infections in all age groups. Viral infections cause

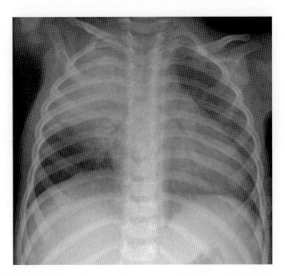

Fig. C3.1 Frontal radiograph shows consolidation of the right upper lobe consistent with lobar pneumonia.

inflammation of the small airways, which results in peribronchial edema and increased peribronchial markings on chest radiographs. These are seen as symmetric, ropelike linear markings radiating from the hila of the lungs. On the lateral view, the hila may appear prominent and the lungs will be hyperinflated (Fig. C3.3).

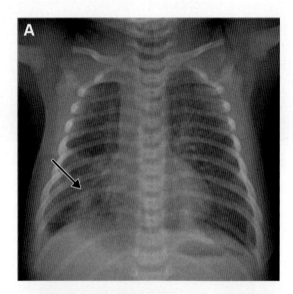

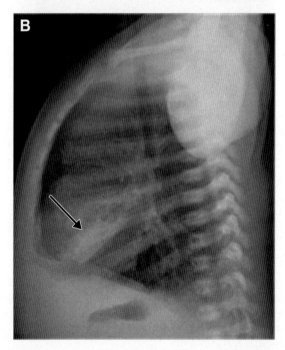

Fig. C3.3 Frontal (A) and lateral (B) radiographs of the chest show typical findings of viral pneumonia with hyperinflated lungs and increased perihilar markings. Note subsegmental atelectasis in the right middle lobe (arrow).

Common complications of pneumonia in children include parapneumonic effusion, empyema, cavitary necrosis, or lung abscess. Chest radiograph is the primary imaging modality for evaluation of these complications, though ultrasound or contrast-enhanced CT may be helpful in further evaluation if chest radiographs do not demonstrate any abnormalities.

DIFFERENTIAL DIAGNOSIS
Clinical Differential

Children with pneumonia most commonly present with cough, fever, and malaise, but may also present with abdominal pain. In the clinical evaluation of a child with cough and fever, differentiation between viral and bacterial infection is important in regard to treatment decisions. Also, consideration of other respiratory tract diseases such as croup, bronchiolitis, and bronchitis should be made.

Imaging Differential

There are several diagnoses that may appear similar to round pneumonia on chest radiograph. A bronchogenic cyst may appear as a round, well-defined soft tissue mass on a chest radiograph and can demonstrate a very similar appearance to round pneumonia (Figs. C3.4 and C3.5).

If the round pneumonia is posterior, it may simulate a posterior mediastinal mass such as neuroblastoma. But round pneumonia will have acute borders rather than obtuse borders with the mediastinum and neuroblastoma may demonstrate rib erosion or destruction. Other differential considerations include congenital pulmonary airway malformations or pulmonary sequestration.

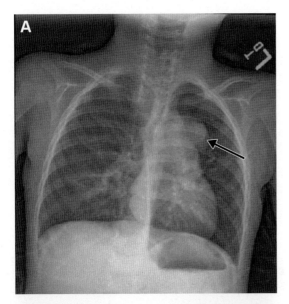

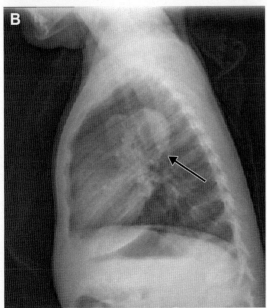

Fig. C3.4 Frontal (A) and lateral (B) views of the chest show a round mass in the left middle mediastinum, mimicking the appearance of a round pneumonia.

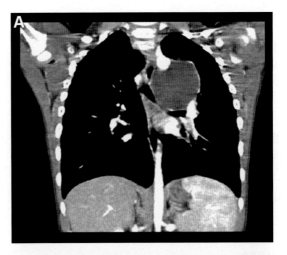

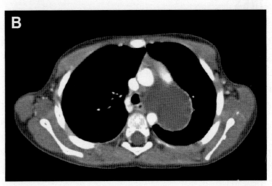

Fig. C3.5 Axial (A) and coronal (B) contrast-enhanced CT images of the chest of the same patient demonstrate a large low-attenuation mass in the middle mediastinum that causes mass effect along the trachea and left main bronchus, consistent with a bronchogenic cyst.

REFERENCES AND SUGGESTED READING

1. Donnelly L. *Pediatric Imaging: The Fundamentals*. 1st ed. Philadelphia, PA: Saunders; 2009.

2. Virkki R, Juven T, Rikalainen H, et al. Differentiation of bacterial and viral pneumonia in children. *Thorax*. 2002;57(5): 438-441.

CASE 4: EPIGLOTTITIS

PATIENT PRESENTATION

A 3-year-old male presents with respiratory distress and drooling. Patient is sitting in a sniffing position and leaning forward with his head and nose tilted upward.

CLINICAL SUSPICION

Epiglottitis

IMAGING MODALITY OF CHOICE

Lateral soft tissue neck radiograph

FINDINGS

Epiglottitis is an acute life-threatening disease that is secondary to infectious inflammation of the epiglottis and surrounding soft tissues. This may result in airway obstruction and may potentially require emergent intubation. *Haemophilus influenzae* is the most common cause of epiglottitis, and since the vaccine for *H influenzae* has become available, the incidence of epiglottitis has significantly decreased. Children with epiglottitis usually develop sudden onset of symptoms and are toxic appearing with high fever, difficulty swallowing, drooling, and shallow breathing with the head held forward.

If the diagnosis is not made on physical examination, a single, lateral, upright view of the neck in extension is frequently diagnostic. Since there may be rapid progression of the condition leading to acute complete obstruction of the upper airway, radiographs should be obtained with minimal manipulation of the neck and with the patient in a comfortable position. Placing the patient supine to obtain a lateral neck radiograph may lead to acute airway obstruction and should be avoided. If the examination cannot be performed with portable equipment, a patient with suspected epiglottitis should be accompanied by someone with equipment readily available to intubate the child and secure the airway in the radiology department.

On lateral plain radiographs of the neck, the normal epiglottis is a thin, curved flap of soft-tissue opacity that is separated from the base of the tongue by air in the vallecula (Fig. C4.1). In epiglottitis, the epiglottis appears swollen and enlarged, with the so-called thumbprint sign, secondary to its appearance similar to a thumb (Fig. C4.2). Additional associated findings may include thickening of the aryepiglottic folds, prevertebral soft tissue swelling, and expansion of the hypopharynx.

The omega epiglottis is an epiglottis with prominent lateral folds and is a normal variant that should not be confused with a truly enlarged and swollen epiglottis. Also, if the epiglottis is imaged obliquely, it can appear falsely wide

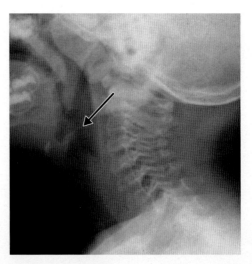

Fig. C4.1 Lateral radiograph of the neck demonstrates normal appearance of the epiglottis (arrow).

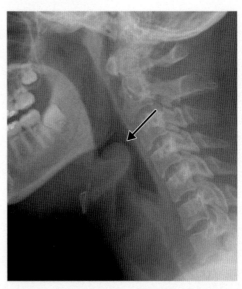

Fig. C4.2 Lateral radiograph of the neck shows diffuse swelling of the epiglottis (arrow), representing the thumb sign in a patient with epiglottitis.

and thickened and may mimic findings of epiglottitis. In these cases, evaluation of the aryepiglottic folds, which remain thin and normal in appearance, may be helpful in making the distinction.

DIFFERENTIAL DIAGNOSIS

Clinical Differential

The most common clinical differential includes croup, bacterial tracheitis, and retropharyngeal abscess.

To help differentiate epiglottitis from croup, consider the age of the patient, prodrome, type of cough, and degree of toxicity. In general, croup occurs in younger children and has a viral prodrome. Children with croup also have a barking cough and rarely appear toxic, as in epiglottitis.

Bacterial tracheitis is characterized by infection of the trachea with exudative membranes on the tracheal wall. Affected children are ill and while uncommon, it is potentially life threatening if a membrane occludes the airway.

Retropharyngeal abscess generally occurs subsequent to upper respiratory tract infection or pharyngitis due to spread to the retropharyngeal lymph nodes.

Imaging Differential

As discussed earlier, it is important to differentiate between true epiglottitis and the omega variant or an epiglottis that is imaged obliquely and appears artifactually thickened.

Findings of epiglottitis on a frontal radiograph may appear similar to the characteristic findings of croup. Croup causes symmetric subglottic narrowing, termed the steeple sign (Fig. C4.3).

Bacterial tracheitis demonstrates intraluminal tracheal membranes or tracheal irregularity on the lateral view of the neck.

Lateral radiograph showing thickening of the retropharyngeal soft tissues may represent retropharyngeal cellulitis or abscess. Visualization of gas on the lateral radiograph may confirm abscess formation, but it may be absent. CT evaluation of abscess demonstrates a rim-enhancing hypoattenuating area within the retropharyngeal soft tissues.

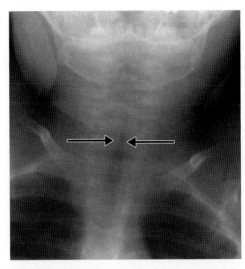

Fig. C4.3 Frontal radiograph of the neck shows a steeple appearance of the trachea (arrows) secondary to symmetric subglottic tracheal narrowing in croup.

REFERENCES AND SUGGESTED READING

1. John SD, Swischuk LE. Stridor and upper airway obstruction in infants and children. *RadioGraphics.* 1992;12:625-643.

2. Donnelly L. *Pediatric Imaging: The Fundamentals.* 1st ed. Philadelphia, PA: Saunders; 2009.

3. Glynn F, Fenton JE. Diagnosis and management of supraglottitis (epiglottitis). *Curr Infect Dis Rep.* 2008;10(3):200-204.

CASE 5: NECROTIZING ENTEROCOLITIS

PATIENT PRESENTATION

Premature infant born after 26 weeks of gestation develops abdominal distention, feeding intolerance, and blood in the stool 2 weeks after birth.

CLINICAL SUSPICION

Necrotizing enterocolitis

IMAGING MODALITY OF CHOICE

Abdominal radiograph

FINDINGS

Necrotizing enterocolitis (NEC) is an idiopathic entity that is predominantly a disease of premature infants and most often occurs in those with extremely low birth weight of less than 1000 g. It generally manifests in the first 3 weeks of life and is likely the result of a combination of infection and ischemia. NEC may occur anywhere throughout the colon, although it most commonly involves the distal ileum and right colon. Symptoms include feeding intolerance, abdominal distention, sepsis, and bloody stool.

Early abdominal radiographic findings of necrotizing enterocolitis range from normal in appearance to findings of bowel distention, paucity of bowel gas in the right lower quadrant, or focal dilatation of bowel that does not change in appearance over time. As the disease process progresses, the presence of pneumatosis intestinalis, or gas within the bowel wall, is a definitive diagnostic finding. This is seen as bubblelike lucencies within the bowel wall mucosa (Fig. C5.1). Also diagnostic is the radiographic

finding of portal venous air, which appears as branching linear lucencies overlying the liver.

Free intraperitoneal air may be seen on abdominal radiographs when bowel perforation has occurred (Figs. C5.2 and C5.3) and is considered an absolute indication for surgical intervention. Multiple radiographic signs of free intraperitoneal air may be seen (refer to Table C5.1). In the absence of free air, treatment of NEC includes bowel rest, nasogastric

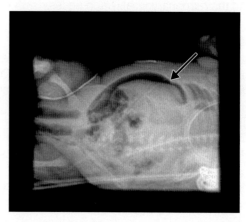

Fig. C5.2 Left lateral decubitus view of the abdomen of a different patient shows a moderate amount of free intraperitoneal air (arrow) tracking down into the inguinal canals due to bowel perforation. There is portal venous gas and pneumatosis intestinalis involving multiple loops of bowel.

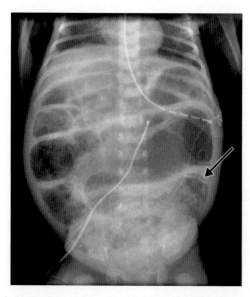

Fig. C5.1 Abdominal radiograph shows dilated bowel loops throughout the abdomen with bubbly lucencies within the bowel wall mucosa (arrow) consistent with pneumatosis intestinalis.

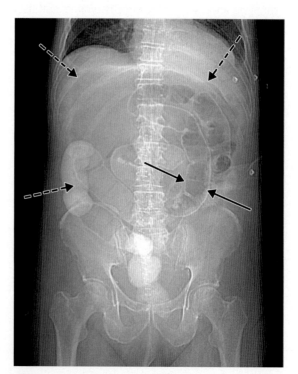

Fig. C5.3 Scout radiograph of the abdomen demonstrates the football sign with increased lucency outlining the entire abdominal cavity (black dotted arrows) and Rigler's sign with visualization of both sides of the bowel wall (black arrows).

Table C5.1 Signs of Free Intraperitoneal Air

1. An overall increased lucency of the abdomen on supine radiographs.
2. Visualization of both sides of the bowel wall, termed Rigler's sign (Fig. C5.3).
3. Visualization of the outline of the intraperitoneal structures such as the falciform ligament, ligamentum teres, umbilical ligaments.
4. Large pneumoperitoneum outlining the entire abdominal cavity, termed the football sign (Fig. C5.3).
5. Pockets of anterior abdominal lucency on cross-table lateral radiographs.

decompression, and antibiotic therapy. The most common complication of NEC is bowel stricture.

In cases of NEC in which the abdomen is distended and gasless, ultrasound may be beneficial. Gray-scale ultrasound may demonstrate thickened or dilated bowel loops and abdominal ascites. The bowel may have increased vascularity due to inflammation or decreased vascularity as a result of ischemia.

DIFFERENTIAL DIAGNOSIS
Clinical Differential

In premature infants demonstrating signs of abdominal distention and diarrhea, etiologies such as systemic and intestinal infections, congenital intestinal obstruction (eg, volvulus, pyloric stenosis, ileal atresia, Hirschsprung's disease), and spontaneous bowel perforation should be considered.

Imaging Differential

The radiographic findings of necrotizing enterocolitis can range from normal to diagnostic. The differential diagnosis can include bowel obstruction or bowel perforation.

Bowel obstruction shows dilated loops of bowel that may include small bowel or large bowel loops depending on the site of obstruction. Air-fluid levels will be seen in the dilated bowel loops on upright abdominal radiographs.

In patients with bowel perforation, most commonly idiopathic, one or more of the previously discussed signs of free intraperitoneal air may be identified.

Other consideration includes nonspecific gaseous distention secondary to bag ventilation or intubation in appropriate clinical settings.

REFERENCES AND SUGGESTED READING

1. Donnelly L. *Pediatric Imaging: The Fundamentals*. 1st ed. Philadelphia, PA: Saunders; 2009.
2. Epelman M, Daneman A, Navarro OM, et al. Necrotizing enterocolitis: review of state-of-the-art imaging findings with pathologic correlation. *RadioGraphics*. 2007;27(2):285-305.

CASE 6: DUODENAL ATRESIA

PATIENT PRESENTATION

Newborn male infant develops bilious emesis on the first day of life. No significant abdominal distention is present on physical examination.

CLINICAL SUSPICION

The differential considerations for bilious emesis include multiple entities such as malrotation with midgut volvulus, duodenal atresia or other anomalies associated with intrinsic or extrinsic duodenum obstruction, and meconium ileus.

IMAGING MODALITY OF CHOICE

Abdominal radiograph is the initial imaging modality of choice. Duodenal obstruction may present as complete or partial obstruction depending on the etiology, but neonates showing evidence of complete duodenal obstruction at abdominal radiography rarely require further radiologic evaluation.

FINDINGS

Duodenal atresia is caused by the failure of recanalization of the duodenal lumen during fetal development resulting in a blind ending duodenum and complete intrinsic obstruction. The duodenum is the most common site of intestinal atresia. Many conditions are associated with duodenal atresia including Down syndrome (approximately 30%), other intestinal atresias, congenital heart disease, imperforate anus, annular pancreas, and renal anomalies.

Infants with duodenal atresia most commonly present with vomiting within hours of birth. The majority of patients have bilious vomiting as the obstruction is mostly distal to the ampulla of Vater. Patients have feeding intolerance and there is usually little or no abdominal distention secondary to the proximal level of obstruction.

Abdominal radiographs in patients with duodenal atresia routinely demonstrate classic findings of a dilated stomach and a dilated proximal duodenum with no gas present distal to the proximal duodenum (Fig. C6.1). This is referred to as the "double-bubble" sign and is diagnostic of duodenal atresia given the appropriate clinical history. With these findings, further imaging with an upper GI series is not indicated, and there is potential hazard of vomiting with barium aspiration if an upper GI examination is performed.

Radiographic findings in patients with partial duodenal obstruction show gaseous distention of the stomach and duodenum with gas in the small bowel. Partial duodenal obstruction may be caused by duodenal stenosis, duodenal web, Ladd bands, malrotation with midgut volvulus, or annular pancreas. If distal bowel gas is present on abdominal radiographs, an upper GI series is indicated to evaluate

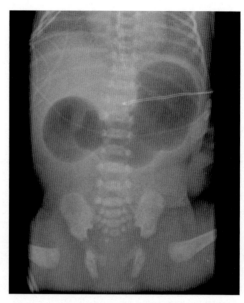

Fig. C6.1 A gas-filled dilated stomach and proximal duodenum are seen with no distal intestinal gas, consistent with duodenal atresia.

and differentiate between the potential causes. In some cases, when there is a very small degree of obstruction, patients may remain asymptomatic or may be incidentally diagnosed during examination for another condition.

Duodenal stenosis and duodenal web are the result of partial canalization of the duodenal lumen during fetal development. A web is usually an obstructing membrane with a pinhole central lumen that is typically at or near the ampulla of Vater. On upper GI exam, duodenal web classically shows a windsock appearance within the duodenal lumen due to ballooning and stretching of the redundant membrane (Fig. C6.2).

Annular pancreas is an anomalous band of pancreatic tissue that encircles the second portion of the duodenum. Annular pancreas cannot be diagnosed at the time of an

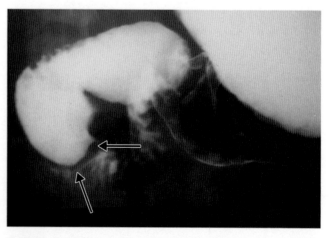

Fig. C6.2 Frontal upper GI spot image shows the classic windsock appearance of a duodenal web.

upper GI exam and may be diagnosed on CT or MRI, which demonstrate pancreatic tissue and an annular duct encircling the duodenum.

Intestinal malrotation is a congenital abnormal position of the bowel within the peritoneal cavity and applies to a wide range of intestinal anomalies. In patients with malrotation, there is abnormal fixation of the small bowel mesentery that results in a short mesenteric base that is prone to twisting. Malrotation of the bowel is associated with a number of syndromes and other anomalies, often occurring in association with other gastrointestinal abnormalities and heterotaxy syndromes. Volvulus due to malrotation occurs when there is twisting of small bowel around the superior mesenteric artery and vein that can result in bowel obstruction and bowel ischemia or necrosis.

Findings of malrotation and midgut volvulus on abdominal radiograph may be normal or may show distention of the stomach and proximal duodenum. A markedly dilated duodenal bulb may be seen in long-standing obstruction from midgut volvulus and may mimic the appearance of duodenal atresia, but will not be seen with acute volvulus. Radiographs may also demonstrate diffuse bowel distention, pneumatosis, portal venous gas, or free peritoneal air from bowel ischemia, necrosis, or perforation.

The upper GI series is the imaging modality of choice for the diagnosis of malrotation with or without volvulus. The diagnosis of malrotation is made by evaluation of the position of the duodenojejunal junction. The normal position of the duodenojejunal junction is to the left of the spine and at the same level as the duodenal bulb on frontal views and posterior, or retroperitoneal, on lateral views.

Patients with bowel malrotation have an abnormal position of the duodenojejunal junction on the upper GI series, and when midgut volvulus is present, the duodenum and proximal jejunum can be seen as Z shaped or corkscrew shaped (Fig. C6.3). CT and ultrasound in malrotation show similar findings with the superior mesenteric vein to the left of the superior mesenteric artery and volvulus indicated by a "swirl" or "whirlpool" sign of twisted mesenteric vessels and bowel (Figs. C6.4 and C6.5). On ultrasound, this is best visualized on color Doppler.

DIFFERENTIAL DIAGNOSIS
Clinical Differential

Differentiation among the causes of bilious emesis in newborns often cannot be made based on clinical history and physical examination. Radiologic evaluation beginning with abdominal radiograph is important in the workup and may help to provide pertinent information that can lead to the correct diagnosis.

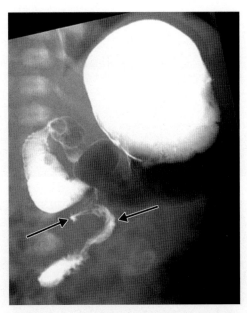

Fig. C6.3 Upper GI series shows malrotation and volvulus. There is abnormal position of the duodenojejunal junction, which terminates below the level of the duodenal bulb and corkscrew appearance of the proximal jejunum (arrows) consistent with volvulus.

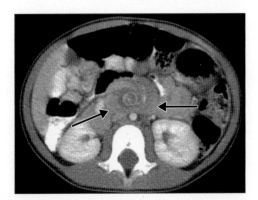

Fig. C6.4 Axial contrast-enhanced CT image shows the swirling or whirlpool appearance of the bowel and mesenteric vessels (arrows) in a case of midgut volvulus.

Imaging Differential

The double bubble sign is the classic radiographic finding of duodenal atresia, but if gas is seen within the distal small bowel, other diagnoses as described earlier should be considered and an upper GI series should be performed to exclude malrotation with midgut volvulus, which is a potentially life-threatening complication.

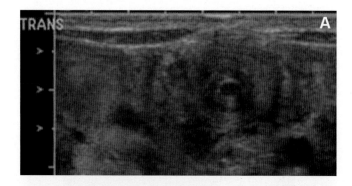

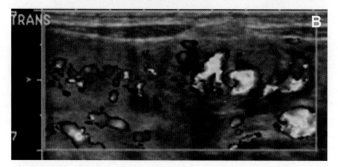

Fig. C6.5 Similar findings of volvulus are seen on gray scale (A) and color (B) Doppler ultrasound images, with a swirling appearance of the bowel and mesenteric vessels.

REFERENCES AND SUGGESTED READING

1. Beroccal T, Torres I, Gutiérrez J, et al. Congenital anomalies of the upper gastrointestinal tract. *RadioGraphics*. 1999;19: 855-872.

2. Mortele K, et al. Multimodality imaging of pancreatic and biliary congenital anomalies. *RadioGraphics*. 2006;2:715-731.

3. Applegate K, et al. Intestinal malrotation in children: a problem-solving approach to the upper gastrointestinal series. *RadioGraphics*. 2006;26:1485-1500.

4. Gilbertson-Dahdal DL, et al. Neonatal malrotation with midgut volvulus mimicking duodenal atresia. *AJR*. 2009;192(5): 1269-1271.

5. Kyung Lee N, et al. Complications of congenital and developmental abnormalities of the gastrointestinal tract in adolescents and adults: evaluation with multimodality imaging. *RadioGraphics*. 2010;30:1489-1507.

CASE 7: HIRSCHSPRUNG'S DISEASE

PATIENT PRESENTATION

Term male infant fails to pass meconium within the first 48 hours of life and has developed abdominal distention.

CLINICAL SUSPICION

Hirschsprung's disease

IMAGING MODALITY OF CHOICE

Abdominal radiograph is the initial imaging modality of choice. If findings on the initial radiographs are abnormal and suggestive of distal bowel obstruction, water-soluble contrast enema is the next step in the evaluation of the colon.

FINDINGS

Hirschsprung's disease is caused by an absence of ganglion cells within the colon that results in a functional obstruction secondary to spasm in the denervated colon. This condition accounts for approximately 15% to 20% of cases of neonatal bowel obstruction. The majority of patients with Hirschsprung's disease present in the neonatal period with failure to pass meconium, but later presentation in childhood or later in life may occur with history of constipation and abdominal distention. Over 90% of cases present within the first 5 years of life, and a very small number may present as adults. Hirschsprung's disease is more common in boys than girls (4:1), and an increased incidence is seen in patients with Down syndrome.

The disease can be classified based on the length of the aganglionic segment, always extending proximally from the anal canal. Short segment disease is most common and involves the rectum and distal sigmoid colon only.

Abdominal radiographs demonstrate findings of distal bowel obstruction including variable gaseous distention of the colon and small bowel, often with air-fluid levels. Performing a water-soluble/barium contrast enema may provide a definitive diagnosis and demonstration of a transition zone between the narrow and dilated portions of the colon.

The rectosigmoid ratio may be helpful in evaluation. In normal newborns, the rectum has a larger diameter than the sigmoid colon, giving a rectosigmoid ratio greater than 1. In Hirschsprung patients, however, the maximal diameter of the rectum is smaller than the maximal diameter of the sigmoid colon, giving a rectosigmoid ratio less than 1. Another finding that may be seen on enema examination is a saw-toothed irregularity of the aganglionic portion of the colon secondary to abnormal peristaltic activity (Fig. C7.1).

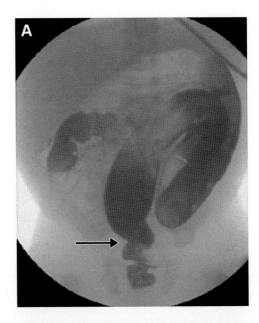

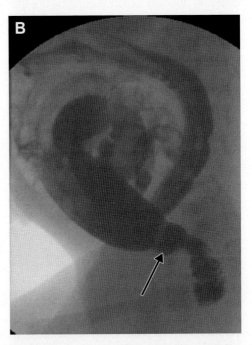

Fig. C7.1 Frontal (A) and lateral (B) images from a barium enema study show poor distention of the rectum with a sawtooth irregularity of the mucosa of the rectum. There is a transition to dilated colon at the rectosigmoid junction (arrow) consistent with Hirschsprung's disease.

DIFFERENTIAL DIAGNOSIS

Clinical Differential

Clinical signs of intestinal obstruction in neonates include failure to pass meconium, progressive abdominal distention, refusal to feed, and vomiting. An extensive differential diagnosis exists in cases of suspected neonatal intestinal obstruction and the combination of the clinical history, physical examination, and radiologic evaluation is required for eventual diagnosis.

Imaging Differential

Differential considerations of low intestinal obstruction include meconium plug syndrome, colonic atresia, meconium ileus, or anorectal malformations such as imperforate anus.

Meconium plug syndrome, also termed small left colon syndrome, is a common cause of distal neonatal bowel obstruction and thought to be related to functional immaturity of the ganglion cells. Findings on contrast enema include small caliber of the left colon extending to the splenic flexure with abrupt transition to dilated proximal colon (Fig. C7.2). Multiple filling defects representing meconium plugs may fill the left colon and may pass during the exam. Unlike Hirschsprung's disease, the rectosigmoid ratio is usually greater than 1.

Meconium ileus occurs in patients with cystic fibrosis with thick meconium that obstructs the distal ileum. Water-soluble enema demonstrates microcolon and filling defects in the terminal ileum representing meconium plugs.

Ileal atresia results from congenital absence or complete occlusion of the ileal lumen thought to be the result of in utero vascular accident. Enema shows a microcolon and contrast may reflux into a normal terminal ileum with obstruction at the site of atresia.

REFERENCES AND SUGGESTED READING

1. Devos AS, Blickman JG, Blickman JG. *Radiological Imaging of the Digestive Tract in Infants and Children.* Berlin: Springer Verlag; 2007.

2. Swenson O. Hirschsprung's disease: a review. *Pediatrics.* 2002;109(5):914-918.

3. Berrocal T, Torres I, Gutiérrez J, et al. Congenital anomalies of the small intestine, colon, and rectum. *RadioGraphics.* 1999;19:1219-1236.

4. Donnelly L. *Pediatric Imaging: The Fundamentals.* 1st ed. Philadelphia, PA: Saunders; 2009.

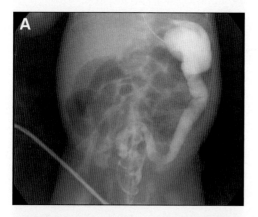

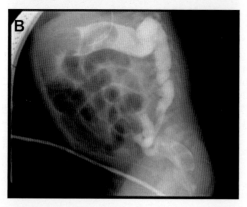

Fig. C7.2 Frontal (A) and lateral (B) contrast enema demonstrates small left colon with a transition to dilated colon at the splenic flexure. Meconium plug is seen in the left colon.

CASE 8: HYPERTROPHIC PYLORIC STENOSIS

PATIENT PRESENTATION

A 1-month-old male newborn presents with nonbilious projectile vomiting. Physical exam demonstrates an olive-shaped mass in the right upper quadrant.

CLINICAL SUSPICION

Hypertrophic pyloric stenosis

IMAGING MODALITY OF CHOICE

Abdominal ultrasound and upper GI series may both be used to diagnose hypertrophic pyloric stenosis, though ultrasound is the examination of choice when hypertrophic pyloric stenosis is suspected. The benefit of ultrasound is that it may provide a rapid diagnosis without radiation exposure. Ultrasound examination also provides direct information on the anatomy of the pyloric canal, and unlike an upper GI series, there is no need for the patient to drink additional contrast material or to await gastric emptying.

FINDINGS

Hypertrophic pyloric stenosis is a condition in which the antropyloric portion of the stomach becomes abnormally thickened and causes gastric outlet obstruction. The clinical presentation varies with the length of symptoms, but infants typically present with nonbilious projectile vomiting in the first 2 to 12 weeks of life secondary to functional obstruction. The vomiting may initially be intermittent, though the frequency will usually increase to follow all feedings and infants may develop weight loss and dehydration.

Ultrasound demonstrates variable distention of the stomach and decreased gastric emptying. On gray-scale ultrasound, the hypertrophied muscle is hypoechoic and there may be hypertrophy of the hyperechoic mucosa. Measurement criteria for the diagnosis of pyloric stenosis include muscle thickness greater than 3 mm and pyloric channel length greater than 15 mm (Figs. C8.1 and C8.2). During dynamic examination, the pylorus does not open and gastric hyperperistalsis without gastric emptying is identified.

On upper GI examination, there is failure of relaxation of the prepyloric antrum, which is typically described as elongated pyloric canal. It may be seen as a string of contrast material through the antropyloric region, termed the string sign. Several linear tracts of contrast material within the canal separated by the intervening mucosa, named the tram track sign, may also be identified.

Other fluoroscopic observations include exaggerated gastric motility resembling a caterpillar, and another sign called the shoulder sign, where the hypertrophied pyloric

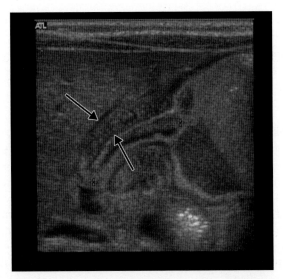

Fig. C8.1 Gray-scale ultrasound images demonstrate typical sonographic findings of hypertrophic pyloric stenosis. There is thickening of the hypoechoic pyloric muscle (arrows), and elongation of the pyloric channel, measuring 18 mm in length.

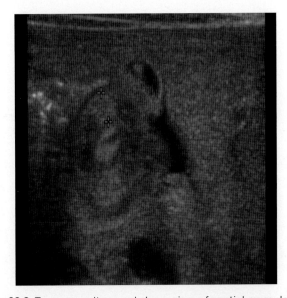

Fig. C8.2 Transverse ultrasound shows circumferential muscular thickening surrounding the central channel filled with echogenic mucosa.

muscle creates an extrinsic impression on the distal antrum. After the examination is performed and a diagnosis is made, excess barium should be removed from the stomach by nasogastric tube to prevent the risk of aspiration.

DIFFERENTIAL DIAGNOSIS

Clinical Differential

The two most common causes of infants presenting with nonbilious vomiting are hypertrophic pyloric stenosis and gastroesophageal reflux. Infants with gastroesophageal reflux may present with irritability, failure to thrive, and nonbilious vomiting.

Other conditions to consider include pylorospasm, hiatal hernia, gastroenteritis, or other causes of gastric outlet obstruction, including preampullary duodenal stenosis.

Imaging Differential

Hypertrophic pyloric stenosis can be diagnosed or excluded by using sonography. Pylorospasm, or failure of relaxation of the antropyloric canal, may be difficult to differentiate from hypertrophic pyloric stenosis. It is more easily evaluated with ultrasound due to the ability to evaluate and measure the pyloric muscle thickness and dynamic evaluation. If the ultrasound demonstrates a normal pylorus, then a search for other causes with an upper GI examination may be warranted.

REFERENCES AND SUGGESTED READING

1. Hernanz-Schulman M. Infantile hypertrophic pyloric stenosis. *Radiology*. 2003;227:319-331.

2. Hernanz-Schulman M, Sells LL, Ambrosino MM, et al. Hypertrophic pyloric stenosis in the infant without a palpable olive: accuracy of sonographic diagnosis. *Radiology*. 1994;193(3):771-776.

3. Cohen HL, Babcock DS, Kushner DC, et al. Vomiting in infants up to 3 months of age. American College of Radiology. ACR Appropriateness Criteria. *Radiology*. 2000;215(suppl):779-786.

CASE 9: MECKEL DIVERTICULUM

PATIENT PRESENTATION

A 14-month-old male child presents with intermittent abdominal pain and currant jelly stool.

CLINICAL SUSPICION

Bleeding Meckel diverticulum

IMAGING MODALITY OF CHOICE

Nuclear scintigraphy with Tc-99m pertechnetate

FINDINGS

Meckel's diverticulum is the result of incomplete obliteration of the omphalomesenteric duct, which is a fetal structure that connects the yolk sac to the portion of the gut that becomes the ileum. Depending on the location, persistence of a portion of this structure may result in cyst, sinus, or fistula formation from the umbilicus to the ileum. The most common malformation, however, is the Meckel's diverticulum.

Meckel's diverticulum most often becomes symptomatic before 2 years of age and may cause symptoms secondary to bleeding, focal inflammation, perforation, intestinal obstruction, or intussusception. The most common presenting symptom is painless rectal bleeding, which may occur as a result of ectopic gastric mucosa. Meckel's diverticulum is usually within 2 ft of the ileocecal valve and may be 5 to 6 cm in length. You may remember the Rule of 2s for Meckel's diverticulum: 2 ft from the ileocecal valve, 2 in long, 2% of the population is affected, 2 types of common ectopic tissue (gastric and pancreatic), 2 years is the most common age for clinical presentation, and boys are 2 times more affected than girls.

In general, findings on abdominal radiographs, ultrasound, CT scan, and barium studies are nonspecific. Abdominal radiographs may be completely normal or may show a right lower quadrant mass, displacement of bowel loops, or bowel obstruction. Ultrasound may be used for evaluation and can demonstrate a fluid-filled structure in the right lower quadrant with the appearance of a blind-ending, thick-walled loop of small bowel. On CT, Meckel diverticulum can be seen as a blind-ending fluid or air-filled structure that communicates with the small bowel (Fig. C9.1).

The imaging modality of choice to detect bleeding Meckel diverticula is a technetium-99m pertechnetate scan, which detects the gastric mucosa within the diverticula. This study will demonstrate focal tracer uptake within the right lower quadrant of the abdomen, with increasing uptake over time (Fig. C9.2). This finding generally appears in the first

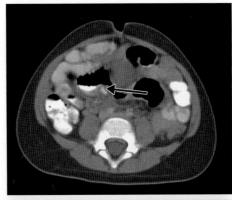
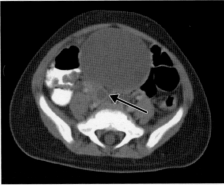

Fig. C9.1 Axial CT images of the abdomen show a dilated, tubular structure (arrow) arising from the terminal ileum with minimal stranding in the adjacent mesenteric fat consistent with Meckel's diverticulum.

30 minutes of the study but may take up to 1 hour to appear. This scan is the preferred method of diagnosis because it is noninvasive, it involves less radiation exposure, and its accuracy is approximately 90%.

Complications of Meckel's diverticulum include inflammation, hemorrhage, intussusception, small bowel obstruction, stone formation, and neoplasm.

DIFFERENTIAL DIAGNOSIS

Clinical Differential

Etiologies that cause symptoms similar to that of Meckel's diverticula include inflammatory bowel disease, intussusception, intestinal duplication containing gastric mucosa, hemangioma, or ovarian pathology.

Imaging Differential

Distinguishing between the above-mentioned pathologies that are in the clinical differential for Meckel diverticulum may be difficult secondary to false positive or false negative results on the Meckel's scan.

False positive results may occur secondary to intussusception, urinary tract activity, various small bowel lesions,

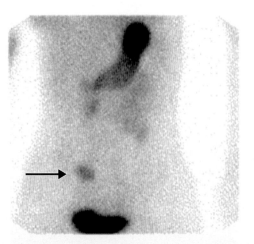

Fig. C9.2 Technetium 99-m pertechnetate image demonstrates abnormal increased activity within the anterior right lower quadrant (arrow).

inflammatory bowel disease, vascular lesions, and infrequently, intestinal duplication cysts containing gastric mucosa.

False negative results have been seen in patients with absent or small amounts of ectopic gastric tissue, malrotation of the ileum, and localized bowel irritability, which increases clearance of the pertechnetate from the area.

REFERENCES AND SUGGESTED READING

1. Levy AD, Hobbs CM. From the archives of the AFIP. Meckel diverticulum: radiologic features with pathologic correlation. *RadioGraphics*. 2004;24(2):565-587.

2. Elsayes KM, Menias CO, Harvin HJ, et al. Imaging manifestations of Meckel's diverticulum. *AJR*. 2007;189,81-88.

3. Guiberteau M, Mettler F. *Essentials of Nuclear Medicine Imaging*. Philadelphia: Saunders; 2006.

CASE 10: BILIARY ATRESIA

PATIENT PRESENTATION

A 3-week-old female infant presents with jaundice, and the laboratory workup shows conjugated hyperbilirubinemia.

CLINICAL SUSPICION

Biliary atresia

IMAGING MODALITY OF CHOICE

Ultrasound is the initial imaging procedure in neonates with jaundice. It can evaluate the hepatic parenchyma, the intrahepatic and extrahepatic biliary ducts, as well as the gallbladder. In the evaluation of biliary atresia, hepatobiliary scintigraphy with 99-m technetium-IDA is also indicated to help differentiate from other liver disease, such as neonatal hepatitis, which is the other most common cause of neonatal jaundice.

FINDINGS

Biliary atresia is secondary to congenital blockage or absence of the extrahepatic bile ducts, which results in neonatal jaundice and progressive conjugated hyperbilirubinemia. Infants with biliary atresia may appear normal and healthy at birth. Symptoms most commonly develop between 2 weeks and 2 months of life and may include jaundice, dark yellow or brown urine, hepatomegaly, and pale or clay-colored stools.

On ultrasound examination in children with biliary atresia, the liver parenchyma is typically normal in echotexture and biliary dilatation is absent. An echogenic triangular structure identified adjacent to the main portal vein is referred to as the triangular cord sign, which represents the fibrotic remnant of the common bile duct. Also, the gallbladder is usually small or absent.

While ultrasound evaluation may help detect other causes of biliary obstruction, distinguishing between biliary atresia and neonatal hepatitis is frequently not possible on ultrasound examination. Imaging with nuclear medicine 99-m technetium-IDA may provide the only clue to diagnosis.

Cholescintigraphy in neonates with biliary atresia without cirrhosis demonstrates uptake within the liver without evidence of biliary or bowel activity in 24 hours (Fig. C10.1). Prior to examination, the patient is given 5 to 7 days of phenobarbital therapy to prime the liver and stimulate better hepatic excretion of the radiotracer and earlier identification of a patent biliary tree.

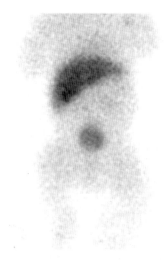

Fig. C10.1 Anterior hepatobiliary scintigraphy at 24 hours shows persistent hepatic activity and bladder visualization without bowel activity, typical of biliary atresia.

DIFFERENTIAL DIAGNOSIS

Clinical Differential

Neonatal jaundice may be the result of "physiologic jaundice," which is secondary to physiologic destruction of red blood cells in the newborn. Prolonged neonatal jaundice that does not clear up with phototherapy should be further evaluated for other causes such as neonatal hepatitis, Dubin-Johnson syndrome, or Alagille syndrome, which is characterized by a paucity of interlobular bile ducts.

Imaging Differential

The two most common causes of neonatal jaundice are biliary atresia and neonatal hepatitis. In comparison to biliary atresia, hepatobiliary scintigraphy in patients with neonatal hepatitis shows liver activity and subsequent excretion of tracer into the bowel. Differentiation between these two entities is important due to differences in management and treatment. Neonatal hepatitis is managed medically, and biliary atresia requires early surgical intervention to prevent biliary cirrhosis.

REFERENCES AND SUGGESTED READING

1. Gerhold JP, Klingensmith WC 3rd, Kuni CC, et al. Diagnosis of biliary atresia with radionuclide hepatobiliary imaging. *Radiology.* 1983;146(2):499-504.

2. Gubernick J, Rosenberg HK, Ilaslan H, et al. US approach to jaundice in infants and children. *RadioGraphics.* 2000;20:173-195.

3. Guiberteau M, Mettler F. *Essentials of Nuclear Medicine Imaging.* Philadelphia: Saunders; 2006.

CASE 11: PRENATALLY DIAGNOSED HYDRONEPHROSIS

PATIENT PRESENTATION

Prenatal ultrasound evaluation of the kidneys demonstrates bilateral hydronephrosis.

CLINICAL SUSPICION

There are a number of causes of hydronephrosis diagnosed in the prenatal period that require further evaluation. Several of the common causes include vesicoureteral reflux, ureteropelvic junction (UPJ) obstruction, and posterior urethral valves.

IMAGING MODALITY OF CHOICE

Given the increasing use and advances in prenatal ultrasound today, the diagnosis and postnatal evaluation of prenatal hydronephrosis is becoming more common. In the postnatal evaluation of hydronephrosis, renal ultrasound and voiding cystourethrogram, or VCUG, are the imaging modalities of choice.

Voiding cystourethrogram is performed fluoroscopically and consists of instillation of contrast into the bladder to capacity and evaluation for ureteral reflux during the filling period and during voiding. This study allows for anatomic evaluation of the bladder for identification of intraluminal abnormalities such as ureteroceles, polyps, or masses, as well as evaluation of the ureters, upper collecting system, and the urethra.

In the case of ureteropelvic junction obstruction, the degree of dilatation of the collecting system and severity of the obstruction may also be evaluated with renal scintigraphy using 99-m technetium-MAG3 with diuretic challenge.

FINDINGS

Vesicoureteral reflux is defined as retrograde flow of urine from the urinary bladder into the ureter toward the kidney. Vesicoureteral reflux is thought to result from shortened or abnormally angulated insertion of the ureter into the bladder, and it may lead to urinary tract infection, acute pyelonephritis, and renal scarring. Diagnosis may be made with VCUG where contrast instilled into the bladder opacifies the ureter and may reach the upper collecting system depending on the degree of reflux.

The grading system is demonstrated in Table C11.1 and Fig. C11.1 and is dependent upon the level to which the reflux occurs within the collecting system, severity of dilatation, and calyceal blunting.

Intrarenal reflux, a phenomenon where contrast refluxes from the calyces into the renal parenchyma in the form of striations, has been underreported and not graded. It can

Table C11.1 Grades of Vesicoureteral Reflux

Grade 1	Reflux into the ureter not reaching the renal pelvis.
Grade 2	Reflux reaching the renal pelvis without blunting of the calyces.
Grade 3	Reflux is associated with mild calyceal blunting.
Grade 4	Progressive calyceal and ureteral dilation.
Grade 5	Presence of very dilated and tortuous collecting system.

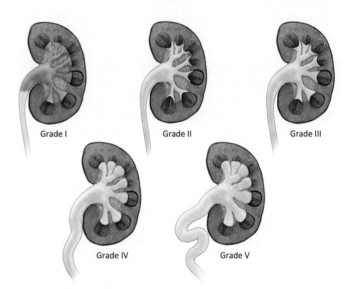

Fig. C11.1 Illustration showing grades of vesicoureteral reflux.

be seen in the settings (5%-15%) of moderate or severe vesicoureteral reflux. These patients are more prone to renal scarring from urinary tract infection.

Ureteropelvic junction obstruction is another common cause of prenatal hydronephrosis and is the most common congenital obstruction of the urinary tract. It is caused by an obstruction of the flow of urine from the renal pelvis into the proximal ureter with the most common cause being narrowing of the ureteropelvic junction (UPJ). Ultrasound examination demonstrates dilatation of the renal pelvicalyceal system without dilatation of the ureter (Fig. C11.2). Renal scintigraphy using 99-m technetium-MAG3 with diuretic (furosemide) challenge may help determine the presence and severity of the obstruction (Fig. C11.3).

Posterior urethral valves occur exclusively in males and result in a varying degree of chronic urethral obstruction due to fusion and prominence of the normal concentric folds of the urethra called plicae colliculi. The severity of obstruction determines the age at presentation and clinical symptoms, although the diagnosis may be made prenatally.

Ultrasound features include a thickened bladder with associated dilatation of the renal collecting systems and

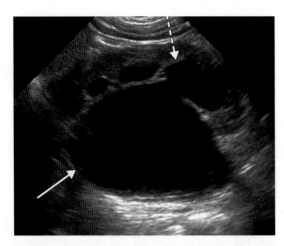

Fig. C11.2 Longitudinal gray-scale transabdominal ultrasound shows a markedly distended renal pelvis (white arrow) communicating with dilated calyces (white dotted arrow). No dilated ureter is seen and findings are consistent with ureteropelvic junction obstruction.

A

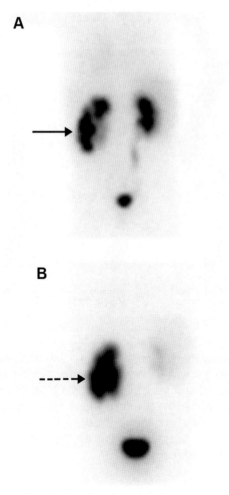

B

Fig. C11.3 (A) Renal scintigraphy with 99-m technetium-MAG 3 demonstrates hydronephrosis of the left kidney (black arrow). (B) There is poor response post Lasix injection and holdup in the left renal pelvis (black dotted arrow) consistent with UPJ obstruction.

ureters. Voiding cystourethrogram is the gold standard for imaging posterior urethral valves and will demonstrate a dilated posterior urethra with an abrupt caliber change to a narrow bulbous and penile urethra (Fig. C11.4). The actual valve tissue may not be visible, but it does not need to be seen to make the diagnosis. Common associated findings include bladder wall trabeculation and vesicoureteral reflux.

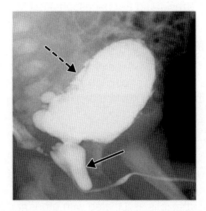

Fig. C11.4 Voiding cystourethrogram shows marked dilatation of the posterior urethra (black arrow) with transition to narrow caliber of the bulbous and penile urethra distal to the valve tissue, which is not seen. There is also irregular bladder wall thickening (dotted arrow).

DIFFERENTIAL DIAGNOSIS

The presence of hydronephrosis at any stage of gestation is generally the first indicator of a potential urinary tract anomaly, and consistent follow-up and postnatal evaluation is needed for further evaluation. In some cases the hydronephrosis may resolve prior to delivery. Other considerations when hydronephrosis is encountered should include primary megaureter, multicystic dysplastic kidney, neurogenic bladder, and ureteropelvic duplication.

REFERENCES AND SUGGESTED READING

1. Pates JA, Dashe JS. Prenatal diagnosis and management of hydronephrosis. *Early Hum Dev.* 2006;82(1):3-8.

2. Fernbach S, Feinstein KA, Schmidt MB. Pediatric voiding cystourethrography: a pictorial guide. *RadioGraphics.* 2000;20:155-168.

3. Berrocal T, Lopez-Pereira P, Arjonilla A, et al. Anomalies of the distal ureter, bladder, and urethra in children: embryologic, radiologic, and pathologic features. *RadioGraphics.* 2002;22:1139-1164.

CASE 12: ESOPHAGEAL ATRESIA AND TRACHEOESOPHAGEAL FISTULA

PATIENT PRESENTATION

Newborn infant with excessive oral secretions and feeding difficulties with choking.

CLINICAL SUSPICION

Esophageal atresia and tracheoesophageal fistula

IMAGING MODALITY OF CHOICE

Frontal and lateral chest radiographs. Radiographic evaluation of the abdomen should also be performed to look for bowel gas in the distal gastrointestinal tract.

FINDINGS

Esophageal atresia and tracheoesophageal fistula is thought to result from a disorder in the formation and separation of the primitive foregut into the trachea and esophagus. Esophageal atresia is associated with other gastrointestinal malformations such as imperforate anus, pyloric stenosis, duodenal atresia, and annular pancreas. It is also most commonly associated with the VACTERL complex (vertebral, anal, cardiac, tracheal, esophageal, renal, and limb anomalies).

Different types of esophageal atresia are identified on the basis of the presence and location, or absence, of a tracheoesophageal fistula (Fig. C12.1). The most common type consists of a blind esophageal pouch with a fistula between the trachea and distal esophagus. Less commonly, the fistula can connect the proximal or both the proximal and distal esophagus to the trachea. The H-type fistula occurs when a tracheoesophageal fistula occurs without atresia.

Esophageal atresia may be suspected prenatally secondary to polyhydramnios or may present at birth with excessive oral and pharyngeal secretions, inability to swallow saliva or milk, difficulty feeding, and failure to pass an enteric tube into the stomach. Children with an H-type fistula may have coughing or choking during feeding or may present with recurrent pneumonia. In some instances, these patients may not be diagnosed for several years.

Frontal and lateral chest radiographs demonstrate an air-filled distended blind pouch of the esophagus. Identification of abdominal bowel gas suggests the presence of a distal tracheoesophageal fistula (Fig. C12.2). The chest radiographs on these patients should also be carefully inspected for evidence of vertebral or cardiac anomalies. An upper GI series is only indicated when the H-type fistula is suspected and should be performed with water-soluble contrast.

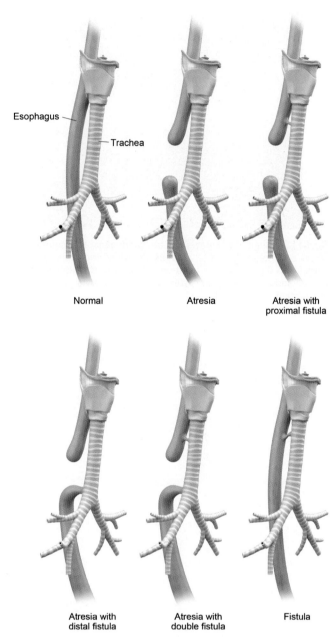

Fig. C12.1 Types of tracheoesophageal fistula.

The treatment of esophageal atresia and tracheoesophageal fistula involves surgical repair. Anastomotic leak is a complication that may occur immediately after repair and may be suggested by an extrapleural fluid collection on chest radiograph. Long-term complications include esophageal stricture, recurrent fistula, esophageal dysmotility, and gastroesophageal reflux.

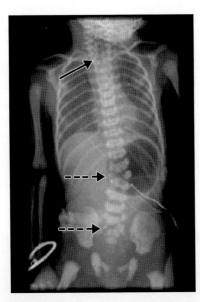

Fig. C12.2 Single view of the chest and abdomen shows the orogastric tube terminating in an air-filled, distended pharyngeal pouch (black arrow) consistent with esophageal atresia. There is a distended stomach bubble without any distal bowel gas in the stomach due to duodenal obstruction. Associated vertebral anomalies of left hemivertebrae at L2 and S2 are present (dashed arrows).

DIFFERENTIAL DIAGNOSIS

Clinical Differential

Differential diagnosis for patients presenting with cyanosis, choking, or coughing during feeding includes laryngotracheal cleft and esophageal stenosis. Laryngotracheal cleft is a congenital defect with communication between the esophagus and airway due to failed closure of the tracheoesophageal septum. Symptoms include feeding difficulties, chronic cough, stridor, and respiratory distress.

Esophageal stenosis may be congenital or acquired due to surgery or gastroesophageal reflux.

In patients presenting with chronic or recurrent pneumonia, considerations should include H-type tracheoesophageal fistula, gastroesophageal reflux with aspiration, aspirated foreign body, cystic fibrosis or other immunocompromised state, or infected congenital lung mass such as congenital pulmonary airway malformation.

Imaging Differential

Frequently, a confirmed diagnosis of esophageal atresia can be made based on the typical findings seen on chest and abdominal radiographs without the need for further imaging, as no other differential diagnosis needs to be considered. The exception to this is in patients suspected of the H-type fistula where an upper GI series is indicated for evaluation.

REFERENCES AND SUGGESTED READING

1. Beroccal T, Torres I, Gutiérrez J, et al. Congenital anomalies of the upper gastrointestinal tract. *RadioGraphics*. 1999;19:855-872.

2. Clark DC. Esophageal atresia and tracheoesophageal fistula. *Am Fam Physician*. 1999;59(4):910-916.

CASE 13: WILMS' TUMOR

PATIENT PRESENTATION

A 3-year-old male presents with abdominal pain with a palpable abdominal mass and hematuria.

CLINICAL SUSPICION

Wilms' tumor

IMAGING MODALITY OF CHOICE

Ultrasonography is usually the initial imaging examination in an infant or child with a palpable abdominal mass. When a solid renal mass is identified on ultrasound examination, contrast-enhanced CT or MR imaging of the abdomen and pelvis is performed for further evaluation of the disease extent, although MRI is preferable to avoid radiation exposure. Also, as the lung is the most frequent location of metastases in case of Wilms' tumor, a chest CT is required for appropriate tumor staging.

FINDINGS

Wilms' tumor, also known as nephroblastoma, is the most common renal malignancy in children and is a malignant tumor of primitive metanephric blastema. Children usually present before 5 years of age, and the peak incidence occurs at 3 years of age. Wilms' tumor can be associated with Beckwith-Wiedemann syndrome, nonfamilial aniridia, congenital hemihypertophy, and other malformations.

On ultrasound, Wilms' tumor appears as a large mass arising from the kidney that is frequently heterogeneous secondary to areas of hemorrhage or necrosis (Fig. C13.1). Color Doppler is useful in determining extension of tumor thrombus into the renal vein or inferior vena cava.

Contrast-enhanced CT examination demonstrates a large, heterogeneous, well-circumscribed renal mass with a surrounding "pseudocapsule" (Fig. C13.2). To help ascertain that the origin of a mass is from the kidney, the "claw sign" may be seen. As the tumor grows in the kidney, the normal renal parenchyma may spread out around a portion of the mass describing this classic sign.

Also, as a Wilms' tumor grows, it displaces surrounding organs and vessels. On the CT, close evaluation of local lymphadenopathy, involvement of the renal vein and inferior vena cava, and careful inspection of the contralateral

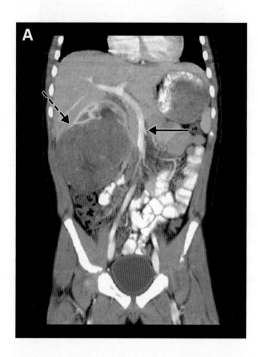

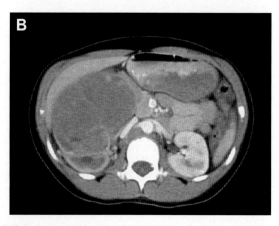

Fig. C13.2 Coronal (A) and axial (B) contrast-enhanced CT images of the abdomen and pelvis show the renal mass is displacing surrounding vessels (black arrow). The CT images also show a classic example of the claw sign with the normal renal parenchyma extending around the mass, indicated the mass is arising from within the kidney (dotted black arrow).

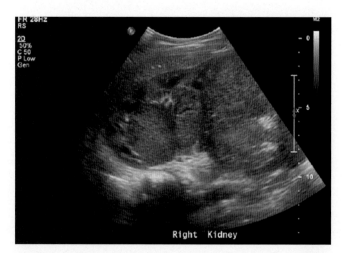

Fig. C13.1 Gray-scale ultrasound image of the right kidney show a large, lobulated heterogeneous mass originating from the lower pole and extending into the collecting structures.

kidney for simultaneous tumor involvement is necessary. Bilateral tumor involvement may be present in approximately 5% of cases.

MRI findings are similar to those of CT and typically show a mass with low signal intensity on T1W and high signal intensity on T2W images, but it may be heterogeneous secondary to hemorrhage within the mass.

DIFFERENTIAL DIAGNOSIS

Clinical Differential

A variety of pediatric renal masses may be differentiated from Wilms' tumor based on age and their clinical and imaging features. The clinical differential diagnosis for Wilms' tumor includes benign processes as well as malignancies. Overall, the most common differential of a pediatric patient presenting with a palpable abdominal mass is neuroblastoma.

Imaging Differential

A few of the differential diagnoses for Wilms' tumor include multilocular cystic nephroma, mesoblastic nephroma, and nephroblastomatosis. On imaging evaluation, neuroblastoma can be differentiated based on its origin from the ad-renal gland or paraspinal neural tissues. The other lesions may be more difficult to differentiate given their similar imaging appearances to Wilms' tumor.

Multilocular cystic nephroma is a benign lesion and is seen as a multiseptated cystic mass on ultrasound, CT, and MRI.

Mesoblastic nephroma is the most common renal mass in infants less than 6 months old, with mean age of diagnosis being 3 months. Ultrasound demonstrates a heterogeneous well-defined solid renal mass, and CT findings include a solid intrarenal mass of variable attenuation.

On imaging, nephroblastomatosis appears as homogeneous peripheral nodular subcapsular masses. These lesions are related to persistent nephrogenic rests in the kidneys and are a precursor to Wilms' tumor.

REFERENCES AND SUGGESTED READING

1. Lowe L. Pediatric renal masses: Wilms tumor and beyond. *RadioGraphics*. 2000;20:1585-1603.
2. Gylys-Morin V, Hoffer FA, Kozakewich H, et al. Wilms tumor and nephroblastomatosis: imaging characteristics at gadolinium-enhanced MR imaging. *Radiology*. 1993;188(2)517-521.

CASE 14: NEUROBLASTOMA

PATIENT PRESENTATION

A 2-year-old male presents with abdominal distention and palpable abdominal mass.

CLINICAL SUSPICION

Neuroblastoma

IMAGING MODALITY OF CHOICE

As discussed previously, initial evaluation of a pediatric patient with a palpable abdominal mass begins with ultrasound evaluation and abdominal radiographs. If findings are suggestive of neuroblastoma, confirmation of the diagnosis and assessment of the disease extent is obtained with CT or MRI. Nuclear scans including MIBG and bone scans are also performed for staging of neuroblastoma.

FINDINGS

Neuroblastoma is the most common solid, extracranial malignancy of childhood and the third most common pediatric malignancy, after leukemia and primary brain tumors. It is a malignant tumor of neural crest cells that most commonly arises in the adrenal gland, but it can occur anywhere along the sympathetic chain. The median age at diagnosis is 22 months, and approximately 90% of patients with neuroblastoma have elevated levels of catecholamines, especially vanillylmandelic acid (VMA).

Abdominal radiographic findings of neuroblastoma may include a nonspecific soft tissue mass, widening of the paraspinal stripe, and enlargement of the intervertebral foramina or erosion of the vertebral pedicles due to intraspinal extension of tumor. The tumor may contain calcifications, and lytic, sclerotic, or mixed bone metastases may be identified.

Neuroblastoma on ultrasound appears as a suprarenal or paraspinal mass that demonstrates varying echogenicity secondary to hemorrhage, necrosis, or cystic degeneration and may contain hyperechoic areas representing calcification. Increased vascularity on color Doppler may also be observed.

On CT, neuroblastoma appears as a lobulated soft tissue mass (Fig. C14.1A,B) that demonstrates an invasive pattern of growth with engulfment rather than displacement of vessels such as the celiac axis, superior mesenteric artery, and aorta. The tumors are often heterogeneous secondary to areas of hemorrhage, and necrosis and calcifications are present in up to 85% of tumors.

On MRI, the tumors tend to have high signal on T2-weighted images and can be heterogeneous in signal due to calcification, hemorrhage, and necrosis. MRI is also extremely helpful in detecting tumor extension into the spinal canal, which is important to identify for surgical management.

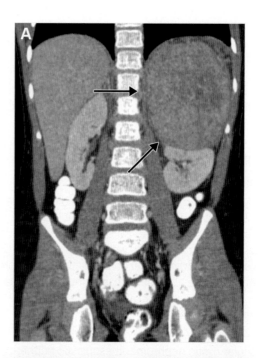

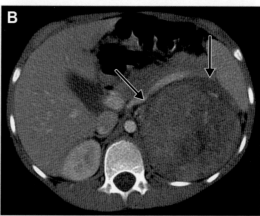

Fig. C14.1 Coronal (A) and axial (B) contrast-enhanced CT images show a large left heterogeneous adrenal mass (arrows) consistent with neuroblastoma.

Table C14.1 Evans Anatomic Staging

Stage	Findings	Prognosis (% survival)
Stage I	Tumor confined to organ of origin	90
Stage II	Tumor extension beyond the organ of origin but not crossing midline	75
Stage III	Tumor extension crossing midline	30
Stage IV	Distal metastasis	10
Stage IVS	Age <1 y, metastatic disease confined to skin, liver, and bone marrow	Near 100

MIBG is a medullary adrenal imaging agent that is taken up by chromaffin cells and is useful for imaging normal and abnormal sympathetic adrenergic tissue, effectively localizing pheochromocytoma and neuroblastoma. The scan can be used to detect adrenal medullary neuroblastoma and its metastases in more than 90% of affected neonates and children. In normal patients, the adrenal gland is only occasionally visualized and is best seen on delayed images. Neuroblastomas and any metastases detected with MIBG present as foci of increased activity. Skeletal metastases may also be identified and are generally best seen on delayed images.

DIFFERENTIAL DIAGNOSIS

Clinical Differential

As discussed previously, the most common differential of a palpable abdominal mass in a pediatric patient is Wilms' tumor and neuroblastoma. While neuroblastoma most commonly presents with a painless abdominal mass, signs and symptoms of neuroblastoma vary with the site of presentation and may even be an incidental finding.

Imaging Differential

The imaging differential considerations for a suprarenal mass in children include neonatal adrenal hemorrhage, pheochromocytoma, and pulmonary sequestration.

Neonatal adrenal hemorrhage can be seen as unilateral or bilateral adrenal masses with areas of high attenuation on CT in the acute stage. Adrenal hematomas gradually decrease in attenuation and size over time.

Pheochromocytomas may demonstrate a wide range of imaging appearances but are characteristically solid, hypervascular masses that are markedly hyperintense on T2-weighted images on MRI.

Extralobar pulmonary sequestration may present as a subdiaphragmatic or suprarenal mass and appears as a solid mass that may demonstrate cystic changes.

REFERENCES AND SUGGESTED READING

1. Lonergan GJ, Schwab CM, Suarez ES, et al. Neuroblastoma, ganglioneuroblastoma, and ganglioneuroma: radiologic-pathologic correlation. *RadioGraphics*. 2002;22(4):911-934.

2. Guiberteau M, Mettler F. *Essentials of Nuclear Medicine Imaging*. Philadelphia: Saunders; 2006.

3. McHugh K, Papaioannou G. Neuroblastoma in childhood: review and radiological findings. *Cancer Imaging*. 2005;5(1):116-127.

4. Donnelly L. *Pediatric Imaging: The Fundamentals*. 1st ed. Philadelphia, PA: Saunders; 2009.

CASE 15: INTUSSUSCEPTION

PATIENT PRESENTATION

A 15-month-old child develops intermittent abdominal pain with vomiting and currant jelly stools. A palpable mass is present in the right abdomen on physical examination.

CLINICAL SUSPICION

Intussusception

IMAGING MODALITY OF CHOICE

Abdominal radiographs are frequently the first test performed.

Ultrasonography and contrast enema examination not only can provide definitive diagnosis of intussusception, but can also aid in treatment.

FINDINGS

Intussusception typically occurs in children between the ages of 3 months and 3 years and is most commonly idiopathic, secondary to lymphoid hyperplasia. Intussusception results from a proximal part of the bowel (the intussusceptum) being pulled into the lumen of a distal part of the bowel (the intussuscipiens) as a result of forward bowel peristalsis. Ninety percent of intussusception in children is ileocolic, involving telescoping of the ileum into the cecum or ascending colon. Small bowel intussusception is less common in children but may occur with lead points such as polyps or Meckel's diverticulum.

Abdominal radiograph findings may include a paucity of bowel gas in the right abdomen (Fig. C15.1), and commonly, a soft-tissue mass that may efface the adjacent

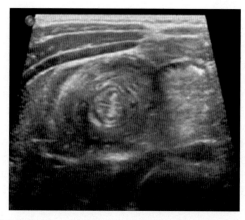

Fig. C15.2 Transverse ultrasound image demonstrates a targetlike mass that has a bowel-within-bowel appearance consistent with intussusception.

hepatic contour is most often seen in the right upper quadrant. Plain radiograph may also detect complications of prolonged intussusception such as bowel obstruction and perforation.

On ultrasound, the intussusception appears as a targetlike mass with alternating rings of hyperechogenicity and hypoechogenicity in the transverse plane (Fig. C15.2). In the longitudinal plane, the intussusception has a pseudokidney appearance with the hypoechoic edematous intussuscipiens surrounding the hyperechoic intussusceptum. If perforation has occurred, ascites with internal echoes or debris may be present with free peritoneal air.

CT findings include a mass with a target appearance with alternating rings of low and high attenuation. Findings of intestinal obstruction with proximal bowel distention and air-fluid levels may also be present.

Image-guided pressure reduction with air or liquid contrast enema is the treatment of intussusception. The appearance of ileocolic intussusception on enema exam is an intraluminal filling defect. With insufflation of air or liquid into the colon under fluoroscopic guidance, the intussusception moves toward the ileocecal valve and successful reduction is reached with resolution of the soft tissue mass and free reflux of air into the small bowel (Figs. C15.3-C15.5).

Contraindications to attempted reduction by air or liquid contrast enema include signs of peritonitis on physical exam and pneumoperitoneum identified on abdominal radiograph. The recurrence rate for intussusception is 5% to 10%, with the majority recurring in the first 72 hours. Surgical intervention is reserved for cases that fail image-guided or noninvasive reduction.

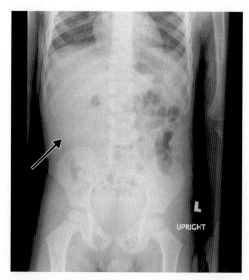

Fig. C15.1 Abdominal radiograph demonstrates a paucity of bowel gas in the right flank (arrow) with a suggestion of mass effect that may represent intussusception.

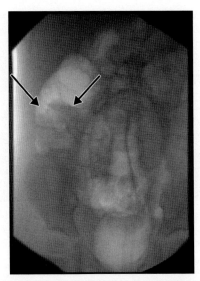

Fig. C15.3 Frontal images of air-reduction of intussusception. Initially, the intussusception is seen as a soft tissue mass near the hepatic flexure (arrows).

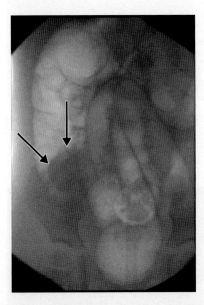

Fig. C15.4 Frontal image from an air enema in the same patient as the previous image shows the intussusception has moved to the region of the ileocecal valve (arrows).

DIFFERENTIAL DIAGNOSIS

Clinical Differential

Several differential considerations include appendicitis, gastroenteritis, intestinal obstruction, and ovarian pathology.

Patients with appendicitis classically present with periumbilical pain that subsequently localizes to McBurney's point in the right lower quadrant with rebound tenderness and fever, nausea, and vomiting.

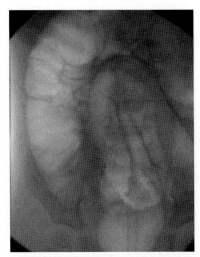

Fig. C15.5 Subsequently, there has been resolution of the soft tissue mass and the intussusception with reflux of air into the small bowel.

Gastroenteritis most commonly causes abdominal pain, nausea, vomiting, and diarrhea.

Abdominal pain in female patients may be attributable to ovarian pathology and should be considered in patients with right or left lower quadrant pain. Ovarian torsion is most important to exclude in those with acute or intermittent abdominal pain, typically in an older age group than those with intussusception.

Imaging Differential

Appendicitis may be suggested by identification of an appendicolith on abdominal radiographs. In case of perforated appendicitis with abscess formation, increased soft tissue opacity may be present in the right lower quadrant on radiographs and can mimic intussusception.

Abdominal radiographs in patients with gastroenteritis can demonstrate prominent bowel loops with air-fluid levels.

REFERENCES AND SUGGESTED READING

1. del-Pozo G, Albillos JC, Tejedor D, et al. Intussusception in children: current concepts in diagnosis and enema reduction. *RadioGraphics.* 1999;19:299-319.
2. Peh WCG, Khong PL, Lam C, et al. Ileoileocolic intussusception in children: diagnosis and significance. *Br J Radiol.* 1997;70:891-896.
3. Donnelly L. *Pediatric Imaging: The Fundamentals.* 1st ed. Philadelphia, PA: Saunders; 2009.

CASE 16: TESTICULAR TORSION

PATIENT PRESENTATION

A 6-year-old male presents with acute pain in the right scrotum.

CLINICAL SUSPICION

Testicular torsion

IMAGING MODALITY OF CHOICE

Scrotal ultrasound. Ultrasound evaluation of the scrotum in patients with suspected testicular torsion is performed with gray-scale and color Doppler imaging. Power Doppler may also be helpful and comparison of the affected testis to the contralateral normal testis should be made.

FINDINGS

Testicular torsion is the spontaneous or traumatic twisting of the testis and spermatic cord within the scrotum, resulting in vascular occlusion and subsequent infarction. There are two types of testicular torsion: extravaginal and intravaginal. The extravaginal type is more common in neonates and is caused by torsion of the spermatic cord proximal to the attachment of the tunica vaginalis at the level of the external inguinal ring. The intravaginal type is the more common type and is secondary to the "bell clapper" deformity in which the tunica vaginalis joins high on the spermatic cord, allowing the testicle to rotate freely within the scrotum.

When the spermatic cord twists, there is initially occlusion of venous flow and then arterial flow. The extent of testicular ischemia depends on the degree of twisting and the duration of the torsion. Most common presenting symptoms are acute testicular pain, redness, and swelling.

In cases of early testicular torsion (within 1-3 hours), the testicular echogenicity may appear normal. Typical findings of torsion include asymmetric enlargement of the testicle and epididymis and homogeneously decreased echogenicity of the affected testis. With progression of ischemia or infarction, the affected testis may become heterogeneous in echogenicity secondary to hemorrhage and necrosis (Figs. C16.1 and C16.2). A worsening appearance of the testis on gray-scale ultrasound correlates with decreased viability.

A definitive diagnosis of complete testicular torsion is made when color Doppler demonstrates blood flow on the normal side and absence of flow on the affected side (Figs. C16.3 and C16.4). If there is incomplete torsion, some arterial flow may persist in the affected testis. Other sonographic findings include twisting of the spermatic cord, reactive hydrocele, and edema of the scrotal wall.

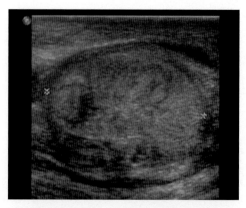

Fig. C16.1 Transverse gray-scale ultrasound image in testicular torsion shows a hypoechoic left testis with heterogeneous echotexture in a patient with testicular torsion.

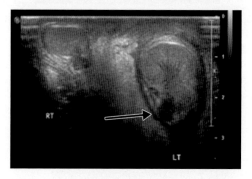

Fig. C16.2 Side-by-side view of the testes on transverse gray-scale ultrasound shows an enlarged left testis with heterogeneous echotexture due to necrosis (arrow) compared to normal right testis.

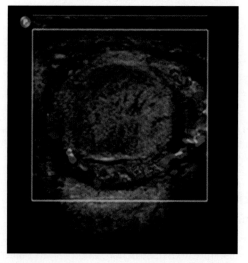

Fig. C16.3 Transverse color Doppler sonogram shows peripheral capsular blood flow with no intratesticular blood flow.

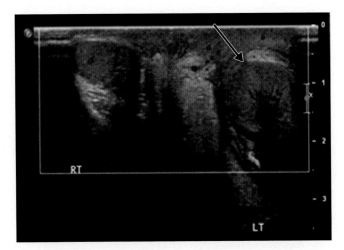

Fig. C16.4 Transverse color Doppler sonogram of testicular torsion demonstrates normal flow to the right testis and absence of flow to the ischemic left testis (arrow).

DIFFERENTIAL DIAGNOSIS

Clinical Differential

The most frequent causes of a patient presenting with the clinical picture of an acute scrotum are acute epididymo-orchitis, testicular torsion, testicular trauma, and torsion of the testicular appendage.

Patients with acute epididymo-orchitis have scrotal pain, swelling, and erythema and may also have urinary symptoms and systemic symptoms with fever.

Torsion of the testicular appendage can present with scrotal swelling, and in some cases a small, firm nodule may be palpable in the scrotum.

Imaging Differential

Ultrasound evaluation in a patient with testicular trauma may show irregular testicular contours, heterogeneous parenchymal echogenicity, and hematocele.

The typical appearance of epididymo-orchitis shows an enlarged hypoechoic epididymis and testis with increased flow on color Doppler. These findings on ultrasound can closely mimic the appearance of a spontaneously detorsed testis with reactive hyperemia.

Torsion of the testicular appendage demonstrates an enlarged appendage, generally located between the upper pole of the testis and epididymis, with surrounding hyperemia.

Also, testicular tumors may present as an enlarged, heterogenous testis that usually demonstrates blood flow, though some areas of the tumor may be necrosed and lack vascularity (Fig. C16.5).

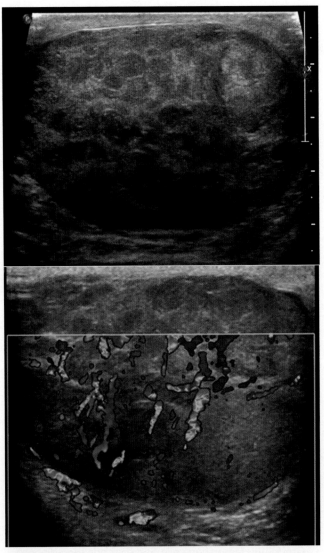

Fig C16.5 Transverse gray-scale ultrasound images shows a diffusely enlarged and heterogeneous testis with increased vascularity secondary to testicular leukemia.

REFERENCES AND SUGGESTED READING

1. Aso C, Enriquez G, Fite M, et al. Gray-scale and color Doppler sonography of scrotal disorders in children. *RadioGraphics*. 2005;25:1197-1214.

2. Dogra VS, Bhatt S. Acute painful scrotum. *Radiol Clin North Am*. 2004;42(2):349-363.

3. Dogra VS, Gottlieb RH, Oka M, et al. Sonography of the scrotum. *Radiology*. 2003;227(1):18-36.

CASE 17: GERMINAL MATRIX HEMORRHAGE

PATIENT PRESENTATION

Premature infant born after 28 weeks of gestation develops seizures in the first week of life.

CLINICAL SUSPICION

Germinal matrix hemorrhage

IMAGING MODALITY OF CHOICE

Brain ultrasound

FINDINGS

Germinal matrix hemorrhage occurs in premature infants and is a significant cause of morbidity and mortality in this population. The germinal matrix is formed early during embryogenesis and is the site of glial and neuronal generation and differentiation and the location from which cells migrate peripherally to form the brain. The germinal matrix is densely vascular as well and subject to hemorrhage. It is generally gone by term, but it remains present in premature infants.

Germinal matrix hemorrhage is most common in the first week of life. Risk factors include infants less than 32 weeks gestation, low birth weight, and disturbances in cardiorespiratory function. There are 4 grades of germinal matrix hemorrhage:

- Grade I: Hemorrhage confined to the caudothalamic groove (Fig. C17.1A,B)
- Grade II: Hemorrhage extends into the ventricle without ventricular dilatation
- Grade III: Hemorrhage fills and distends the adjacent ventricle
- Grade IV: Intraparenchymal hemorrhage (Fig. C17.2)

In general, prognosis depends on the grade and extent of the hemorrhage. Grade I and II hemorrhage have good prognoses, but grade III and IV hemorrhage tend to have poor prognoses with increased mortality.

Brain ultrasound is the examination of choice. The advantage of ultrasound is that it can be performed quickly as a bedside exam and does not use radiation. The examination is performed via the anterior and posterolateral fontanelles. Germinal matrix hemorrhage is seen on sagittal and coronal ultrasound images as an echogenic area close to the caudothalamic groove, which may extend into the lateral ventricles or periventricular brain parenchyma.

Acute blood is echogenic and later becomes isoechoic to hypoechoic. The normal choroid plexus is echogenic and must be distinguished from acute hemorrhage. The choroid plexus terminates at the caudothalamic groove anteriorly and does not extend into the occipital horns.

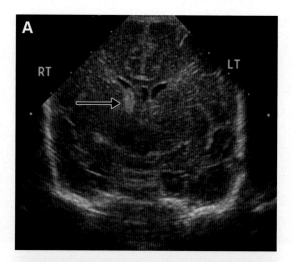

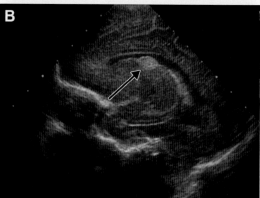

Fig. C17.1 Gray-scale sagittal (A) and coronal (B) images of the brain show a right-sided grade I germinal matrix hemorrhage with an echogenic focus at the caudothalamic groove (arrows), not extending into the ventricle.

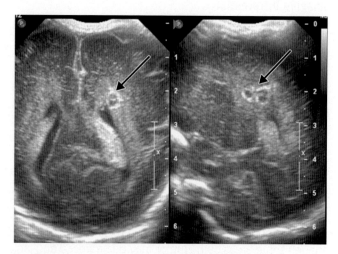

Fig. C17.2 Gray-scale coronal and sagittal images of the brain demonstrate a mixed echogenic focus with cystic changes in the brain parenchyma adjacent to the left lateral ventricle (arrow) consistent with evolving grade IV germinal matrix hemorrhage.

Therefore, echogenicity seen anterior to the groove in the frontal horn or within the occipital horn represents blood. When hemorrhage is identified, the remaining brain should be evaluated for extra-axial fluid collections and congenital anomalies. For larger hemorrhages, CT scan is a better exam and is excellent at detecting parenchymal, subdural, subarachnoid, and intraventricular hemorrhage.

Potential complications of germinal matrix hemorrhage include destruction of the precursor cells within the germinal matrix, hydrocephalus, and infarction of the surrounding tissues.

DIFFERENTIAL DIAGNOSIS

Clinical Differential

Infants presenting with seizures may be the result of epilepsy syndromes, other types of hemorrhage including subarachnoid and subdural hematoma, tuberous sclerosis, or infectious processes such as viral encephalitis or meningitis.

Imaging Differential

Choroid plexus cysts may appear on ultrasound as small cysts that can be differentiated from germinal matrix hemorrhage based on location within the choroid plexus.

Periventricular leukomalacia, which is a white matter disease that affects the periventricular zones and normally results in cavitation and periventricular cyst formation (Fig. C17.3), may initially be seen as hyperechoic areas in the periventricular area, similar to germinal matrix hemorrhage.

Neonates may develop intraventricular hemorrhage that may be confined to the ventricle and not involve the germinal matrix. This diagnosis should be considered in patients who are older than 35 weeks gestation.

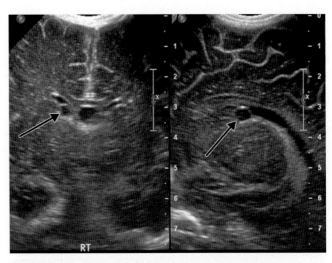

Fig. C17.3 Gray-scale coronal and sagittal brain ultrasound images show a well-defined choroid plexus cyst in the right lateral ventricle (arrows).

Also, ischemia or infarction of the brain may appear hyperechoic in acute and subacute stages, but it tends to occur in different areas of the brain.

REFERENCES AND SUGGESTED READING

1. Roland EH, Hill A. Germinal matrix-intraventricular hemorrhage in the premature newborn: management and outcome. *Neurology Clin*. 2003;21(4):833-851, vi-vii.

2. Donnelly L. *Pediatric Imaging: The Fundamentals*. 1st ed. Philadelphia, PA: Saunders; 2009.

3. Brant W, Helms C. *Fundamental of Diagnostic Radiology*. 3rd ed. Philadelphia: Lippincott Williams and Wilkins; 2007.

CASE 18: AVASCULAR NECROSIS

PATIENT PRESENTATION

A 14-year-old boy with a history of sickle-cell anemia presents with dull right hip pain for 1 month. He denies any trauma, but the pain has not permitted him to play sports at school for over 2 weeks.

CLINICAL SUSPICION

Avascular necrosis of the hip

IMAGING MODALITY OF CHOICE

In concordance with the ACR Appropriateness Criteria, a child who presents with hip pain should initially receive an AP pelvic radiograph and frog-leg lateral views of the symptomatic hip. If the initial radiographs are either normal or equivocal and clinical suspicion is high, then MRI or bone scan should be performed.

FINDINGS

Radiographically, the early findings include sclerosis of the anterior femoral head, which later becomes flattened with repetitive use (Figs. C18.1 and C18.2). There may be accompanying subchondral fractures in patients who do not get early treatment. In patients with sickle-cell disease or chronic corticosteroid use, there is a higher incidence of bilateral disease than from a traumatic origin.

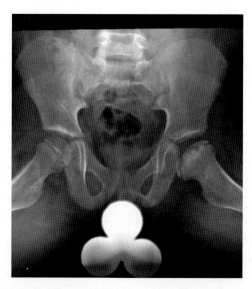

Fig. C18.2 Supine frog-leg lateral view shows epiphyseal sclerosis, fragmentation, and height loss of the left femoral head in another patient with idiopathic left hip avascular necrosis.

The findings are graded on a system from I to VI, I being normal and progressing to advanced degenerative disease with joint space narrowing and flattening of the femoral head. MRI findings include marrow edema in early disease, and on T1WI, a hypointense line outlining an area of marrow edema. On nuclear medicine bone scans, there is decreased scintigraphic activity initially due to lack of blood flow, followed by increased activity if there is revascularization.

DIFFERENTIAL DIAGNOSIS

Clinical Differential

Hip pain in a pediatric patient may be the sequelae of infection, trauma, neoplasm, or osteonecrosis. Large effusions seen on radiographs are more indicative of infection, and aspiration of the joint will help differentiate it from other causes. Some bone tumors are found in radiographs with a history of trauma where a pathologic fracture is the cause of pain.

Imaging Differential

Since avascular necrosis is the end result of many different entities, the differential for the primary cause includes chronic steroid use, sickle-cell disease, developmental dysplasia of the hip, posttraumatic articular abnormality, and rare metabolic diseases. Bone bruise due to repetitive trauma also can look similar to early avascular necrosis on MRI.

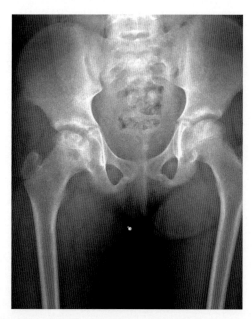

Fig. C18.1 AP view of the hip shows the characteristic femoral head sclerosis and flattening (right greater than left), consistent with bilateral avascular necrosis. This was a teenager with known sickle-cell disease.

REFERENCES AND SUGGESTED READING

1. ACR Appropriateness Criteria. http://www.acr.org/ac.

2. Hayes, Conway WF, Daniel WW. MR imaging of bone marrow edema pattern: transient osteoporosis, transient bone marrow edema syndrome, or osteonecrosis. *RadioGraphics*. 1993;13:1001-1011.

3. Steinberg ME, Hayken GD, Steinberg DR. A quantitative system for staging avascular necrosis. *J Bone Joint Surg Br*. 1995;77(1):34-41.

4. Ito H, Matsuno T, Minami A. Relationship between bone marrow edema and development of symptoms in patients with osteonecrosis of the femoral head. *AJR*. 2006;186:1761-1770.

5. Silverman FN. Lesions of the femoral neck in Legg-Perthes disease. *AJR*. 1985;144:1249-1254.

6. Mitchell MD, Kundel HL, Steinberg ME, et al. Avascular necrosis of the hip: comparison of MR, CT, and scintigraphy. *AJR*. 1986;47:67-71.

CASE 19: CHILD ABUSE

PATIENT PRESENTATION

A 10-month-old boy who has not yet learned to walk presents with leg swelling and tenderness along with failure to thrive. The child also seems to be lagging behind in his developmental milestones.

CLINICAL SUSPICION

Child abuse

IMAGING MODALITY OF CHOICE

With a suspected fracture of the leg, a dedicated lower extremity radiograph series would be the imaging modality of choice. In the situation where child abuse is suspected, and in the absence of focal neurological signs or symptoms, the American College of Radiology recommends a skeletal survey for osseous abnormality screening for children less than 24 months of age.

For children older than the age of 2, skeletal surveys are of less value, and radiographs should usually be tailored to the area of injury. When there is a suspicion of abuse or unexplained injuries, skeletal survey is still indicated in children 2 to 5 years of age. If a skeletal survey does not demonstrate abnormal findings but the clinical suspicion is still very high, a nuclear bone scan is indicated.

When patients subject to suspected child abuse present with neurologic symptoms, head CT without contrast is the most appropriate initial radiologic exam, since most child abuse deaths are due to head trauma (Fig. C19.1). With clinically suspicious nonskeletal chest, abdominal, or pelvic injuries, CT of the respective areas is the first line of imaging. Literature shows that blunt trauma due to child abuse is associated with a sixfold increase in odds of death compared to injuries resulted from other mechanisms.

Skeletal Survey Components

A skeletal survey consists of frontal and lateral views of the skull, lateral views of the cervical spine, lateral views of the thoracolumbar spine, and single frontal views of each long bone, the chest, abdomen, and oblique views of the ribs.

FINDINGS

The most common fractures of child abuse are long bone diaphyseal fractures, which are nonspecific without a proper history. Fractures that are more specific for abuse include rib fractures from squeezing, long bone metaphyseal fractures due to aggressive grabbing and twisting of the extremity, and diaphyseal long bone fractures in a child who is not yet walking (Figs. C19.2 and C19.3). Scapular fractures usually indicate abuse since they require a lot of force but are uncommon. Multiple fractures in separate stages of healing should also alert the clinician to possible abuse (Fig. C19.4).

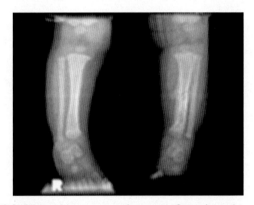

Fig. C19.2 Bilateral lower extremity x-rays. Comminuted transverse left tibial diaphyseal fracture with callus formation and proximal metaphyseal bucket handle fracture.

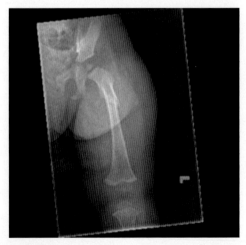

Fig. C19.3 Left femur x-ray shows acute spiral fracture in a child who has not yet started to walk.

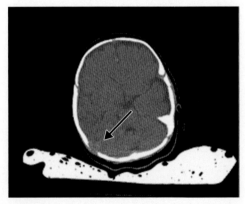

Fig. C19.1 Head CT without contrast shows diastasis of the right lambdoid suture with underlying subdural hemorrhage (arrow).

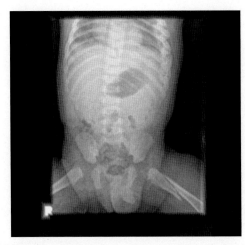

Fig. C19.4 AP view of the abdomen shows multiple rib fractures in various stages of healing along with a spiral fracture of the left femur in a child who has not yet learned to walk.

On CT, solid organ injuries such as liver and splenic lacerations are suspicious in the absence of accidental trauma. Care must be sought to look for a history of rickets, osteogenesis imperfecta, or other rare metabolic diseases as fractures may result from minimal or normal stress to the bone in such conditions and can mimic child abuse.

DIFFERENTIAL DIAGNOSIS

There are a few situations that may mimic child abuse, and they should be sought in the absence or suspicion of the proper history. Newborn children may have birth trauma including clavicle and humerus fractures. In young children less than 6 months, physiologic periosteal reaction may lead to suspicion of a healing fracture but is often symmetric. Patients with osteogenesis imperfecta (OI) have multiple fractures in different stages of healing, although the bones are usually osteopenic. Look for the blue sclerae in children with OI. Clinical suspicion and history will help guide decision making when fractures are present on radiographs.

REFERENCES AND SUGGESTED READING

1. ACR Appropriateness Criteria. http://www.acr.org/ac.
2. Lonergan GJ, Baker AM, Morey MK, et al. From the archives of the AFIP. Child abuse: radiologic-pathologic correlation. *RadioGraphics*. 2003;23(4):811-845.
3. Bulloch B, Schubert CJ, Brophy PD, et al. Cause and clinical characteristics of rib fracture in infants. *Pediatrics*. 2000;105(4):E48.
4. Kleinman PK. Diagnostic imaging in infant abuse. *AJR*. 1990; 155(4):703-712.
5. Ablin DS, Greenspan A, Reinhart M, et al. Differentiation of child abuse from osteogenesis imperfecta. *AJR*. 1990;154:1035-1046.
6. Prosser I, Maguire S, Harrison SK, et al. How old is this fracture? Radiologic dating of fractures in children: a systematic review. *AJR*. 2005;184(4):1282-1286.
7. Kahana T, Hiss J. Forensic radiology. *Br J Radiol*. 1999;72:129-133.
8. Kemp AM, Butler A, Morris S, et al. Which radiological investigations should be performed to identify fractures in child abuse? *Clin Radiol*. 2006;61(9):723-736.

CASE 20: RICKETS

PATIENT PRESENTATION

A 14-month-old boy who has recently emigrated from Turkey presents with bilateral leg bowing since beginning to walk. The mother thinks her son's shots are up to date but is unsure and is unable to provide any records.

CLINICAL SUSPICION

Rickets

IMAGING MODALITY OF CHOICE

Frontal radiographs of the knees and wrists are the appropriate initial exams to order when rickets is suspected. Frontal standing views of the bilateral lower extremities are also performed to evaluate femoral bowing, which may be confused with genu vara and tibia vara.

FINDINGS

The most indicative radiologic clue leading to the correct diagnosis on plain film is physeal widening of long bones with metaphyseal splaying in the background of osteopenia (Figs. C20.1 and C20.2). The normal physis width is less than 2 mm, but in rickets it is widened due to the decreased cartilage matrix calcification. This in turn leads to decreased osteoid matrix with a subsequent increased cartilage width secondary to continued cartilage proliferation. The osteoblasts in the metaphysis continue to make osteoid that cannot calcify and strengthen. Repeated microtrauma due to joint use will subsequently cause metaphyseal splaying.

The increased weight upon the long bones when the child begins to walk will cause them to bow causing short stature (Fig. C20.3). Another finding seen in some patients is delayed closure of the fontanelle. If the disease is not caught early enough, secondary hyperparathyroidism may

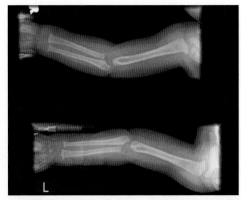

Fig. C20.2 Bilateral upper extremity x-rays show demineralization and metaphyseal flaring in a case of rickets.

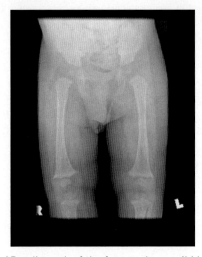

Fig. C20.3 AP radiograph of the femora shows mild bilateral bowing deformity of the femora along with metaphyseal flaring and physeal widening.

develop, causing subperiosteal bone resorption. If a renal cause is suspected, renal ultrasound is recommended.

DIFFERENTIAL DIAGNOSIS

Clinical Differential

Rickets is the common clinical spectrum that can occur if the bones do not have enough calcium, phosphorous, or vitamin D. In patients less than 6 months of age, this is likely due to maternal deficits or renal problems. In children greater than 6 months of age, this is likely due to either malabsorption or nutritional rickets, which is endemic in some parts of the world.

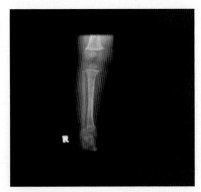

Fig. C20.1 AP radiograph of the right tibia and fibula shows generalized bone demineralization with metaphyseal flaring and physeal widening.

Imaging Differential

The most concerning differential diagnosis is leukemia, which can present with diffuse osteopenia and bending of bones at areas of leukemic infiltration. Congenital syphilis causes destruction of the metaphysis and can mimic rickets. Blount's disease may also present similarly with tibial varus deformity. Clinical history will help guide the proper diagnosis.

REFERENCES AND SUGGESTED READING

1. Wharton B, Bishop N. Rickets. *Lancet.* 2003;362(9393): 1389-1400.
2. Cheema J, Grissom L, Harcke T. Radiographic characteristics of lower-extremity bowing in children. *RadioGraphics.* 2003;23(1):871-880.
3. Swischuk LE, Hayden CK. Rickets: a roentgenographic scheme for diagnosis. *Pediatric Radiol.* 1979;8:203-208.

CASE 21: THYROGLOSSAL DUCT CYST

PATIENT PRESENTATION

A 10-year-old boy presents to clinic with a longstanding soft midline nonpainful neck mass. He recently experienced an upper respiratory infection.

CLINICAL SUSPICION

Thyroglossal duct cyst

IMAGING MODALITY OF CHOICE

Thyroglossal duct cyst is a clinical diagnosis, and imaging is indicated only in those cases in which infection or ectopic thyroid are of clinical concern. The thyroid may be difficult to palpate in children, therefore ultrasound can be utilized to visualize normal thyroid in its proper location. If there is tenderness to palpation, dysphagia, or dysphonia, CT or MRI can demonstrate infected tissue.

Infection and malignancy are the two main complications of thyroglossal duct cysts; the latter is rare and occurs more in adults than in the pediatric population. The differential for neck mass is also broader in adults. CT is therefore essential to look for both malignant features and alternate diagnoses. Ultrasound is also limited in fully evaluating the extent of thyroglossal duct cysts and deep ectopic thyroid tissue.

FINDINGS

A midline neck cystic mass is the most common finding, and the cyst will typically move upward on protrusion of the tongue due its attachment to the embryonic duct. Approximately half are at the level of the hyoid bone, with the other half equally distributed in suprahyoid and infrahyoid locations. On ultrasound, simple thyroglossal duct cysts are anechoic midline neck masses and demonstrate internal echoes with infection or recent hemorrhage (Figs. C21.1 and C21.2). Contrast and noncontrast CT demonstrates a low-attenuation, thin-walled, well-circumscribed midline neck cyst (Fig. C21.3).

The finding of an enhancing mural nodule or irregular calcification raises the concern for malignancy. Although rarely necessary for diagnosis, on MRI it appears hypointense on T1WI with the majority being hyperintense on T2WI. If ectopic thyroid tissue is suspected, preoperative nuclear medicine scintigraphy may be indicated for localization.

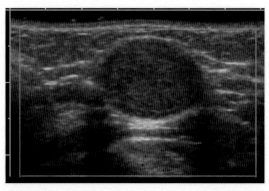

Fig. C21.1 Transverse US image through the neck shows a mildly complex well-defined midline cystic structure between the hyoid bone and tongue base.

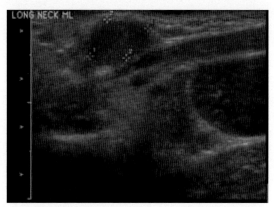

Fig. C21.2 Longitudinal US through the neck shows a midline mass adjacent to the strap muscles.

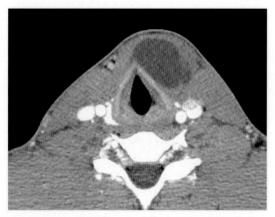

Fig. C21.3 Axial contrast-enhanced CT through the neck in another patient shows a well-defined, thin-walled cystic structure near midline at the level of the hyoid bone.

DIFFERENTIAL DIAGNOSIS

Clinical Differential

There are few midline neck cystic lesions, which include dermoid inclusion cysts, lymph nodes, and cystic hygromas. Branchial cleft cysts are similar clinically to thyroglossal duct cysts but are usually located in the lateral neck. Off-midline thyroglossal duct cysts may be indistinguishable from branchial cleft cysts.

Imaging Differential

Dermoid cysts can be differentiated by the appearance of fat globules within. Lymph nodes can be differentiated if a fatty hilum is seen. Branchial cleft cysts are similar radiographically to thyroglossal duct cysts and are differentiated by their location and connections.

REFERENCES AND SUGGESTED READING

1. Branstetter B, Weissman J, Kennedy T, et al. The CT appearance of thyroglossal duct carcinoma. *AJNR.* 2000;21:1547-1550.

2. Prasad KC, Dannana NK, Prasad SC. Thyroglossal duct cyst: an unusual presentation. *Ear Nose Throat J.* 2006;85(7): 454-456.

3. Dedivitis RA, Camargo DL, Peixoto GL, et al. Thyroglossal duct: a review of 55 cases. *J Am Coll Surg.* 2002;194(3):274-277.

4. Wadsworth DT, Siegel MJ. Thyroglossal duct cysts: variablity of sonographic findings. *AJR.* 1994;163(6):1475-1477.

5. Ahuja AT, King AD, King W, et al. Thyroglossal duct cysts: sonographic appearance in adults. *AJNR.* 1999;20:579-582.

6. Glastonbury CM, Davidson HC, Haller JR, et al. The CT and MR imaging features of carcinoma arising in thyroglossal duct remnants. *AJNR.* 2000;21:770-774.

CASE 22: SALTER-HARRIS FRACTURES

PATIENT PRESENTATION

A 14-year-old boy falls on his right hand after getting tackled during a junior high football game. Patient has point tenderness and swelling over the right distal radius.

CLINICAL SUSPICION

Right wrist fracture

IMAGING MODALITY OF CHOICE

X-ray wrist series according to the ACR Appropriateness Criteria. This initial exam has a relatively low radiation level and is the first line of imaging with acute wrist trauma. A wrist series includes a PA, lateral, and semipronated oblique radiographs of the wrist. Additional semisupinated oblique view may increase yield for distal radius fractures.

For all fractures, if initial radiographs are normal and there is high clinical suspicion for fracture, the next 2 options are equally appropriate in the correct scenario. The first is to cast the extremity and repeat x-ray in 10 to 14 days. If there was an initial fracture that could not be visualized on an earlier radiograph, it will usually manifest itself after 2 weeks on the subsequent radiograph. The other option is an MRI without contrast if there is an immediate need for confirmation or exclusion of fracture.

CT without contrast is less appropriate in the setting of suspected fracture with negative initial radiographs because it usually will not change management. When the radiographs show an intra-articular fracture and surgery is planned, CT without contrast is usually indicated for surgical planning.

FINDINGS

Physeal fractures of all the long bones are stratified using the Salter-Harris classification. Salter-Harris fractures involve the growth plate and are categorized according to their involvement of the metaphysis, physis, and epiphysis (Fig. C22.1).

Salter I fractures only involve the physis and are the mildest fracture involving the growth plate (Fig. C22.2). This usually occurs when a child rolls a wrist or ankle, and since the surrounding ligaments are stronger than the growth plate, it is more likely to fracture. On radiographs, there is usually widening of the physis, but most radiographs are normal.

Salter II fractures involve both the physis and metaphysis (Fig. C22.3). These, like Salter I, usually do not cause bone shortening because they rarely involve the reproductive layer of the physis.

Salter-Harris Classification

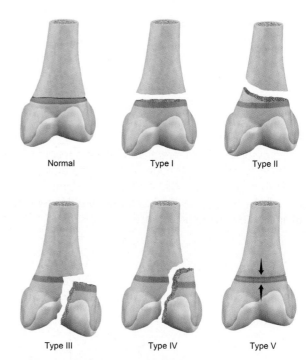

Normal   Type I   Type II

Type III   Type IV   Type V

Fig. C22.1 Salter-Harris classification.

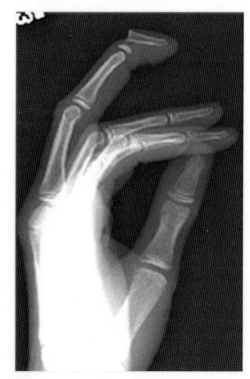

Fig. C22.2 Lateral view of the left hand demonstrates widening of the physis and dorsal displacement of the distal third phalanx, a Salter I fracture.

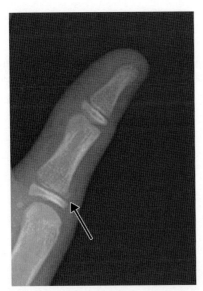

Fig. C22.3 Salter II fracture through the metaphysis and physis (arrow).

Salter III fractures involve both the physis and epiphysis and carry a worse prognosis since both the reproductive layer of the physis and the joint articular surface are involved (Fig. C22.4).

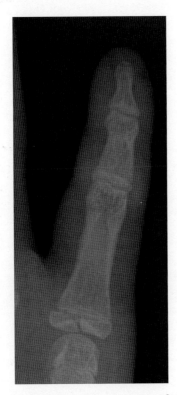

Fig. C22.4 Coned down digit radiograph shows a Salter III fracture through the physis and epiphysis of the base of the proximal phalanx.

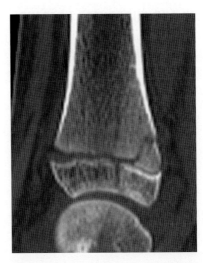

Fig. C22.5 Sagittally oriented CT through the ankle demonstrates a Salter IV fracture through the distal tibial metaphysis, physis, and epiphysis. It carries a high risk of limb shortening.

Salter IV fractures involve all three components: the metaphysis, physis, and epiphysis (Fig. C22.5).

Salter V is a compression fracture of the growth plate without metaphyseal or epiphyseal involvement.

Salter I and II fractures are usually treated without surgery, and III and IV may need surgery depending on the clinical scenario. Arrest of growth can also occur secondary to the formation of a bone bridge traversing the physis and with resulting tethering of the metaphysis and epiphysis.

DIFFERENTIAL DIAGNOSIS
Clinical Differential

The clinical differential diagnosis is limited with acute joint pain after trauma, with straining of the ligaments being first. Also within the differential, especially in young gymnasts or patients doing repetitive tasks, is a stress injury. Stress injuries can cause widening of the distal radial physis and mimic a Salter-Harris I fracture. The history of chronic stress separates these two entities, although there may be an acute fracture in the background of chronic stress injury.

Imaging Differential

Salter-Harris fractures are usually easily recognized using conventional radiography, although some fracture lines may not manifest until 1 to 2 weeks later. Salter I and V fractures may not manifest any radiologic findings, and if they are suspected, comparison radiographs of the opposite side should be obtained. MRI is helpful if there is suspicion of soft tissue abnormalities presenting as acute fracture.

REFERENCES AND SUGGESTED READING

1. Ogden JA. Injury to the growth mechanisms of the immature skeleton. *Skeletal Radiol.* 1981;6(4):237-253.

2. Rogers LF, Poznanski AK. Imaging of epiphyseal injuries. *Radiology.* 1994;191:297-308.

3. Salter RB, Harris WR. Injuries involving the epiphyseal plate. *J Bone Joint Surg.* 1963;45:587-622.

4. Shi DP, Zhu SC, Li Y, et al. Epiphyseal and physeal injury: comparison of conventional radiography and magnetic resonance imaging. *Clin Imaging.* 2009;33(5):379-383.

5. Ecklund K, Jaramillo D. Patterns of premature physeal arrest: MR imaging of 111 children. *AJR.* 2002;178(4):967-972.

6. ACR Appropriateness Criteria. http://www.acr.org/ac.

CASE 23: JUVENILE ARTHRITIS

PATIENT PRESENTATION

An 8-year-old boy presents to clinic for the third time in 2 months for recurring right knee pain and fever. The pain is now in both knees and involves his left ankle.

CLINICAL SUSPICION

Arthritis, either infectious or inflammatory

IMAGING MODALITY OF CHOICE

In line with the ACR Appropriateness Criteria, the initial examination for nontraumatic knee pain in a child is an x-ray of the knee. These are usually done in a series, with an AP, oblique, and lateral views obtained. In the atraumatic setting, it may be necessary to obtain the opposite side for comparison when findings are inconclusive. If referred pain from the hip is suspected, then x-ray of the ipsilateral hip is recommended. Nontraumatic joint pain is rare in children, and a source should always be sought. Therefore, if the initial radiographs are negative or show only a small effusion, an MRI without contrast is the next imaging modality of choice.

FINDINGS

In patients with juvenile idiopathic arthritis (JIA), most initial radiographs will be negative or show a small joint effusion. If the diagnosis is unknown, these nonspecific symptoms may be treated conservatively at first.

If the symptoms do not relieve themselves, become worse, or begin to involve other joints, MRI of the affected extremity can be very valuable. Usually more than one joint is involved. This may be either oligoarthritis with less than five involved joints, or may be polyarthritis with five or more involved joints. The early MRI findings will demonstrate subchondral bone marrow edema, tenosynovitis, and synovial hypertrophy, depending upon classification.

These findings, along with the clinical history, should alert the clinician to an arthritic, infectious, or posttraumatic cause. As the disease process progresses, follow-up radiographs will demonstrate larger effusions, osteopenia, periarticular soft tissue swelling, joint erosions, joint space narrowing, and even growth disturbances due to premature closure of the growth plate (Figs. C23.1-C23.3). Ankylosis of the wrist or spine and scoliosis are other radiographic findings. The same advanced changes are seen on MRI along with the visualization of articular cartilage erosions, complex effusions with joint bodies, and pannus formation.

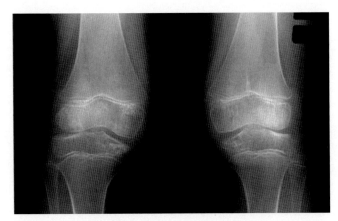

Fig. C23.1 Bilateral knee radiograph shows joint space narrowing, subchondral sclerosis, and lateral subluxation of the tibia.

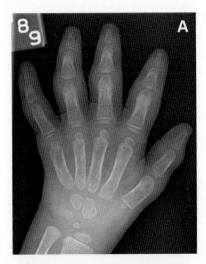

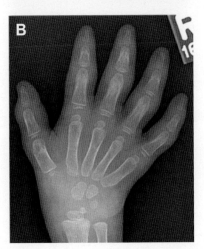

Fig. C23.2 Bilateral hand radiographs in a 3-year-old with early JIA. Symmetric abundant soft tissue swelling is the predominant finding.

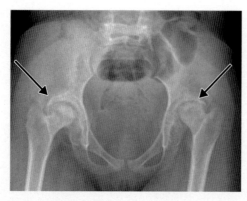

Fig. C23.3 Bilateral hip radiograph in a 12-year-old shows extensive joint space narrowing and remodeling of both hips (arrows) with femoral head and acetabular destruction.

DIFFERENTIAL DIAGNOSIS

The aforementioned findings, along with soft tissue swelling, pain, and decreased range of motion in a patient less than 16 years old leaves a relatively narrow differential. The umbrella term JIA encompasses the juvenile spondyloarthropathies, including ankylosing spondylitis, Reiter's, and psoriatic arthritis, which present similarly and can be distinguished with clinical history and varying lab results.

Referred pain from adjacent joints may be the culprit early on in the disease process before the soft tissue findings are evident. Transient synovitis, pigmented villonodular synovitis, and infectious arthritis may also mimic early juvenile idiopathic arthritis due to their monarticular nature. Continued hemarthrosis due to hemophilia can also present with chronic polyarticular joint pain and effusions.

REFERENCES AND SUGGESTED READING

1. ACR Appropriateness Criteria. http://www.acr.org/ac.
2. Restrepo R, Lee EY. Epidemiology, pathogenesis, and imaging of arthritis in children. *Orthop Clin North Am*. 2012;43(2): 213-225.
3. Jacobson JA, Girish G, Jiang Y, et al. Radiographic evaluation of arthritis: degenerative joint disease and variation. *Radiology*. 2008;248:737-747.
4. Senac M, Deutsch D, et al. MR imaging in juvenile rheumatoid arthritis. *AJR*. 1988;150:873-878.
5. Barbaric ZL, Young LW. Synovial cysts in juvenile rheumatoid arthritis. *AJR*. 116(3):655-660.
6. Sommer OJ, Kladosek A, Weiler V, et al. Rheumatoid arthritis: a practical guide to state-of-the-art imaging, image interpretation, and clinical implications. *RadioGraphics*. 2005;(25): 381-398.

CASE 24: ACHONDROPLASIA

PATIENT PRESENTATION

Newborn infant with short limbs.

CLINICAL SUSPICION

Achondroplasia

IMAGING MODALITY OF CHOICE

Evaluation of the skeletal manifestations of achondroplasia is best performed with a frontal full body radiograph, or "babygram," of the infant. This will demonstrate the abnormalities involving the skull, spine, pelvis, and extremities with limited radiation exposure.

Cross-sectional imaging with CT may be performed of the brain for evaluation of the size of the foramen magnum, as well as of the spine for evaluation of the vertebral bodies and narrowing of the spinal canal. MRI of the brain is recommended for evaluation of cervicomedullary compression at the foramen magnum.

FINDINGS

Achondroplasia is the most common cause of short-limb dwarfism and is a type of rhizomelic dwarfism, meaning that the greatest shortening involves the proximal limbs. It is due to a mutation in the fibroblast growth factor gene 3 (FGFR3), which causes abnormal cartilage formation. Achondroplasia is an autosomal dominant disease, and homozygous achondroplasia is a lethal condition.

Achondroplasia may be diagnosed antenatally and is usually most often evident in the third trimester with short femur length detected on ultrasound. Postnatal radiograph evaluation demonstrates findings in the skull, spine, pelvis, and extremities. Skull radiographs show enlargement of the skull, frontal bossing, midface hypoplasia, and a small foramen magnum (Fig. C24.1).

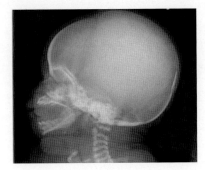

Fig. C24.1 Lateral radiograph of the skull shows enlarged skull with midface hypoplasia.

A characteristic finding that is identified on frontal view of the lumbar spine is progressive decrease of the lumbar interpedicular distance from proximal to distal, opposite of the normal relationship. Lateral view of the spine shows shortening of the pedicles and vertebral bodies with posterior vertebral scalloping. Other findings involving the spine include thoracolumbar kyphosis and scoliosis.

The pelvis demonstrates small squared iliac wings and a flat and broad pelvic inlet, referred to as a "champagne glass" pelvis (Fig. C24.2). The acetabular roof is horizontal and the sacroiliac notches are short. Findings in the chest include flaring of the anterior ribs and anteroposterior shortening of the ribs.

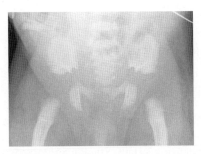

Fig. C24.2 Frontal view of the pelvis shows small squared iliac wings and horizontal acetabular roofs in a patient with achondroplasia.

There is shortening and thickening of the long bones with metaphyseal flaring and cupping, as well as bowing of the lower extremities (Fig. C24.3). The growth plates may be V shaped, and the phalanges are short and broad.

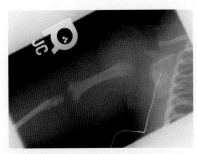

Fig. C24.3 Proximal limb shortening with associated metaphyseal flaring in achondroplasia.

Narrowing of the foramen magnum in patients with achondroplasia predisposes to spinal cord compression. MRI may show stenosis of the foramen magnum with compression of the cervicomedullary junction and increased T2 cord signal due to cord edema. MRI may identify other common findings in the spine of congenital canal stenosis, nerve root compression, and disc herniations. Hydrocephalus, communicating or noncommunicating, may be evaluated with CT or MRI.

DIFFERENTIAL DIAGNOSIS
Clinical Differential

Other clinical considerations for rhizomelic dwarfism include diastrophic dysplasia and thanatophoric dysplasia. Thanatophoric dysplasia is a fatal condition in early infancy commonly due to respiratory insufficiency. These patients have a large head with a prominent forehead, depressed nasal bridge, and small chest.

Patients with diastrophic dysplasia may be differentiated based on frequent findings of micrognathia, cleft palate, hand deformities, and flexion contractures.

Imaging Differential

Imaging differential considerations include thanatophoric dysplasia, diastrophic dysplasia, and osteogenesis imperfecta.

Thanatophoric dysplasia is a lethal skeletal dysplasia characterized by severe flattening of the vertebral bodies with a normal trunk length. Several findings may be similar to achondroplasia, including macrocephaly, frontal bossing with flattening of the nasal bridge, and small squared iliac wings. Thanatophoric dysplasia type I shows a curved, "telephone receiver" femur, and type II may be characterized by the "cloverleaf skull," which describes the appearance of bulging of the different bones of the cranial vault associated with pansynostosis or closure of all of the sutures.

Radiologic manifestations of diastrophic dysplasia include short tubular bones with metaphyseal flaring. Classically, the first metacarpal is rounded in shape and is proximally displaced in relation to the carpal bones, termed hitchhiker's thumb. Findings of the spine may include scoliosis, kyphosis, platyspondyly, and interpedicular narrowing of the lumbar spine. The feet demonstrate abduction of the great toes and clubfoot deformity.

Features of osteogenesis imperfecta vary with the type of disorder. The predominant radiologic findings include generalized osteoporosis, short tubular bones, fractures of long bones and ribs, and bowing deformities. There may also be vertebral fractures, vertebra plana, and kyphoscoliosis.

REFERENCES AND SUGGESTED READING

1. Lachman R, Sillence D, Rimion D, et al. Diastrophic dysplasia: the death of a variant. *Radiology*. 1981;140:79-86.
2. Dighe M, Fligner C, Cheng E, et al. Fetal skeletal dysplasia: an approach to diagnosis with illustrative cases. *RadioGraphics*. 2008;28:1061-1077.
3. Cheema JI, Grissom LE, Harcke HT. Radiographic characteristics of lower-extremity bowing in children. *RadioGraphics*. 2003;23:871-880.
4. Donnelly L. *Pediatric Imaging: The Fundamentals*. 1st ed. Philadelphia, PA: Saunders; 2009.

CASE 25: CLUBFOOT

PATIENT PRESENTATION

Initial physical examination of a newborn demonstrates the right foot is twisted inward.

CLINICAL SUSPICION

Clubfoot or talipes equinovarus

IMAGING MODALITY OF CHOICE

Plain radiographs are the initial imaging modality of choice for assessing alignment disorders of the foot. The technique for proper evaluation includes weight-bearing frontal and lateral views. Simulated weight-bearing views may be obtained in infants or nonambulatory patients. Weight-bearing views are indicated to evaluate the bones in their functional states in both the frontal and lateral views, and the tibia should be perpendicular to the image plane.

FINDINGS

The foot is divided into three compartments: the hindfoot, midfoot, and forefoot. The hindfoot includes the talus and calcaneus; the midfoot is composed of the cuboid, navicular, and cuneiform bones; and the metatarsals and phalanges are considered the forefoot.

Patients with talipes equinovarus, or clubfoot, demonstrate key components of plantarflexion of the calcaneus relative to the tibia, inversion of the hindfoot, and adduction of the forefoot. Plantarflexion of the calcaneus is also termed hindfoot equinus and refers to the anterior portion of the calcaneus abnormally plantarflexed in relation to the posterior calcaneus. This produces an abnormal tibiocalcaneal angle greater than 90 degrees, which is measured on the lateral radiograph as the angle between the long axis of the tibia and long axis of the calcaneus.

Hindfoot inversion can be identified on radiographs as inversion of the plantar aspect of the foot relative to the long axis of the tibia with the lateral radiograph showing near-parallel alignment of the talus and calcaneus (Fig. C25.1). There is resultant decrease of the talocalcaneal angle on both frontal and lateral views, normally measured 30 to 50 degrees on lateral view and 25 to 40 degrees on AP view.

There is also adduction of the forefoot characterized on the frontal view as increased overlap of the metatarsals. On the lateral view, the metatarsals will appear to be one on top of another in a ladderlike arrangement with the fifth metatarsal being most inferior (Fig. C25.2). Initial treatment includes noninvasive measures, such as physical therapy and bracing. If this is unsuccessful, surgical correction may be needed and may include a combination of soft tissue releases, osteotomies, and tendon transfers.

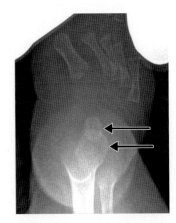

Fig. C25.1 AP radiograph of the foot shows forefoot adduction in clubfoot. There is also near-parallel alignment of the talus and calcaneus (arrows) indicating hindfoot inversion.

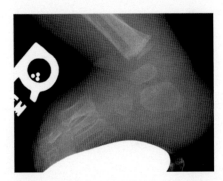

Fig. C25.2 Lateral radiograph of the foot shows stacked appearance of the metatarsals due to forefoot adduction in a patient with clubfoot.

DIFFERENTIAL DIAGNOSIS

Differential considerations include metatarsus adductus and rockerbottom foot. Metatarsus adductus is forefoot inversion without the other findings of clubfoot.

Rocker bottom flatfoot is a congenital anomaly of the foot that is characterized by a hyperextended foot with a convex sole. The calcaneus is in equinus, similar to that of talipes equinovarus, and there is dorsal dislocation of the navicular at the talonavicular joint with vertical talus. Rocker bottom foot can be a surgical complication of over-correction of a clubfoot.

REFERENCES AND SUGGESTED READING

1. Thapa MM, Pruthi S, Chew FS. Radiographic assessment of pediatric foot alignment: review. *AJR.* 2010;194(suppl):S51-S58.

2. Harty MP. Imaging of pediatric foot disorders. *Radiol Clin North Am.* 2001;39:733-748.

Chapter 10

Introduction to Women's Imaging

By Haitham Elsamaloty, Mohammed Al-Natour, Neda Haswah, Stephanie Holz, and Khaled M. Elsayes

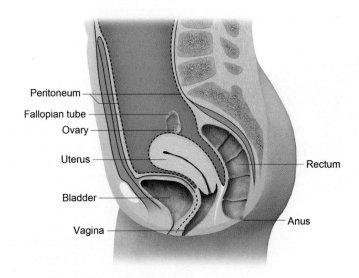

INTRODUCTION TO WOMEN'S IMAGING (FEMALE PELVIS IMAGING)

FEMALE PELVIS

The uterus is a pear-shaped organ located in the female pelvis between the urinary bladder anteriorly and the rectum posteriorly (Figs. 10.1 and 10.2). The average dimensions are approximately 8 cm long, 5 cm across, and 4 cm thick, with an average volume between 80 and 200 mL. The uterus is divided into 3 main parts: the fundus, body, and cervix.

Blood is provided to the uterus by the ovarian and uterine arteries, the latter of which arise from the anterior division of the internal iliac artery. The uterine artery occasionally gives off the vaginal artery (although this is usually a separate branch of the internal iliac artery), which

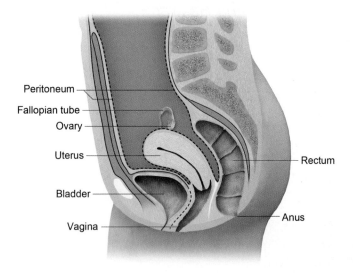

Peritoneum
Fallopian tube
Ovary
Uterus
Rectum
Bladder
Vagina
Anus

Fig. 10.1 Sagittal view of the female pelvis, demonstrating relative positions of the bladder, uterus, and rectum.

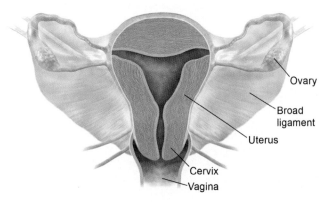

Ovary
Broad ligament
Uterus
Cervix
Vagina

Fig. 10.2 Illustration of the uterus, adnexal structures, and upper vagina.

supplies the upper vagina, and the arcuate arteries, which surround the uterus. It then further branches into the radial arteries, which penetrate the myometrium to provide blood to all layers, including the endometrium.

Once these vessels reach the endometrial level, they branch into the basal arteries and spiral arteries, which support the specialized functions of each layer. The basal arteries are not responsive to hormones; they support the basal endometrial layer, which provides the proliferative cells for endometrial growth. The spiral arteries supply the functionalis layer and are uniquely sensitive to steroid hormones. In ovulatory cycles in which pregnancy does not occur, menses results following constriction of these terminal arteries, causing endometrial breakdown with desquamation of the glands and stroma.

The ovaries are the female pelvic reproductive organs that house the ova and are responsible for the production of sex hormones. They are paired organs located on either side of the uterus within the broad ligament below the uterine (fallopian) tubes. The ovary is within the ovarian fossa, a space that is bound by the external iliac vessels, obliterated umbilical artery, and ureter. The ovaries are responsible for housing and releasing ova, or eggs, necessary for reproduction. At birth, a female has approximately 1 to 2 million ova, but only 300 of these eggs will ever become mature and be released for the purpose of fertilization.

The ovaries are small, oval-shaped, and grayish in color, with an uneven surface. The actual size of an ovary depends on a woman's age and hormonal status; the ovaries, covered by a modified peritoneum, are approximately 3 to 5 cm in length during childbearing years and become much smaller and then atrophic once menopause occurs. A cross section of the ovary reveals many cystic structures that vary in size. These structures represent ovarian follicles at different stages of development and degeneration.

Ultrasound is the imaging modality of choice for the female pelvis. It is widely available, has broad acceptance by patients as a familiar test, and is relatively inexpensive. High-resolution imaging of transvaginal ultrasound provides high diagnostic accuracy for pelvic pathology. However, there are some shortcomings with this modality, such as the limited field of view, obscuration of pelvic organs by the presence of bowel gas, inherent limitations dependent on patient size, and its dependence on the skill and experience of the operator. The American College of Radiology has provided guidelines for when ultrasound is an appropriate imaging tool for the evaluation of the female pelvis (Table 10.1).

For a pelvic sonogram performed transabdominally, the patient's urinary bladder should in general, be distended adequately to displace the small bowel and its contained gas from the field of view. Occasionally, overdistention of the bladder may compromise evaluation. When this occurs, imaging may be repeated after the patient partially empties the bladder.

Table 10.1 Indications for Pelvic Sonography

Indications for pelvic sonography include, but are not limited to:

1. Pelvic pain
2. Dysmenorrhea (painful menses)
3. Menorrhagia (excessive menstrual bleeding)
4. Metrorrhagia (irregular uterine bleeding)
5. Menometrorrhagia (excessive bleeding irregularly)
6. Follow-up of previously detected abnormality (eg, hemorrhagic cyst)
7. Evaluation and/or monitoring of infertile patients
8. Delayed menses or precocious puberty
9. Postmenopausal bleeding
10. Abnormal pelvic examination
11. Further characterization of a pelvic abnormality noted on another imaging study (eg, CT or MR)
12. Evaluation of congenital anomalies
13. Excessive bleeding, pain, or fever after pelvic surgery or delivery
14. Localization of intrauterine contraceptive device
15. Screening for malignancy in patients with an increased risk

For a transvaginal sonogram, the urinary bladder is preferably empty. The sonographer or the physician may introduce the vaginal transducer, preferably under real-time monitoring. When possible, a woman member of the physician or hospital's staff should be present as a chaperone in the examining room if a man is performing the examination.

Ultrasound has high diagnostic accuracy rates for uterine and ovarian abnormalities. MRI should be considered for the evaluation of adnexal pathology when sonographic characteristics are not definitive to determine whether an adnexal mass is ovarian in origin and to determine the likelihood of malignancy. MRI has an established role in the preprocedural and postprocedural assessment for uterine artery embolization, diagnosis of adenomyosis, staging of known endometrial and cervical carcinoma, evaluation of suspected Müllerian ductal anomalies, and presurgical workup for pelvic floor prolapse. Other indications include assessment of the pregnant patient with acute pelvic pain and of fetal anatomy. In most cases, fetal anatomy is well evaluated by ultrasound, but MRI can play a role in problem solving. For cases of acute pelvis and if there is a concern for acute appendicitis, the role of MRI has yet to be established. Beyond the period of organogenesis, CT may be considered. Within the period of organogenesis, however, MRI is a safe alternative, and limited studies to date have shown promising results.

REFERENCES AND SUGGESTED READING

1. Hubert J, Bergin D. Imaging the female pelvis: when should MRI be considered. *Appl Radiol.* 2008;37(1):9-24.
2. Katz VL, Lentz GM, Lobo RA, Gershenson DM. *Comprehensive Gynecology.* 5th ed. Philadelphia: Mosby Elsevier; 2007.
3. Gray H. *Anatomy, Descriptive and Surgical, The Unabridged Gray's Anatomy.* Philadelphia: Running Press; 1999.
4. Chung KW. *Gross Anatomy.* 4th ed. Philadelphia: Lippincott Williams & Wilkins; 2000.
5. ACR–ACOG–AIUM–SRU Practice Guideline for the Performance of Pelvic Ultrasound.

CASE 1: ECTOPIC PREGNANCY

PATIENT PRESENTATION

A 25-year-old woman presents to the ER complaining of pelvic pain and vaginal bleeding. Quantitative urine β-hCG is positive indicating early pregnancy. Patient has history of pelvic inflammatory disease.

CLINICAL SUSPICION

Ectopic pregnancy

IMAGING MODALITY OF CHOICE

Transabdominal and transvaginal pelvic ultrasound (TVS) in addition to color Doppler evaluation. Advantages: readily available, low cost, sensitive, no ionizing radiation, and color Doppler evaluation. The overall sensitivity of TVS to diagnose an ectopic pregnancy is 98.3%, with a specificity of 99.9%, a positive predictive value of 97.5%, and a negative predictive value of 100% [7].

FINDINGS

Ultrasound findings of tubal ectopic pregnancy (Figs. C1.1 and C1.2):

- Endometrium:
  - No intrauterine pregnancy; no gestational sac, no yolk sac, and no fetal pole in the endometrium.
  - Pseudosac that represents fluid centrally located in endometrial cavity with an absent double decidual reaction. Pseudosac is most often irregular in shape or flat (Fig. C1.1A).

- Fallopian tube or adnexa:
  - Echogenic ringlike mass in the right or left fallopian tubes or adnexa that is separate from the ovary. This echogenic region may have a yolk sac, embryonic pole with or without cardiac activity, and blood products (Figs. C1.1 and C1.2).
- Free fluid:
  - The presence of fluid with debris suggesting hemorrhage increases the likelihood of ectopic pregnancy (Fig. C1.2).
- Color Doppler:
  - Ring of color around the echogenic ringlike mass. "Ring of fire" (Fig. C1.2).

Ectopic pregnancy accounts for about 2% of all pregnancies and is the most common cause of pregnancy-related mortality in the first trimester. A history of pelvic pain along with bleeding and abnormal β-hCG levels should always trigger an evaluation for an ectopic pregnancy. The fallopian tube is the most common location for an ectopic pregnancy, accounting for about 95% of cases, though there are other rare types of ectopic pregnancies including interstitial, cornual, ovarian, cervical, scar (Fig. C1.3), intra-abdominal, and heterotopic.

RISK FACTORS FOR ECTOPIC PREGNANCY

- Prior ectopic pregnancy
- History of pelvic inflammatory disease; tubal scarring
- History of gynecologic surgery
- Infertility
- Use of intrauterine device

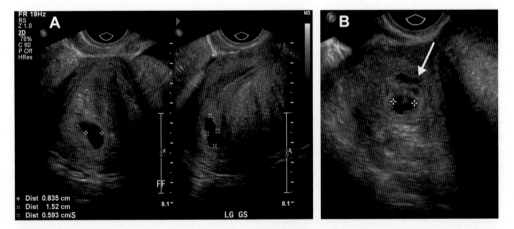

Fig. C1.1 (A) Transverse and longitudinal transvaginal gray-scale ultrasound images of a 26-year-old woman who presented with abdominal pain and positive urine β-hCG show an endometrial cavity full of fluid centrally without evidence of intrauterine pregnancy consistent with pseudosac (calipers). (B) Transverse transvaginal gray-scale ultrasound image of the same patient shows a ringlike mass (arrow) with yolk sac seen outside the uterus in the right adnexa consistent with an ectopic pregnancy.

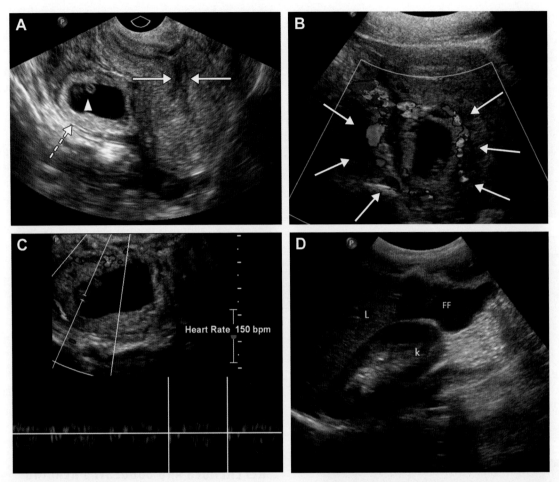

Fig. C1.2 Multiple transabdominal and transvaginal ultrasound images of a different patient with an ectopic pregnancy demonstrating (A) echogenic debris in the endometrial cavity (arrows) and a gestational sac (dashed arrow) with a yolk sac (arrowhead) outside the uterus. (B) "Ring of fire" appearance with prominent blood flow around the echogenic ring of the ectopic pregnancy is also seen (arrows). (C) Cardiac activity is seen in the ectopic pregnancy. (D) Longitudinal view of the right upper quadrant shows free fluid (FF) adjacent to the kidney compatible with a ruptured ectopic pregnancy. Liver (L), kidney (K). Note that "ring of fire" can also be seen with hemorrhagic cysts.

- History of placenta previa
- Use of in vitro fertilization
- Congenital uterine anomalies
- History of smoking
- Endometriosis; increases the risk for tubal scarring from fibrosis
- Intrauterine exposure to diethylstilbestrol

Ectopic pregnancy in a C-section scar is very rare with an incidence of 1:2,000 pregnancies, and it can lead to life-threatening complications such as uterine rupture and massive hemorrhage. Ultrasound guided methotrexate injection is emerging as the treatment modality of choice in stable patients. Subsequent pregnancies may also be complicated by uterine rupture, hence the uterine scar should be evaluated before as well as during those pregnancies.

DIFFERENTIAL DIAGNOSIS

Intrauterine pregnancy with hemorrhagic corpus luteum cyst: Always check for intrauterine pregnancy, which is diagnosed with intradecidual sign, double decidual sac sign, yolk sac, or embryo.

Adnexal cyst will be in the ovary rather than adjacent to the ovary. Although ovaries can be a rare location for an ectopic pregnancy, the cyst wall will be less echogenic than the wall of an ectopic pregnancy, and an anechoic cyst is unlikely to be an ectopic pregnancy. If diagnosis is unclear, a follow up sonogram and β-hCG will be helpful.

Heterotopic pregnancy: Very rare indicating combined intrauterine and extrauterine pregnancy. In such instances pregnancies are typically of similar gestational age.

Tubal cyst: Thin-walled anechoic cyst separate from the ovary.

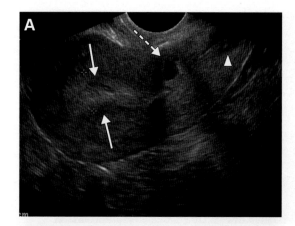

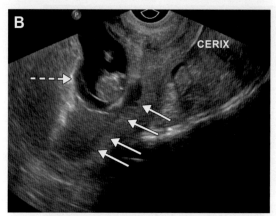

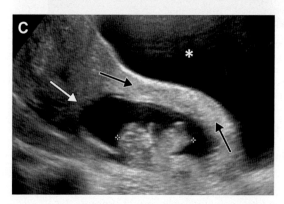

Fig. C1.3 Transabdominal gray-scale ultrasound image of the pelvis in this 32-year-old patient who presented with abdominal pain, positive urine β-hCG, and history of cesarean section 2 years prior to presentation show the rare case of an ectopic pregnancy in a cesarean scar. (A) There is an eccentric gestational sac within anterior myometrium in the lower uterine segment at the site of prior C-section scar (dashed arrow). An empty uterine cavity (arrows) and cervix (arrowhead) are seen. (B) Sagittal transvaginal ultrasound image of the pelvis for the same patient 4 weeks later shows a viable ectopic pregnancy at the site of prior C-section scar (dashed arrow) with an empty uterine cavity filled with blood (arrows). An empty cervix is seen again. (C) Transabdominal ultrasound image shows the eccentric anterior lower uterine gestational sac (white arrow) with thin myometrium (black arrows) between the sac and bladder (asterisk) compatible with scar ectopic pregnancy.

Tubo-ovarian abscess: Cervical motion tenderness when performing transvaginal sonography. Elevated white blood cell count

Exophytic leiomyoma: Broad base attachment to uterus. Usually multiple with similar echogenicity to other leiomyomas.

Instances where a positive pregnancy test is encountered without evidence of pregnancy could be due to early intrauterine or ectopic pregnancy and miscarriages; follow-up ultrasound and β-hCG should be performed. If it is an early pregnancy, follow-up β-hCG levels should show normal doubling in 2 days, while in ectopic pregnancy or miscarriages β-hCG should not rise normally or should decrease, although normal rise could be seen in 21% of ectopic pregnancy cases. Miscarriages can cause retrograde flow of blood into the tube mimicking ectopic pregnancy.

TREATMENT

- Watchful waiting in stable patient for spontaneous abortion.
- Methotrexate in reliable patients with ectopic pregnancy less than 5 cm and no fetal cardiac activity.
- Laparoscopy if patient presents with hemodynamic instability and possible tubal rupture.

REFERENCES AND SUGGESTED READING

1. Lin EP, Bhatt S, Dogra VS. Diagnostic clues to ectopic pregnancy. *RadioGraphics*. 2008;28(6):1661-1671.

2. Levine D. Ectopic pregnancy. *Radiology*. 2007;245(2): 385-397.

3. Mckenna DA, Poder L, Goldman M, et al. Role of sonography in the recognition, assessment, and treatment of cesarean scar ectopic pregnancies. *J Ultrasound Med*. 2008;27(5):779-783.

4. Seow KM, Huang LW, Lin YH, et al. Cesarean scar pregnancy: issues in management. *Ultrasound Obstet Gynecol*. 2004;23(3):247-253. doi:10.1002/uog.974.

5. Rotas MA, Haberman S, Levgur M. Cesarean scar ectopic pregnancies: etiology, diagnosis, and management. *Obstet Gynecol*. 2006;107(6):1373-1381. doi:10.1097/01. AOG.0000218690.24494.ce.

6. Michener C, Dickinson JE. Caesarean scar ectopic pregnancy: a single centre case series. *Aust N Z J Obstet Gynaecol*. 2009;49(5):451-455. doi:10.1111/j.1479-828X.2009.01067.x.

7. Kirk E, Papageorghiou AT, Condous G, et al. The diagnostic effectiveness of an initial transvaginal scan in detecting ectopic pregnancy. *Hum Reprod*. 2007;22:2824-2828.

CASE 2: GESTATIONAL TROPHOBLASTIC DISEASE

CASE PRESENTATION

A 48-year-old Asian woman who is 12 weeks pregnant presents to the emergency department with painless vaginal bleeding and hyperemesis. The patient has never had any primary workup or ultrasound studies during the first trimester. On clinical examination the patient seems to have a uterus that is larger than the expected gestational age and an elevated blood pressure. Laboratory workup shows β-hCG levels of 198,000.

CLINICAL SUSPICION

Complete hydatidiform mole

IMAGING MODALITY OF CHOICE

Transabdominal and transvaginal pelvic ultrasound. Advantages: readily available, low cost, sensitive, no ionizing radiation.

FINDINGS

Ultrasound findings for complete hydatidiform mole:

- Uterine cavity filled with multiple hypoechoic areas of varying size and shapes (vesicles) resembling a "bunch of grapes" that increase in size with gestational age is the best imaging clue (Fig. C2.1).
- Theca lutein cysts secondary to very high beta human chorionic gonadotropin levels (β-hCG) in up to 50% of cases. "Soap-bubble" or "spoke wheel" appearance (Fig. C2.2).
- Color Doppler: very vascular with very high velocity blood flow (Fig. C2.1).

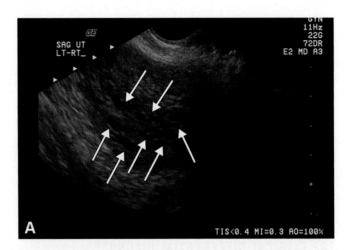

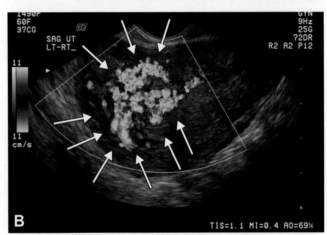

Fig. C2.1 Transvaginal ultrasound showing multiple cystic structures "cluster of grapes" (arrows) filling the uterine cavity, and absence of fetal parts (A). Color Doppler ultrasound shows the lesion to be highly vascular (arrows) (B). Appearance is compatible with complete hydatidiform mole.

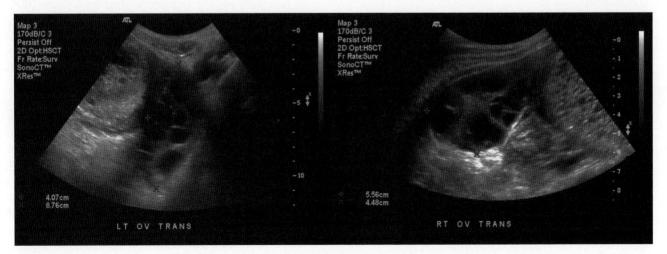

Fig. C2.2 Transabdominal gray-scale ultrasound images shows enlarged bilateral ovaries with replacement of parenchyma with multiple multilocular cysts giving a "soap bubble" appearance consistent with theca lutein cysts, classically seen with molar pregnancy.

- First trimester moles may have a sonographic appearance simulating that of an incomplete abortion.

Ultrasonography has replaced all other means in early screening and is the examination of choice for initial diagnosis. However, CT typically shows an enlarged uterus with central areas of low attenuation, and MRI typically shows a uterine mass of heterogeneously T2 high signal intensity that distends the endometrial cavity. The T2 high signal intensity is mainly due to numerous cystic spaces, which typically show low T1 signal intensity. Foci of T1 increased signal intensity can also correspond to areas of hemorrhage.

TOP CLINICAL DIFFERENTIAL DIAGNOSES

- Multiple gestations
- Invasive mole
- Choriocarcinoma
- Triploidy
- Threatened abortion
- Ectopic pregnancy

TOP IMAGING DIFFERENTIAL DIAGNOSES

Placental hydropic degeneration: This represents hydropic changes without proliferation often seen after failed pregnancy due to fetal demise or anembryonic gestation. This can look similar to complete hydatidiform mole, but it is less vascular and clinically associated with low β-hCG levels rather than high levels as seen with complete moles.

Placental sonolucencies (pseudomole): This is often a normal finding after 25 weeks of gestation, but it could be associated with preeclampsia and intrauterine growth restriction.

Partial mole (also known as triploidy): Similar in appearance to complete mole; however, the presence of fetal tissue is specific to partial moles. Differential diagnosis includes twin gestation, one of which is a complete mole, or placental hemorrhages discussed in Fig. C2.3.

Invasive mole or choriocarcinoma: Those are largely indistinguishable on imaging and look similar to complete moles on ultrasonography. MRI has the ability to demonstrate myometrial and parametrial invasion; however, again invasive mole vs choriocarcinoma is an exclusively histological diagnosis even though the presence of metastasis can suggest choriocarcinoma rather than invasive mole.

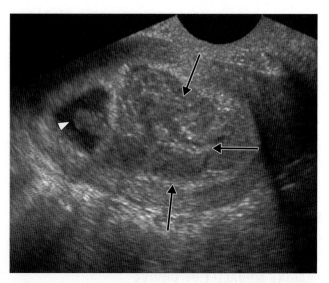

Fig. C2.3 Transvaginal gray-scale ultrasound image shows echogenic material filling the majority of the uterine cavity (arrows). Adjacent to this material is a gestational sac containing an embryo (arrowhead). These findings were due to a pathologically proven partial mole. The differential diagnosis for this appearance includes twin gestation, one of which is a complete mole. Differential also includes a large subchorionic hemorrhage, which can be distinguished on the basis of the β-hCG level and the presence of vascular flow within the molar tissue. No flow would be expected in a hemorrhage.

Used with permission from Elsayes KM, Trout AT, Friedkin AM, et al. Imaging of the placenta: a multimodality pictorial review. *RadioGraphics.* 2009;29:1371-1391.

DISCUSSION

Complete hydatidiform moles are the most common gestational trophoblastic neoplastic tumors and are considered essentially benign. They are mainly due to proliferative growth of trophoblastic tissue and may become invasive in 12% to 15% of cases or develop into choriocarcinoma in 5% to 8% of the cases.

A complete mole is typically formed by a single (90%) or two (10%) sperm combining with an ovum that has an inactive nucleus leading to a 100% paternal genetic makeup, which most commonly has a karyotype of 46, XX. This chromosomal abnormality results in loss of the embryo and proliferation of trophoblastic tissue.

A partial mole on the contrary is typically formed by a normal ovum that is fertilized by two sperms or one sperm that duplicates itself yielding the karyotype of 69, XXX or 69, XXY (triploidy). Fetal tissue is present with partial moles, but fetal growth is often complicated by severe symmetric growth restriction, multiple structural anomalies, and oligohydramnios. Partial moles look similar to complete mole on ultrasound evaluation; however, the presence of fetal tissue is unique for partial moles (Fig. C2.3).

Complete hydatidiform moles have a higher risk of developing into choriocarcinoma than do partial moles.

The incidence of complete moles in the United States is 0.5:1,000 in comparison to 8:1,000 in Asia.

Prognosis for complete mole is overall good. Malignant degeneration to an invasive form or choriocarcinoma can occur; those usually tend to be generally highly chemosensitive and carry a much better cure rate than other comparable malignancies despite their aggressiveness.

RISK FACTORS

- Age: < 20 y (2 fold), > 40 y (10 fold), and >50 y (50% chance).
- Prior molar pregnancy.
- Contraception: Combined oral contraceptive pills have been proved to double the chances of molar pregnancy.
- Previous spontaneous abortion: double the incidence.
- Multiple sexual partners.

TREATMENT

- Suction and curettage followed by metastatic disease workup.
- Hysterectomy advocated by gynecologists in patients over 35 years old who are not interested in preserving fertility.

- After evacuation, β-hCG levels should be monitored weekly until it is undetectable followed by monthly monitoring for 6 to 24 months.
- In women with persistent disease or chemotherapy resistant disease, angiography is useful in workup of myometrial invasion and surgical management.
- Pregnancy should be postponed if desired to avoid confusing the clinical picture while monitoring β-hCG levels.

REFERENCES AND SUGGESTED READING

1. Bertel C, Atri M, Arenson AM, et al. Sonographic diagnosis of gestational trophoblastic disease and comparison with retained products of conception. *J Ultrasound Med.* 2006;25 (8):985-993.
2. Zhou Q, Lei XY, Xie Q, et al. Sonographic and Doppler imaging in the diagnosis and treatment of gestational trophoblastic disease: a 12-year experience. *J Ultrasound Med.* 2005;24: 15-24.
3. Leyendecker JR, Gorengaut V, Brown JJ. MR imaging of maternal disease of the abdomen and pelvis during pregnancy and the immediate postpartum period. *RadioGraphics.* 2004;24(5):1301-1316.
4. Elsayes KM, Trout AT, Friedkin AM, et al. Imaging of the placenta: a multimodality pictorial review. *RadioGraphics* 2009;29:1371-1391.

CASE 3: PLACENTAL PATHOLOGY

PATIENT PRESENTATION

A 40-year-old woman who presents at 30 weeks of gestation with vaginal bleeding.

CLINICAL SUSPICION

Placenta previa, placental abruption

IMAGING MODALITY OF CHOICE

Transvaginal and transabdominal ultrasound. Advantages: readily available, low cost, sensitive, no ionizing radiation.

DIFFERENTIAL DIAGNOSIS

Antepartum hemorrhage is defined as vaginal bleeding between 20 weeks of gestation and delivery, and it is considered a major factor of maternal and fetal morbidity and mortality. Placenta previa and placental abruption are by far the most common causes of antepartum hemorrhage.

Placenta previa refers to an abnormally located placenta in which the placenta is near or covers the cervical internal os. Placental abruption represents separation of the placenta from the uterine wall. While both placenta previa and placental abruption usually present with vaginal bleeding, placental abruption seems to be associated with abdominal/pelvic pain that is sudden in onset. Transvaginal and transabdominal ultrasound are essential for diagnosis.

ACR appropriateness criteria in order of preference for second and third trimester bleeding with or without pain:

1. **US transabdominally.** If cervix and placenta are not visualized transabdominally, further evaluation with transvaginal or transperineal US should be done unless contraindicated as discussed below.

2. **US transvaginal.** Considered safe in patients with placenta previa or placental abruption, even in those who present with vaginal bleeding [9]. This can be done particularly when transabdominal US is inconclusive. If there is evidence of ruptured membranes or open cervix with bulging amniotic sac at or below the external os, transvaginal US is contraindicated.

3. **US transperineal.** This is least preferred.

Placenta Previa

Placenta previa most often presents with painless bleeding, and the diagnosis should never be made before 15 weeks of gestation. There are four types of placenta previa based on position of the placenta in relation to the internal cervical os (Table C3.1). Screening to rule out placenta previa should be done as part of the second trimester anatomic survey examination, and if a complete or central placenta previa

Table C3.1 Subtypes of Placenta Previa

Placenta Previa Subtype	Description
Low-lying placenta (Fig. C3.2)	Lower placental margin is within 2 cm of the internal cervical os.
Marginal previa (Fig. C3.3)	Placenta extends to the edge of the internal os but does not cover it.
Complete previa (Fig. C3.4)	Placenta covers the internal os.
Central previa (Fig. C3.5)	Central placenta is implanted directly over the internal os.

Used with permission from Elsayes KM, Trout AT, Friedkin AM, et al. Imaging of the placenta: a multimodality pictorial review. *RadioGraphics.* 2009;29:1371-1391.

is diagnosed, those will not likely resolve with advancing pregnancy, and appropriate action needs to be made such as bed rest, hospitalization, maternal blood transfusion, and delivery will be likely with cesarean section. However, if marginal or low-lying placenta is seen, a repeat ultrasound at 32 weeks should be done to ensure the placental edge has migrated farther away from the internal os [5]. Advance maternal age (≥35) is associated with increased incidence of placenta previa at time of delivery. Prognosis of placenta previa is excellent if picked up early during antenatal care and subsequently appropriately managed.

US will reliably exclude placenta previa if the lower placental edge is shown to lie >2 cm away from the internal cervical os (Fig. C3.1). This is most often accomplished by transabdominal examination of the cervix and lower uterine segment with the bladder moderately full; but the bladder

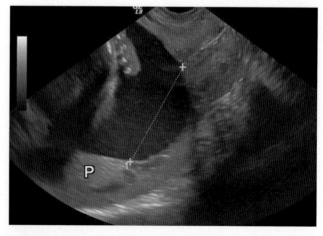

Fig. C3.1 Transvaginal US image obtained at 27 weeks gestation shows a posterior placenta (P) without previa. The most caudal tip of the placenta is nearly 5 cm (cursors) from the internal cervical os. Distances greater than 2 cm are considered normal.

Used with permission from Elsayes KM, Trout AT, Friedkin AM, et al. Imaging of the placenta: a multimodality pictorial review. *RadioGraphics.* 2009;29:1371-1391.

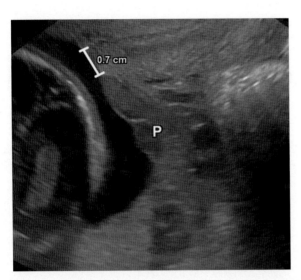

Fig. C3.2 Transvaginal US image obtained at 20 weeks gestation shows a low-lying placenta (P). The placental margin comes to within 0.7 cm of the internal cervical os.

Used with permission from Elsayes KM, Trout AT, Friedkin AM, et al. Imaging of the placenta: a multimodality pictorial review. *RadioGraphics*. 2009;29:1371-1391.

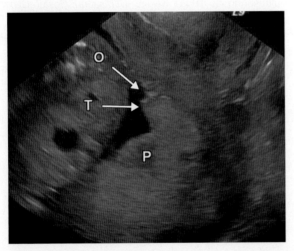

Fig. C3.3 Transvaginal US image obtained at 19 weeks gestation shows marginal placenta previa. The placental tip (T) is located immediately at the internal cervical os (O) but does not cover it. P = body of the placenta.

Used with permission from Elsayes KM, Trout AT, Friedkin AM, et al. Imaging of the placenta: a multimodality pictorial review. *RadioGraphics*. 2009;29:1371-1391.

should not be so full as to artificially elongate the cervix [4]. Focal myometrial contraction can cause the uterine walls to come closer together and falsely show placenta previa; however, this will resolve once contractions resolve.

Placental Abruption

Placental abruption can be diagnosed by ultrasonography by showing placental detachment with an accompanying clot (Fig. C3.6). If gray-scale sonography is challenging,

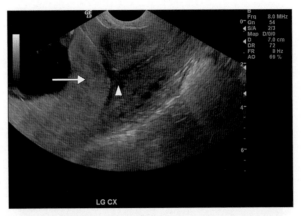

Fig. C3.4 Transvaginal US image obtained at 20 weeks gestation shows complete placenta previa. The placenta (arrow) entirely covers the internal cervical os (arrowhead).

Used with permission from Elsayes KM, Trout AT, Friedkin AM, et al. Imaging of the placenta: a multimodality pictorial review. *RadioGraphics*. 2009;29:1371-1391.

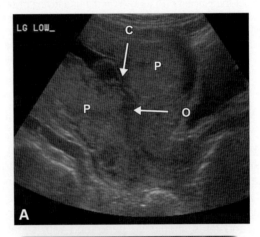

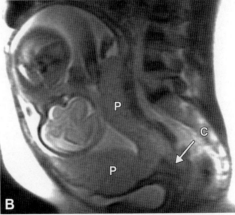

Fig. C3.5 Transabdominal US image obtained at 18 weeks gestation (A) and sagittal SSFSE MR image obtained at 29 weeks gestation (B) show central placenta previa. The placenta (P) entirely covers the internal cervical os (O) in (A). In the case shown in the US image, the umbilical cord (C) in (A) inserts immediately above the os. C in (B) = uterine cervix.

Used with permission from Elsayes KM, Trout AT, Friedkin AM, et al. Imaging of the placenta: a multimodality pictorial review. *RadioGraphics*. 2009;29:1371-1391.

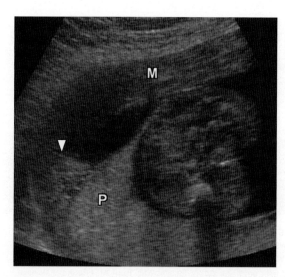

Fig. C3.6 US image shows placental abruption in another patient. A crescenteric collection of predominantly hypoechoic fluid lifts the edge of the placenta (P) away from the underlying myometrium (M). The fluid collection contains layering high-attenuation material (arrowhead), a finding consistent with blood.

Used with permission from Elsayes KM, Trout AT, Friedkin AM, et al. Imaging of the placenta: a multimodality pictorial review. *RadioGraphics.* 2009;29:1371-1391.

color Doppler can be helpful sometimes that shows no flow in blood clot.

Risk factors for developing placental abruption include smoking, blunt abdominal trauma, cocaine use during pregnancy, advanced maternal age, prior C section, leiomyoma, prior placental abruption, and multiparity.

In cases of placental abruption, close monitoring of the mother and fetus should be performed with serial ultrasound follow-up. If there is any evidence of placental insufficiency including bradycardia and increased systolic/diastolic ratio in the umbilical cord, early delivery and even cesarean section in cases of acute distress should be done rather than expectant management.

REFERENCES AND SUGGESTED READING

1. Elsayes KM, Trout AT, Friedkin AM, et al. Imaging of the placenta: a multimodality pictorial review. *RadioGraphics.* 2009;29:1371-1391.

2. Bhide A, Thilaganathan B. Recent advances in the management of placenta previa. *Curr Opin Obstet Gynecol.* 2004;16(6):447-451.

3. Moodley J, Ngambu NF, Corr P. Imaging techniques to identify morbidly adherent placenta praevia: a prospective study. *J Obstet Gynaecol.* 2004;24(7):742-744.

4. Sunna E. Transvaginal and transabdominal ultrasound for the diagnosis of placenta praevia. *J Obstet Gynaecol.*1999;19(2):152-154.

5. Hertzberg BS, Bowie JD, Carroll BA, Kliewer MA, Weber TM. Diagnosis of placenta previa during the third trimester: role of transperineal sonography. *AJR.* 1992;159(1):83-87.

6. Olive EC, Roberts CL, Nassar N, Algert CS. Test characteristics of placental location screening by transabdominal ultrasound at 18-20 weeks. *Ultrasound Obstet Gynecol.* 2006;28(7):944-949.

7. American College of Radiology ACR Appropriateness Criteria: www.acr.org.

8. Kaakaji Y, Nghiem HV, Nodell C, et al. Sonography of obstetric and gynecologic emergencies: part I, obstetric emergencies. *AJR.* 2000;174(3):641-649.

9. Masselli G, Brunelli R, Di Tola M, et al. MR imaging in the evaluation of placental abruption: correlation with sonographic findings. *Radiology.* 2011;259(1):222-230.

10. Sauerbrei EE, Pham DH. Placental abruption and subchorionic hemorrhage in the first half of pregnancy: US appearance and clinical outcome. *Radiology.* 1986;160(1):109-112.

CASE 4: CLUBFOOT

CLINICAL PRESENTATION

A 25-year-old woman who presents at 20 weeks for routine second trimester ultrasound. Sonographer notices an abnormally inward oriented foot.

CLINICAL SUSPICION

Clubfoot

IMAGING MODALITY OF CHOICE

Transabdominal pelvic ultrasound. Advantages: readily available, low cost, sensitive, no ionizing radiation.

FINDINGS

Sonographic findings for clubfoot (Figs. C4.1 and C4.2):

- Normally, in the coronal plane, the long axis of the foot should not be seen in the same plane as the long axis of the lower leg; however, in clubfoot the long axis of the foot and lower leg will be seen in the same coronal plane.
- Clubfoot shows an abnormal orientation of foot and ankle, where the foot is inverted at the ankle and plantar flexed (talipes equinovarus, *equino* = plantar flexed, *varus* = inward orientation).
- 3-D ultrasound may be helpful as well.
- After birth, plain films of neonate with clubfoot will show hind foot deformity with the talus and calcaneus parallel to each other.

DISCUSSION

Clubfoot has a high association with aneuploidy, particularly with trisomy 18, and other entities such as oligohydramnios,

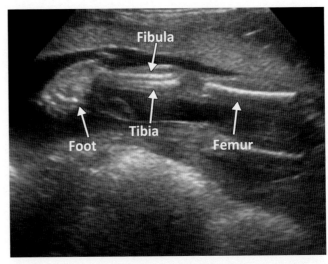

Fig. C4.1 Gray-scale sonographic image from fetal survey showing a clubfoot. Coronal image of the long axis of both the right foot and lower leg (arrows) are seen in the same coronal plane. The foot is inverted and lies at a sharp angle relative to the lower leg.

spina bifida, or a result of intrauterine growth restriction. There is a positive familial correlation. Usually manifests as bilateral (Fig. C4.2) but can be an isolated finding. It is usually found during routine second trimester fetal survey.

DIFFERENTIAL DIAGNOSIS

Rocker bottom foot:

- Convex foot secondary to a vertical talus orientation, which can also have an associated clubfoot.
- Strong association with trisomy 18.

Amniotic band syndrome:

- Abnormal amnion may cause fetal parts to be restricted.
- May result in missing toes and foot deformity.

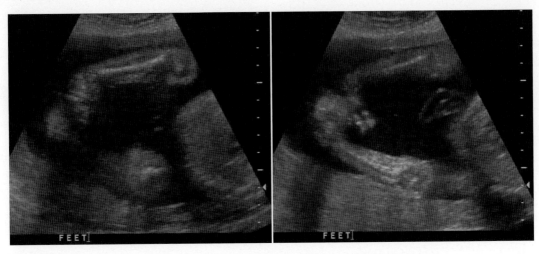

Fig. C4.2 Gray-scale sonographic image of a different patient from a fetal survey shows bilateral clubfoot.

TREATMENT

Surgically corrected based on severity of deformity. Most result in surgical management; however, conservative management as done for nonsevere minority. Decision for surgery is not made until at least 3 months of age postnatal.

REFERENCES AND SUGGESTED READING

1. Ippolito E, Fraracci L, Farsetti P, et al. Validity of the anteroposterior talocalcaneal angle to assess congenital clubfoot correction. *AJR.* 2004;182(5):1279-1282.

2. Mammen L, Benson CB. Outcome of fetuses with clubfeet diagnosed by prenatal sonography. *J Ultrasound Med.* 2004;23(4):497-500.

3. Canto MJ, Cano S, Palau J, et al. Prenatal diagnosis of clubfoot in low-risk population: associated anomalies and long-term outcome. *Prenat Diagn.* 2008;28(4):343-346.

4. Offerdal K, Jebens N, Blaas HG, et al. Prenatal ultrasound detection of talipes equinovarus in a nonselected population of 49 314 deliveries in Norway. *Ultrasound Obstet Gynecol.* 2007;30(6):838-844.

CASE 5: CHIARI II MALFORMATION

CASE PRESENTATION

A 38-year-old woman who is 16 weeks pregnant presents for fetal ultrasound due to abnormal maternal serum screening test showing elevated maternal serum α-fetoprotein (AFP).

CLINICAL SUSPICION

Open neural tube defect (ONTD)

IMAGING MODALITY OF CHOICE

Transabdominal pelvic ultrasound. Advantages: readily available, low cost, sensitive, no ionizing radiation.

OVERVIEW

Chiari II malformation is a fairly common congenital anomaly of the spine and posterior fossa characterized by spina bifida (meningocele/myelomeningocele) and posterior fossa hypoplasia.

The pathophysiology behind Chiari II malformation is thought to be secondary to CSF leakage through open spinal dysraphism during the fourth week of gestation allowing for CSF to flow through the central canal so it is therefore not maintained in the ventricular system. Ventricular distention is the driving force for development of the calvaria, and given its absence, the posterior fossa never fully develops. Later during gestation, the rhombencephalon rapidly develops, forcing the cerebellum cephalad and caudad along with the brainstem due to hypoplasia of the posterior fossa. Ultimately the flow of CSF through the foramina of Luschka and Magendie becomes blocked or impaired by crowding of structures in the posterior fossa explaining the ventriculomegaly and hydrocephalus in Chiari II patients.

FINDINGS

Ultrasound findings for Chiari II malformation:

Posterior fossa compression: Small or obliterated cisterna magna. This is the most common finding, which is seen on routine axial posterior fossa view and considered when the cisterna magna measures less than 3 mm. The cerebellum usually is small and compressed; severe compression of the cerebellum leads to banana sign.

Ventriculomegaly: Normal unilateral transverse lateral ventricle atrial dimension measured in the posterior horns just above the level of the thalami should not exceed 10 mm. Mild ventriculomegaly (10-12 mm) is seen in 50% of fetal ultrasounds for Chiari II malformation. Usually ventriculomegaly progresses during pregnancy with 90% of Chiari II fetuses having ventriculomegaly at birth (Fig. C5.1).

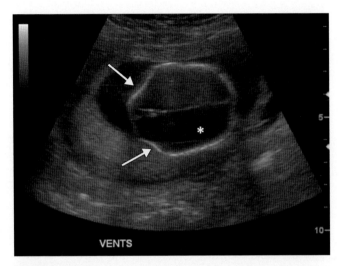

Fig. C5.1 Axial ultrasound image of the head showing a frontal bone concavity leading to the "lemon sign" (arrows). There is enlargement of bilateral ventricles consistent with ventriculomegaly (asterisk).

Triangular shaped ventricle sometimes seen.

Frontal bone concavity, also known as "lemon sign": This sign is nonspecific and can be seen in 1% of all second trimester fetuses. It is usually transient and often seen in the second trimester only (Fig. C5.1).

Dorsal vertebral defect: Eight percent of the defects have an overlying sac. If there is skin covering the defect, this will not be Chiari II malformation. The defect could either contain a meningocele (simple anechoic sac) or a myelomeningocele (heterogenous complex sac). Twenty percent have no sac, also known as myeloschisis. The ONTD is lumbar > sacral > thoracic > cervical (Fig. C5.2).

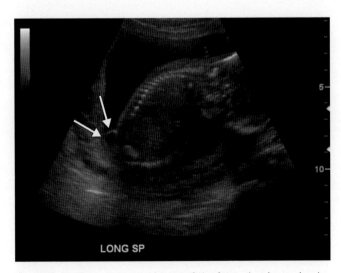

Fig. C5.2 Sagittal ultrasound image of the fetus showing a simple anechoic sac at the dorsal aspect of the lumbar spine consistent with a meningocele (arrows).

- Clubfoot is seen in 24% of Chiari II cases.
- Scoliosis and/or kyphosis are usually seen at the level of the ONTD.

Chiari II malformation is associated with high morbidity and mortality with about 35% of live-born babies dying within the first 5 years.

Clinical symptomatology varies in severity depending on the range of anatomical severity. Common clinical presentations include those of brain stem dysfunction, cranial nerve palsies, neurogenic bladder, those related to myelomeningocele, hydrocephalus, musculoskeletal, and kyphoscoliosis.

Chiari II malformation is associated with trisomy 18 and 13, with slight increase in risk with advanced maternal age.

Folate deficiency and teratogenic anticonvulsants have been related to Chiari II malformation as they are known to cause open neural tube defects.

TREATMENT

An elevated maternal serum α-fetoprotein can trigger antenatal diagnosis. If any suspicious findings are seen on ultrasound, a fetal MRI should be obtained to better detect and characterize the full constellation of findings associated with Chiari II malformation.

Once the diagnosis is established antenatally, arrangement should be made for cesarean delivery at term to decrease risk of meningomyelocele sac rupture and decrease risk of infection. An immediate postnatal ONTD surgery should be done, and almost 80% need ventriculoperitoneal shunting. In utero interventions are evolving.

Preventive treatment with folic acid at the preconception stage can reduce the risk for developing ONTD and decrease recurrence by about 70%.

IMAGING DIFFERENTIAL DIAGNOSES

Differential diagnosis for ventriculomegaly (hydrocephalus):

Aqueductal stenosis: Obstruction of the aqueduct of Sylvius leading to noncommunicating hydrocephalus, which is often severe and progressive. However, in this case, a normal posterior fossa is seen.

Dandy-Walker malformation: Partial or complete agenesis of the cerebellar vermis leading to enlargement of the cisterna Magana. The fourth ventricle is communicating with cisterna magna and often ventriculomegaly is seen.

Communicating hydrocephalus secondary to infection or hemorrhage.

Differential diagnosis for calvarial abnormalities:

Craniosynostosis: Premature suture fusion leading to abnormal calvarial shape and may cause a small posterior fossa however spine is most often normal.

Isolated frontal bone concavity: Seen in 1% of normal fetuses.

REFERENCES AND SUGGESTED READING

1. El Gammal T, Mark EK, Brooks BS. MR imaging of Chiari II malformation. *AJR.* 1988;150(1):163-170.

2. Hadley DM. The Chiari malformations. *J Neurol Neurosurg Psychiatr.* 2002;72(suppl 2):ii38-ii40.

3. Naidich TP, Pudlowski RM, Naidich JB, et al. Computed tomographic signs of the Chiari II malformation. Part I: Skull and dural partitions. *Radiology.* 1980;134(1):65-71.

4. Curnes JT, Oakes WJ, Boyko OB. MR imaging of hindbrain deformity in Chiari II patients with and without symptoms of brainstem compression. *AJNR.* 1989;10(2):293-302.

5. Naidich TP, Mclone DG, Fulling KH. The Chiari II malformation: Part IV. The hindbrain deformity. *Neuroradiology.* 1983;25(4):179-197.

6. Dipietro MA, Venes JL, Rubin JM. Arnold-Chiari II malformation: intraoperative real-time US. *Radiology.* 1987;164(3):799-804.

7. Maixner WJ. *Spina Bifida, Management and Outcome.* Springer; 2008. ISBN:8847006511.

CASE 6: CONGENITAL PULMONARY AIRWAY MALFORMATION

PATIENT PRESENTATION

A 28-year-old woman with abnormal chest findings on anatomical fetal ultrasound at 20 weeks of gestation.

OVERVIEW

Congenital pulmonary airway malformation (CPAM), also known previously as congenital cystic adenomatoid malformation (CCAM), is a lung hamartoma with proliferation of terminal bronchioles and lack of normal alveoli. The hamartomatous lesion communicates with the tracheobronchial tree and is supplied by the pulmonary artery and drained by the pulmonary vein. Terminology has been changed to better reflect the developmental disorder of airway morphogenesis as such a lesion can be neither cystic nor adenomatoid.

CPAM is rare; however, it is considered the most common respiratory tract congenital malformation and accounts for about 75% of fetal lung masses encountered antenatally. The reported incidence rate of CPAM ranges from 1 in 11,000 to 1 in 35,000 live births with a higher incidence in midtrimester ultrasounds due to spontaneous resolution as will be discussed later.

The pathogenesis of such lesions is poorly understood. There are no genetic causes or recurrence risk described; however there is association with other abnormalities in 3% to 12% of the cases, most commonly other lung malformations, including sequestrations, and renal anomalies.

CPAMs are usually discovered incidentally on antenatal ultrasound seen as cystic or echogenic lung mass and usually show greatest growth at 20 to 26 weeks of gestation. Ninety-five percent of those are unilateral and usually affect one lobe without any definite side of predilection.

IMAGING FINDINGS

Ultrasound findings of CPAM (Fig. C6.1):

- Variable appearance from solid (microcystic) to complex cystic mass (macrocystic). There are at least three subtypes of (CPAM) classified based on size of cyst. Type I is the most common one (70%) and has one or more large dominant cysts (3-10 cm). Type II represents about 20% of all CPAM cases and consist of smaller cysts measuring less than 2 cm in diameter. Type III represents about 10% of cases and has only microcysts measuring less than 5 mm in diameter. Type III typically involves an entire lung and has a worse prognosis.
- Color Doppler evaluation shows the mass is supplied by the pulmonary artery and drained by the pulmonary vein; however, this can be difficult to demonstrate.

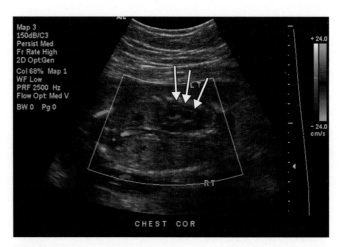

Fig. C6.1 Coronal color Doppler ultrasound image of the posterior chest showing a large multicystic mass in the left lung (arrows). The aorta is seen, and it does not seem to provide any blood supply to the mass in the left hemithorax compatible with CPAM.

- Heart is displaced.
- Stomach is in normal location.
- Hydrops, which is the most important predictor factor for outcomes and occurs in < 10% of cases leading to dismal prognosis.
- Polyhydramnios, which may result from compression of the esophagus and is associated with hydrops.

MANAGEMENT

CPAM has increased risk for developing hydrops fetalis and fetal demise especially if represented by a large dominant cyst or if the CPAM volume ratio (CVR) > 1.6, which can be calculated sonographically (CPAM volume/head circumference).

The majority of CPAM lesion stabilize or regress in utero over the course of pregnancy, and once the diagnosis is suspected antenatally, weekly ultrasound monitoring should be performed until growth stabilizes with special attention to developing hydrops. If CVR > 1.4, betamethasone should be considered, which has been shown to decrease growth. In the case where hydrops is seen, in utero interventions should be considered as almost 100% mortality is seen if untreated. Otherwise excellent prognosis is seen without hydrops even if large at the time of diagnosis.

Postnatally, CPAM patients have increased risk for neonatal complications including air trapping and pneumothorax as well as infection, which can also present later in life. There is a small risk for malignant transformation throughout childhood and adulthood.

Delivery should be done in a tertiary facility capable with dealing with the abovementioned complications, and postnatal workup should be performed for all lesions even if regressed in utero or even in asymptomatic individuals by obtaining CT of the chest with contrast as CXR can fail to identify it. Most authors believe that the risk of infection and malignancy warrants resection, which is usually performed at 1 month of age or later, as early resection can maximize compensatory lung growth.

TOP DIFFERENTIAL DIAGNOSES

Bronchopulmonary sequestration (BPS): Indistinguishable from microcystic CPAM on gray-scale imaging. Feeding vessel is from aorta, and 90% are left-sided with ipsilateral effusion.

Hybrid lesion (CPAM + BPS): Dual pathology has been reported in as many as 50% of echogenic lung mass cases, and such diagnosis should be considered when a systemic vessel supplies a cystic lung mass.

Congenital diaphragmatic hernia: Peristalsis on ultrasonography is pathognomonic with small abdominal circumference due to absent normal fluid-filled stomach and small bowel loops.

Congenital lobar obstruction: Uniformly echogenic and usually in the upper lobes. This is rarely diagnosed in utero and usually manifests postnatally as lobar emphysema.

Teratoma: Solid and cystic components with calcifications, which is the most specific component.

Tracheal atresia: Can be confused for bilateral CPAM. Usually associated with inversion of the diaphragm with fluid-filled trachea and bronchi as well as ascites.

Other cystic masses: These include bronchogenic cyst, esophageal duplication cyst, and neuroenteric cyst. Such lesions are more often seen in the mediastinum rather than the lungs.

REFERENCES AND SUGGESTED READING

1. Rosado-de-Christenson ML, Stocker JT. Congenital cystic adenomatoid malformation. *RadioGraphics*. 1991;11(5): 865-886.

2. Berrocal T, Madrid C, Novo S, et al. Congenital anomalies of the tracheobronchial tree, lung, and mediastinum: embryology, radiology, and pathology. *RadioGraphics*. 2004; 24(1):e17.

3. Gross GW. Pediatric chest imaging. *Curr Opin Radiol*. 1992;4(5):36-43.

4. Collins J, Stern EJ. *Chest Radiology, the Essentials*. Lippincott Williams & Wilkins; 2007. ISBN:0781763142.

5. Evans MI. *Prenatal Diagnosis*. McGraw-Hill Professional; 2006. ISBN:0838576826.

6. Lee EY, Boiselle PM, Cleveland RH. Multidetector CT evaluation of congenital lung anomalies. *Radiology*. 2008;247(3):632-648.

7. Entezami M, Albig M, Knoll U, et al. *Ultrasound Diagnosis of Fetal Anomalies*. Thieme; 2003. ISBN:1588902129.

8. Chen WS, Yeh GP, Tsai HD. et al. Prenatal diagnosis of congenital cystic adenomatoid malformations: evolution and outcome. *Taiwan J Obstet Gynecol*. 2009;48(3):278-281.

9. Ierullo AM, Ganapathy R, Crowley S, et al. Neonatal outcome of antenatally diagnosed congenital cystic adenomatoid malformations. *Ultrasound Obstet Gynecol*. 2005;26(2): 150-153.

10. Tran H, Fink MA, Crameri J, et al. Congenital cystic adenomatoid malformation: monitoring the antenatal and short-term neonatal outcome. *Aust N Z J Obstet Gynaecol*. 2008;48(5):462-466.

CASE 7: FIRST TRIMESTER INCREASED NUCHAL TRANSLUCENCY

PATIENT PRESENTATION

A 40-year-old woman who is 12 weeks pregnant who was referred for fetal ultrasound by her OB-GYN doctor due to abnormal maternal serum screening test.

CLINICAL SUSPICION

Aneuploidy, congenital heart defects, hydrops

IMAGING MODALITY OF CHOICE

Transabdominal ultrasound. Advantages: readily available, low cost, sensitive, no ionizing radiation.

FINDINGS

Ultrasound findings for increased nuchal translucency (Fig. C7.1):

- Nuchal translucency (NT) refers to fluid under the skin in the back of the fetal neck.
- Measurement performed at 11 to 14 weeks of gestational age.
- NT ≥ 3 mm always abnormal.
- Simple fluid without septations.

  Pitfalls: Beware of amnion. Gravity dependent fetus may lie on amnion. Wait for fetus to move away and show amnion and skin on same image to avoid the pitfall.

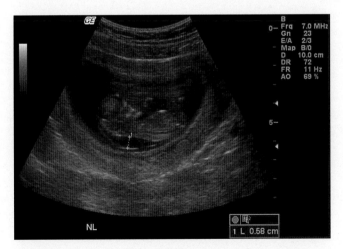

Fig. C7.1 Increased nuchal translucency, with measurements more than 3 mm. Calipers (+) measure the fluid under the skin in the back of the fetal neck. The nuchal translucency is more than 3 mm, which is always abnormal. Calipers are recommended to get accurate measurements.

DISCUSSION

Pregnant patients often are referred by their OB-GYN physician after an abnormal first trimester maternal serum results such as β-human chorionic gonadotropin or pregnancy-associated plasma protein A. However, Nuchal translucency (NT) measurement is now recommended in all 11 to 14 weeks pregnancies. The larger the NT, the worse the prognosis. The normal cutoff is equal to 3 mm or less. If suspected, chorionic villus sampling should be obtained.

Increased NT is found in aneuploidy and congenital heart defect and is associated with hydrops. Trisomies, particularly trisomy 21 (most common), trisomy 18, trisomy 13, and Turners syndrome have increased nuchal translucency. There is approximately 90% detection rate for aneuploidy. Trained ultrasonographers with correct caliper placement are important. Increased maternal age has increased incidence of fetal aneuploidy.

TOP DIFFERENTIAL DIAGNOSES

Top differential diagnoses for increased nuchal fold translucency:

Chorioamniotic separation: Amnion mistaken for fetal skin. Wait for fetus to move away and show amnion and skin on same image to avoid this pitfall.

Cystic hygroma: Large fluid collections with septations behind fetal neck.

Poor measurement technique: Calipers not correctly placed. Skilled sonographers are necessary.

Nuchal fold thickness is a different parameter that is measured during second trimester fetal ultrasound survey (16-22 weeks), and it is not to be confused with nuchal translucency (which is measured in the first trimester as discussed above).

The proposed theory for the cause of increased nuchal fold thickness is edema occurring secondary to congenital heart disease and lymphatic obstruction in association with aneuploidy such as Down (trisomy 21), Edwards (trisomy 18), Patau (trisomy 13), and Turner (monosomy 45, X) syndromes.

Nuchal fold thickness is measured on an axial image through the head at the level of the thalami, cavum septum pellucidum, and cerebellar hemispheres with one caliper at the outer limit of the occipital bone and the other one at the outer aspect of the skin edge (Fig. C7.2). An abnormal value is one that is more than 6 mm.

Most thickened nuchal folds tend to resolve toward the third trimester. However, this doesn't reduce the increased risk for aneuploidy. In fact, a thickened nuchal fold is considered the most sensitive and specific second trimester finding of Down syndrome with a false positive rate as low as 1%.

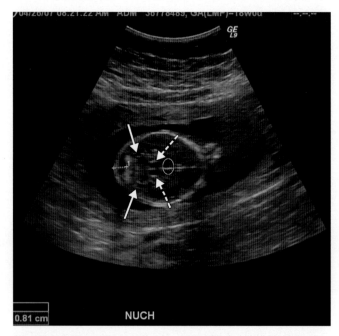

Fig. C7.2 Axial gray-scale ultrasound image of fetal head during the 18th week of gestation, taken at the level of the cavum septum pellucidum (circle), thalami (dashed arrows), and cerebellar hemispheres (arrows) showing thickened nuchal fold measuring 8 mm between the outer aspect of the occipital bone and outer edge of skin as marked by calipers. This fetus was found to have Down syndrome.

REFERENCES AND SUGGESTED READING

1. Avgidou K, Papageorghiou A, Bindra R, et al. Prospective first trimester screening for trisomy 21 in 30,564 pregnancies. *Am J Obstet Gynecol.* 2005;192(6):1761-1767.

2. Souka AP, Von Kaisenberg CS, Hyett JA, et al. Increased nuchal translucency with normal karyotype. *Am J Obstet Gynecol.* 2005;192(4):1005-1021.

3. Nicolaides KH. Nuchal translucency and other first-trimester sonographic markers of chromosomal abnormalities. *Am J Obstet Gynecol.* 2004;191(1):45-67.

4. Locatelli A, Piccoli MG, Vergani P, et al. Critical appraisal of the use of nuchal fold thickness measurements for the prediction of Down syndrome. *Am J Obstet Gynecol.* 2000;182 (1 Pt 1):192-197.

CASE 8: OMPHALOCELE

CASE PRESENTATION

A 20-year-old woman who is 18 weeks pregnant presents for routine screening. The ultrasonographer recognizes abdominal contents herniating within a membranous sac.

CLINICAL SUSPICION

Omphalocele

IMAGING MODALITY OF CHOICE

Transabdominal pelvic ultrasound. Advantages: readily available, low cost, sensitive, no ionizing radiation.

FINDINGS

Ultrasound findings for omphalocele:

- Omphalocele: Midline defect in which extruded abdominal contents, mainly liver, persist beyond 12 weeks of gestation (Fig. 8.1).
- Omphalocele is contained by a sac; small bowel and liver are usually within the herniated sac. Umbilical cord inserts in the center of the sac.
- Size of abdominal wall defect is important:
  - < 5 cm: Minor or small; chromosomal abnormalities more likely
  - 5 cm: Large; usually contains liver; higher rate of cardiac, renal, pulmonary anomalies
- Bowel malrotation is frequent.

DISCUSSION

Physiologic midgut herniation is a normal phenomenon before 12 weeks of gestation that allows for normal physiologic bowel rotation, so omphalocele should never be diagnosed until the gestational age is more than 12. Physiologic rotation, though, doesn't include liver, and if liver herniating through a midline defect before 12 weeks of gestation is encountered, wrong dating should be suspected as this is highly specific for omphalocele. Isolated omphalocele survival rate is 75% to 95%, and most cases are sporadic. The high mortality is mainly due to increased association with chromosomal abnormalities, mainly trisomy 13, 18, and 21, which lead to a poor prognosis. Omphaloceles are also associated with intestinal atresia, tracheoesophageal fistula, bowel malrotation, pulmonary hypoplasia, and congenital heart disease. Not infrequently, omphaloceles can be complicated by rupture, which is associated with very poor prognosis. Polyhydramnios is common with omphaloceles, and amniocentesis for karyotyping should always be performed when diagnosis is made.

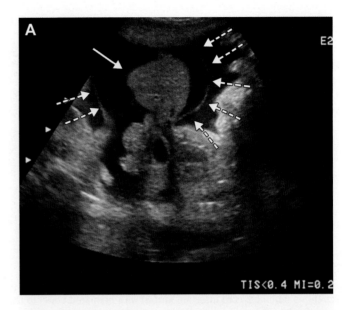

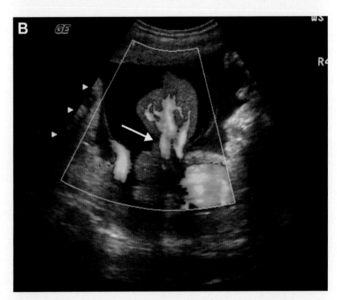

Fig. 8.1 (A) Gray-scale ultrasound image of an omphalocele shows herniation of liver (arrow) through a midline defect which is covered by a thin membrane (dashed arrow). (B) Color Doppler evaluation shows the umbilical cord insertion in midline of the hernia sac (arrow) consistent with omphalocele.

TREATMENT

Treatment for omphalocele:

- C-section for giant omphalocele, otherwise vaginal delivery
- Sac should be covered to prevent fluid loss and to prevent rupture
- Urgent repair is not indicated unless sac ruptures

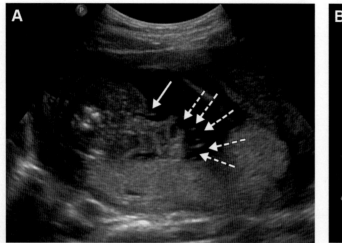 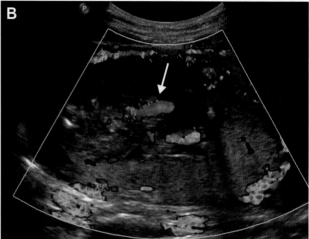

Fig. C8.2 (A) Ultrasound of a midtrimester 18 weeks fetus showing bowel extruded (dashed arrows) to the right of the umbilical cord insertion (arrow). No membrane is covering herniated bowel. Appearance is consistent with gastroschisis. (B) Color Doppler ultrasound image confirms umbilical cord insertion (arrow) with herniated bowel to its right.

TOP DIFFERENTIAL DIAGNOSES

Gastroschisis: Gastroschisis refers to herniation of fetal bowel loops into the amniotic cavity through a right paraumbilical abdominal wall defect. This anomaly doesn't have a membrane covering the hernia, and the abdominal wall defect is anterior on the right side of the umbilical cord insertion (Fig. C8.2). Extruded contents include only bowel and stomach, but not liver as seen with omphaloceles. Gastroschisis on the contrary to omphalocele is not associated with chromosomal abnormalities and has a better prognosis. The only associated abnormalities with gastroschises are bowel related such as malrotation and intestinal atresia.

Umbilical hernia: Small skin-covered midline anterior wall defect. May contain bowel.

Bladder exstrophy: Lower anterior wall defect with bladder involvement.

REFERENCES AND SUGGESTED READING

1. Blazer S, Zimmer EZ, Gover A, et al. Fetal omphalocele detected early in pregnancy: associated anomalies and outcomes. *Radiology.* 2004;232(1):191-195.

2. Hwang PJ, Kousseff BG. Omphalocele and gastroschisis: an 18-year review study. *Genet Med.* 2004;6(4):232-236.

3. Wilson RD, Johnson MP. Congenital abdominal wall defects: an update. *Fetal Diagn Ther.* 2004;19(5):385-398.

CASE 9: COMPLETE SEPTATE UTERUS

PATIENT PRESENTATION

A 26-year-old woman presents with recurrent first trimester pregnancy loss.

CLINICAL SUSPICION

Uterine anomaly leading to infertility

IMAGING MODALITY OF CHOICE

MRI of the pelvis. Although various imaging modalities have been described including hysterosalpingogram and ultrasound, MRI is considered the imaging modality of choice in modern radiological practice for differentiating congenital uterine anomalies with 100% accuracy, 100% sensitivity, and 100% specificity.

A septate uterus is a type of a Müllerian duct anomaly resulting from partial or complete failure of resorption of the urogenital septum after fusion of the paramesonephric ducts. The septum is usually fibrous but can also have various muscular components.

Septate uterus is considered the most common congenital uterine anomaly, and it is the most common anomaly associated with reproductive failure (in about 70% of the cases).

The septum which arises in the midline fundus is considered to be complete when it extends to the external cervical os (Fig. C9.1); otherwise it is called a partial septated

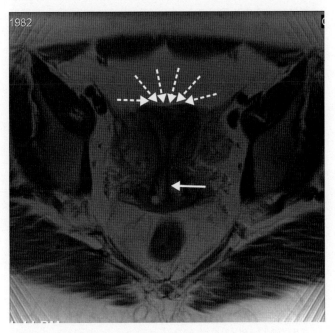

Fig. C9.1 Axial oblique T2WI MR shows a complete septated uterus with a nearly flat fundal contour (dashed arrows) and a septum that extends to the external cervical os (arrow) consistent with a complete septated uterus.

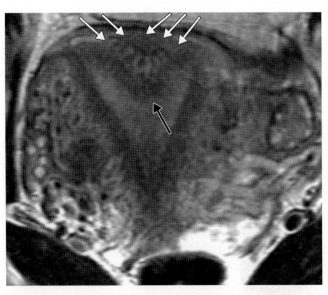

Fig. C9.2 Axial oblique T2WI MR image showing a partial broadly septate uterus. The fundal contour is slightly convex (arrows), and the septum is primarily myometrial (black arrow).

uterus (Fig. C9.2), or if also involving the vagina, septated uterus and vagina. As with other Müllerian duct anomalies, concurrent renal anomalies maybe seen, hence renal evaluation should always be done if encountered.

A complete septate uterus is associated with the worst obstetric outcome of the Müllerian duct anomalies. Patients with septate uteri usually do not have difficulty conceiving, but the pregnancies frequently end in abortion or premature birth, as the miscarriage rate reaches about 90% mainly due to increased contractility, poor decidualization, and/or reduction in endometrial capacity.

FINDINGS

MRI findings of complete septate uterus: T2 weighted sequence is the most accurate way to demonstrate (Fig. C9.1). (All of the following features are based on T2 WI.)

- The external uterine contour may be convex, flat, or mildly concave (< 1 cm indentation). This is important to differentiate from Didelphys uterus, in which complete duplication of uterus is seen.
  - Superior segment of the septum is usually isointense to the myometrium (muscular).
  - Inferior segment of the septum is usually low in signal intensity (fibrous).
  - Symmetric small and narrow endometrial canals.
  - Complete duplication of normal cervix can be seen.
- T1WI + C may help evaluate uterine fundal contour if difficult to identify on T2 WI because of bowel artifact.

TREATMENT

Hysteroscopic resection of septum is considered the best approach. Reproductive outcome has been shown to improve after resection of the septum, with reported decreases in the spontaneous abortion rate from 88% to 5.9% after hysteroscopic metroplasty.

DIAGNOSTIC DIFFERENTIAL

Bicornuate uterus: Nonfusion of fundal myometrium with an intervening cleft > 1 cm. Bicornuate uterus is further subdivided according to the involvement of the cervical canal into:

- Bicornuate unicollis, in which one cervix is present and the myometrial indentation terminating proximal to the internal cervical os.

- Bicornuate bicollis, in which two cervical canals are seen with central myometrial indentation extending to the external os (Fig. C9.3). As with other Müllerian duct anomalies, abnormalities of the renal tract can be also seen.

While infertility is not associated with this type of anomaly as implantation of the embryo is not affected, there is a slightly increased risk for cervical incompetence leading to second trimester pregnancy loss, and hence prophylactic cervical cerclage has been recommended before future pregnancies.

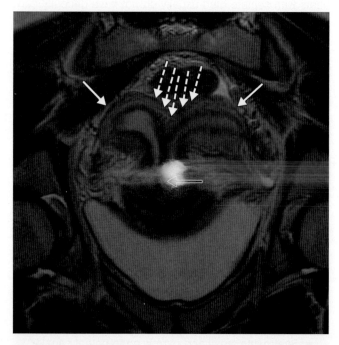

Fig. C9.3 Coronal T2WI MR shows fundal duplication of the uterine horns (arrows) with a septum extending to the level of the cervix (black arrow). There is a wide intervening fundal cleft (dashed arrows) with significant divergence of the uterine horns. Findings are compatible with the diagnosis of bicornuate bicollis uterus.

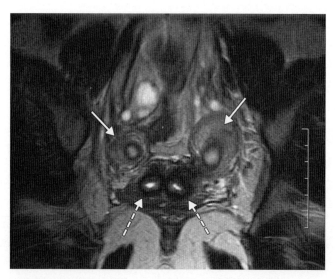

Fig. C9.4 Coronal oblique T2WI MR shows two completely separate corpus uteri (arrows) and cervices (dashed arrows). Note preservation of zonal anatomy. Findings are compatible with didelphys uterus.

Arcuate uterus: Mild indentation of the fundal myometrium on the endometrial cavity.

Didelphys uterus: There is complete duplication of uterus and cervix without communication secondary to failure of fusion of paramesonephric ducts embryologically. Normal zonal anatomy of each corpus and cervix are seen with each hemi-uterus (Fig. C9.4). As with all other Müllerian duct anomalies, there is also an increased risk for renal abnormalities. Didelphys uterus is 75% associated with vaginal septum, which could be transverse and present with unilateral or bilateral hematocolpos, which is associated with increased risk for developing endometriosis. Reproductive outcome data is limited with didelphys uteri, however outcome seems to be better than that seen with complete septate uteri.

Unicornuate uterus with a rudimentary horn: Asymmetric uterine horns.

REFERENCES AND SUGGESTED READING

1. Reuter KL, Daly DC, Cohen SM. Septate versus bicornuate uteri: errors in imaging diagnosis. *Radiology*. 1989;172(3):749-752.

2. Saleem SN. MR imaging diagnosis of uterovaginal anomalies: current state of the art. *RadioGraphics*. 2003;23(5):e13.

3. Troiano RN, McCarthy SM. Mullerian duct anomalies: imaging and clinical issues. *Radiology*. 2004;233(1):19-34.

4. Chaudhry S. AJR teaching file: infertility in a young woman. *AJR*. 2007;189(3):S11-S12.

CASE 10: FAILED FIRST TRIMESTER PREGNANCY

PATIENT PRESENTATION

A 20-year-old woman who presents with painful vaginal bleeding. Last menstrual cycle 8 weeks ago, with a positive home pregnancy test. Beta-hCG is positive but low for gestational age.

CLINICAL SUSPICION

Fetal demise, abortion, ectopic pregnancy, normal early pregnancy

IMAGING MODALITY OF CHOICE

Transvaginal ultrasound (TVUS). Advantages: readily available, low cost, sensitive, no ionizing radiation.

The sequence of events in early pregnancy follows a predictable pattern on transvaginal ultrasound evaluation. In a normal intrauterine pregnancy, the gestational sac is first seen at 5 weeks gestational age and appear as a rounded small cystic fluid collection with no visible contents located in a central echogenic portion of the uterus (the decidua). The yolk sac, a round structure measuring 3 to 5 mm in diameter, appears at about 5½ weeks of gestation. The embryo is usually first seen at 6 weeks of gestation, and at the time a heartbeat is also first seen.

The intradecidual sac sign (IDSS) has been described based on transabdominal ultrasound to be diagnostic for intrauterine pregnancy, however with current transvaginal ultrasound technique this sign appears to be absent in at least 35% of gestational sacs that yield normal pregnancy. So its absence shouldn't be diagnostic for a failed first trimester pregnancy, and a follow-up ultrasound and β-hCG should always be done when encountered.

FINDINGS

Ultrasound findings for early first trimester nonviable pregnancy (Figs. C10.1–C10.4). According to the recently published guidelines by the Society of Radiologists in Ultrasound Multispecialty Consensus Conference on Early First Trimester Diagnosis of Miscarriage and Exclusion of a Viable Intrauterine Pregnancy:

- Mean sac diameter (MSD) size is needed for evaluation, TVUS (preferred).
- Usually cannot evaluate fetal demise until 6 weeks of pregnancy.
- Failed first trimester pregnancy is definite only if TVUS shows:
  - Mean sac diameter (MSD) ≥ 25 mm without visible embryo

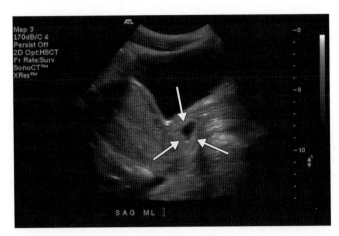

Fig. C10.1 Gray-scale transabdominal ultrasound: Low-lying gestational sac (arrows), which has irregular contours and no embryo, consistent with failed first trimester pregnancy.

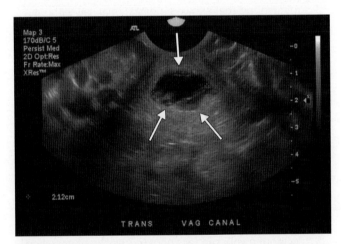

Fig. C10.2 Gray-scale TVUS image showing a low-lying gestational sac in the vaginal canal, which has irregular contours (arrows). No heartbeat detected (not shown). Findings are consistent with a failed first trimester pregnancy.

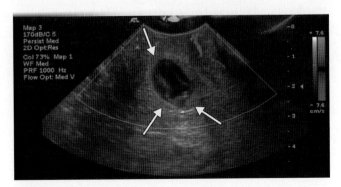

Fig. C10.3 Color Doppler imaging shows fetal demise with poor color Doppler signal around deformed sac without an embryo (arrow).

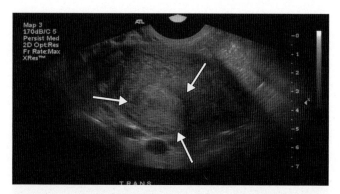

Fig. C10.4 Gray-scale EVUS shows large echogenic region in the endometrial cavity consistent with blood and no viable embryo or yolk sac (arrows).

- Crown-rump length (CRL) ≥ 7 mm without heartbeat
- Absence of embryo with heartbeat 2 weeks after an ultrasound that showed a gestational sac without a yolk sac (at about 7 weeks of gestation)
- Absence of embryo with heartbeat ≥ 11 days after an ultrasound study that showed a gestational sac with a yolk sac (at about 8 weeks of gestation)
- Failed first trimester pregnancy is only highly suggested if:

(a) TVUS:

- MSD of 16 to 24 mm and no visible embryo
- MSD of 8 to 10 mm and no visible yolk sac
- CRL of 5 to 7 mm and no visible heartbeat
- Absence of embryo with heartbeat at 1 to 2 weeks after an ultrasound that showed a gestational sac without a yolk sac (at about 6-7 weeks of gestation)
- Absence of embryo with heartbeat 7 to 10 days after an ultrasound study that showed a gestational sac with a yolk sac (at about 6½-7½ weeks of gestation)
- Absence of embryo ≥ 6 weeks of gestation (6 weeks after last menstrual period)
- Enlarged yolk sac > 7 mm
- Small gestational sac in relation to the embryo (MSD-CRL < 5 mm)

(b) TAS: Technically a diagnosis of failed first trimester pregnancy should only be done based on TVUS, however very rarely a TVUS can't be performed such as in patients who are victims of abuse, or those who have pelvic or perineal trauma. Published data suggests that TAS findings that are highly suggestive of failed first trimester pregnancy are:

- MSD > 20 mm without yolk sac
- MSD > 25 mm without embryo

- Over all a useful rule is the "Alive at 5" rule, which states that if an embryo has a crown-to-rump length of > 5 mm, cardiac activity should be seen in a normal pregnancy; otherwise a failed pregnancy should be suspected and follow-up ultrasound a repeated β-hCG should be performed unless the findings meet the criteria for definite failed pregnancy as discussed above.
- Cardiac activity is evaluated in the M mode.

(c) Color Doppler:

- Fetal demise shows poor color Doppler signal around sac.
- If possibility of normal early gestation is considered, follow-up with gray-scale rather than Doppler is suggested.

- **Other features:** Irregular sac shape, low sac position, thin endometrial echo complex, and if available useful history such as falling β human chorionic gonadotrophin (β-hCG).
- If findings are equivocal, always recommend scheduled US and β-hCG follow-up.

DISCUSSION

Fetal demise most often presents with painful vaginal bleeding. Measuring mean sac diameter and comparing to the normal values is critical for assessment. Equivocal cases should always be followed up by β-hCG and ultrasound if symptoms persist. Most spontaneous abortions occur < 12 weeks due to abnormal chromosomes. Most will spontaneously abort without treatment.

ACR appropriateness criteria recommendations:

1. Transvaginal pelvic ultrasound: correlate findings with quantitative β-hCG.
2. Transabdominal pelvic ultrasound: correlate findings with quantitative β-hCG.
3. US pelvis with Doppler—pulsed Doppler of the embryo should be avoided.
4. M-mode imaging should be used to document embryonic viability.
5. Color and pulsed Doppler US imaging can be extremely useful for abnormalities or findings unrelated to a live embryo, including uterine and adnexal vascular abnormalities, ovarian torsion, retained products of conception, and adnexal masses.

TOP DIFFERENTIAL DIAGNOSES

Very early intrauterine pregnancy: Schedule follow-up at a time when gestational sac should have reached discriminatory threshold. MSD increases by 1 mm per day.

Pseudosac of ectopic pregnancy: Carefully evaluate the fallopian tubes and adnexal regions for ectopic pregnancy.

REFERENCES

1. Jauniaux E, Johns J, Burton GJ. The role of ultrasound imaging in diagnosing and investigating early pregnancy failure. *Ultrasound Obstet Gynecol.* 2005;25(6):613-624.

2. Sohaey R, Woodward P, Zwiebel WJ. First-trimester ultrasound: the essentials. *Semin Ultrasound CT MR.* 1996;17(1):2-14.

3. Bree RL, Edwards M, Bohm-Velez M, Beyler S, Roberts J, Mendelson EB. Transvaginal sonography in the evaluation of normal early pregnancy: correlation with HCG level. *AJR.* 1989;153(1):75-79.

4. Doubilet PM, Benson CB, Bourne T, Blaivas M, for the Society of Radiologists in Ultrasound Multispecialty Panel on Early First Trimester Diagnosis of Miscarriage and Exclusion of a Viable Intrauterine Pregnancy. *N Engl J Med.* 2013;369:1443-1451. October 10, 2013.

CASE 11: ENDOMETRIOSIS/ADENOMYOSIS

PATIENT PRESENTATION

A 25-year-old woman presents to her gynecologist with chronic pelvic pain that is worse with sexual intercourse and around her menses. She has an irregular menstrual cycle and has been trying to get pregnant for the last 2 years without success.

CLINICAL SUSPICION

Endometriosis

DISCUSSION

Endometriosis is a gynecological condition in which functional cells from the endometrium grow outside the uterine cavity, most commonly in the peritoneum overlying the ovary, but other pelvic organs can also be affected by the disease.

Endometrial cells in areas outside the uterus (endometriosis) are influenced by hormonal changes and respond in a way that is similar to the cells found inside the uterus. Symptoms are often worse with the menstrual cycle.

Endometriosis is typically seen during the reproductive years; it has been estimated that endometriosis occurs in roughly 6% to 10% of women. Symptoms may depend on the site of active endometriosis. Its main but not universal symptom is pelvic pain in various manifestations. Endometriosis is a common finding in women with infertility mainly due to excessive inflammatory adhesions.

Pathologically, endometriosis can vary from microscopic foci to multifocal infiltrative lesions. Grossly visible endometriotic cysts (endometriomas, also known as chocolate cysts) can also be a manifestation of the disease process, mainly seen in the ovaries, but endometriomas are not to be confused with endometriosis, as they are only part of a disease spectrum that also includes endometriotic implants, infiltration, and adhesions.

The most accepted theory for how endometriosis occurs is that they are actually metastatic deposits in the peritoneal cavity secondary to retrograde menstruation.

When repeated cyclical hemorrhage happens in a deep implant within the ovaries an endometriotic cyst/endometrioma or chocolate cyst develops, and this can essentially replace the entire ovary involved. The cyst wall is formed from thick fibrous adhesions, and it's usually filled with dark degenerated blood products (hence the name "chocolate cyst").

Imaging evaluation of endometriosis is limited for small foci of endometriotic implants and is mainly used for evaluation of endometriomas and effect of adhesions and fibrosis on surrounding structures, which are usually late features of the disease—which means that if a high clinical suspicion for the diagnosis of endometriosis is present with negative imaging, the diagnosis can't be excluded.

In the next section, we will mainly discuss imaging features of endometriomas and to a lesser extent endometriosis.

IMAGING MODALITY OF CHOICE

Transabdominal and transvaginal pelvic ultrasound. Advantages:

- Quick examination to perform
- Lower cost than MRI
- More accessible and easier to schedule than MRI
- Screening tool to identify pelvic masses that may represent an endometrioma

Disadvantages:

- Visualization of the pelvic anatomy may be distorted from adhesions.
- Presence of bowel gas and stool could limit the field of view.
- Leiomyomas could be present as well, limiting the field of view due to shadowing from calcifications (which can sometimes be seen in leiomyoma).

MRI can be used for problem solving after a pelvic mass is identified by US and the diagnosis of endometrioma is suspected or to quantify the involvement of the adjacent bowel and ureters due to fibrosis secondary to endometriosis.

FINDINGS

Ultrasound findings of endometriosis (Fig. C11.1A, B):

- May present as focal, multifocal, or infiltrative lesions.
- Endometrioma is usually cystic lesion in the adnexa or pelvis that is homogeneously hypoechoic with low-level echoes.
- Some endometriomas demonstrate a fluid-fluid level due to different ages of hemorrhage or peripheral echogenic nodules due to blood clots.
- No internal blood flow is identified with color Doppler imaging of endometrioma.
- With infiltrative lesions, indistinct margins of a hypoechoic mass are seen (relative to uterine myometrium). The infiltrative lesions may contain small cystic areas or bright foci.

MRI findings of endometriosis (Fig. C11.2): MRI is 98% specific in diagnosing an endometrioma due to its ability to detect blood products of different ages.

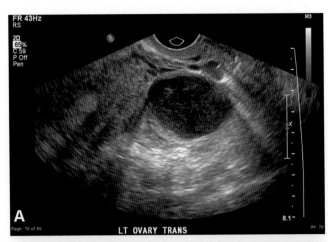

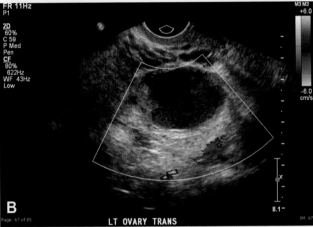

Fig. C11.1 (A) Transvaginal ultrasound image of a left ovarian round, homogeneously hypoechoic mass with low-level echoes and posterior acoustic enhancement. (B) Transvaginal color Doppler image showing no internal vascularity within the mass compatible with an endometrioma.

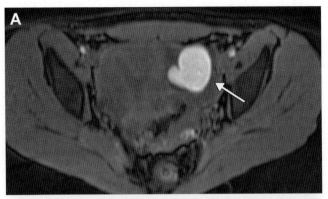

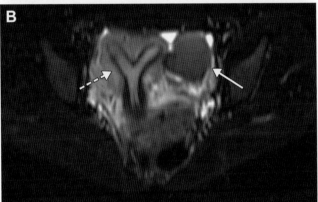

Fig. C11.2 Axial fat-saturated T1-weighted (A) and axial fat-saturated T2-weighted (B) MRI images demonstrating an oval-shaped mass in the left adnexa (arrows) with high signal intensity on T1-weighted images and low-signal intensity on T2-weighted images (T2 shading) compatible with endometrioma. An incidental septate uterus is seen as well (dashed arrow).

On MRI, endometrioma shows as cystic lesion that is hyperintense on T1 weighted fat-suppressed images and can have a variable signal intensity on T2 weighted images, though typically lower in signal intensity than on T1 weighted images, a phenomena known as T2 shading indicating chronicity mainly due to high concentrations of protein and iron (degenerated blood products) in hemosiderin-laden macrophages from recurrent cyclical hemorrhages into a focal nondraining cyst. In fact, when T2 shading is present this indicates that the patient is less likely going to respond to medical treatment.

Grading of the signal within the mass may be seen due to different ages of blood products.

CLINICAL DIFFERENTIAL DIAGNOSIS

- Pelvic adhesions
- Pelvic inflammatory disease
- Pelvic neoplasm

Imaging differential diagnosis for endometrioma:

Ovarian hemorrhagic cyst: Can have a similar appearance to endometrioma on ultrasound; however it will usually resolve on follow-up ultrasound imaging in 2 menstrual cycles.

Ovarian teratoma: More complex appearance with fat and often calcification. If fat can be depicted on MR imaging, this is diagnostic for an ovarian teratoma.

Ovarian malignancy: Have a more complex appearance than endometrioma on US and MRI. On ultrasonography, malignant ovarian neoplasms usually show increased vascularity on color Doppler evaluation and significant postcontrast enhancement on MRI.

TREATMENT OF ENDOMETRIOSIS

First-line treatment is medical targeting hormonal manipulation. Frequently used agents involve oral contraceptive pills, medroxyprogesterone acetate, and gonadotropin-releasing hormone agonists. Medical treatment has proved to be useful in reducing symptoms of pain and decreasing the anatomic extent of the disease.

Surgery is considered for patients with intractable pain refractory to medical treatment, bearing in mind that if the patient is placed on hormonal replacement therapy (exogenous estrogen) endometriosis may recur.

In patients with infertility, conservative surgeries retaining reproductive function have been described by performing lysis of adhesions, which can be helpful but are associated with a high recurrence rate. Advanced reproductive techniques have also been described to restore fertility including intrauterine insemination and ovarian hyperstimulation.

ADENOMYOSIS

Adenomyosis is a condition characterized by the presence of ectopic glandular tissue found in muscle.

Adenomyometriosis refers to the presence of ectopic endometrial glandular tissue (the inner lining of the uterus) within the myometrium (the thick, muscular layer of the uterus).

The cause of adenomyosis is unknown, but it appears to be more common in multiparous women and it has been associated with any sort of uterine trauma that may break the barrier between the endometrium and myometrium, such as a caesarean section, tubal ligation, pregnancy termination, and uterine instrumentation (eg, dilatation and curettage). Adenomyosis differs from endometriosis, and these two disease entities are found together only in 10% of the cases.

Adenomyosis is common in women between the ages of 35 and 50 years, because it is between these ages that women have an excess of estrogen (estrogen dominance).

By ultrasonography, diffuse uterine adenomyosis manifests as a heterogeneously hypoechoic, striated, ill-defined areas in an enlarged or globular uterus (Fig. C11.3A).

Adenomyosis is demonstrated on MRI as thickening of the junctional zone, measuring > 12 mm, with possible myometrial cystic changes (Fig. C11.3B).

The enlarged uterus is felt to be secondary to dysfunctional smooth muscle hyperplasia adjacent to the areas of benign myometrial invasion by the endometrium, which explains why patients with adenomyosis frequently present with dysfunctional uterine bleeding and menorrhagia. In addition, patients with this clinical entity usually complain of dysmenorrhea.

Adenomyosis usually involves a large portion of the uterus, typically the posterior wall. Although the uterus is usually markedly enlarged, its overall contour is usually preserved.

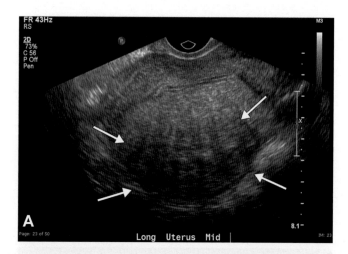

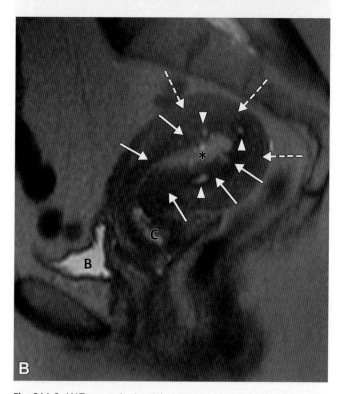

Fig. C11.3 (A)Transvaginal pelvic ultrasound showing an enlarged uterus with heterogeneous appearing, hypoechoic, posterior uterine parenchyma (arrows) in a striated pattern. The endometrial canal is deformed consistent with diffuse adenomyosis. (B) Sagittal T2 weighted pelvic MRI image showing a thickened junctional zone (arrows), which is identified as the band of lower signal between the high signal endometrium (asterisk) and the intermediate signal outer myometrium (dashed arrows). There are also scattered areas of high T2 signal in the uterine parenchyma consistent with cysts (arrowheads) seen in diffuse adenomyosis. The uterus is also retroverted. (B) Urinary bladder, (C) cervix.

IMAGING DIFFERENTIAL DIAGNOSIS

Leiomyomatosis: An enlarged uterus is usually seen on US with a lobular contour and occasionally areas of posterior acoustic shadowing due to calcifications. Leiomyomas ar typically well circumscribed hypointense to myometrium on T2WI, although they can also be hyperintense when they undergo cystic degeneration.

Physiologic thickening of the junctional zone: Occurs early in the menstrual cycle (days 1-2).

Focal myometrial contractions: This can cause thickening of inner myometrium, which can mimic junctional zone thickening; however, this is only a transient finding.

Endometrial hyperplasia: Thickened endometrium is seen (> 15 mm in premenopausal women and > 5 mm in postmenopausal women) mainly due to a prolonged unopposed estrogen effect or treatment with tamoxifen. It is a precancerous condition especially if atypia is seen on sampling.

Endometrial cancer: Endometrial cancer is typically characterized by significantly thickened endometrium; intermediate to high in signal intensity on T2WI and can invade the myometrium.

TREATMENT OF ADENOMYOSIS

Medical treatment targeting cyclic hormonal alteration mainly with gonadotropin releasing hormone analogues can be helpful but not in all cases. Surgery remains the mainstay of treatment. However, minimally invasive interventions such as uterine artery embolization is an emerging procedure for managing adenomyosis, as it has been noticed that adenomyosis decreases in size when uterine artery embolization is done in cases with coexistent fibroids and symptoms (bleeding and pain) seem to accordingly improve.

REFERENCES

1. Chamie L, Blasbalg R, Pereira R, Warmbrand G, Serafini P. Findings of pelvic endometriosis at transvaginal US, MR imaging, and laparoscopy. *RadioGraphics.* 2011;31,E77-E100. doi:10.1148/rg.314105193.

2. Mounsey A, Wilgus A, Slawson D. Diagnosis and management of endometriosis. *Am Fam Physician.* 2006;74(4):594-600. http://www.aafp.org/afp/2006/0815/p594.html.

3. Novellas S, Chassang M, Delotte J, et al. MRI characteristics of the uterine junctional zone: from normal to the diagnosis of adenomyosis. *AJR.* 2011;196(5):1206-1213. doi:10.2214/AJR.10.4877.

4. Tamai K, Tagashi K, Ito T, Morisawa N, Fujiwara T, Koyama T. MR imaging findings of adenomyosis: correlation with histopathologic features and diagnostic pitfalls. *RadioGraphics.* 2005;25:21-40. doi:10.1148/rg.251045060.

CASE 12: DERMOID CYST

PATIENT PRESENTATION

A 30-year-old woman presents to the OB-GYN clinic for evaluation of pelvic mass and fullness. Quantitative urine β-hCG is negative.

CLINICAL SUSPICION

Ovarian mass

IMAGING MODALITY OF CHOICE

Transabdominal and transvaginal pelvic ultrasound. Advantages: readily available, low cost, reasonably sensitive, no ionizing radiation, easy assessment of perfusion to look for associated torsion.

FINDINGS

Ultrasound findings of dermoid cyst (mature cystic teratoma): mature cystic teratomas have a variety of appearances:

- Heterogeneous mass with echogenic component.
- Highly echogenic components due to fat content (Fig. C12.1).
- Fat fluid level.
- Shadowing echogenic mural nodule (sebaceous material) = Rokitansky plug "diagnostic" (Fig. C12.2).
- Hair: Punctate echoes in one plane that elongate to become linear echoes in orthogonal plane, moves through more fluid component with transducer pressure (Fig. C12.3).

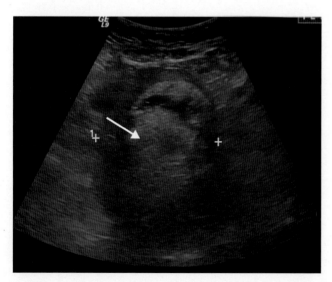

Fig. C12.1 Transverse transabdominal ultrasound showing a left ovarian cystic mass with echogenic component (arrow) consistent with fat.

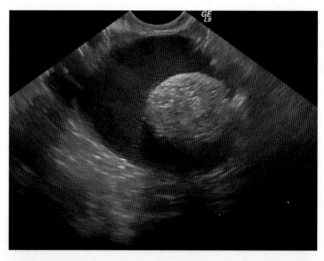

Fig. C12.2 Transverse transvaginal ultrasound showing an ovarian cystic lesion with echogenic nodule projecting into the lumen (Rokitansky nodule or dermoid plug).

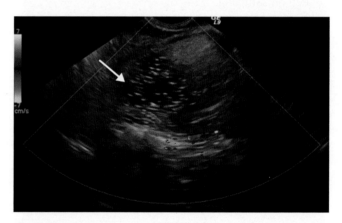

Fig. C12.3 Longitudinal transvaginal ultrasound of the mass shows punctate echoes as well as linear echoes (arrow) from hair.

- Teeth: Highly echogenic focus/foci with distal acoustic shadowing (Fig. C12.4).
- Tip of the iceberg sign = Only leading edge of the mass is identified with posterior acoustic shadowing due to calcification, preventing assessment of deeper edges, the size cannot be measured.
- 10% to 20% bilateral.

Mature cystic teratomas (MCTs) are the most commonly excised ovarian neoplasm and account for about 95% of all ovarian germ cell tumors. They are congenital cystic tumors that are composed of well-differentiated derivatives from at least 2 of the 3 germ cell layers (eg, hair from ectoderm, fat from mesoderm). MCTs are often asymptomatic; however they may undergo torsion especially if > 6 cm in size, May rupture in 1%, or rarely undergo malignant degeneration in 0.2% to 1.4% of cases if they go untreated and are presenting in older patients (sixth-seventh decades).

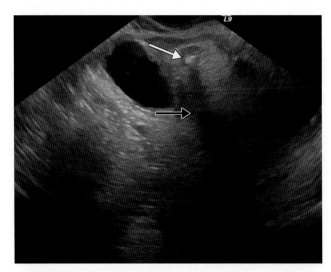

Fig. C12.4 Longitudinal transabdominal ultrasound showing an echogenic focus (arrow) within the mass with posterior acoustic shadowing (black arrow) compatible with calcification "found to be a tooth on gross pathology."

Such lesions are often discovered on CT incidentally or in the setting of evaluation for acute abdomen "torsion." Characteristic appearance on CT is a mass with large irregular solid component containing foci of fat plus coarse calcifications. Hemorrhage is also often present (Fig. C12.5).

MRI is sometimes used for evaluation of ovarian masses that are indeterminate based on transvaginal ultrasound—in particular, to differentiate blood products from fat, T1-weighted imaging should always be acquired with and without fat suppression as the presence of fat is diagnostic for dermoid cyst (Fig. C12.6).

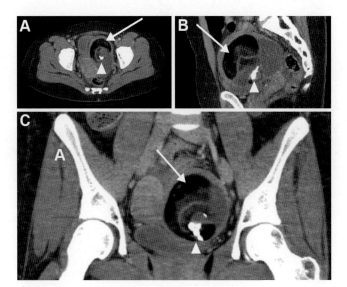

Fig. C12.5 Axial (A), Sagittal (B) and coronal (C) CT images showing a left thick-walled ovarian mass containing fat (white arrows) and calcium "tooth" (white arrowheads).

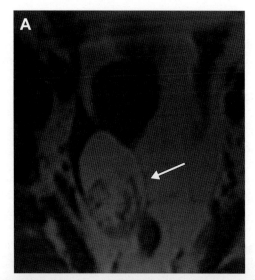

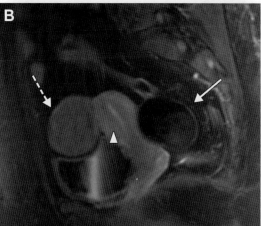

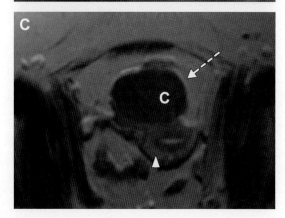

Fig. C12.6 (A) Axial T1 MRI image showing a hyperintense lesion in the right adnexa (arrows). (B) Sagittal T1 fat-saturated plus contrast image of the pelvis shows suppression of the signal intensity in the lesion posterior to the uterus correlating with the lesion in (A). The lesion also doesn't show any significant enhancement. Features are typical for dermoid cyst.

Incidentally noted is a benign exophytic subserosal uterine leiomyoma superior and anterior to the uterine fundus (dashed arrows). The leiomyoma is showing the typical MRI features of benign leiomyoma, generally a well-defined mass arising from the myometrium (arrowheads) and enhancing as much or slightly less on T1 FS postcontrast image (B). Leiomyomas are usually hypointense to the myometrium on T2 weighted sequence as seen in image (C).

IMAGING DIFFERENTIAL DIAGNOSIS

Hemorrhagic cyst: Fine network of fibrin strands rather than floating hair, distal acoustic enhancement rather than acoustic shadowing.

Endometrioma: Rokitansky nodule is not seen, homogenous low-level internal echoes, often history of chronic pelvic pain.

Abscess: Tubo-ovarian abscess or appendicular abscess with appendicolith may be particularly challenging, pain and/or fever should suggest the diagnosis. An infarcted dermoid cyst due to torsion can also become infected with secondary abscess formation.

Torsion: If presenting with torsion, bear in mind that any adnexal mass can act as a lead point for torsion.

Bowel: Large bowel may contain echogenic feces and does not undergo peristalsis as much as small bowel. The use of transvaginal sonography helps differentiate bowel from ovaries.

TREATMENT

Surgical resection is recommended if > 6 cm due to higher risk of torsion.

REFERENCES AND SUGGESTED READING

1. Outwater EK, Siegelman ES, Hunt JL. Ovarian teratomas: tumor types and imaging characteristics. *RadioGraphics*. 2001;21(2):475-490.

2. Tempeman CL, Fallat ME, Lam AM, et al. Managing mature cystic teratomas of the ovary. *Obstet Gynecol Surv*. 2000;55(12):738-745.

3. Ulbright TM. Germ cell tumors of the gonads: a selective review emphasizing problems in differential diagnosis, newly appreciated and controversial issues. *Mod Pathol*. 2005;18(suppl 2): S61-S79.

CASE 13: OVARIAN TORSION

PATIENT PRESENTATION

A 10-year-old girl who presents with acute onset of left-sided pelvic pain.

CLINICAL SUSPICION

Ovarian torsion

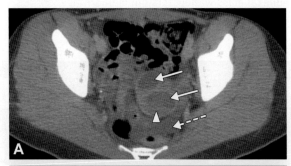

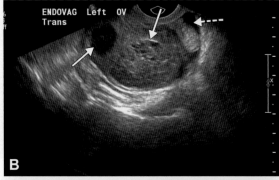

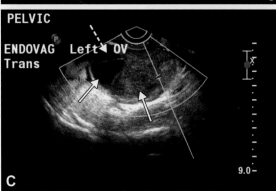

Fig. C13.1 (A) Axial noncontrast CT image of the pelvis in a 38-year-old woman who presented to the ER with left-sided pelvic pain that started suddenly 6 hours prior to presentation. The pain was constant and associated with nausea and vomiting. Patient has history of right-sided oophorectomy and hysterectomy. The image shows free fluid (dashed arrow), 2 cystic lesions in an enlarged left adnexa (arrows); the lesions are located to the left and posterior and have dense contents (arrowheads). (B) Transverse gray-scale ultrasound image of the left adnexa shows the left ovary is enlarged, echogenic with peripherally displaced follicles (arrow). A probably functional cyst is seen as well (large arrow) with minimal adjacent free fluid (dashed arrows). (C) Transverse color Doppler evaluation shows absence of both arterial and venous spectral waveforms consistent with adnexal torsion.

IMAGING MODALITY OF CHOICE

Transabdominal pelvic ultrasound. In an older patient, and if patient is sexually active, additional transvaginal ultrasound should be performed as well (Fig. C13.1). Color Doppler must be performed to asses for viability. Advantages: readily available, low cost, sensitive, no ionizing radiation. Color Doppler to asses for perfusion and viability.

FINDINGS

Ultrasound findings for ovarian torsion:

- Best diagnostic clue: Enlarged ovary on symptomatic side with loss of venous and or arterial flow.
- Asymmetric ovarian enlargement, usually greater than 20 mL (normal ovary size up to 20 mL or $3 \times 4 \times 5$ cm) (Fig. C13.1).
- Peripheral cysts, 8 to 12 mm in diameter (Fig. C13.2).

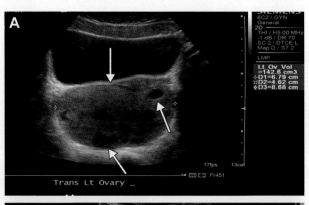

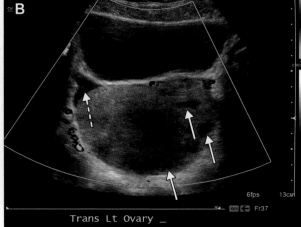

Fig. C13.2 (A) transabdominal gray-scale ultrasound image of the pelvis in this 10-year-old girl who presented with sudden onset left pelvic pain showing the left ovary (large arrow) is very large, echogenic, with peripheral follicles (arrows). (B) Color Doppler evaluation shows no color flow within the ovary, consistent with an avascular torsed ovary. Small amount of adjacent free fluid (dashed arrow). Findings are compatible with ovarian torsion.

- Free fluid.
- Fallopian tube thickening > 10 mm.
- Color Doppler evaluation: Presence of blood flow does *not* exclude torsion. Preservation of venous flow in a torsed ovary correlates with viability (Fig. C13.1).

Ultrasound is the best diagnostic tool in a premeno-pausal woman with acute pelvic pain. Laboratory values, especially β-hCG is critical in the diagnosis of ectopic pregnancy. When the serum test for pregnancy is negative and the patient has an adnexal mass, such findings may be secondary to a complicated ovarian cyst (hemorrhagic, rupture), pelvic inflammatory disease, or ovarian torsion. Appendicitis and right-sided ovarian torsion can present in a similar fashion and adequate history is necessary.

CLINICAL DIFFERENTIAL DIAGNOSIS

Ectopic pregnancy: Elevated β-hCG, echogenic ring or mass, separate from the ovary, ovary is usually normal.

Adnexal mass without torsion: Hemorrhagic corpus luteum—echogenic fluid in the ovary (Fig. C13.3).

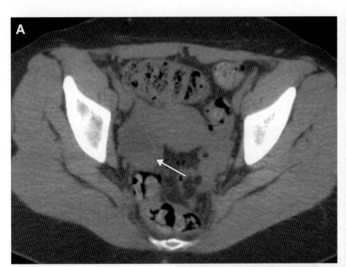
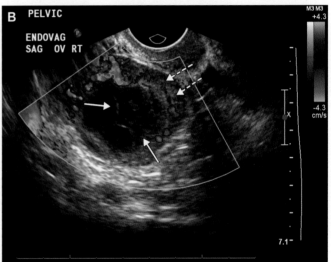
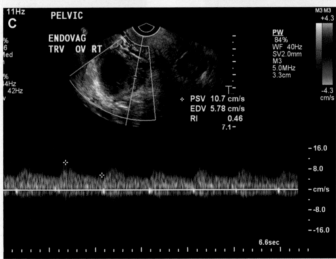

Fig. C13.3 (A) Axial noncontrast CT image without contrast of the pelvis for a 36-year-old woman who presented to the ER with sudden onset of right-sided pelvic pain and negative β-hCG, showing a cystic mass in the right adnexa with dense contents (arrow) (notice the similarity to the prior case). The right ovary also appears large. (B) Endovaginal transverse gray-scale ultrasound image of the right ovary with color Doppler evaluation shows a cystic ovarian lesion with internal linear interdigitating echoes and clumped echoes at the margin of the lesion (arrows) with normal adjacent ovarian tissue (dashed arrow) and normal spectral arterial waveforms in the right ovary (C). Findings are consistent with a hemorrhagic cyst.

Ovarian torsion is caused by spontaneous twist of ovary and fallopian tube. Torsion of normal adnexal structures is more common in pediatric patients than in adults. Mean age is 10 to 11 years, primarily in premenarchal girls. Risk factors include preexisting ovarian masses, rapid uterine expansion such as first trimester, or immediately postpartum.

Appendicitis: Thickened wall, dilated, blind-ending tubular structure, surrounding inflammatory changes.

TREATMENT

Torsion with adequate blood supply

- Laparoscopic "detorsion"
- Resection of any mass

Avascular torsion:

- Laparotomy and salpingo-oophorectomy

REFERENCES AND SUGGESTED READING

1. Rha SE, Byun JY, Jung SE, et al. CT and MR imaging features of adnexal torsion. *RadioGraphics*. 2002;22(2):283-294.
2. Chiang G, Levine D. Imaging of adnexal masses in pregnancy. *J Ultrasound Med*. 2004;23(6):805-819.
3. Anders JF, Powell EC. Urgency of evaluation and outcome of acute ovarian torsion in pediatric patients. *Arch Pediatr Adolesc Med*. 2005;159(6):532-535.
4. Ignacio EA, Hill MC. Ultrasound of the acute female pelvis. *Ultrasound Q*. 2003;19(2):86-98; quiz 108-110.

CASE 14: OVARIAN CANCER

PATIENT PRESENTATION

A 78-year-old woman who presents with lower abdominal/pelvic pain and swelling.

CLINICAL SUSPICION

Ovarian or other gynecological cancer. Symptoms are non-specific, and inflammatory, infectious, or neoplastic process should be considered.

Ovarian cancer is the second most common gynecologic malignancy after endometrial cancer and fifth most common malignancy in women. However, it accounts for more deaths than any other primary gynecologic malignant neoplasm. It is most commonly found in women between the ages of 40 and 65 years. Risk factors include nulliparity, positive family history, genetic susceptibility *BRCA1*, *BRCA2*, Lynch syndrome, and fertility drug use.

Primary ovarian tumors are common and can be classified based on origin into epithelial, germ cell, and sex cord–stromal ovarian tumors. Epithelial ovarian tumors are the most common type of all ovarian neoplasms and form most of malignant tumors arising from the ovary (80%-90%) occurring primarily in adults. Subtypes of ovarian epithelial carcinoma include serous (most common), followed by mucinous, endometrioid, and rarely clear cell. Other rarer forms have been also described.

Patients unfortunately often present late due to nonspecific symptoms, and most ovarian cancer cases have extrapelvic peritoneal disease and/or abdominopelvic lymphatic spread at time of presentation, indicting an advanced stage that reflects their high mortality.

Imaging plays an essential role in evaluating the extent of extrapelvic disease, which determines feasibility of cytoreductive surgery and predicts surgical outcomes.

In general, serous and mucinous ovarian carcinoma, the most common malignant ovarian neoplasms, are indistinguishable based on CT or US imaging features; however, MRI can sometimes distinguish them if mucin is concentrated enough in mucinous ovarian carcinoma to alter MRI signal intensity, mainly on T1 weighted imaging.

MR is the most specific modality, although initial workup includes US and CT. Serum tumor markers (CA-125) are used for follow-up.

IMAGING MODALITY

Initially with ultrasound followed by MRI (for characterization) or CT (for staging). Advantages: ultrasound is readily available, inexpensive, and sensitive. CT and MR are more specific and help detect metastatic foci and peritoneal deposits.

FINDING

Ultrasound findings for most common forms of ovarian cancer (serous and mucinous):

- Large multiloculated complex cystic mass with low-level echoes and anechoic components.
- Thick septations (> 3 mm).
- Echogenic mural nodularity.

Color Doppler:

- Increased color Doppler flow in solid portions is highly indicative of malignancy.
- Spectral Doppler: Low resistive index (RI < 0.4), although this is often unreliable and insensitive

MRI findings of ovarian cancer (CA)—most specific modality:

- T2WI: High signal intensity cystic mass. Thick septations with mural nodularity (Fig. C14.1A).
- Precontrast T1WI: Often demonstrates the cystic areas with low-signal intensity like fluid, and the soft tissue as isointense.
- Increased concentration of mucin can lead to increased signal intensity on T1WI.
- T1WI with contrast: Soft tissue component and mural nodularity shows enhancement (Fig. C14.1B).

CT findings most common forms of ovarian cancer (serous and mucinous):

- Nonenhanced CT: Cystic adnexal mass with thick septa and soft tissue density components.
- Contrast-enhanced CT: Enhancing thick septa and solid mural nodules (Figs. C14.2).
- Size: Initial diagnosis is often late and masses are large.
- Due to late presentation, most patients have metastatic disease (most commonly in the liver), peritoneal carcinomatosis (Fig. C14.3), and ascites. Characteristic calcified peritoneal components are indicative of serous cystadenocarcinoma (although the nodular noncalcified pattern is typical) (Fig. C14.4).

PET/CT:

- Can be useful to asses for metastatic, recurrent, and residual disease.

IMAGING DIFFERENTIAL DIAGNOSIS

Ovarian metastases: Patient with known malignancy with pelvic masses; however, initial presentation may be similar.

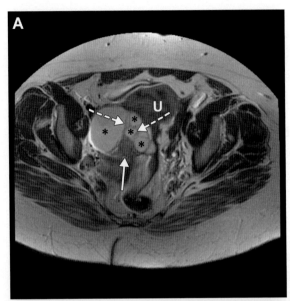

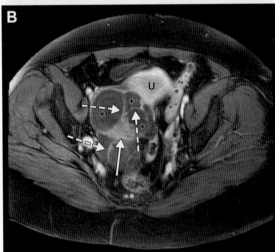

Fig. C14.1 (A) Axial T2 weighted MRI image of the pelvis showing multiloculated cystic mass in the right adnexa (asterisk) with thick septa (dashed arrows) and solid intramural component (arrows). (B) Axial fat-saturated T1-weighted MRI image of the pelvis postcontrast shows enhancement of the septa (dashed arrows) and intramural solid component (arrow). This was found to represent a serous cystadenocarcinoma of the ovary. (U) Uterus.

Ovarian lymphoma: Mostly solid adnexal masses.

Tubo-ovarian abscess: Patients with fever and are acutely sick, adnexal masses and pelvic ascites.

Endometriosis: Chronic painful pelvic masses; high signal intensity on T1WI. Shows low T2WI signal and no enhancement.

Cystic teratoma: Heterogeneous cystic mass with echogenic component, due to fat. Fat/fluid level may be seen.

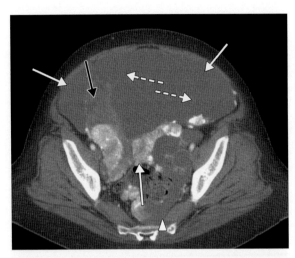

Fig. C14.2 Axial contrast-enhanced CT image of the pelvis in a different patient shows a large complex cystic mass (arrows) with multiple enhancing septa (dashed arrows) and solid component (black arrow). Ascites is also seen layering in the pelvis (arrowhead). This was found to be a serous cystadenocarcinoma.

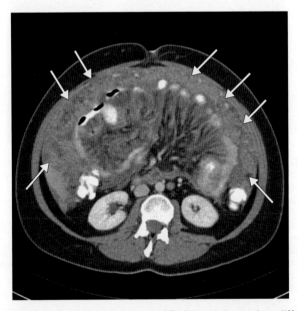

Fig. C14.3 Axial contrast-enhanced CT of the abdomen in a different patient with known history of ovarian cancer shows enhancing nodular thickened omentum (arrows) consistent with peritoneal carcinomatosis.

OVARIAN CANCER STAGING

International Federation of Gynecology and Obstetrics staging system:

- Stage I: Tumor limited to ovaries
- Stage II: Tumor confined to pelvis

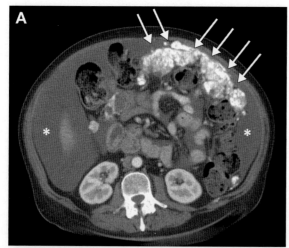

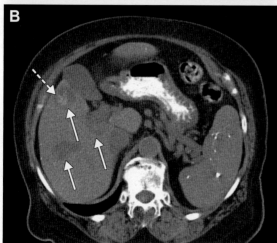

Fig. C14.4 (A) Axial CT scan examination of the abdomen and pelvis with intravenous contrast in a different patient with known history of ovarian papillary serous cystadenocarcinoma shows large nodular calcifications in the peritoneum (arrows). There is also ascites (asterisks). Findings are consistent with peritoneal carcinomatosis. (B) Axial non-contrast-enhanced image of the abdomen in a different patient with known papillary serous cystadenocarcinoma shows multiple areas of metastasis in the liver (arrows). Calcifications are seen in one of the lesions (dashed arrow) characteristic of ovarian serous cystadenocarcinoma metastasis.

- Stage III: Intraperitoneal metastases outside the pelvis, and/or positive retroperitoneal lymph nodes
- Stage IV: Distant metastases

These are the main stages, and there are subcategories not mentioned here for simplification.

TREATMENT

Treatment for stages I-IV includes:

- Cytoreductive surgery: Total abdominal hysterectomy, removal of both ovaries and fallopian tubes, omentectomy, biopsy of lymph nodes and other tissues in the pelvis and abdomen. Young women whose disease is confined to one ovary are often treated by a unilateral salpingo-oophorectomy.
- Chemotherapy: Stages II-IV and high-grade Stage I.
- Radiation: Stages II-IV.

REFERENCES

1. Prat J, for the FIGO committee on Gynecologic Oncology. FIGO Guidelines: Staging classifications for cancer of the ovary, fallopian tube, and peritoneum. *Int J Gynecol Obstet.* 2014;124:1-5.

2. Sohaib SA, Mills TD, Sahdev A, et al. The role of magnetic resonance imaging and ultrasound in patients with adnexal masses. *Clin Radiol.* 2005;60(3):340-348.

3. Agarwal A, Yeh BM, Breiman RS, et al. Peritoneal calcification: causes and distinguishing features on CT. *AJR.* 2004;182(2)441-445.

4. Smith LH, Morris CR, Yasmeen S, et al. Ovarian cancer: can we make the clinical diagnosis earlier? *Cancer.* 2005;104(7):1398-1407.

5. Togashi K. Ovarian cancer: the clinical role of US, CT, and MRI. *Eur Radiol.* 2003;13(suppl)4:L87-L104.

CASE 15: CERVICAL CANCER

PATIENT PRESENTATION

A 30-year-old woman presents with watery vaginal discharge and postcoital vaginal bleeding for 6 months. Recent pelvic exam revealed a cervical mass.

CLINICAL SUSPICION

Cervical carcinoma

IMAGING MODALITY OF CHOICE

MRI of the pelvis (performed for local staging) and PET/CT with intravenous contrast (for systemic staging). MRI Advantages: no ionizing radiation, more readily available in most locations, better soft tissue delineation, can more readily detect parametrial spread, bladder, and rectal involvement.

MRI disadvantages: does not detect lymph node metastases as well as PET/CT since it relies on size criteria, will not detect distant metastatic disease since the whole body is not scanned, may overestimate the presence of parametrial spread in larger tumors.

PET/CT advantages: can detect distant metastatic disease, better at delineating lymph node involvement since it can detect metabolic activity in a normal sized metastatic lymph node.

PET/CT disadvantages: ionizing radiation, may not be readily available in all locations, can have false positive findings from normal physiology especially in premenopausal patients, can have false negative scans in small volume disease, physiologic bladder activity can mask extent of disease in the pelvis.

Cervical cancer is the third most common gynecologic malignancy after endometrial and ovarian carcinoma respectively. It mainly affects women 40 to 45 years old and has an average overall 5-year survival of 67%. If the tumor is detected in an earlier stage, the 5-year survival can reach up to 90%. Risk factors for developing cervical cancer include human papillomavirus (HPV) infection, early onset sexual activity, multiple partners, oral contraceptive pills, and smoking. Cervical cancers are most commonly squamous cell type in 80% to 90% of cases. Cervical carcinomas have a poorer prognosis if they occur in younger patients, if tumor diameter is > 4 cm, if depth of stromal invasion > 5 mm, or if histology is of adenocarcinoma arising from the glandular lining of the endocervical canal rather than the squamous epithelium. Tumors that are entirely within the cervical canal are detected later leading to poor prognosis as well.

Goal of imaging is essentially to help the clinician determine which patients have early disease that can be treated surgically and which patients have advanced disease that will be treated with radiation and possible chemotherapy. This mandates that radiologist should be familiar with the staging system of cervical cancer and how this affects management.

STAGING OF CERVICAL CANCER

- Stage I: Tumor is strictly confined to the cervix (Fig. C15.1).
  - Stage IA: Only diagnosed microscopically based on abnormal PAP smear.
  - Stage IB: Clinically visible tumor < 4 cm (IB1) or >4 cm (IB2).
- Stage II: Tumor invades beyond uterus (not lower third of vagina).
  - Stage IIA: No parametrial invasion.
  - Stage IIB: With parametrial invasion (Fig. C15.2).
- Stage III:
  - Stage IIIA: Tumor extends to lower third of the vagina.
  - Stage IIIB: Tumor extends to pelvic sidewalls or causing hydronephrosis/ nonfunctioning kidney.
- Stage IV: Tumor extends to rectal mucosa or bladder or extends outside true pelvis (Fig. C15.3).
  - Stage IVA: Spread to adjacent organs.
  - Stage IVB: Spread to distant organs.

Overall stages IA and IB1 tumors are treated with local ablation, brachytherapy, or fertility-preserving surgery with simple or modified radical hysterectomy. Stage IB2 and stage and stage IIA tumors are treated with radical hysterectomy and lymph node dissection. There is a trend for increasing use of chemoradiation in conjunction with the abovementioned treatments.

Stage IIB and beyond would not benefit from surgical intervention and are only treated with radiation/chemotherapy.

Recent data are showing that MRI can accurately stage cervical cancer with an accuracy of 94% for stage IB and II, and more important an accuracy of 75% to 95% for evaluating parametrial invasion, which corresponds to stage IIB and makes patients not candidates for surgical intervention.

FINDINGS

MRI Findings of Cervical Cancer

T1 images show the tumor as isointense to the normal cervix (Fig. C15.1).

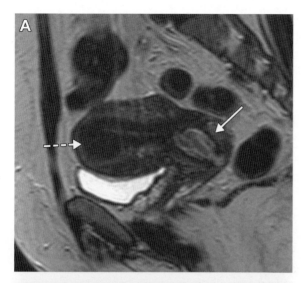

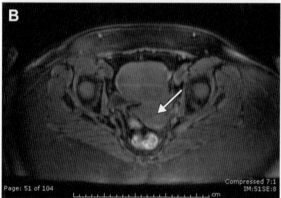

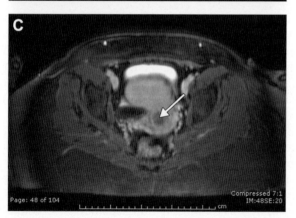

Fig. C15.1 (A) Sagittal T2-weighted pelvic MRI image showing a stage I cervical carcinoma as an area of higher T2 signal adjacent to the lower signal normal cervical tissue (arrow). Incidental intramural uterine leiomyoma partially imaged along the uterine fundus as an area of darker T2 signal (dashed arrow). (B) Axial T1-weighted fat-saturated pelvic MRI image before contrast administration demonstrating that the cervical carcinoma is isointense to normal cervical tissue (arrow). (C) Axial T1-weighted fat-saturated image after contrast administration showing a central area corresponding to cervical carcinoma of decreased enhancement (arrow) when compared to the surrounding normal enhancing cervical tissue.

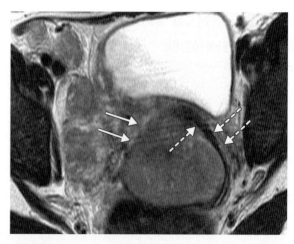

Fig. C15.2 Axial oblique T2-weighted image demonstrates disruption of the low-signal cervical stromal ring (arrows) consistent with parametrial invasion, making the tumor at least stage IIB and ineligible for surgical intervention. The tumor does not involve the left parametrium marked by normal low-signal intensity rim (dashed arrows).

Cervical tumors are best demonstrated on T2 images. Cervical cancer is likely hyperintense on T2-weighted images against the low-signal of normal cervical stroma (Fig. C15.1).

If a rim of low-signal intensity is present around the tumor, it indicates that the tumor is confined to the cervix with no parametrial spread (Fig. C15.1). Any disruption in the low-signal intensity rim is a sign of parametrial invasion (Fig. C15.2).

PET/CT Findings of Cervical Cancer

PET/CT findings of cervical cancer (Figs. C15.4, C15.5):

- PET/CT can show distant metastatic disease even in patients with small primary tumors.
- PET/CT demonstrates lymphadenopathy in the pelvis and the abdomen (paraaortic), which changes radiation therapy planning.
- Primary tumor is iso or hypoattenuating on CT images relative to normal cervical tissue and has moderate to markedly increased metabolic activity.
- Most tumors that are 0.7 cm or larger demonstrate PET activity.
- Due to spatial resolution limitations, PET/CT may not detect small areas of disease involvement near the primary tumor like parametrial spread.
- PET/CT can detect metastatic deposits in lymph nodes that are normal size and may not have been detected by other imaging modalities alone like CT or MRI.

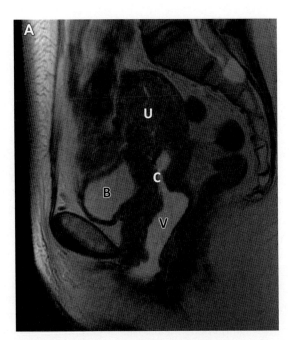
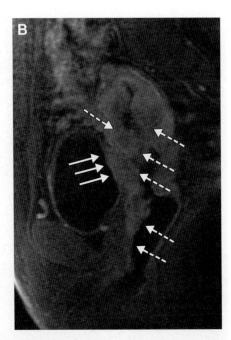

Fig. C15.3 (A) Sagittal T2-weighted image shows an advanced stage IV cervical cancer. The vagina is distended with Gel (V). The tumor extends to the uterus, vagina, and urinary bladder (U). (B) Sagittal T1 fat-saturated postcontrast image shows enhancement of tumor extending to uterus, vagina (dashed arrows). Note that urinary bladder invasion is better delineated on postcontrast images (arrows). B, urinary bladder; C, cervix; U, uterus; V, vagina.

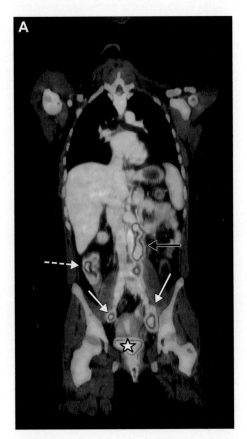
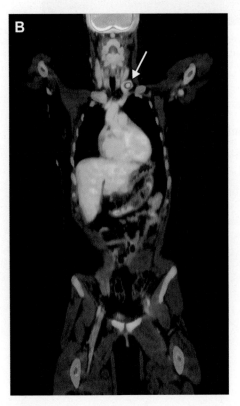

Fig. C15.4 (A) PET/CT coronal image showing activity in the pelvis (star) consistent with cervical carcinoma with bilateral pelvic (arrows) and left paraaortic lymph node activity (black arrow) consistent with metastatic lymphadenopathy. Activity along the right lower abdomen is physiologic colon activity (dashed arrow). (B) Coronal PET/CT image of the same patient with activity in a left supraclavicular lymph node (arrow) later proven to be metastatic cervical carcinoma on fine needle aspiration.

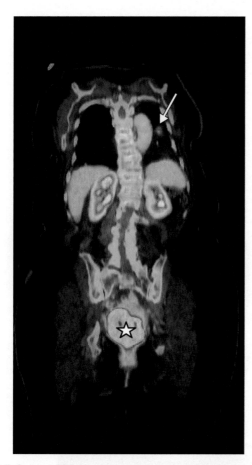

Fig. C15.5 Coronal PET/CT image with pelvic activity from cervical carcinoma (star) and activity in the left mid lung from metastatic pulmonary nodule (arrow). Physiologic bilateral renal activity is also present.

Clinical Differential Diagnosis

- Cervical polyps
- Cervicitis
- Endometrial or vaginal cancer secondarily involving the cervix

IMAGING DIFFERENTIAL DIAGNOSIS

Nabothian cyst: Less complex appearance than cancer on a T2-weighted image and it will not enhance.

Cervical polyp: Histologic differentiation is needed since they appear as a mass with or without cysts filling the endocervical canal.

Endometrial polyp or fibroid: Look for stalk of the mass prolapsing through the cervical canal.

Endometrial or vaginal cancer secondarily involving the cervix: Look for where the mass is centered to suggest the initial origin. Histologic evaluation may be needed to determine original source.

TREATMENT

Hysterectomy for patients where disease is limited to the cervix with no parametrial invasion or metastatic lymphadenopathy. Chemotherapy and radiation for patients with lymph node metastases or parametrial extension.

REFERENCES AND SUGGESTED READING

1. Okamoto Y, Tanaka Y, Nishida M, et al. MR Imaging of the uterine cervix: imaging-pathologic correlation. *RadioGraphics.* 2003;23:425-445.

2. Pandharipande P, Choy G, del Carmen M, Gazelle G, Russell A, Lee S. MRI and PET/CT for triaging Stage 1B clinically operable cervical cancer to appropriate therapy: decision analysis to assess patient outcomes. *AJR.* 2009;192:802-814. doi:10.2214/AJR.08.1224.

3. Sala E, Wakely S, Senior E, Lomas D. MRI of malignant neoplasms of the uterine corpus and cervix. *AJR.* 2007;188:1577-1587. doi:10.2214/AJR.06.1196.

4. Son H, Kositwattanarerk A, Hayes M, et al. PET/CT evaluation of cervical cancer: spectrum of disease. *RadioGraphics,* 2010;30:1251-1268.

CASE 16: UTERINE LEIOMYOMA

PATIENT PRESENTATION

A 37-year-old woman presents with dysfunctional uterine bleeding and recurrent miscarriages.

CLINICAL SUSPICION

Uterine leiomyoma, but symptoms are not specific and endometrial cancer is a consideration.

IMAGING MODALITY OF CHOICE

Transabdominal and transvaginal pelvic ultrasound. Advantages: readily available, low cost, sensitive, no ionizing radiation.

MRI is not usually required for diagnosis except in complex cases or for problem solving. However, MRI is the most sensitive and specific modality in detecting uterine leiomyomas.

Uterine leiomyoma (uterine fibroid) is a benign tumor arising from the myometrium (smooth muscle), and it is considered the most common solid benign uterine neoplasm. Uterine leiomyomas occur in 25% of women in the reproductive age and are more common in the African American population.

Fibroids are typically affected by cyclical hormonal changes (stimulated by estrogen), hence they are rare in prepubertal females, usually grow during pregnancy, and involute with menopause.

Uterine leiomyomas are multiple in 85% of cases, and they vary significantly in size and location. Uterine leiomyomas can be further subdivided based on location into intramural (most common) (Fig. C16.1), subserosal

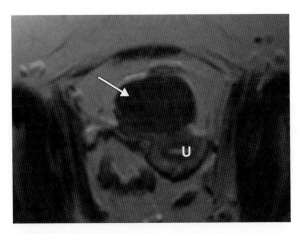

Fig. C16.2 Axial T2-weighted image of the pelvis shows a large exophytic, broad-based hypointense mass (arrow) arising from the uterus (U) consistent with a subserosal leiomyoma.

(Fig. C16.2), and submucosal (least common 10%) (Fig. C16.3).

Uterine leiomyomas are often asymptomatic and discovered incidentally, however the ones of the submucosal subtype are usually symptomatic, causing abnormal uterine bleeding, recurrent miscarriages, infertility, premature labor, and/or fetal malpresentation; this is understandable given the location inside the endometrial cavity. Intramural subtypes are symptomatic only in 25% of cases, and the symptoms usually arise from dysfunctional uterine bleeding. The subserosal subtype are also only symptomatic in 25% of cases; however, symptoms are mainly due to pressure effects and pain.

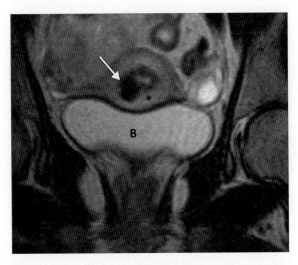

Fig. C16.1 Coronal T2-weighted MRI image of the pelvis shows a hypointense mass (arrow) centered primarily within the myometrium (asterisk) with minimal submucosal extension in the uterine fundus. Findings are consistent with an intramural leiomyoma with mild submucosal extension. (B) Urinary bladder.

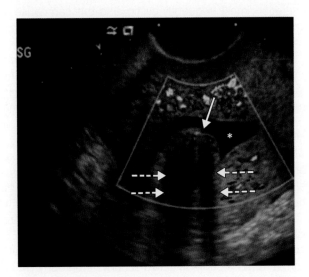

Fig. C16.3 Color Doppler image from a sonohysterography study shows a broad-based, hypoechoic, and well-defined solid mass (arrow) projecting into the endometrial cavity (asterisk). The mass has posterior acoustic shadowing from calcification (dashed arrows). Note the overlying echogenic layer of endometrium confirming subendometrial location consistent with submucosal fibroid.

Only < 0.5% of all leiomyomas can undergo malignant transformation into leiomyosarcomas, and unfortunately no imaging modality can distinguish benign leiomyomas from the rare leiomyosarcomas.

FINDINGS

Sonographic Findings of Uncomplicated Uterine Leiomyoma

- Leiomyomas are usually hypoechoic to normal myometrium.
- Calcification is occasionally seen and causes posterior acoustic shadowing.
- Typically color Doppler evaluation shows increased vascularity unless there is degeneration.

CT Findings of Uncomplicated Uterine Leiomyoma

- Soft tissue mass.
- Coarse calcifications can be seen.
- Usually distort the normal smooth uterine contour.
- Enhancement pattern is variable.

MRI Findings of Uncomplicated Uterine Leiomyoma

- Isointense to slightly increased signal intensity on T1-weighted imaging.
- Low-signal intensity on T2-weighted imaging in comparison to the myometrium.
- Variable enhancement on postcontrast sequences.

Uterine leiomyomas can undergo different types of degeneration, most frequently cystic, and this can cause diagnostic dilemma based on US and CT. However, MRI can be helpful as a problem-solving tool in those instances.

Submucosal leiomyomas are the most common form of symptomatic leiomyomas and can be clinically challenging to differentiate from endometrial polyps. Imaging plays an essential role in differentiating submucosal leiomyomas from endometrial polyps. Sonohysterography can also be utilized for differentiation.

On ultrasound and sonohysterography, submucosal fibroids (Fig. C16.3) are broad based, hypoechoic, well defined, solid masses with posterior acoustic shadowing. They also usually have an overlying echogenic layer of endometrium, which helps confirm their subendometrial location and distinguish it from endometrial polyps (Fig. C16.4). If questionable on regular pelvic ultrasound evaluation, a newer technique called sonohysterography (where saline can be injected to distend the endometrial cavity and better delineate endometrial pathologies) can be used in which the endometrial cavity is filled with fluid to

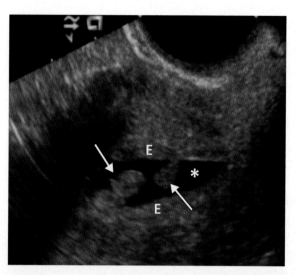

Fig. C16.4 Axial sonohysterogram shows 2 pedunculated echogenic masses (arrows) in the fluid-filled endometrial cavity (asterisk). The masses are in continuity with endometrium (E) but not myometrium. Appearance is compatible with endometrial polyps.

increase contrast and can better delineate mass indenting the endometrial cavity rather than being endometrial in origin. Sonohysterography can also be helpful for presurgical planning as submucosal fibroids can be removed hysteroscopically only if the intraluminal surface is > 50% of total circumference of the mass.

DIFFERENTIAL

Imaging differential diagnosis for uterine leiomyomas:

Uterine leiomyosarcoma: Extremely rare. No imaging modality can differentiate benign leiomyoma from the rare malignant leiomyosarcoma.

Focal adenomyosis: On US, leiomyoma is better defined than adenomyoma and may have a pseudocapsule of compressed adjacent myometrial tissue. MRI is a good modality to distinguish focal adenomyosis from leiomyoma in complex cases.

Ovarian mass: Subserosal leiomyomas can sometimes be confused to be masses that are ovarian in origin on US. MRI is a good imaging tool to differentiate subserosal fibroids from ovarian neoplasms.

Endometrial polyp: Endometrial polyps (Fig. C16.4) do not have a stretched endometrial lining overlying the mass and do not have continuity with underlying myometrium. A single vascular pedicle can also be seen on color Doppler evaluation. On MRI, endometrial polyps have high signal intensity on T2-weighted images (isointense to endometrium).

TREATMENT

Treatment of uterine leiomyoma:

- Surgical:
  - Myomectomy: transabdominal or hysteroscopic (for submucosal fibroids).
  - Total hysterectomy if extensive disease is present.
- Uterine artery embolization is an emerging interventional procedure alternative to total hysterectomy with recent data proving its effectiveness in alleviating symptoms (bleeding, pressure, and pain) in up to 98% of cases. It also causes up to 60% decrease in leiomyoma size after one year of treatment.
- Medical treatment using GnRH analogues: This can be helpful; however, symptoms tend to recur after cessation of medication.

REFERENCES AND SUGGESTED READING

1. Dubinsky TJ. Value of sonography in the diagnosis of abnormal vaginal bleeding. *J Clin Ultrasound.* 2004;32(7):348-353.
2. Ojili V, et al. Uterine artery embolization for the treatment of symptomatic fibroids. *Int J Gynaecol Obstet.* 2004;87(3): 249-251.
3. Murase E, et al. Uterine leiomyomas: histopathologic features, MR imaging findings, differential diagnosis, and treatment. *RadioGraphics.* 1999;19(5):1179-1197.
4. Ueda H, et al. Unusual appearances of uterine leiomyomas: MR imaging findings and their histopathologic backgrounds. *RadioGraphics.* 1999;19 Spec No:S131-S145.
5. Mayer DP et al. Ultrasonography and magnetic resonance imaging of uterine fibroids. *Obstet Gynecol Clin North Am.* 1995;22(4):667-725.
6. Atri M, et al. Transvaginal US appearance of endometrial abnormalities. *RadioGraphics.* 1994;14(3):483-492.

INTRODUCTION TO WOMEN'S IMAGING (BREAST IMAGING)

BREAST ANATOMY

The basic functional unit in the breast is the lobule, also called the terminal ductal lobular unit (TDLU). The TDLU consists of 10 to 100 acini that drain into the terminal ducts.

The terminal ducts drain into larger ducts and finally into the main duct of the lobe or segment, which drains into the nipple. The breast contains 15 to 18 lobes, each of which contains 20 to 40 lobules (Fig. 10.3).

The terminal ductal lobular unit is an important structure physiologically because most invasive cancers arise from it. It is also the site of origin of ductal carcinoma in situ (DCIS), lobular carcinoma in situ (LCIS), fibroadenoma, and fibrocystic changes including cysts, apocrine metaplasia, adenosis, and epitheliosis.

Breast Cancer Screening

Mammography is the only method of screening for breast cancer shown to decrease mortality. Annual screening mammography is recommended starting at:

1. Age 40 for general population.
2. Age 25 to 30 for BRCA (BReast CAncer 1) carriers and untested relatives of BRCA carriers.

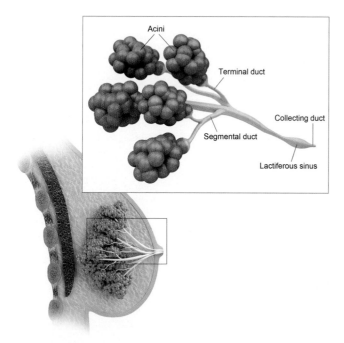

Fig. 10.3 Breast anatomy, demonstrating the acini draining into the terminal ducts and eventually converging into the collecting ducts that terminate in the nipple.

3. Age 25 to 30 or 10 years earlier than the age of the affected relative at diagnosis (whichever is later) for women with a first-degree relative with premenopausal breast cancer or for women with a lifetime risk of breast cancer ≥ 20% on the basis of family history.
4. Eight years after radiation therapy but not before age 25 for women who received mantle radiation between the ages of 10 and 30.
5. Any age for women with biopsy-proven lobular neoplasia, atypical ductal hyperplasia (ADH), ductal carcinoma in situ (DCIS), or invasive breast cancer.

However, mammography alone does not perform as well as mammography plus supplemental screening in certain subsets of women, particularly those with a genetic predisposition to the disease and those with dense breasts. Therefore, supplemental screening is recommended in selected high-risk populations; as such, MRI and mammography combined have a higher sensitivity (92.7%) than ultrasound (US) and mammography combined (52%). In high-risk women for whom supplemental screening is indicated, MRI is recommended when possible. US can be used for patients with contraindications to MRI.

Microcalcifications

Diagnostic mammographic workup (including spot magnifications views in the craniocaudal, mediolateral oblique, and 90° mediolateral projections) remains the optimal initial procedure for evaluating screening-detected calcifications that are not typically benign. Ultrasound should only be performed if the diagnostic mammographic workup demonstrates suspicious microcalcifications with an associated mass/focal asymmetry or in cases of suspicious calcifications with an extensive distribution. This may be useful in determining the method of biopsy guidance, diagnosing invasive disease, and facilitating a single-step surgery (excision and lymph node dissection). Currently, short-term follow-up or biopsy of calcifications directly from screening mammography is not recommended.

Nonpalpable Masses

Screening mammography potentiates the detection of early, clinically occult cancers, with benchmark data demonstrating mean size at diagnosis to be 13 mm, and a detection rate of 4.7/1,000 screening examinations. While most lesions found on screening mammography are benign, a PPV of 33% can be achieved for lesions undergoing biopsy after diagnostic evaluation.

Additional workup, including diagnostic mammography and/or US, may be required to differentiate suspicious findings, such as masses and asymmetries/focal asymmetries, from normal breast tissue. Application of *ACR BI-RADS Atlas* criteria, terminology, and assessments helps guide management and optimizes communication of findings and recommendations.

US is a useful adjunctive tool in evaluating abnormal mammographic findings, but it requires use of good quality, high-frequency equipment and application of strict criteria, as outlined in the *ACR BI-RADS Atlas.*

Breast US can help differentiate cysts from solid masses, aid in characterization of solid masses, and guide percutaneous biopsy. Elastography may improve specificity in the evaluation of solid masses.

Breast MRI may be useful as a problem-solving tool in a small, carefully selected group of patients who have inconclusive results after thorough diagnostic evaluation of mammographically detected noncalcified nonpalpable findings.

Percutaneous biopsy of suspicious lesions can provide accurate tissue diagnosis at decreased cost, precluding the need for surgery in specific benign cases while allowing definitive single-stage surgical treatment in cases returned as malignant. Core needle biopsy, using either stereotactic or US guidance, is preferable to fine needle aspiration cytology, based on sufficiency and accuracy of sampling.

Palpable Masses

Because of inconsistencies in clinical examination, a thorough imaging workup of a palpable mass should be completed prior to biopsy. Diagnostic mammography is the initial imaging modality of choice for evaluating a clinically detected palpable breast mass in a woman age 40 or older.

Breast US is the initial imaging modality of choice for evaluating a clinically detected palpable breast mass in a woman younger than age 30. For women ages 30 to 39, either US or diagnostic mammography may be used for initial evaluation. Correlation between imaging and the palpable area of concern is essential.

Any highly suspicious breast mass detected by imaging should be biopsied, irrespective of palpable findings. Any highly suspicious breast mass detected by palpation should be biopsied, irrespective of imaging findings.

REFERENCES

1. ACR Appropriateness Criteria, Breast cancer screening.

2. Reduction in breast cancer mortality from organized service screening with mammography: further confirmation with extended data. *Cancer Epidemiol Biomarkers Prev.* 2006;15(1):45-51.

3. Duffy SW, Tabar L, Chen HH, et al. The impact of organized mammography service screening on breast carcinoma mortality in seven Swedish counties. *Cancer.* 2002;95(3): 458-469.

4. Hendrick RE, Smith RA, Rutledge JH III. Smart CR. Benefit of screening mammography in women aged 40-49: a new meta-analysis of randomized controlled trials. *J Natl Cancer Inst Monogr.* 1997;(22):87-92.

5. Tabar L, Vitak B, Chen HH, Yen MF, Duffy SW, Smith RA. Beyond randomized controlled trials: organized mammographic screening substantially reduces breast carcinoma mortality. *Cancer.* 2001;91(9):1724-1731.

6. Lee CH, Dershaw DD, Kopans D, et al. Breast cancer screening with imaging: recommendations from the Society of Breast Imaging and the ACR on the use of mammography, breast MRI, breast ultrasound, and other technologies for the detection of clinically occult breast cancer. *J Am Coll Radiol.* 2010;7(1):18-27.

7. Berg WA. Tailored supplemental screening for breast cancer: what now and what next? *AJR.* 2009;192(2):390-399.

8. Brekelmans CT, Seynaeve C, Bartels CC, et al. Effectiveness of breast cancer surveillance in BRCA1/2 gene mutation carriers and women with high familial risk. *J Clin Oncol.* 2001;19(4):924-930.

9. Chart PL, Franssen E. Management of women at increased risk for breast cancer: preliminary results from a new program. *CMAJ.* 1997;157(9):1235-1242.

10. Macmillan RD. Screening women with a family history of breast cancer—results from the British Familial Breast Cancer Group. *Eur J Surg Oncol.* 2000;26(2):149-152.

11. Scheuer L, Kauff N, Robson M, et al. Outcome of preventive surgery and screening for breast and ovarian cancer in BRCA mutation carriers. *J Clin Oncol.* 2002;20(5):1260-1268.

12. Warner E, Plewes DB, Shumak RS, et al. Comparison of breast magnetic resonance imaging, mammography, and ultrasound for surveillance of women at high risk for hereditary breast cancer. *J Clin Oncol.* 2001;19(15):3524-3531.

13. ACR Appropriateness Criteria, Breast microcalcifications—initial diagnostic workup.

14. ACR Appropriateness Criteria, Nonpalpable mammographic findings excluding calcifications.

15. ACR Appropriateness Criteria, Palpable breast masses.

BREAST IMAGING

BI-RADS CLASSIFICATION

BI-RADS stands for the Breast Imaging Reporting and Data System for breast imaging, which was introduced by the American College of Radiology (ACR).

All other systems that were previously used were abandoned because unlike the BI-RADS system, they lacked quantification, used very subjective and undefined terms, and were not evidence-based.

BI-RADS is a quality assurance tool designed to standardize mammography reporting, reduce confusion in breast imaging interpretations, and facilitate outcome monitoring.

It contains a lexicon for standardized terminology (descriptors) for mammography, breast US, and MRI, as well as standard reporting with final assessment categories and guidelines for follow-up and outcome monitoring.

It even helps evaluate the quality of reporting.

Report Organization

The reporting system is designed to provide an organized approach to image interpretation and reporting.

1. Describe the indication for the study.
2. Describe the breast composition.
3. Describe any significant finding.
4. Compare to previous studies.
5. Conclude to a final assessment category.
6. Give management recommendations.

When a breast lesion is described, standard BI-RADS descriptions for mammography, ultrasound, and MRI should be used as described below. If more than one imaging modality is performed, for instance US with mammography or with MRI, an integrated report with assessment based on the highest level of suspicion must be used.

When multiple modalities are used, we always need to make sure that we are dealing with the same lesion. For instance, a lesion found with US does not have to be the same as the mammographic or physical findings. Sometimes repeated mammographic imaging with markers on the lesion found with US can be helpful.

BREAST IMAGING LEXICON

Mammographic breast composition: Mammographic breast composition is described as follows:

1. The breast is almost entirely fat (< 25% glandular tissue)
2. Scattered fibroglandular densities (25%-50%)

3. Heterogeneously dense breast tissue (51%-75%)
4. Extremely dense (> 75% glandular)

Mass: A *mass* is a space-occupying lesion seen in two different projections. If a potential mass is seen in only a single projection it should be called a *density* until its three-dimensionality is confirmed. Masses can be further subdivided into:

1. Circumscribed (well-defined or sharply defined) margins: The margins are sharply demarcated with an abrupt transition between the lesion and the surrounding tissue. Without additional modifiers, there is nothing to suggest infiltration.
2. Indistinct (ill-defined) margins: The poor definition of the margins raises concern that there may be infiltration by the lesion and this is not likely due to superimposed normal breast tissue.
3. Speculated margins: The lesion is characterized by lines radiating from the margins of a mass.

Architectural distortion: The normal architecture is distorted with no definite mass visible. This includes speculations radiating from a point, and focal retraction or distortion of the edge of the parenchyma. Architectural distortion can also be an associated finding.

Focal asymmetry: This is a density that cannot be accurately described using the other shapes. It is visible as asymmetry of tissue density with similar shape on two views, but completely lacking borders and the conspicuity of a true mass. It could represent an island of normal breast, but its lack of specific benign characteristics may warrant further evaluation. Additional imaging may reveal a true mass or significant architectural distortion. Due to confusion of the term *mass* with the term *density*, which describes attenuation characteristics of masses, the term *density* has been replaced with *asymmetry*.

Calcifications:

1. **Amorphous or indistinct calcifications:** These are often round or "flake" shaped calcifications that are sufficiently small or hazy in appearance that a more specific morphologic classification cannot be determined.
2. **Coarse, heterogeneous calcifications:** Irregular calcifications with varying sizes and shapes that are usually larger than 0.5 mm in diameter.
3. **Fine, pleomorphic or branching calcifications:** Fine pleomorphic calcifications are more conspicuous than the amorphous forms. They vary in sizes and shapes and are usually smaller than 0.5 mm. Fine branching calcifications are thin, linear, or curvilinear, may be discontinuous and smaller than

0.5 mm. Their appearance suggests filling in of the lumen of a duct involved irregularly by breast cancer.

4. **Benign calcifications:** Benign calcifications are usually larger than calcifications associated with malignancy. They are usually coarser, often round with smooth margins, and are much more easily seen.

When an abnormality is described (mass, architectural distortion, focal asymmetry, or calcifications), we always use the standard BI-RADS descriptors and mention the lesion size and location.

FINAL ASSESSMENT CATEGORIES

A negative diagnostic examination is one that is negative, with a benign or probably benign finding (BI-RADS 1, 2, or 3). In BI-RADS 3, the radiologist prefers to establish the stability of a lesion by short-term follow-up.

In the evaluation of BI-RADS 3 lesions, the malignancy rate should be < 2%. A positive diagnostic examination is one that requires a tissue diagnosis (BI-RADS 4 and 5). In BI-RADS 4, the radiologist has sufficient concern to urge a biopsy (2%-95% chance of malignancy). In BI-RADS 5, the chance of malignancy should be > 95%.

BI-RADS 0: Needs additional imaging evaluation and/or prior mammograms for comparison. BI-RADS 0 is utilized when further imaging evaluation (eg, additional views or ultrasound) or retrieval of prior films is required. When additional imaging studies are completed, a final assessment is made. This category should always be avoided by immediately doing additional imaging or retrieving old films before reporting. It is even better to have the old films before starting the examination

BI-RADS 1: Negative: There is nothing to comment on. The breasts are symmetric and have no masses, architectural distortion, or suspicious calcifications present.

BI-RADS 2: Benign finding. Like BI-RADS 1, this is negative for malignancy, but here, the interpreter chooses to describe a benign finding in the mammography report. Involuting, calcified fibroadenomas, multiple secretory calcifications, fat-containing lesions such as oil cysts, lipomas, galactoceles, and mixed-density hamartomas, all have characteristically benign appearances and may be labeled with confidence. The interpreter may also choose to describe intramammary lymph nodes, vascular calcifications, implants, or architectural distortion clearly related to prior surgery, while still concluding that there is no mammographic evidence of malignancy.

BI-RADS 3: Probably benign finding—initial short-interval follow-up is suggested. A finding placed in this category should have less than a 2% risk of malignancy. It is not expected to change over the follow-up interval, but the radiologist would prefer to establish its stability. Lesions appropriately placed in this category include:

- Nonpalpable, circumscribed mass on a baseline mammogram (unless it can be shown to be a cyst, an intramammary lymph node, or another benign finding)
- Focal asymmetry that becomes less dense on spot compression view
- Cluster of punctate calcifications

The initial short-term follow-up is a unilateral mammogram at 6 months, then a bilateral follow-up examination at 12 months and 24 months after the initial examination. If the findings shows no change in the follow-up period, the final assessment is changed to BI-RADS 2 (benign) and no further follow-up is needed. If a BI-RADS 3 lesion shows any change during follow-up, it will change into a BI-RADS 4 or 5 and appropriate action should be taken.

BI-RADS 4: Suspicious abnormality—biopsy should be considered. BI-RADS 4 is reserved for findings that do not have the classic appearance of malignancy but have a wide range of probability of malignancy (2%-95%).

BI-RADS 5: Highly suggestive of malignancy—appropriate action should be taken. BI-RADS 5 must be reserved for findings that are classic breast cancers, with a > 95% likelihood of malignancy. A speculated, irregular high-density mass, a segmental or linear arrangement of fine linear calcifications or an irregular speculated mass with associated pleomorphic calcifications are examples of lesions that should be placed in BI-RADS 5.

BI-RADS 5 contains lesions for which one-stage surgical treatment could be considered without preliminary biopsy. However, current oncologic management may require percutaneous tissue sampling as, for example, when sentinel lymph node imaging is included in surgical treatment or when neoadjuvant chemotherapy is administered.

BI-RADS 6: Known biopsy-proven malignancy—appropriate action should be taken. BI-RADS 6 is reserved for lesions identified on the imaging study with biopsy proof of malignancy prior to definitive therapy. This category was added to the classification because sometimes patients are treated with neoadjuvant chemotherapy. During the course of the treatment the tumor may be less visible, while still you know you are dealing with biopsy-proven cancer.

Figs. 10.4 to 10.10 show some BIRADS example cases.

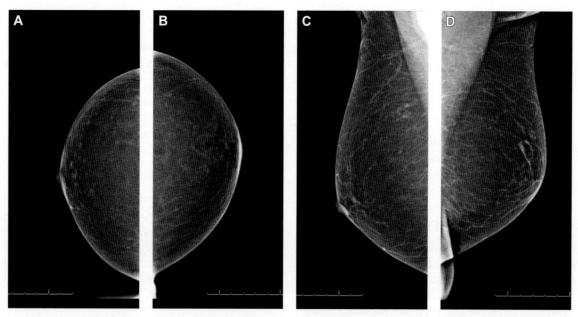

Fig. 10.4 Example 1: Standard craniocaudal (CC) and mediolateral oblique (MLO) veiws of bilateral breasts in a screening mammogram showing negative mammogram (BIRADS 1). Breast stroma is almost completely fatty replaced. Breasts are symmetrical. No mass or architectural distortion. No calcifications or suspicious lymph nodes.

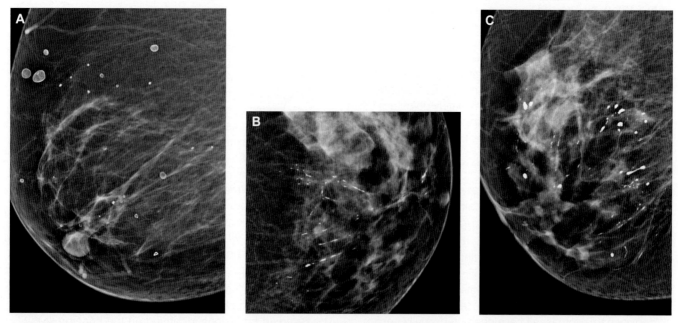

Fig. 10.5 Example 2: Examples of benign findings classified as BIRADS 2. (A) Multiple round and oval-shaped well-circumscribed masses are seen with uniform continous eggshell calcifications consistent with multiple oil cysts that are manifestations of remote posttraumatic fat necrosis. (B) Bilateral dense, thick, continous rodlike calcifications in a ductal pattern radiating from the nipple. Minimal rounded calcifications are seen also. Appearance is typical for secretory calcifications that are benign. Such calcifications occur mainly due to plasma cell mastitis in premenopausal women; specifically those with prior pregnancies. In postmenopausal women they are mainly due to mammary duct ectasia unrelated to prior pregnancies.

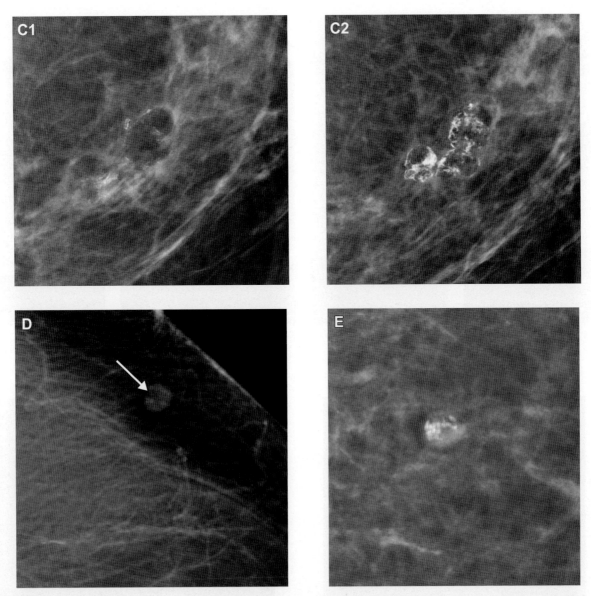

Fig. 10.5 (*continued*) (C) C-1 diagnostic mammography was obtained in this 45-year-old patient who had a papable mass in one of her breasts 2 years after having bilateral breast reduction surgery. A magnified image of the findings seen correlating to the area of palpable mass shows a bilobed lucent mass with curvilinear rim of calcifications. Appearance is typical for fat necrosis. Calcifications typically develop in the area of fat necrosis 1.5 to 5 years after trauma "in this case iatrogenic due to surgical reduction." If surgery was done for tumor resection and calcifications were seen at the site of lumpectomy within the first 1.5 years postsurgery, they are more likely to be due to residual or recurrent tumor rather than fat necrosis, particularly if the original tumor had calcifications. Calcifications due to fat necrosis, and any other benign etiology, usually coarsen over time as seen in Fig. C-2, which is an image taken for the same patient 2 years after C-1. (D) Mammography image shows a well-circumscribed lobulated mass with a fatty lucent hilum (arrow) in the lateral breast. Appearance is typical for a benign intramammary lymph node that was mammographically stable for at least 4 years. (E) Mammography image shows a well-circumscribed lobulated that which has been stable over the course of years with interval development of popcornlike calcifications when compared to prior studies consistent with a degenerating fibroadenoma.

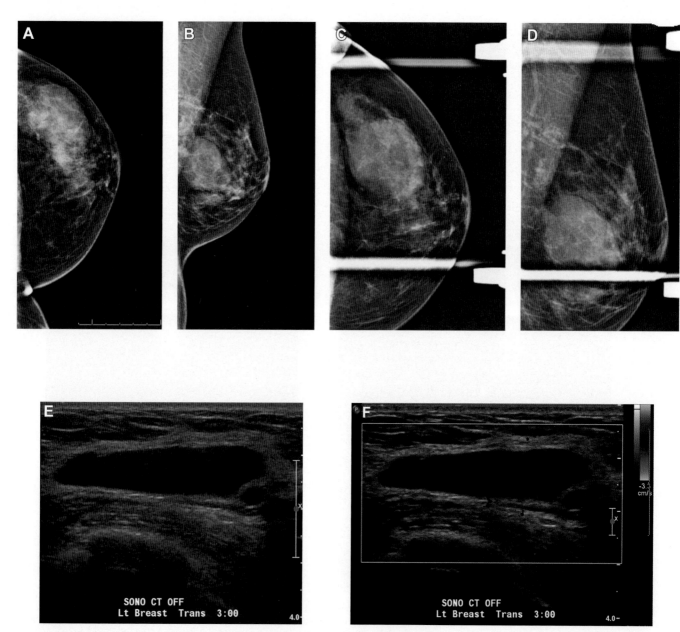

Fig. 10.6 Example 3: (A,B) standard CC and MLO views of the left breast in a base line screening mammogram for this patient who is 40 years old. A large oval mass is seen in the outer deep mid left breast with partially obscured margins; a BIRADS 0 classification was given to this study and the patient was called back for obtaining additional views and/or ultrasound. (C,D) Compression CC and ML views were obtained that showed the mass to have well-circumscribed margins. (E,F) Ultrasound of the mass shows a large, well-circumscribed anechoic oval mass with posterior acoustic enhancement and no increased blood flow. This corresponds to the mammographic finding and is consistent with a simple cyst. A small adjacent simple cyst is also seen. At that point a BIRADS classification of 2 was given.

Simple breast cysts are completely benign and are thought to occur due to duct obstruction. They are the most commonly encountered breast masses and can be difficult to be distinguished from solid masses based on mammographic findings. They can fluctuate in size with menstrual cycle and seem to grow under estrogenic stimulation, maximizing in the premenstrual phase. No treatment is usually required unless they are painful.

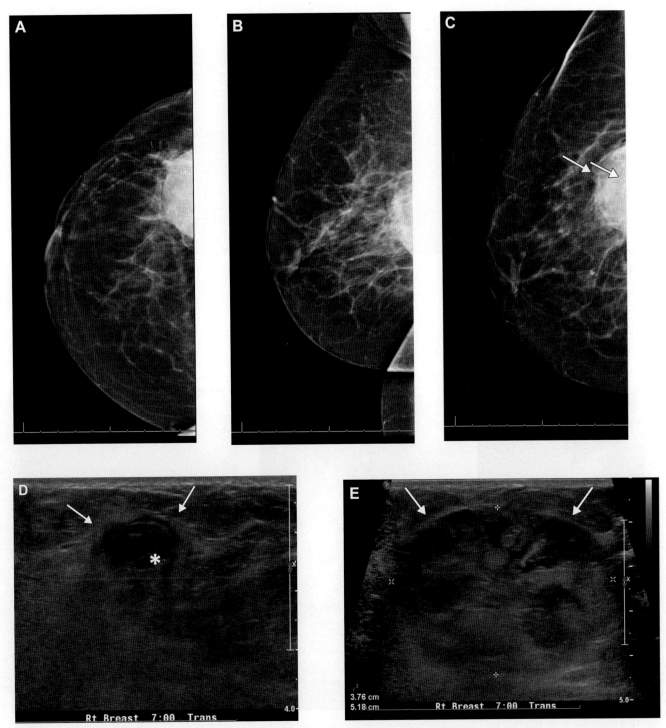

Fig. 10.7 Example 4: (A,B) Standard CC and MLO views of the right breast in this screening mammogram for a 60-year-old woman who never had any prior mammograms. There is a large, dense, partially visualized oval mass in the outer deep mid right breast (arrows), the visualized margins of the mass appear well demarcated (notice the similarity to the mammographic findings on prior study). The study was reported as a BIRADS 0 and the patient was called back for obtaining additional views and/or ultrasound. (C) An exaggerated CC view failed to show the posterior margins of the mass. (D,E,F) US images of the mass shows a corresponding large heterogeneous irregular mass (arrows) invading the pectoralis muscle (asterisk) with posterior acoustic enhancement and focal areas of increased blood flow. At that point and since findings were highly suggestive of malignancy, the BIRADS classification was upgraded to 5 based on ultrasound features and a biopsy was obtained that confirmed mucinous carcinoma of the breast. The posterior acoustic enhancement, although atypical with malignant neoplasm, is seen in this case as a result of the mucinous component. In this case the diagnosis of mucinous carcinoma was suggested based on the typical imaging characteristics prior to pathological diagnosis. (*continued*)

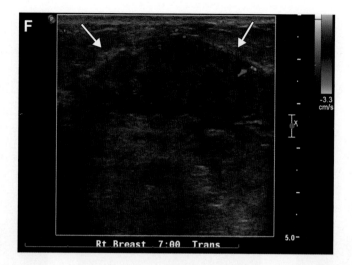

Fig. 10.7 (*continued*)

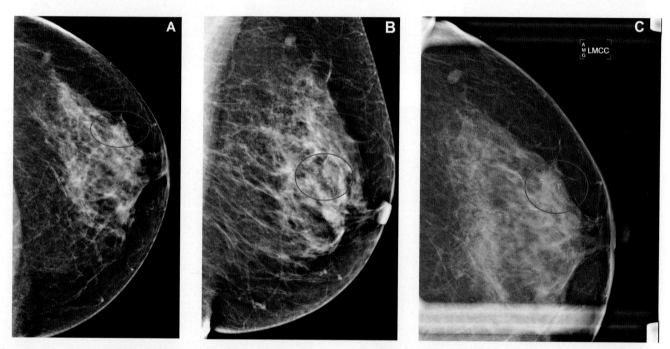

Fig. 10.8 Example 5: (A,B) Standard CC and MLO views of the left breast in a screening mammogram for a 61-year-old woman shows a suspicious new area of fine calcifications in the outer mid left breast (oval shape). The study was reported as BIRADS 0 and the patient was called back for obtaining magnification views to better characterize the calcifications. (C,D) Compression CC and ML views shows the calcifications are pleomorphic and heterogeneous with a linear and slightly branching pattern (oval shape). The appearance is suspicious for malignancy, and hence the classification was upgraded to BIRADS 4 and biopsy was recommended. Vacuum assisted stereotactic biopsy of those calcifications showed a high-grade ductal carcinoma in situ.

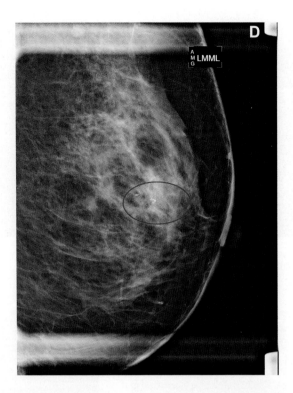

Fig. 10.8 (*continued*)

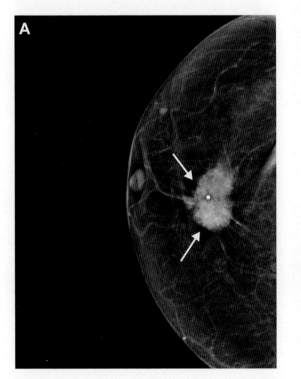

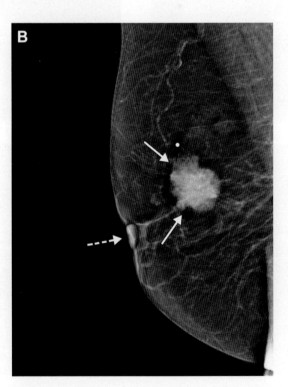

Fig. 10.9 Example 6: (A,B) Diagnostic mammography was obtained in this 70-year-old woman for a palpable mass in the right breast. There is a large speculated, irregular high-density mass (arrows) with fine linear calcifications and nipple retraction (dashed arrows). Findings are highly suggestive of malignancy and are reported as BIRADS 5. (*continued*)

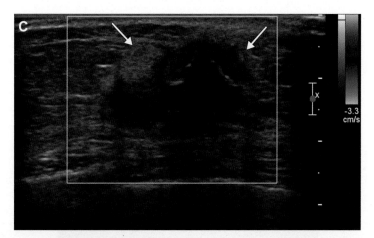

Fig. 10.9 (*continued*) (C) Ultrasound image of the mass also shows an irregular hypoechoic mass with some increased internal blood flow (arrows). The appearance is also highly suggestive of malignancy. US guided biopsy was performed showing invasive ductal carcinoma of the breast.

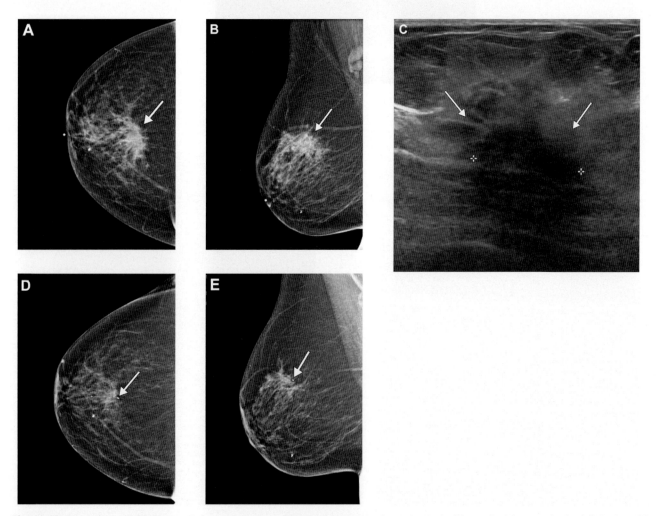

Fig. 10.10 Example 7: (A,B) Diagnostic mammogram in 63-year-old woman who presented with a palpable mass in the left breast. CC and MLO views of the left breast shows a large irregular speculated mass (arrows), which is highly suspicious for malignancy. US study was obtained (C) confirming the highly suspicious features of the mass (arrows) (hypoechoic, irregular, with posterior acoustic shadowing). The study was reported as BIRADS 5 and US guided biopsy was done confirming the diagnosis of an invasive ductal carcinoma of the breast. The patient received neoadjuvant chemotherapy (to reduce the tumor size preoperatively) and a mammogram was obtained after 6 months (D,E) that showed a clip at the site of the mass (arrows), which was left at the time of the biopsy. The mass has significantly shrunken in size in response to chemotherapy and the study was reported as BIRADS 6.

CASE 17: FIBROADENOMA

PATIENT PRESENTATION

A 22-year-old woman presents with a palpable mass in the left breast that was noticed incidentally. On clinical examination the mass appears firm, highly mobile, and painless.

CLINICAL SUSPICION

Fibroadenoma

IMAGING MODALITY OF CHOICE

Give the theoretical increased risk of radiation from mammography and low incidence of breast cancer in women younger than age 30, breast ultrasound should be the initial imaging modality of choice for evaluating a clinically detected palpable breast mass in this age group. If ultrasound demonstrates a suspicious finding, an ultrasound-guided biopsy should be performed and bilateral mammography is recommended to evaluate for additional ipsilateral and contralateral lesions. However, if a benign lesion such as fibroadenoma is demonstrated on ultrasound in this age group, sonographic surveillance may be an acceptable alternative to traditional biopsy.

Note: mammography has diminished sensitivity in detecting breast lesions in younger females due to denser breast tissue.

FINDINGS

Ultrasound findings of fibroadenoma (Fig. C17.1):

- Circumscribed oval or gently lobulated hypoechoic to isoechoic mass.
- Long axis parallel to skin surface.
- Length to depth ratio typically > 1.4.

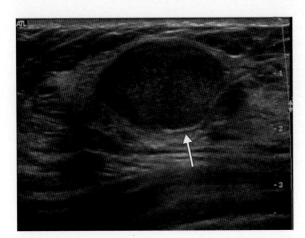

Fig. C17.1 Ultrasound shows a large, circumscribed, oval hypoechoic solid mass with a hyperechoic pseudocapsule (arrow).

- Homogenous, low level, internal echogenicity.
- It can be isoechoic with fat.
- Adjacent tissue may be compressed leading to a hyperechoic pseudocapsule.
- Associated calcifications may be seen indicated by echogenic foci with posterior shadowing typically in degenerating fibroadenomas seen in older patients.
- It could contain, in 2% to 4% of cases, small cystic foci, which is more in favor of phylloides tumor.
- Color Doppler may show internal septal vessels.

Fibroadenomas are benign fibroepithelial tumors that represent the most common solid mass in women of all ages. The mean age at diagnosis is 25 years old. The vast majority of such tumors are self-limited and involute spontaneously following menopause.

DIAGNOSTIC DIFFERENTIAL DIAGNOSIS

Phylloides tumor: 23% show cysts, especially if malignant.

Malignant neoplasms: May mimic fibroadenomas especially in old age groups.

Other benign lesions: Fat lobule, complicated cyst, lactating adenoma, and fibroadenomatoid change.

TREATMENT

- Clinical and sonographic follow-up is adequate for most of the cases.
- Biopsy if new, enlarging or suspicious features.
- Complete excision is curative.
- If growth > 20% in diameter in 6 months, this highly suggests phylloides tumor and surgical excision is recommended.

REFERENCES AND SUGGESTED READING

1. Graf O, Helbich TH, Fuchsjaeger MH, et al. Follow up of palpable circumscribed noncalcified solid breast masses at mammography and US: can biopsy be averted? *Radiology*. 2004;233(3):850-856.
2. Gordon PB, Gagnon FA, Lanzkowsky L. Solid breast masses diagnosed as fibroadenoma at fine-needle aspiration biopsy; acceptable rates of growth at long-term follow-up. *Radiology*. 2003;299(1):233-238.
3. Donegan WL. Evaluation of a palpable breast mass. *New Engl J Med*. 1992;327(13):937-942.

CASE 18: BREAST MASSES

PATIENT PRESENTATION

A 50-year-old woman presents with a palpable breast mass.

CLINICAL SUSPICION

Breast neoplasm

IMAGING MODALITY OF CHOICE

Diagnostic mammography is the initial imaging modality of choice for evaluating a clinically detected palpable breast mass in a woman age 30 or older.

Following the detection of a clinically palpable mass by mammography, an ultrasound study should be obtained to differentiate cystic from solid lesions. Moreover, ultrasound might further characterize the lesion in terms of shape, margins, and internal matrix as well as provide guidance for biopsy, aspiration, or localization if needed.

It is reported that when mammography and ultrasound are negative or benign in the evaluation of a palpable breast mass, the negative predictive value is very high reaching over 97%.

In Table C18.1, we will discuss the classic imaging characteristics on different imaging modalities for breast cancer, benign fibroadenoma, and cystic lesions in three different patients. All of them are 50 years old and presenting with a palpable breast mass.

Table C18.1 Classic Imaging Characteristics of Different Breast Masses

Imaging Modality	Breast Cancer (Figs. C18.4-C18.6)	Fibroadenoma (Figs. C18.1-C18.3)	Cystic Lesions (Figs. C18.7-C18.8)
Mammography	Irregular mass with speculated margins (Fig. C18.4). Architectural distortion. Skin or nipple retraction.	Oval, macrolobulated, or rounded mass. Partly obscured margins (Fig. C18.1). Clustered coarse heterogenous calcifications if involuting. May mimic malignancy.	Often circumscribed. Thick-walled cystic masses may be indistinctly marginated (Fig. C18.7). Mammography is not typically diagnostic and ultrasound study should always be obtained.
Ultrasound	Irregular or lobulated hypoechoic mass (Fig. C18.5). Thick echogenic rim or halo. Posterior shadowing. Vertical orientation. May be thick-walled cystic mass.	Circumscribed oval or gently lobulated hypoechoic to isoechoic mass. Long axis parallel to skin surface (Fig. C18.2). Homogenous internal echogenicity. Calcifications with posterior shadowing if involuting.	Mass with anechoic (cystic) ± hypo/hyperechoic (solid) components depending on complexity. Thick septations. Complex cysts should always be aspirated and biopsied for possible malignancy (Fig. C18.8).
MRI	Speculated or lobulated heterogenous mass. Rim enhancement. Rapid washout. Usually hypointense on T2WI FS but could be hyperintense centrally due to central necrosis (Fig. C18.6).	Oval or macrolobulated smooth enhancing mass. May have nonenhancing internal septations. Variable enhancement patterns that vary from rapid intense to no enhancement if densely hyalinized. Typically isointense with parenchyma on T2WI FS (Fig. C18.3).	Cystic component hypointense on T1WI. Cystic component hyperintense on T2WI.

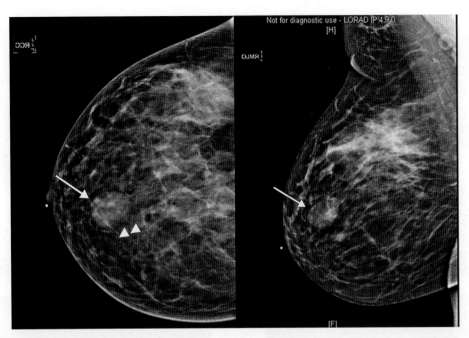

Fig. C18.1 CC and MLO views of the right breast in this 50-year-old woman show a well-circumscribed mass that is isodense to breast parenchyma (white arrows) and has a partially obscured margin laterally (arrowheads).

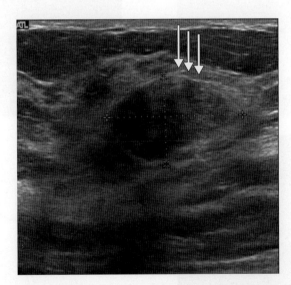

Fig. C18.2 Gray-scale ultrasound image corresponding to the lesion noticed on mammography show a circumscribed oval hypoechoic to isoechoic mass with a long axis parallel to the skin. Hyperechoic pseudocapsule is noticed as well (arrows). Findings are consistent with benign fibroadenoma.

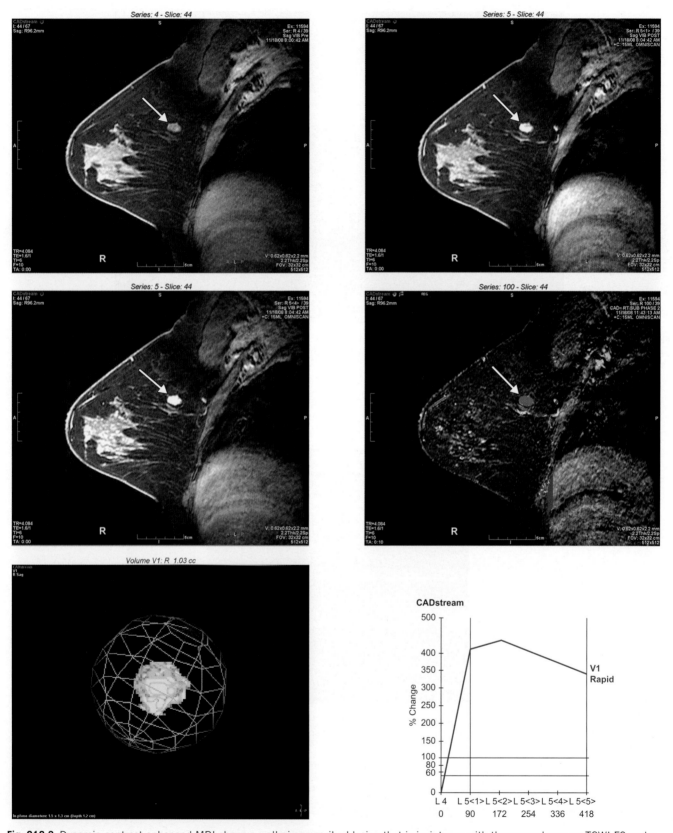

Fig. C18.3 Dynamic contrast enhanced MRI shows a well-circumscribed lesion that is isointense with the parenchyma on T2WI FS and a type 2 washout curve (arrows). The findings are highly suggestive of benign etiology. However, given the age of patient at presentation and the type 2 washout curve noticed, a biopsy was performed confirming the diagnosis of fibroadenoma, which might have variable enhancement patterns based on its degree of hyalinization and involution.

Size:
In-plane diameters: 1.5 x 1.3 cm (Depth 1.2 cm)
Angio volume: 1.0 cc

Enhancement composition:

Initial rise	41% Rapid	59% Medium	
Delayed phase			
Persistent	41%	58%	
Plateau	1%	0%	
Washout	0%	0%	

Curve peak: 114 % (Rapid washout)

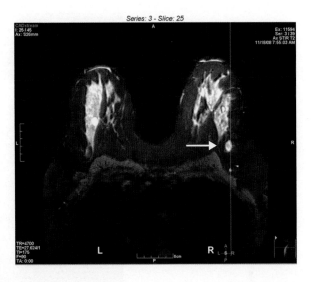

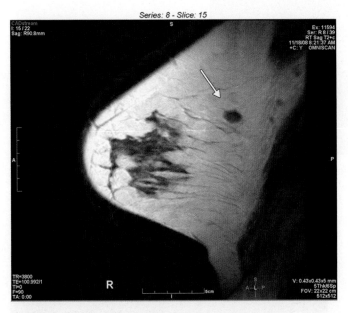

Fig. C18.3 (*continued*)

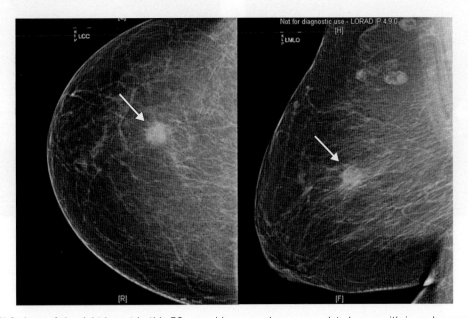

Fig. C18.4 CC and MLO views of the right breast in this 50-year-old woman show a speculated mass with irregular margins highly suspicious for malignancy (arrows).

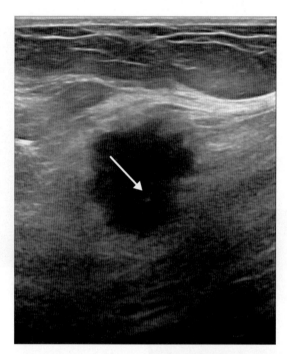

Fig. C18.5 Gray-scale ultrasound image corresponding to the lesion noticed on mammography show an irregular hypoechoic mass with some degree of posterior acoustic shadowing and microcalcification (arrow). This appearance is typical for a malignant process.

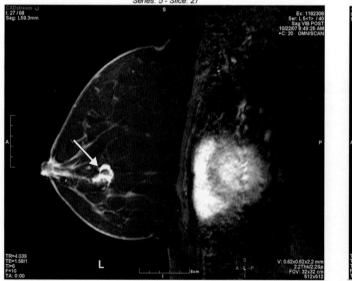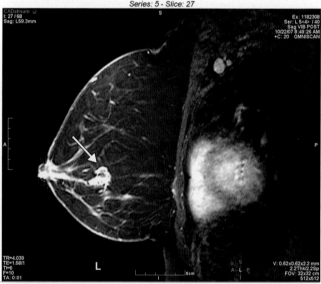

Fig. C18.6 Dynamic contrast enhanced MRI shows an irregular lesion in the breast that shows rim enhancement and central necrosis with rapid type 3 washout curve (arrows). The appearance is typical for malignancy.

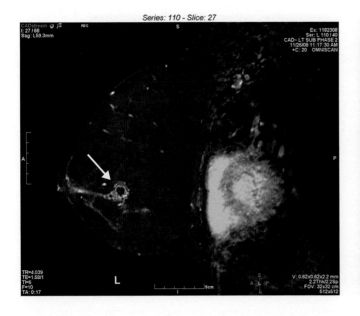

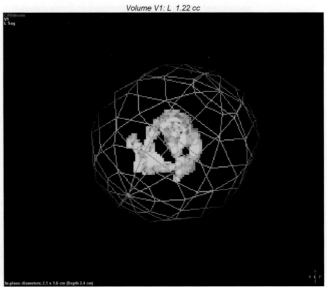

Size:
In-plane diameters: 2.1 x 1.6 cm (Depth 2.4 cm)
Angio volume: 1.2 cc

Enhancement composition:

Initial rise	62% Rapid	38% Medium
Delayed phase		
Persistent	25% ■	35% ■
Plateau	15% □	2% □
Washout	22% ■	1% ■

Curve peak: 413 % (Rapid washout)

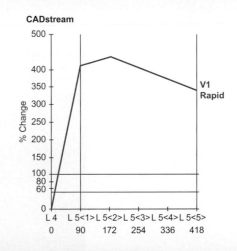

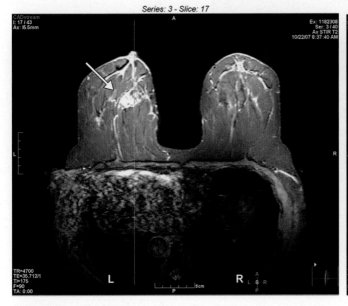

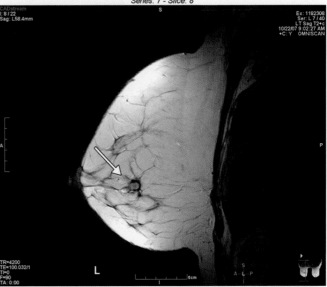

Fig. C18.6 (*continued*)

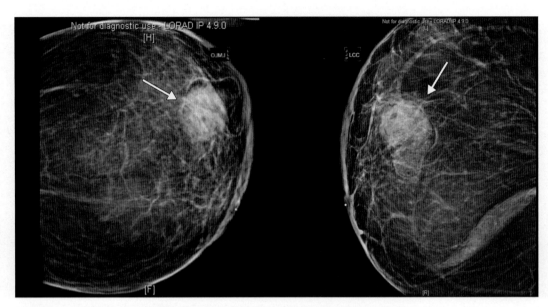

Fig. C18.7 CC and MLO views of the right breast in this 50-year-old woman show a mostly circumscribed hyperdense mass with focal area of indistinctive margins (arrows).

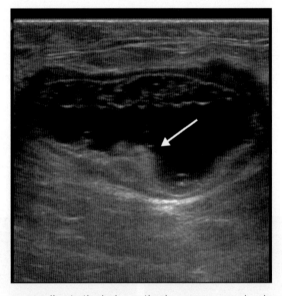

Fig. C18.8 Gray-scale ultrasound image corresponding to the lesion noticed on mammography show a complex cystic mass with mural nodule (arrow) and low-level internal echoes. Due to the complexity of the lesion it was further investigated by performing ultrasound-guided aspiration and turned out to be a benign abscess.

REFERENCES AND SUGGESTED READING

1. Graf O, Helbich TH, Fuchsjaeger MH, et al. Follow up of palpable circumscribed noncalcified solid breast masses at mammography and US: can biopsy be averted? *Radiology.* 2004;233(3):850-856.

2. Gordon PB, Gagnon FA, Lanzkowsky L. Solid breast masses diagnosed as fibroadenoma at fine-needle aspiration biopsy: acceptable rates of growth at long-term follow-up. *Radiology.* 2003;299(1)233-238.

3. Donegan WL. Evaluation of a palpable breast mass. *N Engl J Med.* 1992;327(13):937-942.

4. Macura KJ, Ouwerkerk R, Jacobs MA, et al. Patterns of enhancement on breast MR images: interpretation and imaging pitfalls. *RadioGraphics.* 2006;26(6):1719-1734.

5. Lee SG, Orel SG, Woo IJ, et al. MR imaging screening of the contralateral breast in patients with newly diagnosed breast cancer: preliminary results. *Radiology.* 2003;226:773-778.

6. Kuhl C. The current status of breast MR imaging. Part I. Choice of technique, image interpretation, diagnostic accuracy,

and transfer to clinical practice. *Radiology*. 2007;244(2): 356-378.

7. Kuhl C, et al. The current status of breast MR imaging. Part II. Clinical applications. *Radiology*. 2007;244(3):672-691.

8. American College of Radiology appropriateness criteria.

9. Cardenosa G. Ultrasound of cysts, cystic lesions, and papillary lesions. *Ultrasound Clinics*. 2006;1(4):617-629.

10. Berg WA, Sechtin AG, Marques H, et al. Cystic breast masses and the ACRIN 6666 experience. *Radiol Clin North Am*. 2010;48(5):931-987.

11. Elsamaloty H, Elzawawi MS, Mohammad S, et al. Increasing accuracy of detection of breast cancer with 3-T MRI. *AJR*. 2009;192(4):1142-1148.

CASE 19: DCIS

PATIENT PRESENTATION

A 65-year-old woman presents with abnormal mammographic calcifications detected in the left breast on screening mammography. Patient was asymptomatic and on clinical examination and no definitive masses or lesions were identified.

CLINICAL SUSPICION

Ductal carcinoma in situ (DCIS)

IMAGING MODALITY OF CHOICE

The incidence of contralateral breast DCIS is about 6%, hence bilateral diagnostic mammography is recommended. This further facilitates the detection of multifocal and multicentric tumors. Magnification views as well as other special views should be performed for the areas of concerning calcifications to further characterize the calcifications and their extent.

Ultrasonography should be performed with special attention to the area of concern as it can localize solid components in areas of mammographic calcifications. If a solid component is identified in ultrasonography, an ultrasound-guided biopsy can be performed.

If ultrasonography fails to detect a solid component which is the case in most low to intermediate grade DCIS, vacuum assisted stereotactic biopsy should be performed and followed by specimen radiography to confirm retrieval of calcifications. Pathology results for such biopsies can yield one of three options: Benign, atypical ductal hyperplasia, or DCIS. Eighteen percent of atypical ductal hyperplasia cases were found to be malignant; mainly DCIS, after surgical excision, so they should be treated with surgical excision.

The role of MRI is yet to be established in the initial diagnosis of DCIS and mainly preserved for evaluation of local recurrence.

FINDING

Mammographic findings of DCIS (Figs. C19.1-C19.3):

- Mammographic calcifications remain the best diagnostic clue with 70% to 80% sensitivity.
- Pleomorphic calcifications; 20% to 40% are due to DCIS, any grade.
- Amorphous calcifications: 20% malignant, of which 90% are due to DCIS which are usually low grade.
- Fine linear or branching calcifications are highly suggestive of high-grade DCIS.
- Clustered calcifications: the most common pattern with exclusion of smooth > 1 mm calcifications.
- Linear or segmental distribution of any calcification pattern suggests DCIS.
- Regional distribution of calcifications has an intermediate suspicion index.

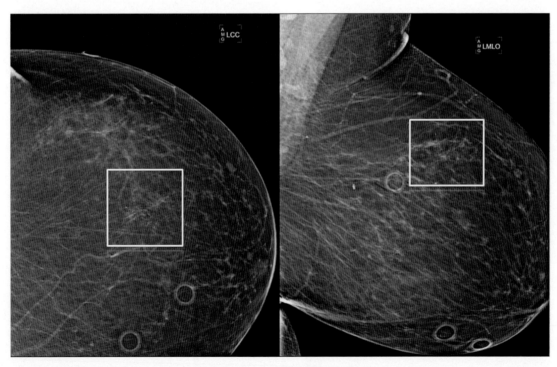

Fig. C19.1 Craniocaudal and mediolateral oblique mammographic images of the left breast show fine linear casting calcifications (white boxes) suggesting filling of a duct and its branches.

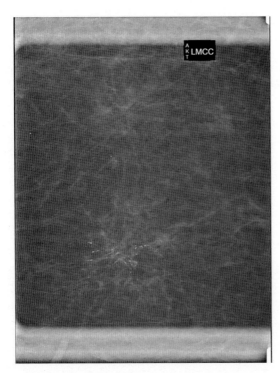

Fig. C19.2 Magnification craniocaudal view show fine microcalcifications in linear branching distribution highly suggestive of DCIS.

- Mass with calcifications.
- Mass with asymmetry favors an invasive component.

Ultrasonographic findings: 50% sensitivity to suspect DCIS:

- Dilated ducts, indistinct walls, and echogenicity.
- Hypoechoic mass with calcifications.

- Isolated calcifications.
- Intracystic or circumscribed mass, mainly seen with papillary DCIS.
- Increased vascularity on Doppler evaluation.

    MRI findings:

- Focal area or regional clumped enhancement.

DIFFERENTIAL DIAGNOSIS

- Invasive carcinoma
- Atypical ductal hyperplasia
- Sclerosing adenosis: usually punctate amorphous calcifications with an oval mass
- Fibroadenoma: usually well-defined mass with early pleomorphic or amorphous calcifications

TREATMENT

Treatment is based on assessment of histologic grade, margin status, and extent of disease.

- Lumpectomy: wide local excision with negative margins combined with radiation therapy.
- Mastectomy may be recommended in the case of multicentric disease or extensive high-grade DCIS.
- Tamoxifen for ER+ tumors.
- Sentinel lymph node biopsy followed by axillary dissection in case biopsy was positive.

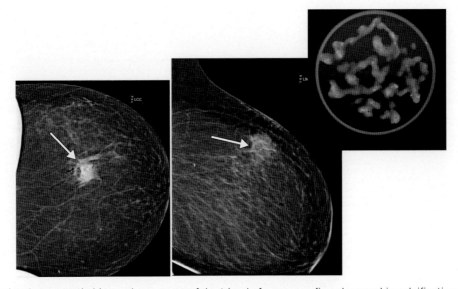

Fig. C19.3 Vacuum assisted stereotactic biopsy shows successful retrieval of numerous fine pleomorphic calcifications. Histopathology showed high-grade DCIS. Notice the developing density at the site of the biopsy consistent with biopsy-related hematoma (arrows). A clip has been placed to easier localize the area in the future prior to surgery.

REFERENCES AND SUGGESTED READING

1. Burstein HJ, Polyak K, Wong JS, et al. Ductal carcinoma in situ of the breast. *N Engl J Med.* 2004;350(14):1430-1441.

2. De Roos MA, Pijnappel RM, Post WJ, et al. Correlation between imaging and pathology in ductal carcinoma in situ of the breast. *World J Surg Oncol.* 2004;2(1):4.

3. Kessar P, Perry N, Vinnicombe SJ, et al. How significant is detection of ductal carcinoma in situ in a breast screening programme? *Clin Radiol.* 2002;57(9):807-814.

4. ACR-ACS-CAP-SSO practice guideline for the management of ductal carcinoma in situ of the breast (DCIS).

5. Dershaw DD, Abramson A, Kinne DW. Ductal carcinoma in situ: mammographic findings and clinical implications. *Radiology.* 1989;170:411-415.

CASE 20: BREAST CANCER EVALUATION AFTER NEOADJUVANT CHEMORADIOTHERAPY

PATIENT PRESENTATION
A 45-year-old woman presents for evaluation of an incidentally discovered left breast mass after a mild trauma.

CLINICAL SUSPICION
Breast cancer

IMAGING MODALITY OF CHOICE
Diagnostic mammography followed by ultrasonography and/or MRI based on mammographic findings (Figs. C20.1-C20.4).

A diagnostic mammography was obtained in this case that showed a large, dense, poorly circumscribed mass in the mid to lateral portion of the left breast highly suspicious for a locally advanced breast cancer. This was then followed by ultrasonography, which further confirmed the aggressive imaging characteristic features of the mass, and an ultrasound-guided core biopsy was performed revealing a pathology of triple receptor negative (ER, PR, HER 2/NEU) poorly differentiated infiltrating ductal carcinoma. Sonography of the left axilla revealed multiple enlarged lymph nodes with benign features; the largest lymph node was biopsied under ultrasound guidance and revealed reactive changes without evidence of metastasis.

Given the large size of the mass and poorly differentiated pathology, further evaluation of this lesion was mandated for determination of local extent of the disease and as baseline for follow up after neoadjuvant chemotherapy as the patient has opted for breast conservative approach. A dynamic contrast enhanced breast MRI study showed the mass more conspicuously with evidence of some architectural distortion and rapid washout curve.

Neoadjuvant chemotherapy was initiated and follow-up studies after 4 cycles of chemotherapy showed almost complete resolution of the mass by mammography and it was no more appreciated by ultrasonographic imaging (Fig. C20.5). Dynamic contrast-enhanced MRI of the breast at that time showed significant improvement in terms of decrease in size of the lesion, which was successfully down staged and localized under MRI guidance (Fig. C20.6) and locally excised.

Contrast breast MRI may detect abnormalities that are not evident clinically, mammographically, or sonographically. It is basically too sensitive with higher rates of false positive results and lower specificity for detection of breast cancer. So what are the indications for breast MRI?
Indications for contrast enhanced breast MRI:

- Screening of high-risk patients.
- Screening of contralateral breast in patients with a newly diagnosed breast malignancy. Rates ranging between 3% and 5% have been reported in the literature of occult malignancy in contralateral breast of newly diagnosed breast cancer patients.
- Evaluation of patients with silicone or saline implants and/or free injections with silicone, paraffin, or polyacrylamide gel in which mammography is typically difficult.
- Extent of disease and the presence of multifocality and multicentricity in patients with invasive carcinoma and ductal carcinoma in situ.
- Presurgical evaluation for deep tissue invasion and relationship of the tumor to the fascia and its extension into adjacent muscles.
- Evaluation of residual disease in patients with pathology close or positive margins.
- Breast MRI may be useful before, during, and after neoadjuvant chemotherapy to evaluate treatment response prior to surgical treatment.
- Evaluation for breast cancer recurrence; MRI can better distinguish cancer recurrence from residual scar tissue.
- MRI may be useful in patients presenting with metastatic disease and/or axillary adenopathy and no mammographic or physical findings of primary breast carcinoma.
- Lesion characterization when other imaging modalities such as ultrasound and mammography are inconclusive.
- Evaluation for recurrence in patients with suspected cancer recurrence and tissue flaps.
- MRI guided biopsy and/or wire localization for lesions that are demonstrable only on MRI and are occult on mammography and ultrasound.

FINDINGS
MRI findings for breast carcinoma:

- Morphologic criteria: Irregular or speculated margins of a focal mass, rimlike enhancement, heterogonous internal enhancement, and enhancing internal septa within a lesion, moderate or marked degree of non-mass regional enhancement, regional enhancement with a micronodular (stippled) pattern "although could be seen with benign fibrocystic disease," clumped, heterogeneous, and homogenous enhancement, segmental distribution of cancer.
- Focal perilesional edema: Demonstrated by focal are of hyperintense T2-weighted signal near a lesion.
- Architectural distortion.
- Skin thickening.
- Axillary lymphadenopathy.

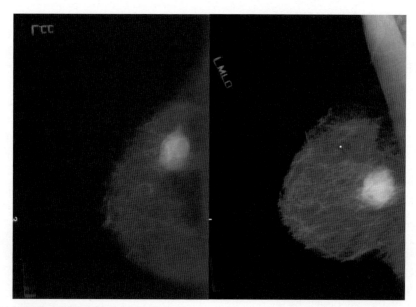

Fig. C20.1 CC and MLO views of the left breast show a large, dense, poorly circumscribed mass in the mid to lateral portion of the left breast.

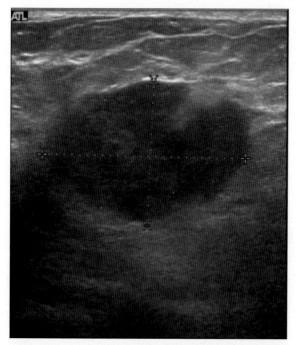

Fig. C20.2 Corresponding sagittal sonography for the mass identified on mammography confirms a solid heterogeneous irregular mass.

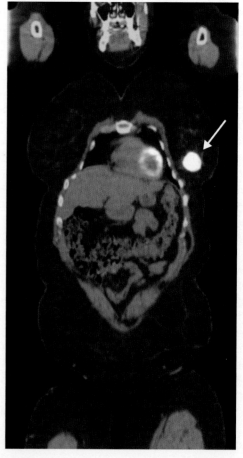

Fig. C20.3 PET-CT shows increased FDG-18 avidity in the mass seen in the left breast (arrow) consistent with malignancy without evidence of distant metastasis or pathological lymphadenopathy

- Enhancement kinetics: Type I is a pattern of progressive enhancement with a continuous increase in signal intensity on each successive contrast enhanced image, this pattern is associated with benign findings in 83% of cases and malignancy in less than 9% of the cases. Type II is a plateau pattern in which an initial increase

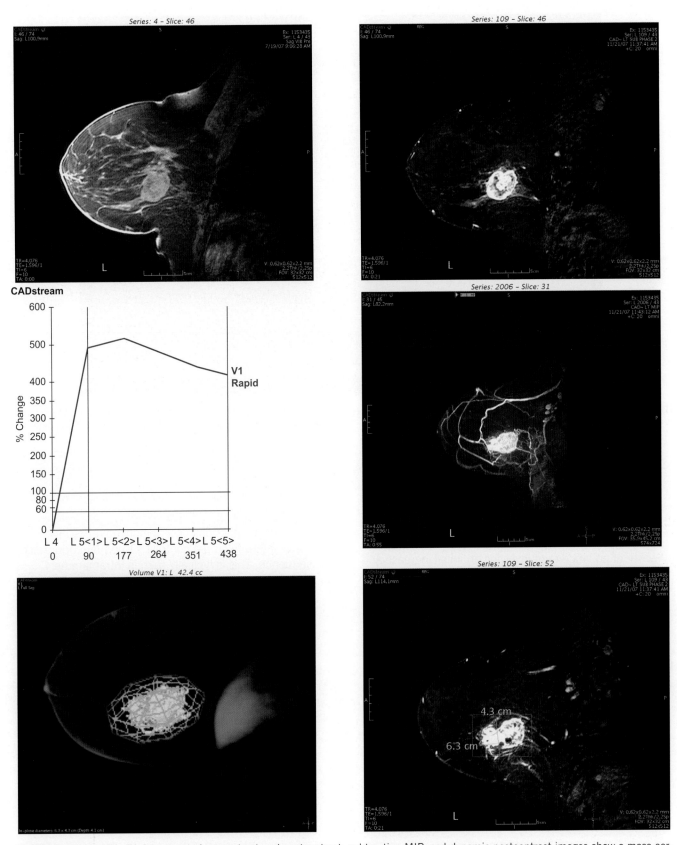

Fig. C20.4 Sagittal T1, T1 fat-saturated precontrast and postcontrast, subtraction MIP, and dynamic postcontrast images show a mass corresponding to the finding seen on mammography, which measures 6.3 × 4.3 × 4.3 cm. The mass of concern has some specular architectural distortion and extension along its borders, particularly along the anterior and lateral borders. The mass demonstrates a type III rapid washout. Increased vascularity to the mass can also be noticed on MIP image. The findings are consistent with a malignant neoplasm.

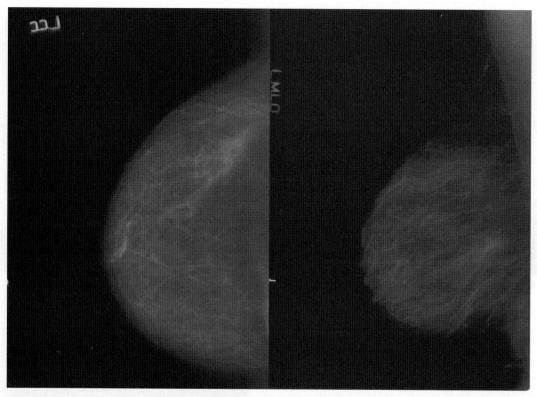

Fig. C20.5 CC and MLO views of the left breast after 4 cycles of neoadjuvant chemotherapy show nearly complete resolution of the previously seen large mass in the left breast of known malignancy. The mass was no more appreciated on ultrasonography at this stage.

in initial signal intensity is followed by a flattening of the enhancement curve; this pattern has a sensitivity of 42.6% and specificity of 75% for the detection of malignancy. Type III is a pattern in which there is a washout enhancement involving an initial increase and subsequent decrease in signal intensity; this pattern is highly specific in ruling out benign etiology and is reported to be associated with malignancy in 76% of the cases.

DIFFERENTIAL DIAGNOSIS

- Fibroadenomas, which typically have benign morphologic features, nonenhancing septations, and type I curve.
- Cysts, which typically have a high signal on T2 fat-suppressed images and usually don't enhance after injection of gadolinium and show as filling defects or demonstrate a thin enhancing rim.
- Fat-containing lesions best demonstrated by high signal intensity on pre contrast T1 non-fat-suppressed sequence. This is typically seen in intramammary lymph nodes, fat necrosis, and hamartomas. These lesions typically appear hypointense on fat-suppressed T1-weighted images with gadolinium.
- Colloid carcinoma, which represents an exception to the rule that all bright signal on T2 fat-suppressed images are benign.
- Adenoid cystic carcinoma, which typically presents as an irregular enhancing mass.
- Metaplastic carcinoma, which could present as lesion with rim enhancement.

CADstream

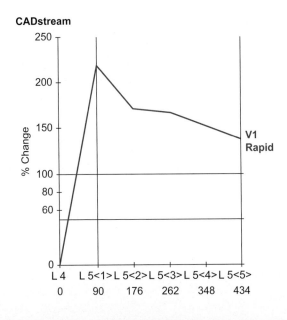

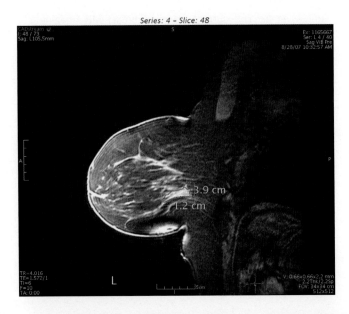

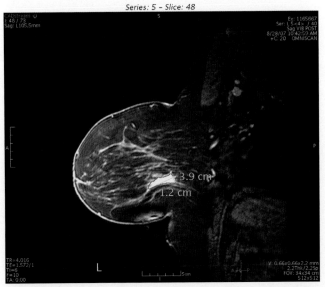

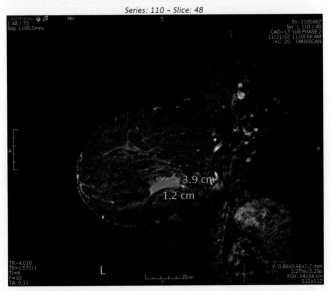

Fig. C20.6 Sagittal T1-weighted, T1-weighed with Fat saturation and dynamic postcontrast T1-weighted images show significant improvement after neoadjuvant chemotherapy manifested by decrease in size to 3.9 × 1.2 × 1.2 cm from 6.3 × 4.3 × 4.3 cm; however, the visualized lesion still demonstrates abnormal type III washout compatible with residual active tumor.

REFERENCES AND SUGGESTED READING

1. Graf O, Helbich TH, Fuchsjaeger MH, et al. Follow up of palpable circumscribed noncalcified solid breast masses at mammography and US: can biopsy be averted? *Radiology.* 2004;233(3):850-856.

2. Gordon PB, Gagnon FA, Lanzkowsky L. Solid breast masses diagnosed as fibroadenoma at fine-needle aspiration biopsy: acceptable rates of growth at long-term follow-up. *Radiology.* 2003;299(1)233-238.

3. Donegan WL. Evaluation of a palpable breast mass. *N Engl J Med.* 1992;327(13):937-942.

4. Macura, KJ, Ouwerkerk R, Jacobs MA, et al. Patterns of enhancement on breast MR images: interpretation and imaging pitfalls. *RadioGraphics.* 2006;26(6):1719-1734.

5. Lee SG, Orel SG, Woo IJ, et al. MR imaging screening of the contralateral breast in patients with newly diagnosed breast cancer: preliminary results. *Radiology.* 2003;226: 773-778.

6. Kuhl C. The current status of breast MR imaging. Part I. Choice of technique, image interpretation, diagnostic accuracy, and transfer to clinical practice. *Radiology.* 2007;244(2):356-378.

7. Kuhl C, et al. The current status of breast MR imaging. Part II. Clinical applications. *Radiology.* 2007;244(3): 672-691.

8. American College of Radiology appropriateness criteria.

9. Cardenosa G. Ultrasound of cysts, cystic lesions, and papillary lesions. *Ultrasound Clinics.* 2006;1(4):617-629.

10. Berg WA, Sechtin AG, Marques H, et al. Cystic breast masses and the ACRIN 6666 experience. *Radiol Clin North Am.* 2010;48(5):931-987.

11. Elsamaloty, Elzawawi MS, Mohammad S, et al. Increasing accuracy of detection of breast cancer with 3-T MRI. *AJR.* 2009;192(4):1142-1148.

Index

Note: Page numbers in italics refer to figures; page numbers followed by *t* indicate tables.